Clinical Practice Guide
for Midwifery & Women's Health

FOURTH EDITION

Nell L. Tharpe, CNM, CRNFA, MS

Adjunct Faculty, Midwifery Institute at Philadelphia University
Philadelphia, Pennsylvania

Adjunct Faculty, Birthwise Midwifery School
Bridgton, Maine

Faculty and Program Coordinator, Midwifery at Green Landing
East Boothbay, Maine

Cindy L. Farley, CNM, PhD, FACNM

Faculty, Midwifery Institute at Philadelphia University
Philadelphia, Pennsylvania

Clinical Midwife, Midwifery Services of Pomerene Hospital
Millersburg, Ohio

Robin G. Jordan, CNM, PhD, FACNM

Course Coordinator of Antepartum Care
Frontier Nursing University
Petoskey, Michigan

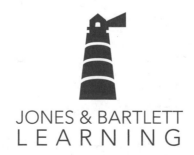

JONES & BARTLETT
LEARNING

World Headquarters
Jones & Bartlett Learning
5 Wall Street
Burlington, MA 01803
978-443-5000
info@jblearning.com
www.jblearning.com

Jones & Bartlett Learning books and products are available through most bookstores and online booksellers. To contact Jones & Bartlett Learning directly, call 800-832-0034, fax 978-443-8000, or visit our website, www.jblearning.com.

Substantial discounts on bulk quantities of Jones & Bartlett Learning publications are available to corporations, professional associations, and other qualified organizations. For details and specific discount information, contact the special sales department at Jones & Bartlett Learning via the above contact information or send an email to specialsales@jblearning.com.

Clinical Practice Guidelines for Midwifery & Women's Health is an independent publication and has not been authorized, sponsored, or otherwise approved by the owners of the trademarks or service marks referenced in this product.

Some images in this book feature models. These models do not necessarily endorse, represent, or participate in the activities represented in the images.

The authors, editors, and publisher have made every effort to provide accurate information. However, they are not responsible for errors, omissions, or for any outcomes related to the use of the contents of this book and take no responsibility for the use of the products and procedures described. Treatments and side effects described in this book may not be applicable to all people; likewise, some people may require a dose or experience a side effect that is not described herein. Drugs and medical devices are discussed that may have limited availability controlled by the Food and Drug Administration (FDA) for use only in a research study or clinical trial. Research, clinical practice, and government regulations often change the accepted standard in this field. When consideration is being given to use of any drug in the clinical setting, the healthcare provider or reader is responsible for determining FDA status of the drug, reading the package insert, and reviewing prescribing information for the most up-to-date recommendations on dose, precautions, and contraindications, and determining the appropriate usage for the product. This is especially important in the case of drugs that are new or seldom used.

Production Credits
Publisher: Kevin Sullivan
Acquisitions Editor: Amanda Harvey
Editorial Assistant: Sara Bempkins
Associate Production Editor: Sara Fowles
Associate Marketing Manager: Katie Hennessy
V.P., Manufacturing and Inventory Control: Therese Connell
Composition: Cenveo Publisher Services
Cover Design: Scott Moden
Cover Image: © newphotoservice/ShutterStock, Inc.
Printing and Binding: Edwards Brothers Malloy
Cover Printing: Edwards Brothers Malloy

Library of Congress Cataloging-in-Publication Data
Tharpe, Nell, 1956
  Clinical practice guidelines for midwifery & women's health/Nell L. Tharpe, Cynthia L. Farley, Robin G. Jordan.—4th ed.
      p. ; cm.
  Includes bibliographical references and index.
  ISBN 978-1-4496-4575-5 (pbk.)
  I. Farley, Cindy L. II. Jordan, Robin G., 1954- III. Title.
  [DNLM: 1. Midwifery—methods—Practice Guideline. 2. Genital Diseases, Female—Practice Guideline. 3. Pregnancy Complications—Practice Guideline. 4. Women's
  Health—Practice Guideline. WQ 165]
  618.2—dc23
                                   2012006817

6048
Printed in the United States of America
16 15 14   10 9 8 7 6

This edition of *Clinical Practice Guidelines for Midwifery & Women's Health* is dedicated to all midwives who persevere in bringing compassionate personalized care to women from all walks of life, in every birth and practice setting, in the face of social, cultural, and medical barriers. Midwifery offers women more than health care; the practice of midwifery seeks to engage with what is central to women's lives, so as to offer women opportunities to care for and about themselves within the communities where they live.

Many thanks to my friends and colleagues, Cindy Farley and Robin Jordan, for joining me in revising this edition. This is a journey I could not have made without their compassionate support. It is with deep gratitude that I pass the baton to Cindy and Robin and move forward into the next phase of my life.

—Nell L. Tharpe, CNM, CRNFA, MS

I am grateful for the love and support of my mother, Carol; my sister, Becky; my son, Kyle; my daughter, Katy; and my loving companion, Larry, through this and all my endeavors in life. It is always a pleasure to work with Nell and Robin, who are exceptional midwife educators and authors. Nell, Robin and I will draw inspiration from your devotion to the discipline of midwifery as we move your work forward in the future.

—Cindy L. Farley, CNM, PhD, FACNM

My heartfelt thanks to my loving companion, Larry Liebler, who has supported me with love and understanding during my long hours spent on this text. I am honored to have participated in this venture with Cindy and Nell—treasured colleagues and friends, who made it all much more fun than I could have imagined.

—Robin G. Jordan, CNM, PhD, FACNM

Contents

Chapter 3   Care of the Pregnant Woman with Prenatal Variations............................. 83

Preface

The fourth edition of *Clinical Practice Guidelines for Midwifery & Women's Health* represents a broad range of clinical practice from a wide variety of sources that include evidence-based, traditional, and empiric care. Both the American College of Nurse–Midwives (ACNM) and the Midwives Alliance of North America (MANA) recommend that midwives utilize written policies and/or practice guidelines. *Clinical Practice Guidelines for Midwifery & Women's Health* has grown out of the need for a concise reference guide to meet that recommendation. Of course, no text on midwifery and women's health can possibly be an all-inclusive reference; thus there are additional safe and reasonable practices that are not addressed in this book. Midwifery practice is a dynamic enterprise, with elements that are timeless, such as providing comfort to women in labor, and elements that evolve as evidence deepens our knowledge base and broadens our practices, such as providing primary care to women in their menopausal years. It is the responsibility of the individual midwife to develop the best plan of care for and with the individual woman, relying on the midwife's accumulated knowledge and experience of midwifery practice, knowledge of the individual woman, and interpretation of current evidence within a framework of midwifery hallmarks of care.

Clinical Practice Guidelines for Midwifery & Women's Health, fourth edition, has been thoughtfully updated to reflect current and emerging practice and provide support and guidance for day-to-day clinical midwifery and women's health practice with diverse populations. Regional differences in practice styles occur; therefore the guidelines are broadly based and reflect current practice and literature to accommodate these differences. Midwives are encouraged to apply the content of the *Guidelines* within the framework of client or patient preferences and their own scope of practice; regional recommendations; local, state, and national standards; and mindful midwifery care.

This book is written for all the midwives, wherever they practice, and the women, children, and families they serve.

Acknowledgments

The authors gratefully acknowledge the following contributors to the fourth edition of *Clinical Practice Guidelines for Midwifery & Women's Health:*

Susan Jacoby, DNP, CNM
Lead Midwife
Central Maine Medical Center
OB/GYN/Midwifery Department
Lewiston, Maine

Deborah Karsnitz, DNP, CNM
Course Coordinator, Postpartum & Newborn Series
Frontier Nursing University
Louisville, Kentucky

Jalana Lazar, CNM, MS, MPH
Staff Midwife, Lifestages
Yellow Springs, Ohio

Amy Marowitz, DNP, CNM
Course Coordinator, Intrapartum Series
Frontier Nursing University
Maple City, Michigan

Elizabeth A. Parr, CNM, MSN
Senior Midwife Tutor, Midwifery Institute of Philadelphia University
Staff Midwife, Allentown Gynecology Associates
Emmaus, Pennsylvania

Joan Slager, DNP, CNM, CPC, FACNM
Director, Nurse-Midwifery
Bronson Women's Service
Kalamazoo, Michigan

Tanya Tringali, CNM, MS
Midwife Tutor, Admissions Assistant
Midwifery Institute of Philadelphia University
Locum Tenens Midwife, Full Circle Women's Health
New Rochelle, New York

Donna Walls, RN, BSN, IBCLC, ICCE
President, Mother Earth Sundries
Master Herbalist, Certified Aromatherapist
Lactation Consultant
Dayton, Ohio

Midwifery Institute of Philadelphia University student contributors to the fourth edition of *Clinical Practice Guidelines for Midwifery & Women's Health* include the following individuals:

Kristen L. Allen, BA, BSN

Tamara Baumann, BS, RNC, WHNP

Kristin Beermann, BA, BSN

Tina C. Bias, RN, BS

Kierston Bocquin, BSN

Nichole Boyce, BSN

Nicole Christian, RN, BSN

Esther Diamond, RN, BA

Colleen Donovan-Batson, CNM, BSN

Kitan Ellerson, RN, BSN

Anne Gilbertson, BA, BSN

Elaine Greene, BSN, CNM

Jade Groff, RN, BSN

Debbie Hamilton, BSN, WHNP, CNM

Leela J. Joy, RN, BSN

Pamela Kelly, BSN, CNM

Traci A. Labreck, RN, BSN

Jane Letushko, RN, BSN

Sarah Ludlow, RN, BSN

Lucinda Manges, RN, BA

Michelle A. Mitchell, BSN, MA, LPC

Amanda Molter, RN, BS

Christie Morris, RN, BSN

Christian Orburn, RN, BSN

Karen M. Owens, CNM, BSN, RDMS

Mari C. Oxenberg, RN, BS

Amy Perilman, BSN, WHNP

Ramona G. Poticher, RN, BSN

Lorraine M. Searle, RN, RM, BSc

A Short History of the Clinical Practice Guidelines for Midwifery & Women's Health

Clinical Practice Guidelines for Midwifery & Women's Health grew out of an idea that germinated in the mind of Nell Tharpe and blossomed in the fertile soil of isolated midwifery practice in rural Maine.

As a new midwife practicing in a small coastal community in the days before widespread computer access and remote from healthcare resources or colleagues, Nell relied on a handful of dog-eared texts and well-marked copies of the *Journal of Nurse–Midwifery* for her clinical information. She longed for a quick-reference text that would guide her through the clinical challenges that women presented in her diverse full-scope practice and provide a means to keep current with the state of midwifery and women's health.

Over the years, Nell collected a file of resources and a wealth of experience (at one point, for more than 3 years, she was the sole birth attendant at her local 17-bed community hospital). Sitting down at her computer, armed with her notes and her vast array of experiences, Nell wrote the first draft of what would become the *Clinical Practice Guidelines for Midwives* in one very full week. She printed and sold it one copy at a time.

The response was immediate: Midwives clamored for this type of reference book. Over the next 6 years, Nell wrote 2 additional editions that were professionally printed and bound before deciding that the business of running a publishing business was more than she could continue to do well while maintaining a practice. Jones & Bartlett Learning was approached and happily took over book sales and contracted for the next edition of what was now titled *Clinical Practice Guidelines for Midwifery & Women's Health*.

In the meantime, Nell completed her MS in midwifery through Philadelphia University, where she thrived under the mentorship and superb teaching of midwife Cindy Farley. As Nell was writing the next edition of the practice guidelines, she realized that the text would benefit from an infusion of fresh ideas. She immediately thought of Cindy and invited her to work collaboratively on the following edition.

Cindy had become aware of Nell's clinical practice guidelines at an American College of Nurse–Midwives (ACNM) annual meeting, long before Nell was her student. She was delighted to know that a midwife was providing a needed service to support midwives in practice. Cindy believed that midwives in practice would benefit from guidelines for care for selected, commonly encountered clinical conditions. Such a text would allow midwives to focus their energies into the creative and interpersonal aspects of providing midwifery care and running a practice.

In 2000, Cindy opened a new midwifery practice, and she purchased her first copy of Nell's clinical practice guidelines. She was particularly impressed with the alternative therapies section and the suggestions for further diagnostic testing as being very midwife-friendly. Additionally, she found the guidelines helpful in meeting local and national ACNM criteria for practice guidelines and peer review.

Cindy had enjoyed working with Nell during her master's program, where the two formed a bond of mutual respect and friendship. Cindy was eager to become involved in the revision of a book she so admired. Additionally, as an educator Cindy continually seeks out real-world experiences for her master's in midwifery students that combine academic course objectives and research critique skills through projects with relevance to practicing midwives. Updating the evidence base and revising selected clinical practice guidelines became a perfect class research project for her students.

In contemplating the revision work needed for the fourth edition of the book, Nell and Cindy realized that even more assistance was needed—due to their own limited time because of their already full schedules, the expanding role of midwifery in primary care, and the volume of information that is now available through the Internet. Cindy immediately thought of her friend, colleague, and former doctoral student, Robin Jordan, as the right person to join them. Robin is an outstanding midwifery educator and experienced author, and her skill set made for a wonderful fit for Nell and Cindy during the complex revision process. She contributed additional and valuable perspectives as the three discussed current midwifery issues and the best ways to present them in this newest edition of *Clinical Practice Guidelines for Midwifery & Women's Health*.

What has been very apparent during this revision is that the computer age is changing how we are accessing and processing information, both personally and professionally. It also promises to change the way we present material in this book in the future. Our goal as authors is to critically review the amazing amount of information available and to synthesize that information into concise, clinically relevant guidelines that are useful to midwives in practice.

Nell, Cindy, and Robin continue to strive to make this ongoing work-in-progress as helpful and user-friendly as possible. If you have any suggestions for additions or improvements for the next edition of this book, please e-mail Nell at tharpen@philau .edu, Cindy at farleyc@philau.edu, or Robin at Robin.Jordan@frontier.edu.

Essential Midwifery Practice

Midwifery is a discipline that melds science with art; it is a humanistic approach to providing quality health care to women, newborns, and their families that recognizes the sacredness of the individual and of the processes of fertility and birth, and that honors women across the life span.

Exemplary midwifery practice is woman oriented and focuses on excellence in the processes and provision of women's health care, with a primary goal of improving maternal and child health (Kennedy, 2000). Exemplary midwives promote the discipline of midwifery through professional actions that benefit women and their families, while allowing adequate personal time for reinvigoration for this important work.

Midwives are blessed with a passion for their work. It is the thoughtful and skilled expression of this passion that women under midwives' care so appreciate and that has helped the discipline of midwifery to thrive.

This book, *Clinical Practice Guidelines for Midwifery and Women's Health*, is designed with the practicing midwife in mind. The text condenses and outlines clinical care, highlighting the art and science behind the midwifery model of care. It is the authors' goal that this book support your professional practice as a resource by allowing you to focus on the women who come to you for care rather than on the administrative task of creating practice-specific clinical practice guidelines.

PURPOSE OF CLINICAL PRACTICE GUIDELINES

The goal of *Clinical Practice Guidelines for Midwifery and Women's Health* is to provide, in a standardized format, a brief, succinct, critically appraised, and referenced synthesis of current midwifery practice including evidence-based, traditional, complementary and alternative medicine (CAM), and empiric options for care. Clinical practice guidelines are used to describe, define, and delineate parameters for evaluation, diagnosis, and care in specific clinical conditions.

Box 1-1 Philosophy of the American College of Nurse–Midwives

We, the midwives of the American College of Nurse–Midwives, affirm the power and strength of women and the importance of their health in the well-being of families, communities, and nations. We believe in the basic human rights of all persons, recognizing that women often incur an undue burden of risk when these rights are violated.

We believe every person has a right to:

- Equitable, ethical, and accessible quality health care that promotes healing and health
- Health care that respects human dignity, individuality, and diversity among groups
- Complete and accurate information to make informed health care decisions
- Self-determination and active participation in health care decisions
- Involvement of a woman's designated family members, to the extent desired, in all health care experiences

We believe the best model of health care for a woman and her family:

- Promotes a continuous and compassionate partnership
- Acknowledges a person's life experiences and knowledge
- Includes individualized methods of care and healing guided by the best evidence available
- Involves therapeutic use of human presence and skillful communication

We honor the normalcy of women's life cycle events. We believe in:

- Watchful waiting and nonintervention in normal processes
- Appropriate use of interventions and technology for current or potential health problems
- Consultation, collaboration, and referral with other members of the health care team as needed to provide optimal health care

We affirm that midwifery care incorporates these qualities and that women's health care needs are well served through midwifery care.

Finally, we value formal education, lifelong individual learning, and the development and application of research to guide ethical and competent midwifery practice. These beliefs and values provide the foundation for commitment to individual and collective leadership at the community, state, national, and international level to improve the health of women and their families worldwide.

Source: American College of Nurse–Midwives [ACNM], 2004.

These *Guidelines* present a utilitarian practice tool that reflects up-to-date evidence presented in an easy-to-follow format addressing conditions frequently seen in clinical midwifery and women's health practice.

How clinical practice guidelines are applied in midwifery or women's health practice is influenced by a number of factors, such as the accepted standards of the midwife's or women's healthcare provider's professional organization(s), local and regional styles of practice, the practice setting, and individual practice preferences. State laws, in the form of both statutes and regulations, affect the scope of practice, as do hospital bylaws, birth center rules and regulations, health insurance contracts, and liability insurance policies.

Each individual midwife determines her or his scope of practice within these legal and professional boundaries based on the individual's philosophy of midwifery practice, educational preparation, experience, and skill level; the community need; and the specific practice setting. A midwife's scope of practice is dynamic and may vary from one practice location to another; it also evolves over time and throughout the individual's career.

Every woman who comes to a midwife for care has a right to information regarding the midwife's scope of practice, usual practice location(s), and indications and provisions for access to specialty medical or obstetric care. Development of professional relationships with multidisciplinary community and regional health-related resources, such as pharmacists, physicians, social service personnel, clergy, and other relevant community organizations, is a valuable asset in fostering continuity of care and ensuring access to comprehensive services for the women whom midwives serve.

Knowledge of evidence-based practice is an expectation in today's healthcare environment. Midwifery, as a discipline, includes domains of knowledge that are quite amenable to evidence-based investigation. At the same time, however, midwifery includes and values knowledge that is not so easily gained from this approach. Midwifery recognizes the importance of considering the "whole" person in a sociocultural–biological context and calls for continuing traditional high-touch, low-tech midwifery care—a perspective that is not typically reflected in current medical research questions, designs, and methodologies. The research evidence base primarily rests on quantitative research methods. This paradigm is often criticized because it reduces phenomena to numerical representations—an approach that does not support holistic understanding. Likewise, this approach does not adequately explore outcomes of midwifery care that are not easily measured with a laboratory test or a Likert scale, such as emotional experiences and spiritual awakenings that result from fundamental life-defining moments such as can occur during labor and birth.

Other valuable types of midwifery knowledge are informed by empiric and traditional midwifery care. Traditional midwifery care includes practices that

have evolved through generations of women providing care to women, whose knowledge and skills have been passed down through centuries and across cultures. Empiric care is care based on observation or experience, and for decades it has formed the basis of most medical decision making. Recommendations for care based on how one was taught and one's experience are examples of empiric care. The practitioner should be aware that a lack of evidence neither invalidates nor supports the effectiveness of empiric or traditional midwifery care practices; rather, it merely indicates that at the present time scientific studies examining the specific practice are lacking.

Midwifery as a discipline applies the domain of midwifery knowledge and the health-related sciences to clinical care using a humanistic approach. Fundamental to midwifery is the honoring of women throughout the life span through recognition of the sacredness of the individual and of the processes of life, fertility, and birth. This recognition is embedded in the language used in *Clinical Practice Guidelines for Midwifery and Women's Health* and is an underlying premise of midwifery literature.

Evidence-based practice is described as "the explicit, judicious and conscientious use of current best evidence from health care research in decisions about the care of individuals and populations" (Sackett, Richardson, Rosenberg, & Haynes, 1997). The process of applying an evidence-based approach to clinical midwifery practice requires the clinician to consider the evidence in light of the specific patient-population served, current recommendations for care and treatment, and the cultural background and unique preferences of individuals by doing the following:

- Asking clinically focused questions specific to the evaluation, diagnosis, and treatment recommendations for specific clinical conditions
- Conducting a focused published literature review using quality peer-reviewed sources
- Critically appraising this literature in light of each study's rigor and adherence to the scientific principles underlying the methodologic decisions

- Appling the results of this appraisal to clinical practice, offering the individual adequate information to make informed decisions and participate in creation of an individualized healthcare plan that recognizes standardized recommendations and treatment (Lydon-Rochelle, Hodnett, Renfrew, & Lumley, 2003)

Various evidence-based resources are available that summarize and synthesize the latest information for busy practitioners, such as the Cochrane Database and the regular feature on evidence-based practice in *Journal of Midwifery & Women's Health*. Nevertheless, the analytical practitioner should be cautious and judicious in applying new evidence in practice. Evidence, as well as our philosophy, beliefs, knowledge and skills, should guide and inform us as we go about the daily business of providing midwifery care to women and their families.

> Scientific evidence is developed with clearly defined populations of patients in narrowly focused areas and is expressed in terms of numerical probabilities; our care is delivered to one woman at a time in the context of her specific life situation and is expressed in terms of hopeful possibilities.

All midwives are encouraged to be lifelong learners and reflective practitioners. Reflection in practice involves methodically evaluating our experiences, connecting with and integrating our feelings about these experiences and our role in them, and comparing our clinical practices with our theories-in-use. Reflective practice entails continually building new understandings to inform our actions during situations as they unfold, while remaining aware of the potential for bias and its effect on our thinking (Schon, 1983).

The old adage of "See one, do one, teach one" has lost favor in the recent past, as it is now perceived as an inadequate method for educating and training skilled and competent health professionals. Within reflective practice, however, this adage can be reinterpreted for the twenty-first century as a motto to remind us of the importance of the following steps:

- Developing and refining clinical judgment through the continual processes of observation, practice, and teaching. From this perspective, the practitioner is encouraged to avoid clinical isolation by seeking opportunities to observe the techniques and practices of peers and colleagues (See One).
- Maintaining clinical skills through deliberate attention to practice, clinical training and simulation; reading of the literature; and application of new knowledge and techniques in the clinical setting (Do One).
- Expanding the individual's skill set and knowledge base beyond the basics to the level necessary to effectively and skillfully teach or mentor new clinicians (Teach One).

Clinical expertise is developed over time and with thoughtful attention to practice. New practitioners and novices are encouraged to maintain heightened awareness of their evolving expertise and to set safe boundaries of practice for themselves. Experienced practitioners are encouraged to remain current in their knowledge and skills and to protect their passion for this work by avoiding the complacency or cynicism that sometimes occurs when practicing midwifery in low-resource settings, in settings hostile to midwifery, or with challenging populations.

WOMEN FIRST

Midwives and other women's health professionals practice within a healthcare system that is increasingly complex. Midwifery and women's health is first and foremost concerned with caring for and about women.

Every individual woman deserves to receive care that is safe and satisfying, that fosters self-determination and her ability to care for herself. Such care, to be effective, addresses the individual's personal, cultural, and developmental needs. Women look to their healthcare provider to give guidance consistent with the individual's real and perceived health needs and internal beliefs.

As midwives caring for women in our country's diverse communities, the ability to listen and to integrate women's concerns into the care provided is an integral component of midwifery practice. The aim is to provide care based on the woman's expressed and identified needs through a personalized plan of care that is mutually developed and supported by both the woman and the midwife, and that reflects the midwife's awareness and sharing of national, regional, and local expectations and recommendations for care.

Sometimes, women do not have an adequate frame of reference to formulate clear questions regarding their health. Teasing out the health concerns that are important to an individual woman requires skill in directed inquiry and active listening, sensitivity to cultural issues, and knowledge of common health practices, procedures, and preferences. Meeting women's health needs requires consideration of the myriad of options for care or treatment available and necessitates cultivation of a broad-based network of interdisciplinary professional and collaborative relationships.

Traditional midwifery care is based on providing care that fosters the physiologic processes of labor and birth. Modern midwifery and women's health care builds on this physiologic noninterventionist foundation to include interventions only as necessary and as indicated by the individual woman's condition and preferences. Determining which interventions are "necessary" and when they are "indicated" defines our individual practice as midwives, yet can also be a function of the environment of care in which the midwife practices.

The midwife–woman relationship can be developed and nurtured in every environment of care. In a situation of trust, clients whose primary point of reference is mainstream medical care can be supported to embrace noninterventionist care for normal labor and birth. Through development of a trusting relationship with her midwife, a client whose primary orientation is toward complementary and alternative care can be guided toward mainstream medical care when it is indicated. The potential for the client to derive comfort and feelings of safety is influenced by both the quality of the midwife–client relationship and the environment of care.

ENVIRONMENT OF CARE

The environments where care is obtained and provided affect each individual's health practices and outcomes. The Environment of Care includes the physical location where care is provided, the sociocultural milieu, and the prevailing attitudes evident during caring efforts provided by attending practitioners. A woman's autonomy and her sense of control over her circumstances are shaped by her environment.

The power dynamics between client and provider and between providers varies in different environments. In fact, a woman's physiologic response can be affected by changes in the environment of care; release of powerful stress hormones is mediated by the individual's sense of safety and confidence in her ability to cope with her present circumstances. These physiologic effects can be particularly striking in the environments where labor and birth occur (Lothian, 2004).

Midwives practice in many different environments, such as hospitals of various acuity levels, offices, birth centers, clinics, and homes. Across the globe, some midwives find themselves practicing in impoverished and low-resource settings. While the practice principles may remain the same regardless of the environment of care, the services and procedures offered often vary based on sociocultural factors and on access to resources, equipment, and qualified personnel. Within the ideal supportive healthcare system, midwives will have access to the full range of services, environments of care, and providers necessary for their client's care, including opportunities for collaborative practice focused on meeting the needs of the client.

No matter where clinicians stand on the continuum of healthcare practices, and regardless of the wide range of environments of care in which they practice, it remains imperative that practitioners understand the broad range of services that are available to the women who come to them for care. The women who seek out midwives for care—our clients—do not live in the healthcare world. Their awareness of which services are available is influenced by issues of access, the effects of advertising and Internet-based information, social and cultural beliefs, the experiences of their friends or relatives, and the ever-present popular media. Practitioners who are knowledgeable of the many options available to clients are prepared to listen and understand which healthcare choices women are making, thereby increasing their effectiveness in addressing women's needs.

HOW TO USE THIS BOOK

You may find it convenient to have several copies of this text: one for your exam room(s), one for your birth setting, and another by the phone at home. These comprehensive *Guidelines* have been formulated to stimulate critical thinking processes and are just one of many references available to inform clinical practice.

Guidelines evolve over time; it has been estimated that 20% of practice recommendations change over a 3-year period (Tillett, 2009). Thus guidelines are inevitably updated on a regular basis. Nevertheless, it remains the professional's responsibility to keep abreast of emerging evidence and recommendations for care, and to determine how to best incorporate clinical practice guidelines and recommendations into practice.

When used in lieu of practice-specific practice guidelines, this text may be individualized by including dated and initialed written additions and deletions, highlighting, and so on. A dated reference copy allows the practitioner to refer back to historical practice parameters should there be a need to describe one's practice at a future date.

Clinical Practice Guidelines for Midwifery and Women's Health uses a system of organization consistent with the way most healthcare providers are taught to gather, interpret, and act on the data obtained during an individual client encounter. Through this format, the *Guidelines* promote a methodical and consistent approach for client assessment, problem identification, and treatment or referral. Clear identification of documentation essentials and practice pitfalls act as reminders to the busy professional. Although the term "midwife" is frequently used throughout this book, the content and recommendations are equally relevant for other women's healthcare professionals.

Use of a systematic approach is indispensable to providing optimal women's health care in today's busy healthcare environment. A consistently applied method of approach and organization is central to providing women with comprehensive health care that meets each client's need in a thorough and satisfying manner.

Use of Symbols

Symbols are used throughout this text to indicate key areas that require particular attention. The purpose of the symbols is to heighten awareness, stimulate critical thinking in areas that are potentially problematic, and encourage comprehensive record keeping and interdisciplinary communication.

 Cultural Awareness

Use of this symbol highlights a need for cultural awareness. The world is fast becoming a global society. No matter where we practice, it is likely that each of us will provide care to women who come from different countries, or from cultures different from our own, or from locations other than where we obtained our primary midwifery education clinical experience.

Cultural sensitivity and humility are essential to ensure quality care of women in our multicultural world. We need to consider each woman as an individual who exists not only in our practice settings but also in the context of her own life circumstances and background. Cultural influences affect birth choices, birth control methods, sexual identity, self-care preferences, and more.

Cultural awareness includes consideration of the client's race, religion, ethnic heritage, age, generation, geographic factors, and cultural mores. Additionally, we need to remember that not everyone from a particular culture embraces the typical beliefs and behavior patterns associated with that culture, and that people can be members of several different subculture groups, some with conflicting beliefs. A client's health beliefs and cultural traditions should be explored and verified as the plan of care is being developed.

 ### Risk Management

Use of this symbol highlights a need to determine whether an identified risk is modifiable through action on the part of the client or the midwife. For risks that are inherent in the client or care practice, careful attention to risk/benefit information and detailed documentation are in order.

Risk management includes thoughtful consideration of factors that can increase risk to the mother or baby, to the well woman, or to the midwife providing care. Identification of those factors that contribute to risk is the first step in reducing their potential impact on outcomes. Risk management as applied to midwifery practice includes careful documentation of care provided, consultations, and case review. Integral components of the midwifery risk management plan are discussed later in this chapter.

 ### Clinician Resources

Use of this symbol denotes a web-based link or application in the Clinician Resources list at the end of each chapter. These resources have been carefully screened and selected for their clinical relevance and usefulness to practice. Each Clinician Resources feature identifies sites providing national practice recommendations, clinical assessment tools, drug resources, screening or testing information, and other essentials critical to keeping the busy midwife up-to-date.

 ### Consultation or Referral

Use of this symbol is a cue to consider whether a client might be best served by the involvement of other professionals in her care, such as dieticians or social workers; whether her condition requires additional expertise to supplement midwifery care through consultation and collaboration; or whether her needs are best met by referral to specialty care for treatment of a specific condition or transfer for continued care.

Consultations and referrals provide for continuity of care when problems develop or when additional expertise is required. Consultations range from informal conversations to detailed problem-oriented evaluation of the client by the consultant. When midwives consult with obstetric/gynecologic (OB/GYN) physicians, they need to remember that the physician practices a different specialty and may employ a different approach to the problem than that taken by the midwife. Consultation requests are documented in the client's medical record. The requesting care provider documents phone consultations, while an in-person consultation is documented by the consultant.

 ### Documentation

Use of this symbol highlights a need for careful documentation practices in accordance with institutional standards and national documentation recommendations. For those midwives or students who seek to improve documentation skills, additional recommendations for documentation are addressed later in this chapter (in Table 1-4, Documentation Standards).

Documentation of care is the basic building block of practice that illuminates and describes midwifery practice. Documentation skills are an essential component of midwifery practice and are the critical means used to describe and validate quality midwifery care and demonstrate differences between the disciplines of midwifery, medicine, and nursing.

A brief description of the categories used in the *Guidelines* can be seen in Table 1-1. Comprehensive

Table 1-1 Clinical Practice Guidelines Format
Key Clinical Information
Client History and Chart Review: Components of the history to consider
Physical Examination: Components of the physical exam to consider
Clinical Impression: Differential diagnoses to consider
Diagnostic Testing: Diagnostic tests and procedures to consider
Providing Treatment: Therapeutic measures to consider
Providing Treatment: Complementary and alternative measures to consider
Providing Support: Education and support measures to consider
Follow-up Care: Follow-up measures to consider
Multidisciplinary Practice: Consider consultation, collaboration, or referral

descriptions of the categories of information that might be obtained during client assessment, evaluation, and development of a midwifery management plan are provided next in the format that you will find throughout the *Guidelines*.

The Clinical Practice Guideline Format

Clinical Practice Guidelines for Midwifery and Women's Health is designed to stimulate critical thinking about clinical topics using a standardized quick-reference format. Each Clinical Practice Guideline offers a multitude of options for the clinician's consideration based on the following aspects of the case: the needs of the individual woman; the clinician's findings, philosophy, and style of practice; and the practice setting or environment of care. The primary intent is to enhance the clinician's ability to provide safe, satisfying care to women while avoiding unintentional omissions in evaluation, diagnosis, or treatment that can result in harm to women, their babies, and, by extension, the profession of midwifery.

Key Clinical Information

This section provides background information to inform the clinician's interpretation of the content of the Clinical Practice Guideline.

Client History and Chart Review: Components of the History to Consider

This section details information useful to developing a database sufficient to drive clinical decision making. Sources of this information include, but are not limited to, patient or family interviews, chart review, interval history, consultation requests, information from cultural interpreters, and dialogue with other health professionals (case review).

The client history is commonly divided into various categories based on the nature of the encounter, the environment of care, the scope of the practitioner, and the goal or objective of the client visit. Categories can include a comprehensive health history, an interval history, and a problem-oriented or event-specific history. The comprehensive health history can be further subdivided into the client's past medical and surgical history, social history, and family medical history. These subtypes of the history can be again subdivided to allow for focus on specific areas of concern, such as menstrual history, obstetric history, or genetic history.

The review of systems is a review of the major body systems with the client to determine the presence or absence of signs and symptoms of health conditions, illness, or disease. This comprehensive review includes the following systems: constitutional symptoms (weight loss, fever, malaise, fatigue); eyes, ears, nose, mouth, and throat; skin; respiratory; cardiovascular; gastrointestinal; genitourinary; musculoskeletal; endocrine; lymphatic/hematologic; immunologic/allergic; psychiatric; and neurologic systems (American Medical Association [AMA], 2010).

Identifying which components of the history to further explore with the client is a skill that can assist the midwife in efficiently identifying problems or concerns and in developing a working list of potential differential diagnoses. Components of the history that are included in the client interview are documented, including, when applicable, the client's stated attitude and observed affect or emotional state. The skilled diagnostician is an active listener who can discern which client responses are pertinent and use directed inquiry to elicit further information.

Review of the medical record is an integral part of the client's health history. Many clients provide a limited and necessarily subjective accounting of their health history. The medical record serves to provide an objective overview of the client's health status and can reveal essential details omitted during the client interview. Be aware, however, that the medical record is an imperfect data source that can contain errors and omit or condense a great deal of important information relevant to understanding the client's healthcare needs.

Physical Examination: Components of the Physical Exam to Consider

This section offers suggestions for broadening or narrowing the focus of inquiry and examination once the history has elucidated the indication for the visit and possible working diagnoses are developed.

Every body system has both general and specific elements that may be evaluated during the physical examination. Thorough evaluation of the area(s) of concern is an integral part of client or patient evaluation. Which components are included during the physical examination depends on the nature of the presenting problem or health condition and the individual midwife's scope of practice. Although many midwives care predominantly for women during the childbearing year, others provide comprehensive women's health care, including evaluation and treatment of gynecologic and/or primary care problems and conditions, examination and care of the infant, and evaluation and treatment of sexually transmitted infections in male sexual partners.

Both performance and documentation of the physical examination are most frequently organized in a head-to-toe fashion. Using a consistent technique allows for systematic client evaluation and comprehensive documentation of results and facilitates review of pertinent information. Standard medical terms are used to describe the presence or absence of findings in an objective manner consistent with the anatomic area under evaluation. "Normal" is a vague descriptor because the range of normal varies widely from client to client. Descriptive terms are used when necessary to enhance the narrative and present a comprehensive report of clinical findings.

Standard terminology is used to identify areas of note (i.e., right lower quadrant, periumbilical, substernal). "Left" and "right" are clearly identified when applicable. Instruments and tests used during the physical examination are identified when necessary to describe the technique used for evaluation—for example: "A speculum was inserted in the vagina to expose the cervix" or alternatively, "Speculum exam demonstrated ...."

The language should be clear and descriptive, and identify clinical findings and, when indicated, client response to the examination. Notes reflect the midwife's critical thinking process during the examination (italicized in the example that follows): "The left breast was noted to have an irregular fixed mass in the upper outer quadrant, extending into the axillary tail. The mass is approximately 2 × 3 cm, with bluish discoloration over the area, *which may represent increased vascularity*. The mass is firm but not hard; however, it is fixed to the chest wall and accompanied by palpable axillary lymph nodes. *The clinical picture is highly suspicious for breast cancer in spite of a negative mammogram last week*."

Clinical Impression: Differential Diagnoses to Consider

This segment is designed to aid the practitioner in considering the wide range of diagnoses that are possible with any given set of symptoms and physical findings. The working diagnosis will drive the choices for testing, treatment, and involvement of additional multidisciplinary, collaborative team members.

The clinical impression may be more familiar under the name of "assessment" or "diagnostic impression."

The differential diagnoses list is a brief summary of diagnoses under consideration given the client's presenting symptoms or condition. Differential diagnoses are often documented in the medical record as a running list from most to least important or likely. More than one diagnosis is possible due to shared symptomatology, such as the dual diagnosis of bacterial vaginosis and *Trichomonas* infection in the presence of vaginal discharge, pruritus, and foul odor.

The clinical impression identifies the midwife's assessment of the client's health status using standardized terms and billing codes based on the client history, physical examination, and any testing performed on-site. The clinical impression and differential diagnoses then direct discussion with the client and development of the midwifery plan of care, which can include further evaluation and testing, plans for continued care, and indications for consultation or referral. The plan of care reflects and is consistent with the differential diagnoses noted. A firm diagnosis can be deferred until the results of diagnostic testing have been reviewed, making testing part of the overall midwifery plan.

The documented clinical impression is also used for coding and billing purposes. The *International Classification of Diseases, Ninth Revision, Clinical Modification* (ICD-9-CM) has been the official system of assigning codes to diagnoses and procedures associated with hospital utilization in the United States. However, it is due to be retired in the next few years (Centers for Medicare & Medicaid Services [CMS], 2010c), when it will be replaced with the *International Classification of Diseases, Tenth Edition, Clinical Modification/Procedure Coding System* (ICD-10-CM/PCS). The ICD-10-CM is intended for use in all U.S. healthcare settings. Each code in this system consists of three to seven digits, rather than the three to five digits used in the ICD-9-CM. The ICD-10-PCS is intended for use in all U.S. in-patient hospital settings; each of its codes consists of seven alphanumeric digits, rather than the three to four numeric digits used under the ICD-9-PCS. The ICD-10-CM/PCS system has been in use for years in other nations; however, the complexity of the U.S. healthcare and payer system has hampered its adoption here. The ICD-10 system offers more detailed data about patient conditions and procedures and reflects current medical practice and nomenclature.

Although useful to document the clinician's thinking, the term "rule out" is not acceptable for coding purposes. Nevertheless, it remains a useful way of clarifying indications for diagnostic testing to confirm or eliminate ("rule out") a specific listed differential diagnosis under consideration. For example, the differential diagnosis of "urinary urgency" can be accompanied by the phrase "rule out urinary tract infection," when infection has not yet been diagnosed pending laboratory confirmation.

Coding decisions are complex and establish the medical necessity for the services provided. The midwife must use the code that best describes the unique situation of the individual patient. Midwives and other clinicians are responsible for accurately coding the services they provide to their clients. Providers and their billers are required to obtain and use the version of the coding structure in current use. This issue will be especially important during the upcoming transition from the ICD-9-CM/PCS to the ICD-10-CM/PCS slated to occur in the next few years. Always check a current resource to obtain the most up-to-date codes. Codes can be obtained from the following site: http://icd9data.com/ or http://www.icd10data.com/.

Establishing medical necessity is vital to getting paid—if codes do not make sense, are not supported by documentation in the client's medical record, or are nonspecific, the unhappy result may be payment downgrades or payer denials. There is a difference between coding and billing. You can always find a code, but billing rules may prohibit its use—such is the case with some diagnoses that are used in the presence or absence of pregnancy.

Diagnostic Testing: Diagnostic Tests and Procedures to Consider

This section offers a range of testing options related to the most common working diagnoses. In some instances, reference ranges have been included to guide clinical decision making. Please note that the reference ranges for the laboratory performing the test may vary from those published here; the specific laboratory's reference ranges should always be considered when reviewing test results.

Diagnostic testing includes tests or procedures performed to elicit additional information to accurately diagnose a clinical problem, to verify a health condition, and to evaluate or monitor an ongoing treatment plan. Testing is documented in a brief and straightforward manner, with additional explanations being provided in unusual situations. Testing is often documented as a numbered list using standard terminology. Each test ordered must be clearly identifiable by other healthcare professionals. One area in which confusion can occur is when diagnostic or screening panels are ordered, the names or components of which are not consistent from facility to facility. For example, the panel "PIH labs" (pregnancy-induced hypertension or preeclampsia panel) can include different arrays of tests at different locations. This can become problematic when a transfer of care is necessary and test results are pending.

Test results should be reviewed and clearly documented or filed in an easy-to-find location, especially when they pertain to ongoing care of a problem. Test results come under the heading of "Objective Findings" when writing or dictating a note in the medical record. Anticipatory thinking regarding potential diagnostic test results is documented in the record to support continuity of care when another clinician is responsible for providing continued care, such as occurs in group practice settings, or with a transfer of care.

Providing Treatment: Therapeutic Measures to Consider

This segment details the most common and accepted options for treatment based on the literature and current clinical practice for the select diagnoses. Every effort is made to include well-documented therapeutic options that had previously been considered "alternative" and are now considered "evidence based"

according to the literature. Examples include vaginal birth after cesarean, hydrotherapy in labor, the Gaskin maneuver, fetal heart rate (FHR) auscultation in labor, and physical therapy for low back strain.

Therapeutic measures include the administration, ordering, or prescription of medications and accepted therapeutic treatments. Documentation of medications includes the medication name, indication for use, dosage, timing, and route of administration. Review of medication instructions, known side effects, and adverse effects is an integral part of the prescriptive process. Care is taken to use pictograms or standardized foreign-language handouts when necessary to ensure women have the information needed to understand and properly execute medication recommendations. When off-label medication use is prescribed, it is documented as such, with documentation of relevant discussions with the client regarding clinician recommendations for off-label medication use and informed consent when indicated. Other treatment modalities, such as physical therapy, chiropractic manipulation, and respiratory therapy treatments, are documented as ordered, including the indication for the treatment.

Providing Treatment: Complementary and Alternative Measures to Consider

This section offers treatment options that are less well documented in the literature, that are less common in mainstream women's health practice, for which there is only empiric evidence, or that are generally considered "complementary and alternative medicine" when compared to commonly accepted mainstream women's health practice. Commonly accepted practices that the literature does not address are included in this category.

Alternative treatment measures include CAM therapies such as acupuncture, acupressure, homeopathy, herbal remedies, and massage. Many CAM treatments are not considered to be "prescribed" because they are available to clients for self-treatment. In contrast, other CAM therapies, such as custom compounding of hormones, do require a prescription.

The midwife should be aware of the wide range of therapies available as treatment options, note current evidence regarding the safety and effectiveness of these treatments, and provide advice for their use. Ideally, sources should be cited for suggested measures, and client instruction and pertinent discussion regarding alternative, traditional, and empiric treatments documented.

Lack of randomized controlled trials can limit recommendations for complementary and alternative measures in some practices, whereas in other practices these time-honored methods of caring for women continue to be discussed on a regular basis. Ethical midwifery practice requires discussion of known risks and benefits of therapeutic measures as well as the limits of our knowledge and documentation of the same. Consider the following example:

> Client, G3, P2002, inquired about use of castor oil to stimulate labor at 41½ weeks. The FHR was reactive today; cervix is soft and 1 cm. We discussed her options: expectant care, herbal or homeopathic remedies to stimulate cervical change, and the parameters for use of medications for cervical ripening and/or induction of labor. She expressed interest in castor oil and was provided with information and instructions for use of P.O. castor oil for cervical ripening (Knoche, Seltzer, & Smolley, 2008). She was instructed to call with the onset of labor or return to the office in the A.M. if no labor ensues for monitoring of maternal/fetal well-being.

Providing Support: Education and Support Measures to Consider

This section details ways in which the clinician can enhance self-care and knowledge of the individual. Of particular concern in this section are suggestions or recommendations for means to enhance the woman's commitment to the treatment plan, promote self-care, and encourage healthy choices.

Client education and support are integral elements of midwifery practice and, as such, should be clearly documented. Use of standardized client education materials can make documentation of education simpler and less time consuming. Maintaining a master file of regularly used client education materials allows the midwife to refer back as needed to see which materials were used during a specific time period. Documentation in the medical record describes patient education content, pertinent discussion, and recommendations for support measures; it also indicates whether patient education and support measure recommendations were provided verbally, in writing, or both. Use of an interpreter or foreign-language handouts is noted. A teaching checklist provides an efficient means to document standardized teaching. The use of written instructions or recommendations allows the client to refer to them after the visit and to refresh her memory regarding instructions or information provided at the visit.

Client support can include coordination of recommended care, such as scheduling of diagnostic tests and coordination of referrals; recommendations for social, psychological, educational, economic, or other resources; and access to off-hours services. Although review of diagnostic test results and clinical planning based on those results fall under the category of follow-up, interaction with the client that includes information about test results, options for care, discussion of alternatives, and a compassionate listening ear occurs within the client support and education framework.

Follow-up Care: Follow-up Measures to Consider

This section details the recommendations for continued care, testing, consultation, or referral that are supported by the literature and/or inclusive of providing thorough, quality, compassionate care. In addition, this section addresses areas of midwifery practice or documentation that enhance positive health and practice outcomes.

Follow-up after a client encounter includes the actual process of documenting care that has been provided, including anticipatory thinking, and recommendations for future care. This documentation also clearly indicates the timing of recommended appointment(s) for further care or testing. This serves to ensure that the midwife, as well as other clinicians, has a clear impression of the client visit, the care provided, and the anticipated next steps in the ongoing care of this individual.

Identification of expectations for the client's next visit(s) and interval self-care are critical elements to include when documenting the midwifery plan of care. Clients who are informed and aware of what is expected of them, and who agree with the treatment plan, are most likely to follow through with recommendations for care. Follow-up can include events such as returning for a scheduled visit (i.e., a routine prenatal visit) or telephone contact from the midwife after receipt of a test result (i.e., a mammogram performed on a client with a suspicious breast mass). Follow-up also includes reminders to call or present for care if mild symptoms at the time of the examination persist or worsen (i.e., nasal congestion that develops into a productive cough with fever, or scant vaginal spotting that turns bright red and heavy), along with instructions on how to reach on-call personnel during off-hours and where and when to present for urgent or emergency care.

When a deviation from normal or unexpected findings occurs, a detailed plan for follow-up care is developed and documented. In the earlier example of a woman with a breast mass, the documentation might include the date on which results were received; discussion with the client about her options for care; referral to a breast specialist; the date and time of the specialist appointment; documentation of the consult request, including records transferred to the specialist with written client consent; and initiation of a mechanism to verify client follow-through with these recommendations and appointments.

Tracking of clients who are receiving ongoing treatment for unresolved problems is an integral part of the midwifery risk management plan. For the many midwives who provide comprehensive women's health care, an organized follow-up system, such as a file or database, can be useful to track the ongoing care of clients requiring scheduled follow-up. In this instance, documentation in the client medical record that the follow-up system has been implemented can help with tracking. Depending on patient volume and the complexity of the clinical issues requiring follow-up care, the follow-up system can be a calendar, a notebook, a cross-referenced index card file, or a software program that automatically generates reminders, identifies no-shows, and provides a comprehensive record of problems and follow-up messages sent to the individual requiring care.

Multidisciplinary Practice: Consider Consultation, Collaboration, or Referral

This section addresses midwifery care as part of a multidisciplinary system of care in which midwives consult with, collaborate with, and refer to various other health providers and services such as OB/GYN physicians, nurse-practitioners, pediatric care providers, and other specialty care providers.

Consultations or referrals are made by midwives for many types of services, including counseling, smoking cessation, nutritional evaluation, psychiatric care, substance abuse treatment, and alternative therapies. Such services can be provided by a wide array of individuals, such as pharmacists, physical therapists, social workers, dieticians, herbalists, acupuncturists, chiropractors, or clergy, based on the needs and wishes of the individual and the midwife's scope of practice.

A consultation comprises any request for collaboration with another healthcare professional to provide care for a client for a specific indication. Documentation of a consultation or referral in the client's medical record includes the name and specialty of the provider, the means by which the contact was made (e.g., phone, letter, or directly by the client), the indication for the consultation or referral, and expectations for care.

Written and telephone consultation or referral requests include a brief history of the problem, essential information about the client, the type of service for which the client is being referred, and expectations regarding care. Providing information about expectations for care allows the midwife to be clear to the consultant about the client's desired course of evaluation or treatment, and to determine whether any conflict in style of practice or management of clinical conditions exists. The goal of a consultation or referral is to obtain appropriate problem-specific care that is acceptable to the client. In some instances, however, differences in philosophy or style of practice are unavoidable; in this scenario, the midwife's primary goal is to obtain best care for the client.

A copy of a written consultation request is maintained in the client's medical record. Documenting information about scheduled consultation or referral appointments can be helpful when following up on diagnosis or treatment of problems. When a consultation is obtained, the consultant's opinion is documented in the client's medical record. When the consultant provides this service via telephone, the midwife requesting the consultation is responsible for documenting the content of the conversation, the consultant's recommendations for care, and the relevance or application of those recommendations to the midwifery plan of care. When the consultant evaluates the client in person, the consultant is responsible for documenting his or her opinion and any care rendered.

This accepted systematic approach to client evaluation and care allows the clinician to collect and present data in an organized fashion. The midwife can then focus on documenting the information collected, care provided, and midwifery management plan in a manner that is reflective of the midwifery model of care. Documentation that reflects the midwifery model of care allows practitioners, researchers, and others to gain a greater understanding of the practice of midwifery.

DOCUMENTATION OF MIDWIFERY CARE

Thoughtful documentation can highlight inherent differences between the midwifery and medical models of providing women's health care. This recognition, in turn, encourages research that demonstrates positive processes and outcomes for clients cared for by midwives, as shown in seminal midwifery care studies described by Farley (2005). The recommendations that follow provide a general guideline for documenting midwifery care (see Table 1-4).

The "midwifery management plan" reflects an overall plan of care in which the intended course of action for evaluation, diagnosis, treatment, follow-up, and client understanding of that plan is clearly documented and logically follows from the indication for the visit. The midwifery management plan is a comprehensive plan that includes recommendations for diagnostic testing; indications for therapeutic measures or treatments, and which modalities were prescribed; client education and support; plans for continued care or follow-up; and consultations or referrals.

Careful and complete documentation serves as the midwife's legal record of events that have occurred. Standardizing the documentation format frees the midwife to concentrate on the content of the client encounter and documentation or note. The client's medical record lives on long after entries about the care provided to this woman are completed, and over time this information may pass through many hands. Some examples of people who read or review the health record to see which care was provided during the encounter with the client include other providers caring for the client at a later date, billing and coding personnel, quality improvement officers, The Joint Commission, peer reviewers, and perinatal morbidity and mortality reviewers.

The ideal medical record provides the reader with a clear view of the client's presentation, the midwife's evaluation process, and the implementation and results of treatment or recommendations. Meticulous documentation also allows other professionals to follow the course of care provided and to gain insight into the client's response. Client health records are an essential communication tool in a group practice and during consultation or referral. This section explores the process of documentation from several points of view:

- Documentation as a reflection of the midwifery model of care; describing care that reflects the philosophy and standards of the practice of midwifery
- Documentation using current procedural terminology (CPT) evaluation and management (E/M) criteria; a method of documentation developed by the American Medical Association (AMA) that reflects the complexity and level of care provided to meet current reimbursement criteria
- Documentation as an essential communication tool; a method of recording events and findings for future reference that follows accepted standards
- Documentation as a means of demonstrating application of risk management and collaborative practice processes

Documentation of the Midwifery Model of Care

As professionals, midwives continually work toward the goal of educating both their clients and their colleagues about how midwifery differs from medicine and nursing. Midwifery educators strive to ensure that these differences are reflected in midwifery education programs and in the clinical experiences of those learning midwifery (American College of Nurse–Midwives [ACNM], 2008). Midwifery encompasses the belief that birth is essentially normal, that women have the right to be listened to and heard, and that birth and well-woman care are important events in the lives of women. These beliefs translate into subtle and overt behavioral differences in maternity and women's health practice that should be reflected in the client's medical record.

While sharing a number of practices in common with other healthcare providers, midwives need to clearly reflect through documentation how midwifery care is unique. Although many of the behaviors that a midwife, a physician, a nurse practitioner, or a physician's assistant demonstrate when providing women's health care may be similar, the origins, attitudes, and client perception of the care may be substantially different. Documentation of midwifery care should reflect the essence of midwifery: woman-oriented care focused on excellence in the processes of providing care with attentiveness to outcomes.

Evaluation and Management Criteria

The CPT system lists codes for services provided by clinicians using specific criteria that must be present in the documentation of care provided. Evaluation and management (E/M) codes are based on the level of service provided. The level of E/M services provided is determined by the amount of history, physical examination, medical decision making (critical thinking), counseling and coordination of care (client education and support), nature of the presenting problem, and the amount of time required to provide care. Accurate coding practices are essential for receiving appropriate reimbursement for services.

As this book went to press, a major transition was occurring in the United States regarding how health visits are coded. Box 1-2 illustrates the upcoming changes as billing codes shift from the ICD-9 system to the ICD-10 system. To obtain more information on how this change may affect your practice, use the link provided in the Clinician's Resources feature at the end of this chapter.

The AMA publishes the CPT handbook and offers online CPT assistance (AMA, 2011). These useful products and services can assist the healthcare provider in choosing a code for a service or procedure based on the documentation of the service or procedure during coding and billing. Midwives should become familiar with these resources as well as with ICD-9 or ICD-10 coding resources because they are important for fiscally responsible practice (ICD9Data.com, 2012). A brief overview of the required components for the level of care provided is offered here.

The history and physical examination and the complexity of critical thinking are the key components used to determine the level of E/M service

---

Box 1-2   Examples of Differential Diagnoses and Code Groups: Comparison of ICD-9 and ICD-10

ICD-9 Codes

V70: Preventive health visit, not otherwise specified (NOS)

788.1: Dysuria

788.41: Urinary frequency

788.63: Urinary urgency

V22: Normal pregnancy, 10 weeks' gestation by last menstrual period (LMP)

611.72: Lump or mass in breast

V22.2: Pregnancy (incidental to presenting complaint) and

789.03: Right lower quadrant pain

Rule out:

   Round ligament pain

   Appendicitis

   Ectopic pregnancy

   Ovarian cyst

ICD-10 Codes

Z00: Encounter for general examination without complaint, suspected or reported diagnosis

R30: Dysuria

R35: Urination, frequent

R31.95: Urgency of urination

N39.9: Disorder of urinary system, unspecified

Z34.01: Supervision of normal first pregnancy, first trimester

Z34.81: Supervision of other normal pregnancy, first trimester

N63: Unspecified mass in breast

Z33.1: Pregnant state, incidental

R10.31: Right lower quadrant pain

Rule out:

   Round ligament pain

   Appendicitis

   Ectopic pregnancy

   Ovarian cyst

Source: ICD9data.com, 2012.

---

provided. The nature of the presenting problem, along with the provision of client education and support, are considered contributory, whereas time spent is considered separately. Time criteria used in E/M are based on the time spent during the face-to-face client visit, whereas the time required for review of diagnostic testing, follow-up, and coordination of care is factored into the time component (AMA, 2011; CMS, 2010b).

The E/M evaluation considers four types of history and physical examination (see Table 1-2). The complexity of clinical decision making required reflects the complexity of reaching a diagnosis and/or of formulating a management plan. The more health records, tests, or other information to be reviewed,

the more complex the evaluation becomes. The greater the number of differential diagnoses and potential plans to be considered, the more complex the management decision making becomes. The higher the risk of complications, morbidity, mortality, or comorbidity related to health problems or recommended testing, the more complex the management decision making becomes. Decision making is evaluated as being straightforward or of low, moderate, or high complexity (AMA, 2010).

Standards for Documentation: Transition to Electronic Health Records

Documentation standards for paper-based health records have been developed to allow use of the

Table 1-2   E/M Categories of History and Physical Examination

TYPE OF VISIT	VISIT COMPONENTS
Problem-focused visit	Brief history of the reason for the encounter and an examination that is limited to the affected area
Expanded problem-focused visit	Adds a pertinent system review and examination of additional body systems that might be affected by the presenting problem
Detailed visit	Adds pertinent history related to the reason for the encounter and a thorough examination of the affected area and related organ systems
Comprehensive visit	Adds a complete review of systems, comprehensive review of the client history and risk assessment, and either a comprehensive physical examination or thorough examination of a single organ system

client's medical record as an effective means of communication between professionals, verification of services provided for billing and reimbursement purposes, and analysis of care provided for quality and appropriateness. Many of these standards will apply as the nation's healthcare information infrastructure transitions to use of a computerized documentation system. It is important to understand that the electronic health record (EHR) is not just a scanned version of the written patient record (CMS, 2010a). Rather, EHRs hold the promise of functions that cannot be achieved by a paper record, such as immediate availability, currency, and completeness of client health information. Computing functions can link the EHR to educational resources specifically tailored to the client's needs. Error reduction, particularly with regard to medication errors, is possible through computer cross-checking of a patient's medications with known allergies, dosing regimens, and potential adverse interactions with other medications the client is taking. Decision support capabilities, such as context-sensitive alerts and eligibility determination for particular therapeutic regimens, can assist clinicians in formulating diagnostic and management plans; Table 1-3 provides some examples of these decision support (and other) apps.

As this edition of this book went to press, federal initiatives were in place to assist healthcare professionals and institutions in the adoption of technologies to convert to an EHR system (CMS, 2010b). Widespread transitions are actively evolving our understanding of the benefits and challenges of EHR. What is clear is that today's midwife will have to embrace and master the skills required to effectively interface with a variety of EHR systems and platforms to ensure that documentation of midwifery care is accurate, complete, and well represented in the record in service of the client's healthcare needs.

The term "app" is short for "application" and refers to a computer software application that relies on common web browsers to render the application executable. While this term has been used by those in the computer industry for years, it became newly popular with the emergence of smartphones and tablet computers. These smaller computer devices can easily accompany the midwife for use at the point of care. Decision support for the clinician is provided through ready access to up-to-date information, calculators designed for specific healthcare purposes, visual illustrations, and algorithms for diagnosis and treatment decisions. Apps are a rapidly expanding market, particularly in healthcare applications with the potential for enhancing practice.

Table 1-3   "There's an App for That"

APPLICATION	PURPOSE
Examples of Decision Support Applications for Clinicians	
Epocrates	Drug reference
My Natural Healer	Complementary and alternative therapies reference
Perfect Wheel	Gestational age calculator
Pocket Lab Values	Medical laboratory test reference
LactMed	Effects of medications on the nursing couplet
STD2010	CDC guidelines for STD treatment
BishopScore	Bishop's score calculator
Diagnosaurus DDX	Differential diagnosis reference
EFM Glossary	Electronic fetal monitor terms and illustrations
NeoTube	Guide for endotracheal intubation of the neonate
Examples of Apps for Client Use and Education	
iperiod	Tracking of menstrual and fertility indicators
BabyCenter	Pregnancy and prenatal care resource
Baby Namer	Name selection reference
ikegel	Guide for pelvic floor exercises
Baby Motion	Fetal movement tracker
Birth Buddy	Timer and graph for contractions
Baby Checklist	Baby supplies organizer
Breast Feeding Friend	Tracks feedings
iNew Mommy Postpartum Adjustment	Screening quiz for postpartum depression

Documentation as Communication: Skills and Techniques

Thorough documentation provides midwives and other healthcare professionals with a clear view of each woman's individual presentation, concerns, and preferences for care. The client record also serves as a means of following the midwife's thought processes regarding development of the working diagnosis and ongoing plans for continued client care. Clear, concise documentation is the key to validating quality care and is an integral part of the midwife's risk management program.

The goal of each note is to present a record of care provided and other essential information to guide the midwife and other healthcare professionals in the event of a transfer of care, such as might occur after problem-oriented referral, transfer to physician care for a high-risk condition, or simple cross-coverage arrangements. Table 1-4 summarizes the standards that must be met in regard to documentation.

In the event of legal action, the ideal medical record provides a clear picture of the client presentation, concerns, participation in care decisions, and response to care or treatment. The medical record identifies the midwife's assessment process and working diagnoses; it also includes her or his anticipatory thinking and planning for diagnosis, treatment, and continued or ongoing care. The midwifery plan

Table 1-4   Documentation Standards

STANDARD	PERFORMANCE MEASURES
1. Elements in the client's health record are organized in a consistent manner.	• The client record is organized in a clear and systematic fashion. • Records are entered in chronologic order.
2. Client health records are maintained and secured in a manner that protects the safety of the records and the confidentiality of the information.	• All health records are stored out of reach and accessible only to authorized persons, or are encrypted and available only to authorized users. See the related standard on maintenance, disclosure, and disposal of confidential information.
3. Client name or identification number is on each document in the record.	• The client name or identification number is found on each document in the record.
4. Entries are legible.	• Handwritten entries are legible. • Notes use a consistent standardized format and language that allows the reader to review care without the use of separate legend/key.
5. Entries are dated.	• Each entry in the record is dated. • Entries generated by an outside source (e.g., referrals, consults) are also dated when reviewed. • Notes related to client encounters or phone calls are placed in the record within 72 hours or 3 business days of occurrence.
6. Entries are initialed or signed by their author.	• Author identification may be a handwritten signature, unique electronic identifier, or initials. This applies to practitioners and members of the office staff who contribute to the record. • When initials are used, there is a designation of signature and status maintained in the office. • Entries generated by an outside source (e.g., referrals, consults) are also initialed or signed when reviewed.
7. Personal and biographical data are included in the record.	• Information necessary to identify the client and his or her insurer and to submit claims is included. • Information is included regarding client need for a language or cultural interpreter or other communication mechanisms as necessary to ensure appropriate client care. • The name of the client's primary care provider is clearly indicated in the record.
8. A. Initial history and physical examinations of new patients are performed within 12 months of a patient first seeking care or within three visits, whichever occurs first.	• A. Documentation for all clients includes an initial comprehensive history and physical examination performed within 12 months of the first visit or within three visits, whichever occurs first. If applicable, written evidence is created that the practitioner advised the client to return for a physical examination. The documentation of such a complete history and physical, included in the health record and done within the past 12 months by another practitioner, is acceptable. Well-child exams meet this standard.

(continues)

Table 1-4 Documentation Standards (continued)	
STANDARD	**PERFORMANCE MEASURES**
B. Past medical history is documented and includes serious accidents, operations, and illnesses.	• A and B. The history and physical documentation contains pertinent information such as age, height, vital signs, past medical and behavioral health history, preventive health maintenance and risk screening, physical examination, diagnostic impression, and documentation related to the ordering of appropriate diagnostic tests, procedures, and/or medications. Self-administered client questionnaires are an acceptable way to obtain baseline past medical history and personal information. Written documentation explains gaps in information contained in the health record regarding the history and physical (e.g., poor historians, patient's inability or unwillingness to provide information).
C. Family history is documented.	• C. The patient record contains immediate family history or documentation that it is noncontributory, unavailable, or unknown.
D. Birth history is documented for patients aged 6 years and younger.	• D. Infant records should include gestational and birth history and should be age and diagnosis appropriate.
9. Allergies and adverse reactions are prominently listed or noted as "none" or "NKA."	• Medication allergies or history of adverse reactions to medications are displayed in a prominent and consistent location or noted as "none" or "NKA." (Examples of where allergies may be prominently displayed include on a coversheet inside the chart, at the top of every visit page, or on a medication record in the chart.) • When applicable and known, there is documentation of the date when the allergy was first discovered, related symptoms, and previous treatments required.
10. Information regarding social history is recorded.	• The client record includes documentation regarding social history relevant to the purposes of the health encounter, such as sexual preferences and behaviors and use of tobacco, alcohol, or illicit drugs (or lack thereof) in clients 12 years of age and older who have been seen three or more times. • Cultural and developmental issues are clearly documented when present. • Family situation, living arrangements, and social support systems are noted. • Healthcare habits and preferences are noted, including use of alternative therapies, herbal remedies, and dietary supplements.
11. An updated problem list is maintained.	• A dated problem list, which summarizes the status of important client health information, such as major diagnoses, past medical and/or surgical history, and recurrent reports of symptoms, is documented and maintained. • The problem list is clearly visible and accessible. • Continuity of care between multiple practitioners in the same practice is demonstrated by documentation and review of pertinent health information.

Table 1-4 Documentation Standards (continued)	
STANDARD	**PERFORMANCE MEASURES**
12. The client's chief complaint or the purpose of the visit is clearly documented.	• The client's description of symptoms or the purpose of the visit is recorded as stated by the client. • Documentation supports that the client's perceived needs and expectations were addressed. • The documented history and physical examination are relevant to the client's reason for visit. • Telephone encounters relevant to health issues are documented in the health record and reflect practitioner review, including phone triage handled by office staff, and after-hours communication handled by on-call staff.
13. Working diagnoses or clinical impressions are consistent with the health history and physical examination findings.	• The health history and physical examination are documented and correspond to the client's stated symptoms, purpose for seeking care, and/or ongoing care for chronic illnesses. • The documentation supports the working diagnoses or clinical impressions.
14. The midwifery action or treatment plan is consistent with diagnosis(es).	• Proposed treatment plans, therapies, or other regimens are documented and logically follow previously documented diagnoses and clinical impressions. • The rationale for treatment decisions appears appropriate and is substantiated by documentation in the record. • Follow-up diagnostic testing is performed at appropriate intervals for diagnoses.
15. There is evidence that risk to the client associated with any diagnostic or therapeutic procedures is addressed.	• The health record shows clear justification for diagnostic and therapeutic measures. • Risk related to all diagnostic and therapeutic measures is discussed with the client using accepted parameters for informed consent and clearly documented in the record.
16. Unresolved problems from previous visits are addressed in subsequent visits.	• Continuity of care from one visit to the next is demonstrated when documentation of a problem-oriented approach to unresolved problems from previous visits occurs in subsequent visit notes.
17. Follow-up instructions and a time frame for follow-up or the next visit are recorded as appropriate.	• Recommendations for the client's return to the provider's office in a specified amount of time is recorded at the time of the visit or following consultation, laboratory, or other diagnostic reports. • Follow-up is documented for clients who require periodic visits for a chronic illness and for clients who require reassessment following an episodic illness. • Client participation in the coordination of care is demonstrated through documented client education, follow-up, and return visits.

(continues)

Table 1-4   Documentation Standards (continued)

STANDARD	PERFORMANCE MEASURES
17. Follow-up instructions and a time frame for follow-up or the next visit are recorded as appropriate. *(continued)*	• Implementation of a standardized plan for follow-up contact with the client is documented for individuals with critical test values or acute conditions who do not return for care as recommended. Such a plan is described in the practice's risk management policy.
18. Current medications are documented in the record, and notes reflect that long-term medications are reviewed at least annually by the practitioner and updated as needed.	• Information regarding current medications is readily apparent from a review of the record. • Changes to the client's medication regimen are noted as they occur. When medications appear to remain unchanged, the record includes documentation of an annual review by the practitioner. • Documentation addresses medication, herbal, or dietary supplement interactions, side effects, or adverse effects when indicated by the agent, or the individual's health status or genetic make-up.
19. Healthcare education is noted in the record and periodically updated as appropriate.	• Education is age, developmentally, and culturally appropriate. • Education may correspond directly to the reason for the visit, may pertain to specific diagnosis-related issues, may address client concerns, or may clarify recommendations. • Education provided to clients, family members, or designated caregivers is documented. • Examples of patient divergence from the plan of care are documented.
20. Screening and preventive care practices are offered in accordance with current recommendations from national standards-setting organizations.	• Each record includes documentation that preventive services were ordered and performed or that the practitioner discussed preventive services with the client and the client chose to defer or refuse them. • Current immunization and screening status is documented. • Practitioners may document that a patient sought preventive services from another practitioner (e.g., family practitioner).
21. An immunization record is completed for clients 18 years and younger, and vaccines offered and administered to adults are documented.	• The record includes documentation of immunizations administered from birth to present for clients 18 years and younger. • When prior records are unavailable, practitioners may document that a child's parent or guardian affirmed that immunizations were administered by another practitioner and the approximate age or date the immunizations were given. • For clients older than age 18, the record reflects discussion of current adult vaccine recommendations and documents any vaccine administration.

Table 1-4   Documentation Standards (continued)

STANDARD	PERFORMANCE MEASURES
22. Requests for consultation are consistent with clinical assessment/physical findings.	• The clinical assessment supports the decision for a referral. • Referrals are provided in a timely manner according to the severity of the patient's condition. • Referral requests and expectations are clearly documented.
23. Laboratory and diagnostic reports reflect practitioner review.	• Results of all laboratory tests and other diagnostics are documented in the health record. • Records demonstrate that the practitioner reviews laboratory and diagnostic reports and makes treatment decisions based on report findings. • Reports within the review period are initialed and dated by the practitioner, or another system of ensuring practitioner review is in place and clearly delineated in the practice's policies and procedures.
24. Client notification of laboratory and diagnostic test results and instruction regarding follow-up, when indicated, are documented.	• Clients are notified of abnormal laboratory and diagnostic results and advised of recommendations regarding follow-up or changes in treatment. • The record documents patient notification of results. A practitioner may document that the client is to call regarding results; however, the practitioner is responsible for ensuring and documenting that the client is advised of any abnormal results and recommendations for continued care.
25. There is evidence of continuity and coordination of care between primary and specialty care practitioners or other providers.	• Consultation reports reflect practitioner review. • Primary care provider records include consultation reports/summaries (within 60–90 days) that correspond to specialist referrals or documentation that there was a clear attempt to obtain reports that were not received. Subsequent visit notes reflect results of the consultation as may be pertinent to ongoing client care. • Specialist records include a consultation report/summary addressed to the referral source. • When a client receives services at or through another provider, such as a hospital, emergency care, home care agency, skilled nursing facility, or behavioral health specialist, there is evidence of coordination of care through consultation reports, discharge summaries, status reports, or home health reports. The discharge summary includes the reason for admission, the treatment provided, and the instructions given to the client on discharge.

Source: Adapted from American Cancer Society, 2010; American Health Information Management Association (AHIMA), 2008; CareFirst BlueCross BlueShield, 2009; National Heart, Lung, and Blood Institute, 2011; National Institutes of Health, 2011; U.S. Preventive Services Task Force, 2011.

for follow-up care and evaluation includes relevant parameters for initiation of multidisciplinary practice when indicated or applicable.

The American College of Nurse–Midwives (ACNM, n.d.), American Association of Birth Centers (AABC, 2007), and the Midwives Alliance of North America (MANA, 2010b) all offer clinical data sets that can be used as tools to evaluate the adequacy of standardized client record forms used in midwifery practice and that contribute to a national database to document and describe midwifery care. These data sets have been developed to provide standardized and validated tools for collecting data about the care midwives provide. Midwives seeking to improve their documentation skills may also use these clinical data sets as a self-evaluation instrument by performing retrospective chart or medical record audits to determine process or documentation strengths and weaknesses and to identify areas needing improvement.

Thorough and complete documentation is concise and focused; rarely is it necessary to provide lengthy notes. Handwritten notes must be legible to the average reader. Notes may be entered on a form that provides a preset format, such as a labor flow sheet, or written on a blank sheet of paper, such as a progress note. Some notes are dictated and transcribed. All practices are moving toward the transition to computer charting.

Notes should reflect pertinent findings and the critical thinking that occurs during the care of each client. All notes should contain, at a minimum, the following information:

- Client identification: Name, date of birth, and medical record number where applicable.
- Date of service: Date and time are necessary for time-sensitive situations such as labor care or during newborn resuscitation.
- Reason for encounter: Often described in the client's own words (e.g., "I think my water broke") or as a simple statement (e.g., "onset of labor").
- Client history: An expansion of the reason for the encounter, commonly known as the "chief report" or the "history of present illness"; it includes all relevant history and subjective information provided by the client or family, including, as applicable, the review of systems, past history (chart review), family history, and social history.
- Objective findings: Includes the results of the physical examination, mental status evaluation, and/or laboratory work, ultrasound, or other testing as indicated by the history and physical. Depending on the level of access to the client's EHR from remote locations, notes pertaining to off-site phone encounters with the client may not include these findings.
- Clinical impression: Also known as the "assessment" or "working diagnosis"; it may include several differential diagnoses under consideration pending laboratory or testing results. These findings may be documented as "primary symptoms" or "conditions" with differential diagnoses listed to validate testing and communicate anticipatory thinking.
- Midwifery plan of care: May be subdivided into several categories; it essentially outlines all diagnostic, therapeutic, and educational measures initiated at the visit, along with further actions anticipated based on potential results and specific needs of the client. The plan of care should end with a recommendation for the timing of the next visit.

Documentation as Risk Management

Exemplary midwifery practice includes understanding and implementing essential components of a risk management program to enhance midwifery care and client outcomes. Thorough documentation using a standardized format allows for objective evaluation of the care provided. Each note should be written from the objective outside observer point of view. Thorough but concise documentation is the ideal. Use of fill-in-the-blank forms or drop-down menus can be a useful way to quickly record essential information, particularly for routine encounters; a common example of this practice is the prenatal flow sheet. These notes are best supplemented with a narrative note whenever there are unusual circumstances or findings.

The problem list is a convenient way to highlight ongoing acute or chronic problems. It should be kept in an easily seen location, thereby enabling all clinicians caring for the client to identify at a glance potential factors that may influence the care provided. Creation of and reference to such a list decreases the potential for a problem to be missed and focuses providers on important current and resolved health issues for this client. The medication list is often placed adjacent to the problem list. Risk may be reduced by reviewing and updating both lists at each visit.

A follow-up file or software is a useful way to track clients with problems that require future care. Although not part of the client medical record per se, such tracking comprises a significant part of the midwife's risk management plan. When notification of abnormal results is documented in the medical record, a plan must be formulated. The follow-up file system tracks whether clients return for recommended care and generates reminders to document clinician notification of clients who have not returned for care as recommended. The midwife's risk management plan should describe the follow-up process and clearly indicate the procedure for utilizing that follow-up system.

Documenting Culturally Competent Care

Midwives and other health professionals have a legal and moral obligation to provide culturally competent care (Office of Minority Health, 2010). Cultural competence is the ability to step outside of your own culture and obtain the vision and skills necessary to provide care in a context that is appropriate for the women whom you serve.

The attitudes and behaviors needed to become culturally sensitive and provide culturally competent care include a sincere interest in other cultures, the ability to communicate effectively across cultural and language barriers, and a demonstrated sense of honor for the customs of others. On a more practical level, the ability to access interpreter services is a key behavior that is both essential and legally mandated. Each midwife is expected to obtain or to have access to information regarding specific healthcare problems that are racially or ethnically mediated. Each midwife should become familiar with historical events and cultural practices that may also affect health in the populations served. Each of these components should be addressed in the client's health record when they are applicable.

Documentation of cultural competence can include a detailed description, such as when the informed consent process is provided through an interpreter before surgery or a procedure. It may be culturally appropriate to excuse the father from the birth room or to ensure a family member is present as a chaperone during intimate examinations. Documentation of cultural indications for changes to or variations from usual care serves to validate the midwifery care provided while reinforcing the need for respect and awareness of cultural differences. Some women may belong to cultural groups characterized by very limited access or availability of health care and accept whatever care is provided. Other women can have a strong need to direct their health care and mandate their active participation in all health-related decisions. Most women fall somewhere between these two extremes.

The essential characteristic of the culturally competent midwife is an ability to embrace diversity while retaining one's sense of personal cultural identity. To do so, it may be necessary to relinquish control in select client encounters. Feelings of discomfort, failure, fear, frustration, anger, or embarrassment can serve to indicate a need for the midwife to examine her or his personal viewpoint and consider thoughtful and deliberate examination of challenging intercultural exchanges as a means to foster personal growth.

Awareness of and sensitivity to cultural practices and beliefs can enhance client satisfaction and build a trusting professional relationship. Cultural diversity encompasses a wide range of reference points, which may include social and emotional development, age, race, religion, sexual orientation, ethnic heritage, country of origin, geographic location, and cultural beliefs and mores. Becoming culturally competent involves a certain level of interest, inquiry, and awareness of cultural differences. It involves not only sensitivity to the customs of the social groups to which the woman belongs, but also an awareness that she may not conform to the common perceptions of those groups' behaviors and beliefs.

Cultural differences can be considered cross-cultural, meaning the midwife and the client come from different ethnic or racial backgrounds, or they may be intercultural, where the midwife and the client come from similar ethnic or social backgrounds but have developed disparate views and beliefs, especially with regard to health care. Examples include the home birth midwife whose client reveals she wants access to pharmacologic pain relief for labor or the hospital-based midwife whose client calls to request an in-home examination for possible labor.

Cultural competence requires that the midwife remains open-minded, cultivates active listening and observational skills, and evaluates each woman's needs according to the environment of care with an attitude of cultural sensitivity and humility. Access to culturally competent interpreters to translate language, social customs, and mores related to women's health care is extremely helpful. Literal translation, however, does not always provide correct or accurate information. Individualizing care also involves taking into account the woman's chronologic age, her developmental stage, emotional development, sexual orientation and preferences, cultural background, and other social factors.

Developmental Considerations

Attention to developmental changes throughout a woman's life is essential to address the concerns that may be most pressing to her. The needs of adolescent women are very different from those of women of childbearing age, which are in turn different from those of the woman who is past menopause—even when each type of client presents for the same type of

visit. Midwives who frequently care for the medically underserved should remember that the effects of poverty, abuse, low self-esteem, or marginal nutrition may adversely impact a woman's developmental growth.

Adolescent Women

Young women in their teens may present at various developmental stages based on age, emotional development, ethnicity, and other social and cultural factors. Developing a mutually acceptable plan of care is frequently an issue, as authority may be challenged and the young woman seeks to explore the boundaries and limits of her situation. Parental presence and involvement may indicate support and guidance for the teen and her choices, or they may reflect the presence of dysfunctional parent–teen dynamics.

Adult Women

The adult phase of life encompasses the concerns of the young adult woman, the mid-life woman, and the gracefully aging woman. Milestone events that affect health and life obligations can include educational and occupational endeavors, development and maintenance of intimate and family relationships, and childbearing and child rearing. After the childbearing years have passed, women often experience a change of focus from reproductive health care to concerns surrounding general health and well-being. Many women celebrate the freedom of mature adulthood. They may explore new attitudes, become more adventurous, and find that their confidence flourishes. Many older women live alone, by choice or by circumstances. Women, more than men, are affected as they age by increasing poverty and diminished resources to cope with illness or disability.

Mentally Challenged Women

Women who struggle with mental challenges may require coordination of specialized services so that they are provided with appropriate reproductive health care. Intimate examinations may require extra time and patience to avoid emotional trauma, especially in the mentally challenged woman with a history of sexual abuse. Sedation or anesthesia for intimate exams can be considered in selected cases.

Physically Challenged Women

Physically handicapped women may or may not have developmental delays depending on the cause of the physical challenge. Individual assessment is necessary to determine the client's developmental level and provide developmentally appropriate services. Examinations may be made more challenging by physical limitations, and ample time should be scheduled to allow for this possibility.

Immigrant and Refugee Women

Women raised in other countries may have culturally mediated variations in development, which may make interpretation of their developmental stages more challenging. Accessing resources to learn about cultural variations may aid in appropriate client assessment and effective coordination of services.

Socioeconomic Challenges

Various socioeconomic challenges may influence the rate and progression of a woman's physical, emotional, and social development. Additionally, a woman's health insurance status (or lack of insurance) will affect covered healthcare services and out-of-pocket expenses. Considering services that might best meet a woman's needs in the context of her socioeconomic resources is an important aspect of caring for vulnerable women.

Informed Consent

Informed consent is a specific process designed to ensure that clients receive the full, unbiased information necessary to actively participate in their healthcare decision making regarding a recommended treatment or procedure (Kuczkowski, 2005). The midwife is expected to recommend a course of action and share her or his reasoning process with the client. Client understanding of the information provided is as important as the information itself. Discussion should be carried on in layperson's terms, and client understanding should be assessed along the way.

Complete informed consent includes discussion of the following elements:

- Indications for the recommended procedure, medication, or treatment
- Accepted or experimental use of the proposed procedure, medication, or treatment
- Potential or anticipated benefits, actions, or effects of the proposed course of action
- Potential risks, harms, and adverse effects of the proposed course of action
- Potential risks, harms, and adverse effects of declining the proposed course of action
- Any urgency to undergoing the proposed course of action
- Alternatives to the proposed course of action, including potential effectiveness, risk, and benefit
- Client understanding of discussion, best demonstrated by the client paraphrasing information received and documented by direct quote (e.g., "You're going to try to turn my baby so she isn't butt first")
- Client choice regarding the recommendation based on participation in the informed consent process

Ideally, the midwife and client signatures will be witnessed by a third party. The informed consent process can also be used to present information on the midwife's practice; indications for consult, collaboration, or referral; and birth options or settings. It provides an opportunity for questions, discussion, and documentation of client participation in decisions.

In most cases, it is clear whether the client is competent to make her own decisions. The midwife should assess the client's ability to understand the nature of the problem, to understand the risks associated with the problem and the recommended course of action, and to communicate her decision based on that understanding.

Competent clients have the right to decline testing or treatment after going through the informed consent process. This right may be limited when the client is pregnant and her decision affects her unborn child. The stress and pain of labor raise interesting questions regarding informed consent and competence during labor.

Components of Common Medical Notes

When documenting care provided using a standardized format, each category noted on the form should be addressed, using either appropriate details or the phrase "not applicable." This practice serves two purposes: It maintains the expected format of the note, and it clearly indicates which clinical components the midwife included while caring for the client. Some electronic health records have automatic fill-in functions that default to a normal finding; this places the midwife in the position of being a careful editor of the client record, rather than being a careful author of the client record.

Office Visit or Progress Note

The office visit/progress note format is typically used for problem-oriented and well-woman office visits as well as for progress notes during labor and postpartum. Standardized prenatal care forms typically vary from this format; however, it becomes useful during evaluation of a problem or complication during pregnancy. Many electronic health record systems have set up their documents using the SOAP format:

- Subjective: Client interview, history, and record review
- Objective: Physical examination and diagnostic or screening test results
- Assessment: Differential or working diagnosis
- Plan: Evaluation, treatment, education, and follow-up care, including coordination of care, consultations, and/or referrals

Procedure Note

The procedure note is used to provide detailed information about a procedure such as endometrial biopsy, intrauterine device insertion, colposcopy, external cephalic version, or circumcision. This format is appropriate to use to document a procedure regardless of location or environment of care and includes the following information:

- Procedure performed
- Indication for procedure: Include diagnosis and any relevant history of present problem
- Informed consent: Include any relevant discussion
- Anesthesia, if used
- Estimated blood loss, in milliliters; a notation of "minimal" is accepted for an estimated blood loss less than 10 mL
- Complications: Describe, along with treatment rendered and the client response to that treatment
- Technique: Describe techniques used, including instruments, anesthesia technique and amount used, sequence of events, and rationale for technique choices, when appropriate
- Findings: Describe clinical findings, specimens collected and disposition of same, and client status post procedure

Medical Consultation or Referral

The purpose of the formal consultation or referral request is to provide the consultant with adequate information about the client in advance, thereby allowing the consultant to focus on the problem or condition. Referral requests may be verbal, written (commonly in letter format), or electronic, and often include the following elements:

- Client introduction: Name, date of birth, and indication for consult or referral
- History of present problem or illness
- Type of consultation requested
- Brief client history: Allergies, medications, illnesses, surgeries, and relevant social history
- Expectation for care: Advises the consultant of any client education provided regarding the problem or illness; appropriate to advocate for the client's preferences when stating expectations for care

Admission History and Physical Examination

The admission history and physical examination format is typically used when admitting a client to the hospital with an obstetric, gynecologic, or medical problem. However, it is also appropriate to use when admitting a client to midwifery care in labor in any environment of care. It includes the following elements:

- Admission diagnosis
- History of present condition or illness
- Past pregnancy and gynecological history
- Past medical history
- Past surgical history
- Current medications
- Allergies
- Social history
- Family history
- Review of systems
- Physical findings
- Diagnostic testing
- Client's preferences for labor and birth (birth plan)
- Midwifery plan of care
- Anticipated course of care based on current findings and maternal preferences
- Indications for consultation, collaboration, or referral
- Plan for reevaluation

Labor Progress Note

Labor progress is typically documented in a SOAP format in the progress notes. Most practitioners document labor progress in notes written every 2 to 4 hours and when notable events or changes occur, including the following elements in the note:

- Date and time: Noting the time is essential during labor
- Interval history since previous note
  - Maternal status: Labor progress, maternal well-being and activity, response to labor, emotional status, and labor preferences
  - Fetal status: Fetal well-being and means of evaluation

  - Labor status: Frequency and duration of contractions, cervical status if applicable, fetal position and station, assessment of maternal and fetal well-being in relation to phase of labor, evaluation for variations or complications of labor
- Assessment: Clinical evaluation of labor phase and progress, and presence of indications for consultation, collaboration, or referral
- Plan of care: Anticipated course of action (including watchful waiting or active intervention, consultation, collaboration, or referral), discussions with client regarding course of labor, and plan for reevaluation

Birth Note

The birth note is designed to summarize the pregnancy, labor, and birth in a brief but comprehensive overview of the pregnancy and labor, including detailed information about the birth and immediate postpartum and newborn periods. A typical birth note includes the following elements:

- Brief review of prenatal course
- Admission status
- Course of labor
  - Length of each stage
  - Rupture of membranes: Time, color, and fetal heart rate
  - Maternal and fetal response during labor
  - Labor events or interventions
  - Complications and treatment
- Birth information
  - Time, date, and location
  - Route and method of birth
  - Maternal and fetal position
  - Techniques or interventions used with indication:
    - Anesthesia, type, and dose
    - Episiotomy or laceration
    - Type of suture and technique of repair if done
    - Medications if used
    - Complications and treatment, including client response

- ▪ Evaluation of placenta
- ▪ Estimated blood loss
- ▪ Maternal status post delivery
- Newborn information
  - ▪ Gender
  - ▪ Resuscitation, if indicated
  - ▪ Apgar score
  - ▪ Weight
  - ▪ Bonding
  - ▪ Feeding, voiding, and stooling
  - ▪ Newborn status post delivery

Discharge Summary

The discharge summary is an appropriate format to use after a hospital admission but may also be used for summarizing a birth center admission or home birth. It includes the following information:

- Admission diagnosis
- Discharge diagnosis
- History of present condition or illness
- Past medical history
- Past surgical history
- Current medications
- Allergies
- Social history
- Family history
- Review of systems
- Physical findings
- Diagnostic testing
- Treatments and procedures
- Hospital or postpartum course
- Complications
- Discharge medications
- Discharge instructions
- Condition on discharge
- Plan for continued care

Documentation is an essential skill for midwifery and women's health practice that should be mastered with the same care and attention given to other components of clinical practice. Meticulous documentation accurately reflects the scope and nature of midwifery care and enhances communication among health professionals who care for and about women.

The information contained within the client's medical record forms a basis for planning continued care, and continuity of care is enhanced through the interdisciplinary documentation of care and services provided. This includes communication between the midwife and the client, and between the midwife and other health professionals contributing to the client's care. Other uses of the medical record, such as internal hospital audits for quality assurance purposes and for protection of the legal interests of the client and healthcare professionals who provided care, are addressed in the next section on risk management.

RISK MANAGEMENT

Risk management is a dynamic process based on assessing probabilities of untoward outcomes or events and on developing strategies to reduce or manage these events. In health care, this term is often used to refer to health risks to the client, health or professional risks to the practitioner, or financial risks to the institution or practice. Application of sound risk management principles to midwifery and women's health practice includes providing and monitoring quality health care to the women whom the midwife serves while practicing in a manner that protects the midwife from undue risk, whether it be from infectious disease, malpractice litigation, or financial insolvency. This section identifies ways to safeguard practice while providing quality care in our litigious society.

Developing a Collaborative Practice Network

Midwives do not practice in isolation. Every midwife, regardless of practice location, needs a network of contacts to help provide ongoing care and services. The collaborative practice model allows for a wide variety of professional relationships that range from informal to highly structured arrangements.

Development of professional relationships with physicians and other healthcare providers in your area begins with you. Make arrangements to meet at a convenient time and introduce yourself. Bring practice brochures or business cards so that these providers and their office staff members understand which services you offer and how to reach you. Present yourself as a competent, skilled, professional colleague. Your goal is to initiate a relationship so that when you have a client who needs care, your credibility has been established. It is not required that you agree on philosophy of care or management styles, but it is important that you establish a good working relationship. It is also good practice to nurture your relationship with the office staff for those times when you may need them to prioritize your requests for assistance during office hours.

Determining in advance which type of consult is indicated affects which information you provide to the consultant provider. Present the consultation request in terms that advocate for the type of care you are seeking for your client. If you do not provide this direction, the physician will likely manage your client as she or he would her or his usual patients.

The AMA *Evaluation and Management Services Guidelines* state "A consultation is a type of evaluation provided by a physician at the request of another physician or appropriate source to either recommend care for a specific condition or problem, or to determine whether to accept responsibility for ongoing management of the patient's entire care or for the care of a specific condition or problem" (AMA, 2010). Forms of consultation that the midwife may use include the following types:

- **Informational:** "Just letting you know that Mrs. B is here in labor. She is a G3, P2002 at term and is at 5 cm after 1 hour of labor. The fetal heart rate is in normal range with good variability, estimated fetal weight is 7½ pounds, and I expect a spontaneous vaginal birth shortly." In this instance, you have already established a professional relationship with a defined collaborating individual that includes notification in specific circumstances or as indicated according to your professional judgment. This may also include proactive consultation to provide information when there is potential for an emergency that may require additional support or expertise.

- **Request for information or opinion:** "Ms. K has atypical glandular cells on her most recent Pap smear. I've never seen this before. What do you recommend for her follow-up?" In this instance, you are looking for information from your consultant physician to guide your client's care when you have reached the limits of your experience and knowledge. This is a good time to discuss future management of such patients and to determine your own needs for continuing education.

- **Request for evaluation:** "I'm sending Mrs. S to you for evaluation of her enlarged uterus. She is a 47-year-old G2, P2002 who has had severe menorrhagia for the past 5 months. We have discussed potential treatments, and she is interested in exploring endometrial ablation to treat her menorrhagia." In this instance, the client has a problem that requires evaluation and treatment, but that care is not within your scope of practice. Clearly stating previous discussions, client preferences, and your expectations for care can influence the care provided to the client. The expectation is that the client will return to you for care once the problem has resolved or been treated. As this is a more formal consultation, a consult form or letter, as well as patient permission for release of supporting clinical documents, should be initiated.

- **Transfer of care:** "Mrs. R has a large lesion consistent with cervical cancer. I am transferring her to you for care of this problem." In this instance, the client has a problem that necessitates ongoing physician management. Transfer of care means that the client is released from midwifery care and the consultant is expected to assume responsibility for her ongoing medical care. In an emergency (e.g., "Ms. P has a postpartum hemorrhage. I believe she has retained placental parts. Her EBL is currently at 1000 mL. Please come to L & D immediately."), the nature of the problem requires immediate action on the part of the consultant. Expectations for immediate physician evaluation of a client must be clearly stated. For those midwives who provide labor and birth care in the out-of-hospital setting, calling the labor and delivery staff, OB/GYN physician, or pediatrician on-call may be needed in addition to calling emergency medical services (EMS), 911, or the emergency room. If you have an established working relationship, a direct admission to a maternity unit prepared for your client's arrival may be possible.

- **Other multidisciplinary practice relationships:** Primary care providers commonly care for clients in the event of a general medical problem such as hypertension, diabetes, or heart disease. Although some midwives have expanded their practice to include primary care services, this care may be limited by the practice setting to treatment of acute minor conditions, such as back pain and upper respiratory infections. Many midwives initially manage selected chronic conditions, such as mild depression, and refer the patient if no improvement occurs with standard measures, or they may continue management of selected stable chronic conditions, such as asthma, and refer the patient if the condition destabilizes.

Every practitioner caring for women, regardless of her or his scope of practice, should develop a network of multidisciplinary care providers such as physicians, chiropractors, naturopaths, acupuncturists, dieticians, mental health professionals, social service personnel, clergy, support and self-help groups, local emergency services, homeless shelters, and addiction centers. This network provides the mechanism by which midwives can address the varied needs of the women who come to them for care.

A key element to providing woman-oriented care is to connect women with essential services they may not know how to access. This can include a combination of mainstream medical care, alternative or complementary modalities, and nonmedical services. The role of the midwife is to listen to women, clarify their needs, and facilitate meeting those needs in a caring and nonjudgmental manner. The foundational philosophy of midwifery guides the care that midwives provide.

Collaborative practice connects midwives with additional health professionals who provide ongoing or specialty care outside the midwife's scope of practice. Along the way, these other specialists become aware of the services midwives offer to women and, in turn, may serve as a source of referrals to the midwifery practice. Women's health care forms a continuum that extends from home birth and alternative care, through general medical and community-based medicine and midwifery, to high-tech tertiary care and specialty services.

Collaborative practice means that a working relationship is formed between the attending midwife and the physician or other multidisciplinary care provider. Each discipline has distinct and different services to offer. Midwives function as an integral part of the healthcare system. Clear discussion of the parameters of midwifery practice within the practice location(s), practice scope guided by collaborative relationships, clinical practice agreements, and clinical options of midwifery care (including privileges) are all useful tools in evaluating whether a particular midwifery practice is appropriate for the individual client. Midwives have a responsibility to provide access to services as indicated by the individual woman's health, her preferences, and the midwife's scope of practice. Not all services are appropriate for all women. The primary goal of the collaborative relationship is accessing the best care for each client as needed. The ACNM joint statement with the American College of Obstetricians and Gynecologists includes the following assertion, which reinforces this principle:

> The American College of Obstetricians and Gynecologists and ACNM believe health care is more effective when it occurs in a system that facilitates communication across health care settings and among providers. OB/GYNs and CNMs/CMs [Certified Nurse-Midwives/Certified Midwives] are experts in their respective fields of practice and are educated, trained, and licensed independent providers who may collaborate with each other based on the needs of their patient. (ACNM, 2011)

Several proactive practice habits are essential to risk management in any clinical setting. The first is quality assurance and improvement. This continuous process can be accomplished by defining clinical standards, analyzing and monitoring clinical practice and practice systems, and adjusting to reduce risk and provide quality care (American Academy of Family Physicians [AAFP], 2008). The second is clear and thoughtful documentation of the care encounter. Orderly, precise, and legible documentation of care is not only the basic tool for monitoring and evaluating a client's progress, but also the best protection against malpractice claims (Nissen, Angus, Miller, & Silverman, 2010). Lastly, a vital component of risk management is building a client–provider relationship that encompasses the qualities of trust and respect. The establishment of trust is essential if the client is to have confidence in the midwife's diagnostic and therapeutic abilities. No single approach to client relationships is appropriate for all providers; however, one common element comprises maintaining a respectful demeanor toward every client.

Risk to the Client

Quantification of risk for an individual is a difficult task and requires careful counseling that avoids absolutes. When a client is "at risk," it is important to specify which condition or complication she is at risk for and why, and to then give a probability of both its occurrence and its nonoccurrence. For example, if a woman undergoing amniocentesis has a 1 in 100 chance of rupture of membranes during the procedure, then she has a 99/100 chance of no rupture during the procedure. Providing women with information on *attributable risk* for a condition (the actual number of additional adverse outcomes attributable to the risk factor) can provide a balanced perspective on the condition risk (Jordan & Murphy, 2009). Using visual tools such as the Paling Palette, a visual tool that displays risk of a condition without numbers, can help women of all languages understand risk for a condition better than just stating numerical risk (Risk Communication Institute, 2011).

New data are continually being compiled and published about risks associated with race, ethnicity, genetics, lifestyle, behaviors, and other factors. By keeping abreast of new data, critically evaluating those data, and incorporating them into your knowledge base, you will then be able to provide clients with information relevant to healthcare decisions and options that are appropriate for them. Frank discussions about the relative risk of options for care should include the potential for unexpected outcomes, the unpredictability of individual response, the consequences of watchful waiting, and the impact and importance of self-determination.

Risk to the Unborn and the Newborn

Calculating risk to the unborn, and by extension to the newborn, is also difficult and fraught with emotions as parents try to make the best decisions possible on behalf of their child. Pregnant women and their families look to their midwives as skilled professionals with the ability to identify potential problems, discuss the various options open to them, involve them in decision making, and take corrective action to safeguard their babies in the womb.

How information is presented during pregnancy and women's healthcare visits may influence the client's attitude about her body, the safety of birth, the ability of the healthcare system to meet her and her baby's needs, and her ability to parent. Risk should be addressed in a realistic fashion that is supportive of women and birth and that does not undermine traditional, alternative, or mainstream medical providers. You can foster the concept that childbearing is a normal and healthy physiologic process while still addressing the fact that there are no guarantees of perfect outcomes, and that access to basic and advanced medical services is available.

Risk to the Midwife

Each midwife needs to determine what is included in her or his own individual scope of practice. Not every midwife provides every service. A scope of practice is a dynamic entity—one that changes with experience, practice location, fatigue, staffing, and distance to specialty care, among other factors. Each midwife must manage her or his individual professional risk by constantly assessing the scope of her or his midwifery practice and determining whether it meets the midwife's needs as well as those of the community of women served.

Identification of a woman with risk factors may influence midwifery management of risk in a number of respects: It may result in a transfer of care, a consultation, or continued independent management of the woman's care. The outcome depends on the midwife's expertise and self-determined scope of practice, state laws regarding midwifery practice, and the midwife's comfort in caring for the particular risk factor in this individual, healthcare setting, community, and legal climate.

Standards of practice define the expected knowledge and behaviors of the midwife according to her education, certification, and licensure status. Midwives are held accountable to national, state, and local standards. Each midwife should maintain familiarity with the professional standards, state laws, and rules that govern her or his midwifery practice. Professional standards are defined by ACNM, MANA, and the International Confederation of Midwives (ICM). Each of these organizations requires that the midwife have knowledge of the following:

- Midwifery practice standards and recommendations
- Pathophysiology and treatment of commonly encountered conditions
- Indications for and access to medical consultation

Risk Management Plan

A risk management plan is designed to outline strategies that reduce and minimize the possibility of loss (AAFP, 2008). Such a plan is a helpful way to organize essential information about the various components needed to identify and manage risk in midwifery practice. A comprehensive and realistic midwifery practice risk management plan demonstrates that

the midwife seeks to provide care that is consistent with best practice, is cognizant of the risk involved in this profession, and has taken reasonable steps to limit that risk. It should include practice policies and procedures that address topics such as the following (Greenwald, 2004; Maine Association of Certified Nurse Midwives, 2009):

- Written practice description
- Philosophy of practice
- Location(s) of practice
- Practice guidelines and standards
- The role and scope of practice for each midwife
- Health record documentation standards
- Documentation forms that reflect care provided
- Informed consent policy and process
- Client autonomy in decision making
- Provisions for practice coverage
- Indications for consultation or referral
- Collaborative practice relationships
- Plan for transfer of care or client when indicated
- Requirements for continuing education
- Education requirements for expanded scope of practice
- Peer review and outcomes-based evaluation of care
- Review process for client or practice-related complaints or concerns
- Licensing and professional practice issues as legally defined by state or professional organization
- The nature and extent of midwifery professional liability coverage
- Malpractice claims procedures

When Bad Things Happen

Midwives vary tremendously in the amount of risk they are willing to live with on a day-to-day basis. Some may prefer to work in settings where there is a physician available at all times, whereas others may practice in isolated settings where the nearest physician is located miles away. Increased midwife autonomy may be associated with increased midwife risk, as can practicing in a setting that is antagonistic to midwives,

Table 1-5	Steps for Living with Bad Outcomes in Practice
DO'S	**DON'TS**
Understand the emotional nature of the events for you and your client.	Do not delay in honest communication with your client.
Continue to provide excellent midwifery care with clear concise documentation.	Do not alter the medical record; however, a late entry that is documented as such is acceptable.
Contact your risk management department and liability insurance company immediately after an occurrence or event in case a suit is filed.	Don't write any written reports or narratives of the events unless directed to do so by risk management or your liability insurance company.
Take care of yourself physically and emotionally. Avoid the emotional isolation associated with litigation by sharing your feelings.	Do not discuss the details of the event with colleagues, family, or friends.
Know that you are not alone. All midwives experience poor outcomes during a lifetime of practice; many become involved in legal proceedings in the aftermath of a poor or unexpected outcome.	

regardless of midwives' legal status as certified or licensed professionals.

Even with thorough documentation of excellent care and a healthy, actively involved client, things can still go awry. Wherever there is life, there is also the possibility of death, illness, or injury. Most midwives encounter bad outcomes in caring for their clients from time to time in the course of their careers (Guidera, McCool, Poell, & Stenson, 2007). Such a result is devastating to the client and her family, as well as to the midwife involved. Midwives' reactions after poor outcomes in practice can range from sorrow to departure from practice (Table 1-5).

Allow yourself time to grieve this event with your client and on your own, but also be prepared to take practical steps that protect your ability to continue to practice and to recover emotionally. Midwives have reported that formal debriefing with a counselor, attorney, midwife partners, or morbidity and mortality committee members have been helpful strategies to promote personal and professional recovery (McCool, Guidera, Delaney, & Hakala, 2007).

Review the chart with a midwife practice partner or your physician consultant—someone with legitimate rights to access the chart and the ability to evaluate the care. Some charts are automatically reviewed for certain key events in the hospital; for example, the occurrence of neonatal seizure or maternal death is discussed at a perinatal morbidity and mortality review. In contrast, women's health care provided in the outpatient setting may not have such a review mechanism. It is important to extract the learning value from these difficult situations while maintaining client confidentiality.

Most malpractice suits in midwifery are initiated for poor neonatal outcomes from events such as shoulder dystocia or fetal distress, misinterpretation of fetal heart rate tracings, or delay in consultation (Angelini & Greenwald, 2005). If errors were made by you or your staff, it is best to be honest and compassionate with your client in a timely fashion. You can apologize without implying guilt or blame, such as "I am sorry this complication occurred" or "I am so sorry this happened to you." Compared to the "deny and defend" stance of traditional risk management, open and honest communication with families and genuine apology when warranted can result in significant reduction in malpractice claims (Agency for Healthcare Research and Quality, 2010). Continue providing support to your client, just as you would before the event, and document your ongoing care and the client's response.

It is always appropriate to share empathy and sorrow with your client. Understand, however, that although midwives pride themselves on delivering excellent relationship-based care, this is only one of many considerations in a client's decision to take legal action.

ETHICAL MIDWIFERY PRACTICE

Ethical midwifery practice is based on a human rights framework (Thompson, 2004). This framework includes four foundational ethical principles:

1. Autonomy: The human right to personal independence and the capacity to make decisions and act on them
2. Justice: The human right to be treated fairly and with reasoned care
3. Beneficence: The human right to be treated with intent to do good
4. Nonmalfeasance: The human right to be treated with intent to avoid harm, the classic "First do no harm" directive attributed to Hippocrates

These guiding ethical principles are reflected in midwifery's philosophical tenets and have also been codified specifically for midwives by several midwifery organizations, including ACNM (2004, 2008), MANA (2010a), and ICM (2008).

For these ethical principles to have any meaning, they must be a touchstone for your practice decisions. Ethical problems are not always clear-cut issues. Sometimes, it is a matter of choosing between what is right and what is easy. Ethical dilemmas are inherent in midwifery care, and they are sometimes embedded in the simple day-to-day provision of care. An example is the client who says to you, "I'll do whatever you think I should," after you provide information on genetic screening options. The reflective practitioner will examine and learn from decisions made and actions taken in the clinical setting from an ethical perspective. Midwifery is a morally important endeavor that promotes women's optimal health, and the ethics of clinical care are worthy of your continued and thoughtful consideration.

EXEMPLARY MIDWIFERY PRACTICE

Optimal midwifery care occurs when the midwife is able to support the physiologic processes of birth and well-woman care while at the same time remaining vigilant for the unexpected (Kennedy, 2000). Remaining attuned to small details that might subtly indicate a significant change in maternal, fetal, or the well-woman's status provides the midwife with the opportunity to identify problems early and initiate treatment geared toward improving outcomes promptly. Midwifery encourages care that is individualized for each woman and each birth. Patience with the birth process is a hallmark of midwifery care. Midwives' compassionate and attentive care reinforces women's belief in their ability to give birth and care for themselves. By utilizing interventions and technology only when necessary, midwives bridge the chasm between medicine and traditional healing.

Exemplary midwives demonstrate professional integrity, honesty, compassion, and understanding. They are able to communicate effectively, remain open-minded and flexible, and provide care in a nonjudgmental manner. When these attributes are coupled with excellent clinical skills, they result in attentive and thorough assessments, excellent screening and preventive health counseling processes, and infinite patience with the process of labor and birth.

Finally, midwives provide personalized care that is tailored to the individual and her present circumstances. Regardless of the clinical practice setting or the client's educational background, midwives endeavor to create an environment that engenders mutual respect and focuses primarily on meeting the needs of the woman or mother and family. Recognition of individual variation is tempered by a thorough grounding in both normal and pathologic processes. This broad scope provides the midwife with a clear view of the continuum of health and allows more accurate assessment and personalization of care.

The midwife who holds as an ideal the provision of exemplary midwifery care must actively create a balance between the professional life as a midwife and the needs and demands of the individual's personal

---

Box 1-3　Web Resources for Clinicians

- Review of systems form: http://www.fammed.ouhsc.edu/forms/FMC_ROS_Form.pdf
- American Cancer Society, Guidelines for the Early Detection of Cancer: http://www.cancer.org/docroot/PED/content/PED_2_3X_ACS_Cancer_Detection_Guidelines_36.asp?sitearea=PED
- ICD-9 Codes: http://icd9data.com/
- Institute of Medicine: http://www.iom.edu/Reports.aspx
- Risk Communication Institute, Paling Palettes: http://riskcomm.com/paling_palettes.htm
- National Institutes of Health, National High Blood Pressure Education Program: http://www.nhlbi.nih.gov/guidelines/hypertension/
- National Institutes of Health, National Guidelines Clearinghouse: http://www.guideline.gov/index.aspx
- National Heart, Lung, and Blood Institute, Clinical Practice Guidelines: http://www.nhlbi.nih.gov/guidelines/
- U.S. Preventive Services Task Force: http://www.ahrq.gov/clinic/epcix.htm

---

life. Time off to refresh and rejuvenate is as necessary to quality practice as is ongoing professional education. Personal relationships nourish the midwife and provide emotional sustenance. All midwives must remain attentive to their own needs to bring their best to midwifery.

Midwives strive to provide exemplary midwifery and women's health care. This demands the development of excellent clinical skills and the determination and persistence to couple them with sound clinical judgment. Each midwife is called on, time and again, to make critical decisions and to act on them in a way that is appropriate for the setting in which the midwife practices while demonstrating respect and honor for the uniqueness of each woman and family in her or his care.

Exemplary midwifery practice, according to Kennedy (2000), encompasses several key concepts. One of these concepts is the basic philosophy of midwifery and its active expression through the individual midwife's clinical practice. Each midwife's philosophy of care is reflected in her or his choice and use of healing modalities, the quality of her or his caring for and about women, and her or his support for midwifery as a profession. Throughout this book, the driving philosophy is of the midwifery philosophy articulated by the ACNM (2004) (see the feature "Philosophy of the American College of Nurse–Midwives" earlier in this chapter).

SUMMARY

Defining one's personal expression of midwifery philosophy in practice is one of the joys of midwifery. What constitutes "best care" for women, mothers, and infants is determined individually at the point of care with the woman herself, with standards of care and practice guidelines being used as guides along the way. Clinical judgment is the heart and soul of midwifery care. A mindful approach to practice reduces client and midwife risk, improves outcomes, and fosters collaborative relationships. This provides the opportunity for the exemplary midwife to rest better at night and to continue a career of service to women and their families for decades.

REFERENCES

Agency for Healthcare Research and Quality. (2010). Full disclosure of medical errors reduces malpractice and medical claim costs for health care system. Retrieved from http://www.innovations.ahrq.gov/content.aspx?id=2673

American Academy of Family Physicians (AAFP). (2008). Risk management and medical liability. Retrieved from http://www.aafp.org/online/etc/medialib/aafp_org/documents/about/rap/curriculum/risk_management_and.Par.0001.File.tmp/Reprint281.pdf

American Association of Birth Centers (AABC). (2007). AABC uniform data set. Retrieved from http://www.birthcenters.org/data-collection/features.php

American Cancer Society. (2010). Screening recommendations. Retrieved from http://www.cancer.org/docroot/PED/content/PED_2_3X_ACS_Cancer_Detection_Guidelines_36.asp?sitearea=PED

American College of Nurse–Midwives (ACNM). (n.d.). ACNM datasets. Retrieved from http://www.midwife.org/publications.cfm

American College of Nurse–Midwives (ACNM). (2004). *Philosophy of the American College of Nurse–Midwives.* Silver Spring, MD: Author. Retrieved from http://www.midwife.org/philosophy.cfm

American College of Nurse–Midwives (ACNM). (2008). *Core competencies for basic midwifery practice.* Silver Spring, MD: Author. Retrieved from http://www.midwife.org/siteFiles/education/Core_Competencies_6_07.pdf

American College of Nurse–Midwives (ACNM). (2011). *Joint statement of practice relations between obstetrician-gynecologists and certified nurse midwives.* Silver Spring, MD: Author. Retrieved from http://www.midwife.org/ACNM/files/ccLibraryFiles

American Health Information Management Association (AHIMA). (2008). Quality data and documentation for EHRs in physician practice. Retrieved from http://library.ahima.org/xpedio/groups/public/documents/ahima/bok1_039546.hcsp?dDocName=bok1_039546

American Medical Association (AMA). (2010). *Current procedural terminology.* Chicago, IL: Author. Retrieved from http://www.ama-assn.org/ama1/pub/upload/mm/362/cpt-consultation-services.pdf

American Medical Association (AMA). (2011). CPT. Retrieved from http://www.ama-assn.org/ama/pub/physician-resources/solutions-managing-your-practice/coding-billing-insurance/cpt.shtml

Angelini, D., & Greenwald, L. (2005). Closed claims analysis of 65 medical malpractice cases involving nurse–midwives. *Journal of Midwifery & Women's Health, 50,* 454–460.

CareFirst BlueCross BlueShield. (2009). Medical record documentation standards. Retrieved from http://www.carefirst.com/providers/attachments/BOK5129.pdf

Centers for Medicare & Medicaid Services (CMS). (2010a). Electronic health records at a glance. Retrieved from http://www.cms.gov/apps/media/press/factsheet.asp?Counter=3788&intNumPerPage=10&checkDate=&checkKey=&srchType=1&numDays=3500&srchOpt=0&srchData=&keywordType=All&chkNewsType=6&intPage=&showAll=&pYear=&year=&desc=&cboOrder=date

Centers for Medicare & Medicaid Services (CMS). (2010b). Evaluation and management services guide. Retrieved from https://www.cms.gov/MLNProducts/downloads/eval_mgmt_serv_guide-ICN006764.pdf

Centers for Medicare & Medicaid Services (CMS). (2010c). The ICD-10 transition: An introduction. Retrieved from http://www.cms.gov/ICD10/Downloads/ICD10IntroFactSheet20100409.pdf

Farley, C. L. (2005). Midwifery's research heritage: A Delphi survey of midwife scholars. *Journal of Midwifery & Women's Health, 50,* 122–128.

Greenwald, L. (Ed.). (2004). *Perspectives on clinical risk management.* Boston, MA: Risk Management Publications, ProMutual Group.

Guidera, M., McCool, W., Poell, J., & Stenson, M. (2007). What to do if you are named in a lawsuit: The professional liability handbook. In *Professional liability resource packet.* Silver Spring, MD: American College of Nurse–Midwives. Retrieved from http://www.midwife.org/professional_liability.cfm

ICD9Data.com. (2012). Free 2012 ICD-9 medical coding data. Retrieved from http://www.icd9data.com/

International Confederation of Midwives (ICM). (2008). International code of ethics for midwives. Retrieved from http://www.internationalmidwives.org/Documentation/CoreDocuments/tabid/322/Default.aspx

Jordan, R., & Murphy, P. (2009). Risk assessment and risk distortion: Finding the balance. *Journal of Midwifery & Women's Health, 54*(3), 192–200.

Kennedy, H. P. (2000). A model of exemplary midwifery practice: Results of a Delphi study. *Journal of Midwifery & Women's Health, 45,* 4–19.

Knoche, A., Selzer, C., & Smolley, K. (2008). Methods of stimulating the onset of labor: An exploration of maternal satisfaction. *Journal of Midwifery & Women's Health, 53,* 381–387.

Kuczkowski, K. M. (2005). Context and process of informed consent for labor analgesia: A legal standard or an enhancement of peripartum care? *Journal of Midwifery & Women's Health, 50,* 65–66.

Lothian, J. A. (2004). Do not disturb: The importance of privacy in labor. *Journal of Perinatology Education, 13,* 4–6. Retrieved from http://www.pubmedcentral.nih.gov/articlerender.fcgi?artid=1595201

Lydon-Rochelle, M. T., Hodnett, E., Renfrew, M. J., & Lumley, J. (2003). A systematic approach for midwifery students: How to consider evidence-based research findings. *Journal of Midwifery & Women's Health,* 48(4), 273–277.

Maine Association of Certified Nurse Midwives. (2009). Certified nurse–midwifery practice in Maine: An initiative to implement standard procedures and practices allowing hospital admission by CNM's of maternity patients. Retrieved from www.mainemidwives. org/2009%20Initiative%20Final%209-09.pdf

McCool, W., Guidera, M., Delaney, E., & Hakala, S. (2007). The role of litigation in the professional practice of midwives in the United States: Results from a nationwide survey of certified nurse–midwives/certified midwives. *Journal of Midwifery & Women's Health,* 52(5), 458–464.

Midwives Alliance of North America. (2010a). MANA statement of values and ethics. Retrieved from http:// mana.org/valuesethics.html

Midwives Alliance of North America. (MANA). (2010b). MANA statistics project. Retrieved from https://www. manastats.org/help_public_about

National Heart, Lung, and Blood Institute. (2011). Clinical practice guidelines. Retrieved from http://www.nhlbi. nih.gov/guidelines/

National Institutes of Health. (2011). National Guidelines Clearinghouse. Retrieved from http://www.guideline. gov/index.aspx

Nissen, K., Angus, S., Miller, W., & Silverman, A. (2010). Teaching risk management: Addressing ACGME core competencies. *Journal of Graduate Medical Education,* 2(4), 589–594.

Office of Minority Health (OMH). (2010). Think cultural health. Retrieved from https://www.thinkculturalhealth. hhs.gov/

Risk Communication Institute. (2011). The Paling Palettes. Retrieved from http://riskcomm.com/paling_palettes .htm

Sackett, D. L., Richardson, W. S., Rosenberg, W., & Haynes, R. B. (1997). *Evidence-based medicine: How to practice and teach EBM.* New York, NY: Churchill Livingstone.

Schon, D. A. (1983). *The reflective practitioner: How professionals think in action.* New York, NY: Basic Books.

Thompson, J. B. (2004). A human rights framework for midwifery care. *Journal of Midwifery & Women's Health,* 49, 175–181.

Tillett, J. (2009). Developing guidelines and maintaining quality in antenatal care. *Journal of Midwifery & Women's Health,* 54, 238–240.

U.S. Preventive Services Task Force. (2011). Topic index A–Z. Retrieved from http://www.uspreventiveservices-taskforce.org/uspstopics.htm

CHAPTER 2

Care of the Woman During Pregnancy

Prenatal care provides an opportunity to deliver meaningful health care at a transformative time in a woman's life within the context of a continuing and nurturing relationship.

As midwives, we are privileged to witness and support the growth and development of mother and fetus during pregnancy. Prenatal care is a comprehensive ongoing program of care that addresses the biophysical, psychosocial, and educational needs of the pregnant woman and her family. The content and structure of prenatal care follow a typical pattern of scheduled visits and tests, but this standard package of care is easily modified to meet the needs and preferences of the individual women we serve.

The purpose of prenatal care is to provide primary preventive health care to pregnant women and to identify that small but significant number of women whose pregnancy will deviate from the wide range of normal in a manner that may jeopardize maternal or fetal well-being. For those women with conditions that fall outside of normal variations of pregnancy, the midwife can consult with, collaborate with, or refer to an appropriate specialist. For the pregnant client, an obstetrician or a perinatologist is the most common consultant needed. Of course, pregnant women are susceptible to all the same ills and injuries as anyone else, so the services of other healthcare professionals, such as a dermatologist, endocrinologist, or physical therapist, may also be required.

Provision of the basic components of prenatal care is included in the core competencies of midwifery practice. For further information, the midwife is encouraged to compare the standards for basic midwifery practice that have been developed by the American College of Nurse–Midwives, the Midwives Alliance of North America, and the International Confederation of Midwives. By reviewing the core documents produced by these organizations (all available online by accessing the respective organizations' websites), one can gain an understanding of the expected standards for midwifery practice in the United States. Additionally, each midwife's practice is shaped by state and local regulations, resources, and standards of practice.

Midwives are concerned with the structure, process, and outcomes of prenatal care and the intrinsic characteristics of the clients they serve. All of these components are important in developing a model of care and service delivery that is responsive to women's needs and that ensures ongoing quality assessment and improvement. The most typical schedule of prenatal care is rendered by a provider or group of providers structured in 12 to 13 visits scheduled every 4 weeks until the 28th week of pregnancy, every 2 weeks until the 36th week of pregnancy, and then weekly until birth. A reduced visit schedule may also be well suited for low-risk women (Walker, Day, Lirette, Mooney-Hescott, McCully, & Vest, 2002).

The Centering Pregnancy® model of group prenatal care has become more popular in recent years. In this model, groups of 8 to 12 women of similar gestational ages meet in 10 sessions throughout pregnancy for health assessment, education, and support. This format capitalizes on pregnant women's need to share their concerns, reactions, and experiences with others and their openness to learning about childbirth. In the group prenatal care approach, the midwife's role shifts from authority figure to facilitator. The women as a group determine the topics addressed at each visit, participate in physical assessments, share self-care strategies, and provide social support to one another. Research has demonstrated improved perinatal health outcomes using this model of prenatal care (Ickovics et al., 2007).

Every woman has unique, yet universal needs during pregnancy. This period is a time of many changes and adjustments of a physical, psychological, and social nature. Caring for a woman during this time of transition can foster individual autonomy and enhance self-care practices. As such, it may improve her ability to care for her child and to develop her strengths as a woman and a mother.

Many of the women midwives see are unfamiliar with the expectations of the healthcare system and need some guidance to navigate the system or to negotiate for care that is appropriate to their needs. Building a warm, caring, and professional relationship allows for mutual trust to develop. Trust, in turn, fosters active maternal participation in healthcare decisions. A woman who trusts her midwife is more

likely to accept the recommendations of the midwife if challenges or complications occur. The midwife's ethical obligation, then, is to behave in a trustworthy manner by providing care during pregnancy that includes respecting each woman's individual desires in relation to the preferred type of healthcare provider, the amount of active participation in her care that she desires, her planned and preferred location of labor and birth, and the methods to access medical services should they be needed. Each midwife is responsible for outlining to the pregnant client the scope of her or his practice and the usual parameters for prenatal, labor and birth, and postpartum care services.

The amount and types of testing performed during pregnancy are determined by indications for testing or evaluation, current recommendations for practice, and discussion with the client regarding the risks, benefits, and alternatives to testing or evaluation processes. It is important to share information regarding the costs of tests and procedures so the client is aware of any expenses that may be incurred. A method to clearly document a woman's decision to decline or refuse an offered or recommended test or procedure is an essential mechanism to have in place.

Maternal participation in prenatal care encourages self-determination and can enhance a woman's confidence in her ability to labor and give birth in a manner that helps her to feel safe and successful. The process of participation builds trust and fosters resilience in the face of unexpected or unfortunate events. Ongoing dialogue with the client demonstrates the multitude of potential situations and options that are possible in childbirth and encourages strength and flexibility on the part of both the mother-to-be and the midwife to deal with whatever circumstances come their way.

DIAGNOSIS OF PREGNANCY

Key Clinical Information

The diagnosis of pregnancy should be entertained when caring for any woman of childbearing age. Early-gestation pregnancy may be discovered by the clinician as an incidental finding during a well-woman visit. Many women make the diagnosis of pregnancy themselves with affordable and easy urine-based home pregnancy tests.

Pregnancy is the most common cause of secondary amenorrhea in women in this life stage. Its signs and symptoms are classified as follows: presumptive, meaning those changes that the mother can perceive; probable, meaning those changes that can be detected by the examiner; and positive, meaning those changes that can be directly attributed to the fetus (Varney, Kriebs, & Gegor, 2004).

The diagnosis of pregnancy may be a welcome event or devastating news. Many women have mixed feelings about the changes that pregnancy will bring to their lives. Ambivalence is common as the newly pregnant woman adjusts her self-image to include a baby that is more an abstraction than a reality in the early days of pregnancy. The diagnosis of pregnancy should be shared and explored in a private setting in a straightforward and kind manner. This openness allows the woman to express a wide range of emotions, and the midwife can then take her cues from the woman's response.

Client History and Chart Review: Components of the History to Consider

(Varney et al., 2004)
- Reproductive history
  - Gravity, parity (G, P TPAL)
  - Last menstrual period
  - Method of birth control
  - Conception issues
    - Known or suspected date of conception
    - Assisted reproductive technologies or treatments
  - Symptoms of pregnancy
    - Breast tenderness
    - Fatigue
    - Fetal movement
    - Nausea and/or vomiting
    - Urinary frequency
  - Birth history

- Signs or symptoms of complications
  - Pain or cramping
  - Bleeding
- Interval history since last menstrual period
  - Drugs or herbs taken
  - Illness or fever
  - Significant family, social, or lifestyle changes
- Relevant social history
  - Client intent and feelings about possible pregnancy
  - Living situation, sex of partner, marital status
  - Information about the father of the baby
  - Support systems
  - Employment situation and environment
  - Socioeconomic status
- Relevant medical/surgical history
  - Allergies
  - Medications
  - Medical conditions
  - Surgeries
  - History of sexually transmitted infections (STIs)
- Review of systems

Physical Examination: Components of the Physical Exam to Consider

- Vital signs
- Skin changes
  - Darkening of pigmented skin
  - Vascular spiders
  - Palmar erythema
  - Striae
- Breast changes
  - Enlargement
  - Increased nodularity
  - Increased vascularity
- Abdominal examination
  - Fetal heart tones
  - Fundal height
  - Palpable fetal movement
  - Abdominal tenderness and consistency
- Pelvic evaluation
  - Uterine sizing
  - Consistency of uterus and cervix

- Color of cervix
- Cervical motion tenderness
- Vaginal or cervical discharge
- Adnexal tenderness

Clinical Impression: Differential Diagnoses to Consider

(ICD9data.com, 2012)

- Pregnancy examination or test, positive result
- Also consider:
  - Ectopic pregnancy
  - Other unwanted pregnancy (see the "Unplanned Pregnancy" section)
  - Threatened abortion
  - Molar pregnancy
  - Blighted ovum
- Secondary amenorrhea (see the "Amenorrhea" section)

Diagnostic Testing: Diagnostic Tests and Procedures to Consider

- Urine or serum human chorionic gonadotropin (HCG)
- Quantitative β-HCG
- Abdominal or vaginal ultrasound

Providing Treatment: Therapeutic Measures to Consider

- Prenatal or other vitamin supplement with folic acid
- Treatment of any underlying condition as indicated

Providing Treatment: Complementary and Alternative Measures to Consider

These measures are intended to supplement—not replace—regular prenatal care:

- Natural prenatal vitamin supplement
- High-folate foods
- Red raspberry leaf tea

Providing Support: Education and Support Measures to Consider

- Pregnancy options counseling as indicated
- Initial nutrition assessment and counseling

- Prenatal care
  - Prenatal testing as indicated
  - Family involvement
- Practice information
  - Providers
  - Medical affiliations
  - Billing arrangements
  - Birth options
    - Location(s)
  - Philosophy of care
  - [www] Patient rights and responsibilities

Follow-up Care: Follow-up Measures to Consider

- Document
  - Expected due date (EDD)
  - Relevant history
  - Clinical findings
  - Clinical impression
  - Discussion and client preferences
  - Midwifery plan of care
- Return for continued care
  - Between 6 and 12 weeks' gestation for initial prenatal visit
  - As soon as possible if more than 12 weeks' gestation
  - Prenatal testing as indicated and desired

Multidisciplinary Practice: Consider Consultation or Referral

- Maternity care services
  - Genetic counseling
  - Genetic diagnostic testing
  - Adoption services
  - Abortion services
  - Specialty care
  - Nutritional services
- Social services
  - Pregnancy verification statement for various agencies:
    - Women, Infants and Children
    - Medicaid
- For diagnosis or treatment outside the midwife's scope of practice

INITIAL ASSESSMENT OF THE PREGNANT WOMAN

Key Clinical Information

The initial assessment of the pregnant woman provides the basis for ongoing prenatal care. Careful attention to client interaction, client history, family history, and physical examination allows the midwife to develop a comprehensive, yet dynamic midwifery plan of care with the client and alerts the midwife to sensitive concerns that may require further investigation or follow-up over time. Gentle touch, coupled with an organized, systematic, yet unhurried manner, is ideal during the first visit. Careful documentation of all information is essential to allow for clear communication with other healthcare team members and to serve as a foundation of information for the busy midwife. This client encounter builds on the information obtained in the pregnancy diagnosis office visit. Some practices routinely separate the various activities and assessments done at the initial evaluation of the pregnant woman into two shorter office visits, because there is a lot to accomplish at this visit. This is a time-intensive visit, but it is well worth the investment of time and energy to establish a good rapport with the pregnant woman and her family and to co-create an optimal plan of care for the individual woman and her baby.

Client History and Chart Review: Components of the History to Consider

- Cultural and demographic information
- OB/GYN history
  - Present pregnancy history
    - LMP, interval, and flow
    - Signs and symptoms
  - G, PTPAL, pregnancy information, and complications
  - Gynecologic disorders or problems
  - Sexual history
  - Contraceptive history
- Risk assessment (see "Assessment of Health Risks in the Pregnant Woman")
- Past medical/surgical history
- Family history
- Social history
- Interval history since last menstrual period
  - Drugs or herbs taken
  - Illness or fever
  - Significant family, social, or lifestyle changes
- Review of systems (ROS)

Physical Examination: Components of the Physical Exam to Consider

- Vital signs
- Observation of general status
- Head, eyes, ears, nose, and throat (HEENT)
- Skin
  - Striae
  - Scars, tracks, or bruises
  - Body art, piercings, or tattoos
- Cardiorespiratory system
- Breasts
- Abdomen
  - Fundal height
  - Fetal heart rate (FHR)
  - Fetal lie and position
- Gastrointestinal system
- Genitourinary system
  - External genitalia
    - Vulvar varicosities
    - Scars, lesions
  - Speculum examination
    - Vagina
    - Cervix
    - Collection of laboratory specimens
  - Bimanual examination
    - Uterine size, contour
    - Tenderness
    - Pelvimetry
  - Rectal examination as needed
    - Presence of hemorrhoids
- Musculoskeletal system
  - Varicosities

Clinical Impression: Differential Diagnoses to Consider

- Pregnancy, normal
- High-risk pregnancy
- Secondary diagnoses related to other findings as indicated by
    - History
    - Physical examination
    - Diagnostic testing

Diagnostic Testing: Diagnostic Tests and Procedures to Consider

(Frye, 2007; Institute for Clinical Systems Improvement, 2006)

- Pregnancy testing if needed
    - Urine or serum HCG
    - Quantitative β-hCG
- STI testing
    - Chlamydia and gonorrhea
    - Venereal Disease Research Laboratory (VDRL) or rapid plasma reagin (RPR)
    - Human immunodeficiency virus (HIV)
    - Hepatitis B surface antigen
- Pap smear with reflex human papillomavirus (HPV) testing
- Hematology evaluation and titers
    - Hemoglobin and hematocrit or complete blood count (CBC)
    - Blood type, Rh factor, and antibody screen
    - Rubella titer
    - Varicella antibody screen
- Fetal and genetic screening and testing
    - All genetic screening offered with full informed consent
        - First-trimester screening
            - Serum screen done between 9 and 13 weeks' gestation
            - Nuchal translucency done at 10 to 13 completed weeks' gestation
            - Screens for Down Syndrome
            - Does not detect neural tube defect (NTD)
        - Second-trimester screening
            - Quad serum screen
            - Done between 15 and 22 weeks' gestation
            - Screens for Down Syndrome and NTD
        - Integrated screening
            - First- and second-trimester serum markers
            - Nuchal translucency done between 10-13 completed weeks, gestation
            - Detects Down Syndrome and NTD
            - Highest sensitivity (95%) with lowest false-positive rate (2%)
        - No screening is offered as an equal option
    - Cystic fibrosis screen offered
    - Ultrasound, vaginal or abdominal
        - Establish or confirm dates
        - Fetal viability
        - Fetal anatomical survey
- Urinalysis, with culture as indicated by history
- Group B *Streptococcus* culture at 35 to 37 weeks' gestation (Centers for Disease Control and Prevention [CDC], 2010a)
    - Swab lower vaginal vault and rectum
    - Self or provider swab
- For selected high-risk populations or individuals, consider
    - Ultrasound for nuchal translucency
    - Amniocentesis or chorionic villus sampling
    - Thyroid-stimulating hormone
    - Sickle cell screen or hemoglobin electrophoresis
    - Blood lead screening
    - One-hour glucose challenge test
    - Wet prep for bacterial vaginosis, candidiasis, and trichomoniasis
    - Tuberculosis testing: purified protein derivative (PPD)
    - History of positive PPD or bacillus Calmette-Guérin (BCG) vaccine, consider chest x-ray

Providing Treatment: Therapeutic Measures to Consider

- Prenatal vitamins with folic acid
- Seasonal influenza vaccination (CDC, 2010b)
- Regular mild to moderate exercise
- Adequate rest
- Stress management techniques
- Social support networks
- Dietary sources of nutrients:
  - Folate
  - Iron
  - Calcium
  - Omega-3 fatty acids DHA and EPA
  - Fiber
  - Whole unprocessed food, organic when possible
- Continue or modify treatment of existing conditions in light of pregnancy diagnosis as indicated

Providing Treatment: Complementary and Alternative Measures to Consider

These measures are intended to supplement—not replace—regular prenatal care:

- Prenatal yoga
- Meditation and relaxation therapies
- Pregnancy massage therapy
- Childbirth education classes
- Prenatal exercise classes

Providing Support: Education and Support Measures to Consider

Discuss the following topics:

- Diet and exercise recommendations
- Lifestyle modification recommendations
- Danger signs and when to call
- How to access care providers
- Typical return visit schedule
- Recommended prenatal visits
- Recommended pregnancy, childbirth, and parenting classes
- Recommended and optional prenatal testing

- Birth options
  - Location of birth
  - Water birth/hydrotherapy availability
  - Vaginal birth after cesarean (VBAC) counseling as needed
- Multidisciplinary medical providers

Follow-up Care: Follow-up Measures to Consider

- Document
  - Pregnancy status
  - Risk assessment with plan for care
  - Informed consent as applicable
- Schedule return for prenatal visits
  - Every 4–6 weeks through 28–32 weeks' gestation
  - Every 2–3 weeks through 32–36 weeks' gestation
  - Weekly from 36 weeks' gestation to onset of labor
  - More or less frequent visits based on risk assessment
  - www. Centering Pregnancy© group starting in second trimester
- Vaginal birth after cesarean (VBAC) or planned repeat cesarean section
  - Obtain and review operative notes to verify type of uterine incision
  - Surgical and or anesthesia consultation

Multidisciplinary Practice: Consider Consultation or Referral

- OB/GYN services
  - Per practice standards
  - Genetic or other counseling
  - Other specialists as indicated by secondary diagnoses or findings
- Social services
  - Women, Infants, and Children (WIC) program
  - Medicaid
- Dietary counseling
- For diagnosis or treatment outside the midwife's scope of practice

Out-of-hospital birth—either in the home or in a free-standing birth center setting—is a safe option for women who meet and maintain the criteria of low risk during pregnancy and who arrange care with a skilled provider (Janssen, Saxell, Page, Klein, Liston, & Lee, 2009; Johnson & Davis, 2005). There are no universally endorsed selection criteria for home birth candidates in the United States (American College of Nurse–Midwives [ACNM], 2004). The information presented here is a brief overview of considerations for labor and birth for the woman who chooses an out-of-hospital birth.

The woman should have a strong preference for birth in an out-of-hospital setting and demonstrate the following characteristics:

- Low risk for perinatal complications/high risk for normal birth and healthy baby
- Maintenance of positive health habits and prenatal care
- Preparation of birthing environment and supportive others
- Spontaneous progressive labor
- Willingness to transfer during labor or postpartum if complications develop
- Plans in place for urgent or emergency transfer of care to a hospital setting

The woman should also have the following psychosocial attributes:

- Understand the shared responsibility for care and outcome
- Have adequate social support for her choice
- Have a strong commitment to labor and birth without drugs
- Agree to the screening criteria of this specific out-of-hospital practice
- Have open and clear communication with the midwife

The interested reader is encouraged to access ACNM, MANA, and AABC documents regarding the safe provision of out-of-hospital care.

American Association of Birth Centers: http://www.birthcenters.org/

American College of Nurse–Midwives: http://www.midwife.org/

Midwives Association of North America: http://mana.org/

ASSESSMENT OF HEALTH RISKS IN THE PREGNANT WOMAN

Key Clinical Information

One of the important elements of prenatal care is the identification of health risks that can be modified or diminished through timely assessment, diagnosis, and treatment. Health risks have the potential to affect the health of the mother, her unborn baby, or her newly born infant. Health risks can be related to lifestyle, diet, social habits, genetic heritage, environmental exposures, and cultural or ethnic background and practices. Prenatal assessment and identification of health risks offer the opportunity to diagnose or treat actual or potential conditions or to provide parents with information and support to help them cope with unexpected outcomes.

Many risk factors for pregnant women are associated with habitual or addictive behaviors, such as dietary habits and smoking. The midwife can start addressing these modifiable behaviors with the client by assessing her readiness to change. For those clients who test positive for substance use, or who demonstrate other lifestyle behaviors with negative health effects, using a direct and woman-centered counseling style, assessing the client's readiness to change, and demonstrating empathy and reflective listening can significantly modify behavior (Rubak,

Sandbaek, Lauritzen, & Christensen, 2005) www Motivational interviewing principles should be used during client encounters discussing lifestyle issues to facilitate behavior change and positive outcomes.

Client History and Chart Review: Components of the History to Consider

- Maternal demographic information
  - Age
  - Partner status
  - Education
  - Socioeconomic status
  - Ethnic/racial background
  - Employment status
  - Religious preference
  - Sexual orientation
- Review of personal medical history
  - Diseases or health disorders
  - Medication use, over the counter or prescription
  - Surgeries
  - Use of complementary and alternative therapies
    - Herbs
    - Homeopathy
    - Acupuncture
- OB/GYN history
  - Prior pregnancy conditions or complications
    - Prior pregnancy losses
    - Birth defects
    - Infertility
  - STIs
  - Previous gynecologic procedures
    - Loop electrosurgical excision procedure (LEEP)
    - Myomectomy
    - Hysterosalpingogram
- Review of family medical history
  - Ethnic heritage
  - Hereditary or genetic health conditions
  - Cultural health habits or conditions
- Pregnancy-related risks
  - Review of health habits
  - Smoking, alcohol, and/or drug use
  - Signs or symptoms of concern

- Nutritional status
  - Diet history
  - Caffeine use
    - 200 mg or less per day recommended (March of Dimes, 2010)
- Physical activity
- Review of environmental exposures (Arnesen, 2006)
  - Cats or raw meat (toxoplasmosis)
  - Paint and pipes in older homes and various household items (lead)
  - High-mercury fish consumption
  - Soft cheeses, packaged meats (listeriosis)
  - Household cleaning chemicals
  - Household pesticides
  - Occupational exposures
- Review of social situation and support
  - Presence of caring partner or support
  - Number and relationship of people in the home
  - Anticipated cultural practices during pregnancy
  - Economic situation and resources
  - Intimate-partner violence screening
  - Barriers to prenatal care
- Psychosocial evaluation
  - Depression screening
- Review of systems

Physical Examination: Components of the Physical Exam to Consider

- Physical assessment:
  - Vital signs
  - Weight
  - Height
    - Body mass index (BMI)
- Evaluate for evidence of the following:
  - Illness
  - Malnutrition
  - Exhaustion
  - Abuse
- Skin examination
  - Needle tracks
  - Bruising

- Burns
- Petechia
- Lesions
- Olfactory evidence
  - Tobacco or alcohol use
  - Ketosis
  - General hygiene

Clinical Impression: Differential Diagnoses to Consider

(ICD9data.com, 2012)

- Pregnancy, normal
- Pregnancy at risk
  - Health habits, specify
  - Genetic disorders
  - Maternal age
  - Health conditions, specify
  - Prior uterine or cervical surgery
  - Infection
  - Abuse
    - Physical
    - Sexual
    - Emotional
  - Substance abuse
  - Poor social support
  - Occupational hazards
- Noncompliance secondary to the following issues:
  - Communication
  - Transportation
  - Limited resources
  - Psychological issues
  - Self-determination
  - Knowledge deficit
- Other diagnoses as noted

Diagnostic Testing: Diagnostic Tests and Procedures to Consider

- Drug screening
- HIV testing
- Hepatitis B and C testing
- Sickle cell prep
- Serum screening for neural tube defect and/or aneuploidy

- Group B *Streptococcus* testing
- STI testing
- Ultrasound
  - Fetal anatomy
  - Nuchal translucency
- Amniocentesis
- Chorionic villus sampling

Providing Treatment: Therapeutic Measures to Consider

- Prenatal or multivitamin with folic acid and omega-3s DHA and EPA as needed
- Brief behavioral therapy
  - Assess client readiness to change problem behavior in stages of change model
    - Pre-contemplation (not ready to change)
    - Contemplation (thinking about changing)
    - Preparation (ready to change)
    - Action (changed)
    - Maintenance (staying changed)
    - Relapse (back to previous problem behavior)
- **WWW** Five "A"s of smoking cessation: ask, advise, assess, assist, arrange (American College of Obstetricians and Gynecologists [ACOG], 2010a)
- Five "R"s of smoking cessation for those who continue smoking: relevance, risk, rewards, roadblocks, repetition (ACOG, 2010a)
- Nicotine replacement therapies, bupropion, and varenicline to be avoided during pregnancy (ACOG, 2010a)
- Other medications or treatments based on diagnosis

Providing Treatment: Complementary and Alternative Measures to Consider

- Nutritional support
- Hypnosis to change health habits
- Support groups
- Other treatments based on diagnosis

Providing Support: Education and Support Measures to Consider

- Allow private time to encourage disclosure
- Provide information about risks and/or benefits:
  - Current lifestyle behaviors
  - Prenatal tests and other offered tests
  - Genetic screening and testing options
  - Treatment options
- Genetic counseling
- Drug and alcohol screening policy
- Social support services
- Develop plan for safety as indicated by history
- Cultural support services
  - Translation services
- Diagnosis-related support groups

Follow-up Care: Follow-up Measures to Consider

- Document
- Return visits
  - Factors determining frequency:
    - Client condition
    - Gestational age
  - Allow adequate time:
    - Develop a cooperative relationship
    - Observe for risk-related behaviors
  - Serial drug or STI testing as indicated

Multidisciplinary Practice: Consider Consultation or Referral

- Maternity care services
  - Genetic counseling and testing
  - Nuchal translucency, amniocentesis, or chorionic villus sampling
  - OB/GYN consultation, collaboration, or referral
- Medical services
  - As indicated for medical or specialty care
- Social services
  - As indicated by lifestyle and social indicators
  - Inpatient or outpatient drug rehabilitation program

- Counseling or therapy
- Women's shelter/safe house
- For diagnosis or treatment outside the midwife's scope of practice

ONGOING CARE OF THE PREGNANT WOMAN

Key Clinical Information

The "routine" prenatal visit is anything but routine for most pregnant women. This visit is each woman's opportunity to have her needs met and her concerns addressed while being evaluated for the well-being of herself and her child. Prenatal care provides an opportunity to look for subtle signs or symptoms that can indicate a deviation from normal.

Prenatal care began in the early 1900s as a method to screen for signs and symptoms of preeclampsia, but over the years it has evolved into a platform for teaching and testing. Follow-up activities by the midwife allow women to fully realize the benefits of prenatal care and foster an ongoing interaction that builds trust and understanding between the client and the midwife. Follow-up on laboratory and test results, on behavioral changes, and on teaching highlights the value placed on these measures. The group prenatal care model capitalizes on the social support and compassion provided by a cohort of peers—women from diverse backgrounds who meet on the common ground of childbearing. The overarching goal of prenatal care is a safe and satisfying pregnancy, with optimal outcomes given the circumstances of the mother's life and health during her pregnancy.

Client History and Chart Review: Components of the History to Consider

(Davis, 2004; Varney et al., 2004)

- Review relevant aspects of chart before client visit
- Interval history since last visit
  - Gestational age
  - Maternal well-being
    - Nutrition
    - Sleep

- ◆ Activity and exercise
- ◆ Bowel and bladder function
  - Presence of common discomforts
    - ◆ Relief measures used and effectiveness
  - Signs or symptoms of
    - ◆ Preterm labor
    - ◆ Pregnancy-induced hypertension
    - ◆ Urinary tract infection
    - ◆ Vaginal bleeding or discharge
    - ◆ Exposure to infectious disease
  - Fetal movement
- Concerns
  - Questions
  - Plans related to pregnancy, labor, and birth

Physical Examination: Components of the Physical Exam to Consider

- Blood pressure (BP), other vital signs as indicated
- Interval weight gain or loss
- Assessment of general well-being
- Abdominal examination
  - Fundal height
  - Fetal heart tones
  - Estimated fetal weight
  - Fetal lie, presentation, position, and variety
- Costovertebral angle (CVA) tenderness
- Examination of extremities
  - Edema
  - Varicosities, phlebitis
  - Reflexes
- Additional components as indicated by history

Clinical Impression: Differential Diagnoses to Consider

(ICD9data.com, 2012)

- Pregnancy
  - Low risk
  - At risk—specify
- Additional diagnoses based on
  - History
  - Physical examination
  - Diagnostic testing

Diagnostic Testing: Diagnostic Tests and Procedures to Consider

- Dip urinalysis for women with signs or symptoms of the following (Institute for Clinical Systems Improvement, 2006):
  - Hypertension
  - Rapid weight gain
  - Preeclampsia
  - Gestational diabetes
- Urine culture
  - History of asymptomatic bacteriuria
  - Sickle cell trait
  - History of pyelonephritis
  - Urinary symptoms
  - Positive dip urinalysis
    - ◆ Many bacteria
    - ◆ Positive nitrite with positive leukocytes
- Glucose challenge test
  - First trimester
    - ◆ Previous gestational diabetes
    - ◆ High risk for gestational diabetes (see the "Gestational Diabetes" section)
  - 24 to 28 weeks' gestation
    - ◆ Selective or universal screening protocol
    - ◆ Repeat testing in high-risk women with prior negative screen
- Blood type and antibody screen
  - Initial prenatal laboratory values
  - 24 to 28 weeks' gestation for Rh-negative mothers
- Hematocrit and hemoglobin
  - Initial prenatal labs
  - 24 to 28 weeks' gestation as needed
  - Every 4–6 weeks to evaluate iron replacement therapy
- Repeat STI testing as indicated
- Repeat wet prep as indicated
- Group B *Streptococcus* testing (CDC, 2010a)
  - 35 to 37 weeks' gestation
  - Signs or symptoms of preterm labor
- Ultrasound evaluation as indicated:
  - Pregnancy dating
  - Genetic evaluation/amniocentesis

- Fetal growth and development
- Placental location
- Biophysical profile
- Amniotic fluid index
- Cervical length measurement
- Additional testing as indicated:
  - CBC with reticulocytes, total iron-binding capacity (TIBC), serum iron, serum ferritin
  - Thyroid-stimulating hormone, free T_4, thyroid antibodies
  - Three-hour glucose tolerance testing
  - Fetal fibronectin
  - CBC with differential, renal and liver function studies, serum uric acid, 24-hour urine for protein
  - Other tests as indicated by findings

Providing Treatment: Therapeutic Measures to Consider

- Encourage appropriate weight gain (Institute of Medicine [IOM], 2009) (see "A Nutritional Primer" at the end of this book)
  - BMI < 18.5: gain 28–40 lb
  - BMI = 18.5–24.9: gain 25–35 lb
  - BMI = 25–29.9: gain 15–25 lb
  - BMI ≥ 30: gain 11–20 lb
- Eat regular meals that include a variety of foods
  - Organic foods when possible
  - Whole, nonprocessed foods
- Prenatal vitamins with folic acid
- Adequate omega-3's: DHA and EPA (Jordan, 2010)
  - Two coldwater fish meals/week for DHA and EPA
    - Low-mercury fish choices
    - Fish oil supplements if fish not eaten
      - Barleans liquid or tablets: 200–300 mg/day
- Iron from dietary sources (see "A Nutritional Primer") with supplementation as needed:
  - Ferro-sequels 1–2 PO daily
  - Floridix 10 mL BID
  - Niferex 150 mg 1–2 PO daily

- Ferrous gluconate 1–2 PO daily
- Other supplement of choice
- Calcium from dietary sources (see "A Nutritional Primer") with supplements as needed:
  - Citracal: 200–400 mg BID
  - Tums: 500 mg, one to two tablets daily
  - Os-cal: one tablet, two to three times daily
- **www.** Influenza vaccine in the fall and winter months (CDC, 2010b)
- Immunization update if at significant risk or traveling abroad
- Preterm birth prevention for women with risk of preterm birth
  - **www.** Weekly IM progesterone (17p) beginning at 16–20 weeks until 36 weeks (ACOG, 2008)

Providing Treatment: Complementary and Alternative Measures to Consider

(Romm, 2010; Walls, 2009)

- Pregnant belly massage
  - Jojoba oil
  - Shea or cocoa butter
  - Calendula infusion
- As indicated by symptom or condition
- Third-trimester herbal support
  - Red raspberry leaf
  - Chamomile
  - Nettle
  - Cranberry
  - Primrose oil gelcaps 500–1000 mg BID after 37 weeks, PO or intravaginally

Providing Support: Education and Support Measures to Consider

- Pregnancy discussion
  - Planned schedule of prenatal visits
    - Offer group prenatal care if available
  - Expectations related to care
    - Client/family expectations
    - Midwife/practice expectations
  - Anticipated testing
  - Fee and payment information

- Health education
  - Midwife call system
    - When and how to call
  - Importance of the following issues:
    - Fetal movement patterns
    - Nutrition and appropriate weight gain for BMI
    - Regular exercise
  - Management of common discomforts
  - Feelings about pregnancy, birth, and family
    - Relationship changes
    - Sexual relations in pregnancy
- Social services available
- Labor discussion
  - Preterm labor and birth education until 37 weeks
  - Planned location of birth
  - Preparation for labor
  - Signs and symptoms of labor
  - Anticipated labor care and birth options
    - Labor support
    - Pain relief
      - Hydrotherapy/water birth
      - Birth ball
      - Heated rice packs
      - Massage
      - Positioning
      - Acupressure
      - Medication options
    - Perineal support (see the "Perineal Massage" section)
    - Episiotomy indicators
    - Transport/consult indicators
  - Physician coverage for needed care or emergencies
  - Anticipated infant care
    - Vitamin K options
    - Ophthalmic prophylaxis
    - Planned method of infant feeding
    - Transport indicators
    - Circumcision options
    - Newborn evaluation at home

- Anticipated postpartum care
  - Based on location of birth
  - Cultural practices after birth
  - Planned help at home, resources
  - Postpartum method of birth control
- Anticipated visits for follow-up care
  - Home visits
  - Mother postpartum visits
  - Infant evaluation

Follow-up Care: Follow-up Measures to Consider

- Review with client
  - Previously performed laboratory results
  - Client education and expressed needs
  - Behavioral and lifestyle changes
  - Healthy lifestyle maintenance or improvement
    - Diet
    - Exercise, activity, and rest
    - Stress management
- Midwifery plan of care
  - Identify
    - Alternative providers and/or location for birth
    - Client risk factors and anticipated management
    - Preferred newborn care provider(s)
  - Anticipated return visit schedule
    - Every 4–6 weeks until 28–32 weeks' gestation
    - Every 2–3 weeks from 30 to 36 weeks' gestation
    - Weekly from 36 weeks' gestation until birth occurs
    - Various scheduling as needed; specify indication
  - Informed consent or consultation, as indicated:
    - Planned out-of-hospital birth
    - VBAC
    - Cesarean birth
    - Postpartum tubal ligation

- Document
  - Findings and updated problem list
  - Discussions with client/family
  - Client preferences for labor and birth
  - Plan for continued care
  - Informed consent forms

Multidisciplinary Practice: Consider Consultation or Referral

- Health education
  - Pregnancy and/or childbirth education classes
  - Diabetes education and diet counseling for the gestational diabetic
  - Pregnancy yoga or exercise program
- Social services
- OB/GYN consultation, collaboration, or referral
  - Complications or problems during pregnancy
  - Surgical consultation
- Anesthesia services
  - Preoperative evaluation
- For diagnosis or treatment outside the midwife's scope of practice

CARE OF THE PREGNANT WOMAN WITH BACKACHE

Key Clinical Information

Backache is pain in the upper or lower back. It affects most pregnant women to some degree, whereas an estimated 15% of pregnant women will have severe back pain (Blackburn, 2007). As pregnancy progresses, a woman's center of gravity shifts and postural compensations are made for this change. Kyphosis of the cervical spine accommodates the growth and weight of the breasts, while lordosis of the lumbar spine accommodates the distention of the abdomen. These changes combine with hormonal influences that loosen ligaments and joints and lead to backache for many pregnant women. Client posture, body mechanics, and muscle tone all influence the amount of strain on the back from the pregnant woman's growing belly.

Other causes of backache during pregnancy deserve thoughtful evaluation, as this general symptom is frequently the only indication of preterm labor, pyelonephritis, or renal calculi, or may represent referred pain from the liver or gallbladder. Additionally, back pathology, such as disc disease or muscle strain, is included in the differential diagnosis when pain is severe or not ameliorated by typical treatments.

Client History and Chart Review: Components of the History to Consider

- Gestational age
- Onset, duration, severity, and location of backache
- History of backache
  - Precipitating event, if any
  - Timing
  - Activities that exacerbate backache
  - Medications or self-help measures used and relief obtained
- Presence of other associated symptoms
  - Presence or absence of contractions
  - Urinary symptoms
    - Frequency
    - Flank pain
  - Presence of neurologic signs or symptoms
  - Sciatica
- Past medical history
  - Back injury or disease
  - Kidney stones or pyelonephritis
- Potential contributing factors
  - Body mechanics
  - Lifting at work or home
  - Physical activity
  - Physical abuse, trauma, or injury

Physical Examination: Components of the Physical Exam to Consider

- Vital signs, including weight
- Abdominal examination
  - Abdominal muscle tone
  - Uterine size
  - Suprapubic tenderness
  - Upper abdominal tenderness

- Back examination
  - Mobility
  - Point tenderness
  - Posture, presence of lordosis, kyphosis, or scoliosis
  - CVA tenderness
  - Presence of muscle spasm
- Pelvic evaluation
  - Backache accompanied by contractions
  - History suggestive of preterm labor
  - Evaluation of cervical status
- Evaluation of neurologic status
  - Muscle tone
  - Strength
  - Coordination
  - Reflexes
- Signs of physical abuse
  - Bruising
  - Burns
  - Partner presence for entire visit

Clinical Impression: Differential Diagnoses to Consider

(ICD9data.com, 2012)

- Backache of pregnancy
- Muscle strain or sprain, lumbar
- Also consider:
  - Pyelonephritis
  - Renal calculi
  - Herniated disc
  - Irritable bowel syndrome
  - Rheumatoid arthritis
  - Pregnancy-induced hypertension
  - Gallbladder disease

Diagnostic Testing: Diagnostic Tests and Procedures to Consider

- Urinalysis
- Urine culture in the patient with a history of urinary tract infections
- Fetal/uterine monitoring
- Ultrasound

- Kidneys if renal calculi suspected
- Upper abdomen if gallbladder disease suspected
- Pregnancy-induced hypertension screening; see "Care of the Pregnant Woman with Prenatal Variations"

Providing Treatment: Therapeutic Measures to Consider

- Abdominal binder designed for pregnancy
- Heat application
  - Hot compresses or packs
  - Warm bath
- Pain relief (King & Brucker, 2011)
  - Acetaminophen (Tylenol)
    - 325–650 mg every 4–6 hours
    - Pregnancy Category B
    - Maximum dose is 4 g daily
    - Best choice for pain relief during pregnancy
  - Naproxen (Aleve, others)
    - 200–800 mg every 4–12 hours
    - Increase in miscarriage risk in early pregnancy (Nakhai-Pour, Broy, Sheehy, & Berard, 2011)
    - Avoid in early and late pregnancy
  - Ibuprofen (Advil, Motrin, others)
    - 400, 600, or 800 mg TID
    - Pregnancy Category B in first and second trimesters
    - Avoid in late pregnancy
- Muscle spasm
  - Flexeril
    - 10 mg TID
    - Pregnancy Category B
- As appropriate for other confirmed diagnosis

Providing Treatment: Complementary and Alternative Measures to Consider

(Romm, 2010; Walls, 2009)

- Massage
  - Arnica-infused oil
  - Peppermint-infused oil
  - Capsaicin salve or ointment

- Adequate calcium and magnesium intake
  - Calcium
- Herbals
  - Chamomile tea
  - Cramp bark tincture

Providing Support: Education and Support Measures to Consider

(Pennick & Young, 2007)

- Use of good body mechanics
  - Low-heeled shoes
  - Posture to minimize lordosis
  - Bend knees to lift using leg muscles
  - Avoid lifting with back
  - Avoid bending or turning from waist
- Planned back care program
  - Pelvic tilt
  - Stretching
  - Swimming
  - Yoga
- Supportive sleep environment
  - Firm mattress
  - Pillows between knees
- Mechanical support measures
  - Well-fitting supportive bra
  - Prenatal abdominal cradle
  - Lumbar support in chair/car
  - Footstool to raise knees above hips

Follow-up Care: Follow-up Measures to Consider

- Document
- Return for care
  - As scheduled for gestation
  - With worsening symptoms
    - ◆ Pain
    - ◆ Numbness or tingling
  - Signs of preterm labor
  - Urinary symptoms

Multidisciplinary Practice: Consider Consultation or Referral

- Acupuncture/acupressure therapy (Pennick & Young, 2007)
- Osteopathic manipulation

- Chiropractic manipulation (Pennick & Young, 2007)
- Physical therapy
  - For evaluation
  - For symptom management
  - For exercise training
  - For mobility aids
- OB/GYN consultation, collaboration, or referral
  - Persistent backache
  - Persistent backache with contractions
  - Development of fever and chills
  - Positive testing for kidney involvement
  - Presence of neurologic symptoms
- Social services
  - Indicators of domestic violence
- For diagnosis or treatment outside the midwife's scope of practice

CARE OF THE PREGNANT WOMAN WITH CONSTIPATION

Key Clinical Information

Constipation represents a change in a person's normal bowel patterns to less frequent or more difficult defecation (Blackburn, 2007). Constipation can occur or be exacerbated in pregnant women due to the decreased motility and increased water reabsorption in the intestine as well as pressure from the enlarged uterus; this condition affects 11% to 30% of women during pregnancy (Blackburn, 2007). Prevention of constipation requires adequate intake of fluid and fiber accompanied by physical activity to stimulate the bowels. Determining acceptable dietary sources of fiber for each client is essential. Candid discussion regarding frequency and consistency of bowel movements is an integral part of evaluation for this common malady.

Client History and Chart Review: Components of the History to Consider

- Gestational age
- Onset of problem
- Bowel habits

- Frequency and consistency of bowel movements
- Straining
- Remedies used and efficacy
- Dietary habits
- Fiber rich foods
  - Fluid intake
- Other associated symptoms
  - Abdominal cramping with bowel movement
    - Nature of abdominal discomfort
    - Location, severity
    - Backache
    - Contractions
  - Presence of blood in the stool
- Potential contributing factors
  - Iron therapy
  - Inactivity
  - Inadequate fluid intake
  - Inadequate fiber intake
  - Narcotic use
- Past medical history
  - Abdominal surgeries (adhesions)
  - Pelvic inflammatory disease (PID)
  - Bowel disorders
  - Status of appendix

Physical Examination: Components of the Physical Exam to Consider

- Vital signs, including temperature
- Abdominal examination
  - Auscultate bowel sounds in all four quadrants
  - Palpate for presence of abdominal pain
    - Location
    - Rebound
    - Guarding
- Pelvic examination
  - Palpate for hard stool in rectum
  - Cervical evaluation if cramping present
- Rectal examination as needed

Clinical Impression: Differential Diagnoses to Consider

- Constipation
- Appendicitis
- Irritable bowel syndrome
- Fecal impaction
- Diverticulitis

Diagnostic Testing: Diagnostic Tests and Procedures to Consider

- Urine for specific gravity
- CBC with differential
- Pelvic ultrasound

Providing Treatment: Therapeutic Measures to Consider

- Increase fiber in diet
  - Dried fruits, prunes, prune juice
  - Whole grains, bran cereals, foods with wheat bran
  - Uncooked vegetables
- Fiber therapy:
  - Citrucel: 1 Tbs in 8 oz fluid, one to three times daily
  - Metamucil: 1 tsp in 8 oz fluid, one to three times daily
  - FiberCon: 1–2 tab with 8 oz fluid, one to four times daily
- Stool softeners:
  - Docusate sodium: 50–100 mg 1 PO QD or BID
  - Docusate calcium: 240 mg 1 PO QD
- Bowel stimulants:
  - Senokot: 1 tablet at bedtime
  - Milk of magnesia: tablet, capsule, or liquid form
- Rectal treatments
  - Glycerin suppositories
  - Fleet enema if stool impacted

Providing Treatment: Complementary and Alternative Measures to Consider

(Romm, 2010)

- Herbal support
  - Senna leaf tea
  - Licorice root
  - Psyllium seed 1 tsp TID
  - Flaxseed meal, 2 Tbs daily added to cereal or yogurt, or mixed with water

- Increase fluid intake
  - 8 cups per day
  - Hot liquid in morning
    - ◆ Herbal teas
    - ◆ Decaffeinated coffee
    - ◆ Hot prune juice
- Increase physical activity
  - Brisk walk after hot drink
  - Follow by toileting
- Bowel retraining
  - Allow regular time for toileting
  - Follow natural urges

Providing Support: Education and Support Measures to Consider

- Walking: helps stimulate natural peristalsis
- Fiber
  - Maintain adequate fiber intake
  - Helps to keep stool soft
  - Must be used with adequate fluid intake
- Stool softeners
  - Bring fluid to the stool to soften it
  - Coat stool with surfactant to help move it
- Bowel stimulants
  - Stimulate peristalsis
  - Should be used with caution during pregnancy
  - May cause cramping
- Suppositories
  - Stimulate evacuation of lower bowel
  - May cause cramping
- Enemas
  - Flush the lower bowel
  - May cause cramping
- Lifestyle recommendations
  - Need for increased fiber and fluid
  - Need for activity to stimulate bowels
  - Hot drink in the morning may stimulate bowels
  - Need for regular time for toileting
- Warning signs of
  - Preterm labor
  - Acute abdomen

Follow-up Care: Follow-up Measures to Consider

- Document
- Return for care
  - As scheduled for gestation
  - Return sooner if symptoms persist or worsen
- For emergency care
  - Symptoms of acute abdomen
  - Obstipation
  - Symptoms of preterm labor

Multidisciplinary Practice: Consider Consultation or Referral

- OB/GYN services
  - Threatened preterm labor
  - Positive occult blood in stool
  - Severe or persistent abdominal pain accompanied by
    - ◆ Fever
    - ◆ Abdominal rigidity or guarding
    - ◆ Obstipation
- For diagnosis or treatment outside the midwife's scope of practice

CARE OF THE PREGNANT WOMAN WITH DYSPNEA

Key Clinical Information

Dyspnea is an unpleasant sense of labored breathing, patient awareness of respiratory discomfort, or shortness of breath. It affects 60% to 70% of women during pregnancy, especially in the first or second trimester (Blackburn, 2007). Physiologic shortness of breath occurs in early pregnancy as the body adjusts to changes in carbon dioxide levels in the blood and its concomitant hyperventilation. Dyspnea again becomes common in the later stages of pregnancy as the uterus pushes against the diaphragm, reducing the functional residual volume of the lungs (Varney et al., 2004). Anemia, cardiac arrhythmias, and poor physical conditioning may also contribute to dyspnea during pregnancy. Additionally, anxiety or panic can precede or exacerbate a dyspneic episode.

Evaluation of shortness of breath during pregnancy is necessary to determine whether it is physiologic or pathologic.

Client History and Chart Review: Components of the History to Consider

- Gestational age
- Timing of onset, duration, and severity of dyspnea
  - With activity or at rest
  - While supine or upright
- Self-help measures or medications used
- Other associated symptoms
  - Fever, chills
  - Cough, dry or productive
  - Syncope
  - Peripheral edema
  - Anxiety or panic symptoms
  - Palpitations
- Cardiopulmonary history
  - Asthma
  - Smoking tobacco or other substances
  - Environmental exposure to allergens, smoke, or fumes
  - Cardiac disorders and/or symptoms
- History of anxiety or panic disorders
- Review of systems

Physical Examination: Components of the Physical Exam to Consider

- Vital signs
- Color
- Auscultation and percussion of the chest
  - Respiratory rate, depth, and volume
  - Cardiac rate and rhythm
  - Lung fields
  - Presence of abnormal breath sounds
- Observe for the following:
  - Respiratory effort
  - Presence of cough, sputum
  - Signs of respiratory distress
  - Edema of the extremities

Clinical Impression: Differential Diagnoses to Consider

(ICD9data.com, 2012)

- Physiologic shortness of breath of pregnancy
- Dyspnea related to the following:
  - Exercise or exertion induced
  - Upper respiratory infection
  - Asthma
  - Anemia
  - Pulmonary embolism
  - Anxiety or panic disorder
  - Other cardiovascular diseases
  - Other respiratory disorders

Diagnostic Testing: Diagnostic Tests and Procedures to Consider

- CBC with differential
- Sputum cultures
- Tuberculosis testing
- Chest x-ray
- Pulmonary function testing

Providing Treatment: Therapeutic Measures to Consider

- Reassurance of normalcy
  - Encourage calm, slow breathing
  - Lean forward or lie down
  - Raise arms to shoulder level
  - Stretch periodically
  - Maintain good posture
- Otherwise as indicated by diagnosis (see the "Care of the Woman with Respiratory Symptoms" section)

Providing Treatment: Complementary and Alternative Measures to Consider

- Maintain slow-paced physical activity
  - Walking
  - Yoga
  - Swimming
- Use pillows as needed for comfort while at rest

Providing Support: Education and Support Measures to Consider

- Review
  - Physiologic basis of shortness of breath
  - Deliberate intercostal breathing
- Comfort measures
  - Loose-fitting clothes
  - Rest periods
  - Avoid lying flat on the back
- Warning signs
  - Flu-like symptoms
  - Productive cough
  - Chest pain, shortness of breath, diaphoresis
  - Anxiety
  - Palpitations

Follow-up Care: Follow-up Measures to Consider

- Document
- Return for care
  - As scheduled for gestation
  - Sooner in the following circumstances:
    - Presence of warning signs
    - Persistence or worsening of symptoms
    - As needed for support

Multidisciplinary Practice: Consider Consultation or Referral

- Medical service
  - Evidence of decompensation
  - History or symptoms of asthma
  - Evidence of respiratory infection or disorder
- Mental health service
  - Anxiety or panic attacks
- For diagnosis or treatment outside the midwife's scope of practice

CARE OF THE PREGNANT WOMAN WITH EDEMA

Key Clinical Information

Edema is abnormal accumulation of excess fluid in the intercellular tissue spaces, most commonly in dependent body parts, such as feet and ankles. Dependent edema is seen in 35% to 80% of pregnant women and becomes more common as pregnancy progresses (Blackburn, 2007). Physiologic edema of pregnancy occurs secondary to fluid retention as the body works to increase and maintain adequate circulating fluid volume. Pressure of the pregnant uterus can cause venous stasis and force fluid out of the circulatory system and into the soft tissue.

Client History and Chart Review: Components of the History to Consider

- Gestational age
- Diet history
  - Fluid intake
  - Sodium in diet
  - Protein intake
- Recent medications
- Onset, location, duration, and severity of edema
  - Precipitating factors
  - Circadian variations in edema
  - Usual fluid intake and urination patterns
  - Self-help measures used and their effects
  - Other associated symptoms
- Symptoms of preeclampsia
- History of
  - Preeclampsia
  - Edema with pregnancy
  - Varicose veins
- Review of systems

Physical Examination: Components of the Physical Exam to Consider

- Vital signs, BP
- Note interval weight changes
- Note presence and pattern of edema
  - Diffuse or localized
  - Presence of pitting edema; time to resolution
  - Bilateral or unilateral
  - Facial, periorbital
- Examination of extremities
  - Deep tendon reflexes
  - Measurement of leg circumference

- Varicosities
- Signs of phlebitis: redness, tenderness, warmth
- Signs of clothing constriction

Clinical Impression: Differential Diagnoses to Consider

(ICD9data.com, 2012)

- Physiologic edema of pregnancy
- Edema related to the following conditions:
  - Preeclampsia
  - Thrombophlebitis
  - Other cardiovascular diseases
  - Other renal disorders

Diagnostic Testing: Diagnostic Tests and Procedures to Consider

- Office urinalysis
  - Proteinuria
  - Specific gravity
- Preeclampsia laboratory values (see the "Care of the Pregnant Woman with Pregnancy Induced Hypertension" section)

Providing Treatment: Therapeutic Measures to Consider

- Rest 1 hour BID with feet higher than heart
  - Suggest elevating foot of bed for gentle overnight elevation
- Prescription support hose
  - Apply with legs elevated to maximize compression

Providing Treatment: Complementary and Alternative Measures to Consider

- Water immersion
- Foot massage, reflexology
- Foot exercises
  - Draw the alphabet with your feet
- Herbal support for fluid balance, two to three cups of tea per day (Walls, 2009)
  - Parsley
  - Dandelion leaf

Providing Support: Education and Support Measures to Consider

- Provide information on:
  - Physiologic basis of edema in pregnancy
  - Warning signs
    - Preeclampsia
    - Phlebitis
- Self-help measures
  - Continue gentle physical activity
  - Rest, elevate extremities, pillow under right hip
  - Increase fluids
  - Add salt to diet to taste if low salt intake
  - Decrease dietary salt if high salt diet intake
- Avoid
  - Constrictive clothing
  - Diuretic medications, foods (asparagus, Brussels sprouts, cabbage), or herbs (juniper berry)

Follow-up Care: Follow-up Measures to Consider

- Document
- Return for care
  - As scheduled for gestation
  - For increasing edema
  - Symptoms of preeclampsia or phlebitis

Multidisciplinary Practice: Consider Consultation or Referral

- OB/GYN services
  - Symptoms of preeclampsia
  - Severe progressive edema
  - Severe varicosities
  - Symptoms of phlebitis or thrombophlebitis
- For diagnosis or treatment outside the midwife's scope of practice

CARE OF THE PREGNANT WOMAN WITH EPISTAXIS

Key Clinical Information

Epistaxis is a nosebleed due to rupture of the nasal blood vessels, which are richly supplied by the internal and external carotid arteries. Frequency of epistaxis is difficult to determine because most episodes resolve with self-treatment and are not reported; however, this condition is thought to occur more frequently during pregnancy. Although nosebleeds are rarely of a serious nature, most women are anxious about the blood loss and may require treatment if the bleeding does not stop promptly. Epistaxis can also be the presenting symptom of labile hypertension. Inhaled drug use can contribute to epistaxis and can rapidly elevate BP and lead to placental abruption or other hypertension-related complications of pregnancy.

Client History and Chart Review: Components of the History to Consider

- Gestational age
- Onset, frequency, duration, and severity of bleeding
  - Precipitating factors or events
    - Allergies or upper respiratory tract infection
    - Use of inhaled drugs (e.g., cocaine, glue)
    - Use of anticoagulant or other medications
    - Trauma
  - Self-help measures used and efficacy
  - Typical nasal hygiene measures
  - Associated signs and symptoms
- Past medical history
  - Epistaxis
  - Bleeding disorder
- Family history
  - Bleeding disorder

Physical Examination: Components of the Physical Exam to Consider

- Vital signs, BP
- Examination of nares
  - Polyps or lesions
  - Trauma
  - Erosion
  - Inflammation
- Observation for bruising

Clinical Impression: Differential Diagnoses to Consider

(ICD9data.com, 2012)

- Epistaxis or secondary to the following conditions:
  - Hypertension
  - Nasal polyps
  - Inhalation drug use
  - Nasal trauma or injury
  - Coagulation defects
  - Seasonal allergies
  - Upper respiratory tract infection

Diagnostic Testing: Diagnostic Tests and Procedures to Consider

- Hematocrit and hemoglobin
  - Persistent, recurrent, copious flow
  - Signs or symptoms of anemia
- Serial BPs
- Drug screen

Providing Treatment: Therapeutic Measures to Consider

- Normal saline nasal spray
- Pressure to nares to stop bleeding
  - Ice with pressure to bridge of nose
  - Pinch bridge of nose
  - Nasal packing

Providing Treatment: Complementary and Alternative Measures to Consider

- Herbal and dietary support:
  - Foods rich in vitamins A, C, and E
    - Deep-green leafy vegetables
    - Onions in diet
    - Parsley
    - Nettle tea
- Treatment
  - Cold compresses of comfrey, yarrow, and/or mullein
  - Plantain and yarrow ointment

Providing Support: Education and Support Measures to Consider

- Reassurance of normalcy
- Provide information on
  - Physiologic basis for epistaxis
  - Nasal hygiene
    - Gentle clearing of nasal debris after bath or shower
  - Self-help measures
    - Avoid vigorous blowing or picking of nose
    - Use humidifier or vaporizer

Follow-up Care: Follow-up Measures to Consider

- Document
- Return for care
  - As scheduled for gestation
  - For bleeding unresponsive to self-help measures

Multidisciplinary Practice: Consider Consultation or Referral

- Ear, nose, and throat (ENT) service
  - Electrocautery of bleeding vessel
  - Nasal polyps or lesions
- Medical services
  - Suspected bleeding disorder
- For diagnosis or treatment outside the midwife's scope of practice

CARE OF THE PREGNANT WOMAN WITH HEARTBURN

Key Clinical Information

Heartburn is a sensation of burning behind the breastbone, resulting from the backflow of stomach contents into the esophagus. Heartburn affects 30% to 70% of women at some point in pregnancy and affects 25% of women daily in their third trimester (Dowswell & Neilson, 2008). The softening influence of the pregnancy hormone relaxin on the lower esophageal sphincter is one contributor to the increased incidence of heartburn noted in pregnancy. As pregnancy progresses, simple mechanical pressure also contributes to heartburn. Women with a history of gastroesophageal reflux disease (GERD) may require treatment during pregnancy. Small meals and a bland diet are often helpful in minimizing this problem.

Client History and Chart Review: Components of the History to Consider

- Gestational age
- Onset, frequency, timing, duration, and severity of heartburn
- Common symptoms
  - Burning epigastric pain
  - Reflux
  - Belching, bloating
- Associated symptoms
  - Palpitations
  - Diaphoresis
- Precipitating factors or events
  - Foods
  - Anxiety
  - Positioning
- Presence of symptoms before pregnancy
- Usual diet
- Self-help measures and efficacy

Physical Examination: Components of the Physical Exam to Consider

- Vital signs
- Interval weight gain or loss
- Abdominal palpation
- Fundal height

Clinical Impression: Differential Diagnoses to Consider

(ICD9data.com, 2012)

- Physiologic heartburn of pregnancy
- Gastroesophageal reflux disease
- Hiatal hernia
- Gastritis
- Gallbladder disease

Diagnostic Testing: Diagnostic Tests and Procedures to Consider

- Consult or refer the client if *Helicobacter pylori* testing is indicated. Both noninvasive and invasive methods of testing are available.

Providing Treatment: Therapeutic Measures to Consider

(King & Brucker, 2011)

- Antacid preparations:
  - Calcium carbonate (Tums) 1–2 tab every 2 hours PRN with full glass of water
  - Magnesium/aluminum combination (Mylanta, Gelusil) 2–4 tsp every 4 hours PRN
  - Aluminum hydroxide (Amphojel) 600–1200 mg between meals and after meals PRN
- Proton pump inhibitors (Pregnancy Category B):
  - Aciphex 20 mg QD
  - Nexium 20 mg QD
  - Prevacid 30 mg BID
- H$_2$ blockers (Pregnancy Category B):
  - Axid 150 mg PO BID
  - Pepcid 20 mg PO BID
  - Tagamet 300 mg PO QID
  - Zantac 150 mg PO BID

Providing Treatment: Complementary and Alternative Measures to Consider

The following herbal remedies may be helpful (Romm, 2010):

- Slippery elm lozenges or tea
- Marshmallow root infusion
- Raw almonds
- Ginger
- Peppermint tea
- Papaya chewable tablets

Providing Support: Education and Support Measures to Consider

- Reassurance of normalcy
- Provide information:
  - Physiologic basis of heartburn
  - Warning signs

- Comfort measures
  - Small, frequent meals
  - Avoid eating before bed
  - Maintain good posture
  - Decrease intake of fatty or spicy foods
  - Take food and fluids separately
  - Elevate head of the bed by 10–30 degrees

Follow-up Care: Follow-up Measures to Consider

- Document
- Return for care
  - As scheduled for gestation
  - Persistent reflux or abdominal pain
  - Indications for referral
    - Persistent severe reflux
    - Abdominal pain
    - Signs or symptoms of ulcer or perforation

Multidisciplinary Practice: Consider Consultation or Referral

- Medical or gastroenterology services
  - Severe symptoms unrelieved by treatment
  - For suspected or documented
    - *H. pylori* infection
    - Hiatal hernia
    - Gastroesophageal reflux disease
    - Gastric ulcer or perforation
- For diagnosis or treatment outside the midwife's scope of practice

CARE OF THE PREGNANT WOMAN WITH HEMORRHOIDS

Key Clinical Information

Hemorrhoids are dilated veins of the hemorrhoidal plexus in the lower rectum. Hemorrhoids are considered common in pregnancy, but their prevalence in pregnancy is unknown. One study found that 85% of women late in their second and third pregnancies had hemorrhoids (Gojnic, Dugalic, Papic, Vidakovic, Milicevic, & Perulov, 2005). Symptoms include irritation, itching, pain, and bleeding. Hemorrhoids are internal when they occur inside the anal canal and external when they occur at the anal opening. Internal hemorrhoids are usually not painful unless they become ulcerated, infected, or project outside through the anus. The pressure of the pregnant uterus on pelvic vessels and constipation both aggravate hemorrhoids, causing bleeding, itching, and burning. Thrombosed hemorrhoids are extremely painful and can require treatment with incision and drainage.

Client History and Chart Review: Components of the History to Consider

- Gestational age
- Prior history of hemorrhoids
- Onset, duration, and severity of hemorrhoids
  - Presence of bleeding, pain, and itching
  - Self-help measures used and their efficacy
- Contributing factors
  - Toileting habits
  - Straining with defecation
  - Low-fiber diet
  - Constipation or diarrhea
  - Medications
    - Iron supplements
    - Stool softeners
    - Enemas

Physical Examination: Components of the Physical Exam to Consider

- Examination and palpation of the rectum for presence of hemorrhoids:
  - External
  - Internal
  - Strangulated
  - Thrombosed
- Anal lesions or masses
- Anal fissures

Clinical Impression: Differential Diagnoses to Consider

(ICD9data.com 2012)

- Hemorrhoids
- Anal fissures
- Anal trauma

- Anal herpes
- Anal fistula
- Rectal polyp
- Rectal malignancy

Diagnostic Testing: Diagnostic Tests and Procedures to Consider

- Stool for occult blood
- Anoscopy

Providing Treatment: Therapeutic Measures to Consider

- AnaMantle HC: topical anesthetic and steroid
  - Pregnancy Category C
  - Apply BID for 7 days
- Anusol-HC: topical steroid in a soothing cream
  - Pregnancy Category C
  - Apply two to four times daily as needed
- Desitin: astringent and protectant
  - Pregnancy Category C
  - Apply two to four times daily as needed
- Manual reduction of hemorrhoids
- Stool softeners as needed
- Ice packs PRN

Providing Treatment: Complementary and Alternative Measures to Consider

- Herbal remedies (Romm, 2010)
  - Bilberry tablets or capsules TID
  - Horse chestnut tea, tincture, or capsules
- Herbal or warm water sitz baths
- Topical applications
  - Witch hazel 10–50% compresses
  - Comfrey compresses
  - Epsom salt compresses
  - Plantain and yarrow ointment
  - Yellow dock root ointment
- Knee-chest position to promote drainage

Providing Support: Education and Support Measures to Consider

- Provide information on:
  - Physiologic basis
  - Increasing fiber and fluids in diet

- ▪ Topical medication use
- ▪ Signs and symptoms necessitating return for care
- Avoid
  - ▪ Straining with defecation
  - ▪ Prolonged sitting on toilet
  - ▪ Constipation (see the section "Care of the Pregnant Woman with Constipation")

Follow-up Care: Follow-up Measures to Consider

- Document
- Return for care
  - ▪ As scheduled for gestation
  - ▪ As soon as possible for thrombosed hemorrhoids

Multidisciplinary Practice: Consider Consultation or Referral

- OB/GYN or surgical services
  - ▪ Evaluation of severe, strangulated, or bleeding hemorrhoids
  - ▪ Blood in stool with no evidence of hemorrhoids or rectal fissure
  - ▪ For incision and drainage of thrombosed hemorrhoids
- For diagnosis or treatment outside the midwife's scope of practice

CARE OF THE PREGNANT WOMAN WITH INSOMNIA

Key Clinical Information

Insomnia is difficulty in initiating or maintaining sleep and can include delays in falling asleep, poor quality of sleep, frequent awakening, and early-morning wakefulness. Most women report alterations in their sleep patterns during pregnancy (Facco, Kramer, Ho, Zee, & Groban, 2010). Chronic or acute sleep deprivation can significantly impair the pregnant woman's ability to function and her body's ability to regenerate and recover from daily stressors. Starting labor with severe sleep deprivation can result in early maternal exhaustion and associated dysfunctional labor patterns. Mood changes can be a primary cause or a result of sleep deprivation (Hensley, 2009).

Client History and Chart Review: Components of the History to Consider

- Gestational age
- Onset, duration, and severity of symptoms
  - ▪ Difficulty falling asleep
  - ▪ Wakefulness
  - ▪ Fitful sleep
  - ▪ Interruptions
    - ◆ Nocturia
    - ◆ Pain or restless leg syndrome
    - ◆ Caretaking responsibilities
    - ◆ Partner/children sleep habits
    - ◆ Environmental noise or disruption
- Sleep habits
  - ▪ Sleep–wake patterns
    - ◆ Bedtime
    - ◆ Naps
  - ▪ Sleep partners
    - ◆ Intimate partner
    - ◆ Children
  - ▪ Total hours of sleep per 24 hours
- Social issues
  - ▪ Emotional response to sleep deprivation
  - ▪ Caffeine intake and timing
  - ▪ Meal patterns and content
  - ▪ Work hours
  - ▪ Anxieties and concerns
  - ▪ Help and support
- Current or prior history of depression or other mood disorders
- Other related symptoms

Physical Examination: Components of the Physical Exam to Consider

- Assess the client for the following conditions:
  - ▪ Nutrition and hydration status
  - ▪ Evidence of sleep deprivation
  - ▪ Physical causes of sleep deprivation
  - ▪ Mood disorders

Clinical Impression: Differential Diagnoses to Consider

(ICD9data.com, 2012)

- Insomnia, or secondary to the following:
  - Anxiety
  - Depression
  - Substance abuse
- Other sleep disorders

Diagnostic Testing: Diagnostic Tests and Procedures to Consider

- Insomnia: diagnosed by:
  - Self-report
  - Sleep studies
  - Other testing: as indicated by symptoms

Providing Treatment: Therapeutic Measures to Consider

- Use only when necessary
- For sleep (King & Brucker, 2011)
  - Ambien (Pregnancy Category B): 5–10 mg at bedtime
  - Ambien CR (Pregnancy Category C): 12.5 mg at bedtime
  - Lunesta (Pregnancy Category C): 2 mg at bedtime
  - Benadryl (Pregnancy Category B): 25–50 mg at bedtime
- For therapeutic sleep for false labor (see the "Care of the Woman with Prolonged Latent-Phase Labor" section)

Providing Treatment: Complementary and Alternative Measures to Consider

(Sarris & Byrne, 2011)

- Sleep hygiene
  - Same time to bed and arising in the morning
  - Avoid watching TV or discussing emotional issues in bed
  - Manage sleep environment
    - Darkened area
    - Sound dampened
    - Use of white noise (e.g., nature tapes, fan)

- Increase vitamin B intake
- L-Tryptophan
- Herbal remedies (Walls, 2009)
  - Chamomile tea
  - Valerian tincture or capsules 1 hour before bedtime
  - Hops tea or tincture (after 20 weeks' gestation)
  - Lemon balm tea
  - Skullcap tincture
  - Passion flower tea, tincture, or fluid extract TID
- Hydrotherapy
- Hypnotherapy
- Acupressure or acupuncture
- Yoga or tai chi
- Aromatherapy: add essential oils to warm bath water or diffuse in room air (England, 1994)
  - Lavender
  - Yling ylang
  - Geranium
- Massage of back, shoulders, and feet

Providing Support: Education and Support Measures to Consider

- Reassurance of normalcy
- Information related to the following topics:
  - Physiologic basis of insomnia
  - Other factors that may interfere with sleep
    - Stress
    - Work hours
    - Caretaking requirements
    - Small children
    - Elderly or ill parents/family
    - Sleep environment
    - Nighttime hunger
- Encourage a positive approach to this difficult problem
- Self-help measures
  - Nap during day to maintain rest
  - Warm bath before sleep
  - Warm milk or comfort foods
  - Massage

- Extra pillows for support
- Regular daily physical activity
- Adequate nutrition
- Limit fluids 2 hours before bedtime
- Avoid or minimize caffeine
- Reinforce abstinence from alcohol
- Stress management techniques
- Welcoming sleep environment

Follow-up Care: Follow-up Measures to Consider

- Document
- Return for care
  - As scheduled for gestation
  - Increased visits as needed:
    - ◆ Evaluation and monitoring of medication use
    - ◆ Emotional support

Multidisciplinary Practice: Consider Consultation or Referral

- Sleep disorder center
- OB/GYN services
  - Maternal exhaustion
- Mental health services
  - Depression
  - Anxiety
- Social services
- For diagnosis or treatment outside the midwife's scope of practice

CARE OF THE PREGNANT WOMAN WITH LEG CRAMPS

Key Clinical Information

Leg cramps are intermittent, painful muscle spasms of the lower leg muscles. A similar condition, known as restless leg syndrome, is characterized by unpleasant sensations in the lower leg ranging from twitching to burning to pain, accompanied by an urge to move the legs when at rest. Leg cramps are estimated to affect 30% to 45% of pregnant women, whereas restless leg syndrome is seen in 10% to 26% of pregnant women (Blackburn, 2007; Hensley, 2009). Leg cramps are a common occurrence during pregnancy and may interfere with a woman's ability to sleep. They are more common during the nighttime hours. Cramping may be related to an imbalance of calcium and magnesium, or it may reflect pressure of the enlarging uterus on pelvic blood vessels or on nerves supplying the lower leg. Other less common causes of leg cramps may be related to duration and type of physical activity, dehydration, and metabolic, vascular, or neurologic disorders.

Client History and Chart Review: Components of the History to Consider

(Hensley, 2009)

- Gestational age
- Onset, frequency, duration, and severity of cramps
  - Timing of cramps
  - Location; bilateral or unilateral pain
  - Precipitating factors
  - Self-help measures used and efficacy
  - Physical activity level
- Other associated symptoms
- History:
  - Back injury
  - Thyroid disease
  - Diabetes mellitus

Physical Examination: Components of the Physical Exam to Consider

(Hensley, 2009)

- Vital signs
- Evaluate foot arch
- Evaluate extremities
  - Color
  - Clonus
  - Muscle spasm
  - Varicosities
  - Calf circumference
  - Pulses

- Muscle strength
- Sensory integrity

Clinical Impression: Differential Diagnoses to Consider

(ICD9data.com, 2012)

- Physiologic leg cramps
- Varicose veins
- Restless leg syndrome
- Thrombophlebitis
- Deep vein thrombosis
- Muscle strain

Diagnostic Testing: Diagnostic Tests and Procedures to Consider

(Hensley, 2009)

- Serial calf measurements
- Venous ultrasound
- Clotting studies
- Serum ferritin

Providing Treatment: Therapeutic Measures to Consider

- Physical manipulation:
  - Dorsiflexion of foot during cramp
  - Hamstring and calf stretching prior to bedtime
- Magnesium supplement: 5 mmol in the morning, 10 mmol at night (King & Brucker, 2011)
- Sleep aids as needed
- Iron supplementation (Hensley, 2009)

Providing Treatment: Complementary and Alternative Measures to Consider

- Dietary sources of calcium and magnesium (see "A Nutritional Primer")
- Acupressure
  - Pressure to posterior mid-calf
- Herbal remedies
  - Raspberry leaf
  - Nettle
  - Dandelion

Providing Support: Education and Support Measures to Consider

- Reassurance of normalcy
- Provide information on
  - Physiologic nature of leg cramps in pregnancy
  - Increasing calcium and magnesium intake (Hensley, 2009)
  - Regular daily activity
    - Walking
    - Yoga
    - Swimming
  - Keep legs warm
- Warning signs
  - Increasing muscle spasms
  - Swelling, pain, or redness in leg

Follow-up Care: Follow-up Measures to Consider

- Document
- Return for care
  - As scheduled for gestation
  - For persistent leg pain or warning signs

Multidisciplinary Practice: Consider Consultation or Referral

- Medical services
  - For non-pregnancy-related cause of leg pain
  - Phlebitis
  - Thrombophlebitis
  - Deep vein thrombosis
- For diagnosis or treatment outside the midwife's scope of practice

CARE OF THE PREGNANT WOMAN WITH NAUSEA AND VOMITING

Key Clinical Information

Nausea is a subjective and unpleasant feeling associated with feeling ill and the urge to vomit. Vomiting is the expulsion of the stomach contents through the mouth as a result of involuntary muscle spasms. Nausea with or without vomiting is a common early-pregnancy symptom—one that is experienced to some degree by an estimated 70% to 85% of pregnant women (Bottomley & Bourne, 2009). Onset is typically at 6 to 8 weeks' gestation and resolution is most common at approximately 12 weeks' gestation, although symptoms can persist until 16 weeks' gestation or later (King & Brucker, 2011).

While nausea and vomiting are considered classic early-pregnancy symptoms, they can cause significant dehydration and contribute to poor nutrition. Approximately 35% of women who experience nausea and vomiting related to pregnancy experience lost time at work or a negative impact on family relationships (Niebyl, 2010). In a small minority of women, nausea and vomiting continue throughout the pregnancy or develop into hyperemesis gravidarum, a condition characterized by persistent nausea and vomiting associated with ketosis and weight loss of greater than 5% from prepregnancy weight (King & Brucker, 2011). For most women, conservative treatment with lifestyle changes and over-the-counter remedies provides adequate relief; however, women

with moderate to severe nausea and vomiting may require medication and intravenous hydration to obtain relief.

Client History and Chart Review: Components of the History to Consider

- Gestational age
- Assess onset, duration, and severity of nausea and vomiting (see Table 2-1)
  - Presence and frequency of vomiting
  - Symptoms of dehydration
  - Other associated symptoms, such as ptyalism
  - Self-help measures used and results
- Assess other factors:
  - Nutritional intake
  - Effect on activities of daily living (ADL)
  - Bowel and bladder patterns
- Past medical history
  - Thyroid disorders
  - Eating disorders
- Review of systems

Table 2-1   Pregnancy–Unique Quantification of Emesis (PUQE) Scale

1. In the last 12 hours, how many hours have you felt nauseated or sick to your stomach?

> 6 hours	4–6 hours	2–3 hours	≤ 1 hour	Not at all
(5 points)	(4 points)	(3 points)	(2 points)	(1 point)

2. In the last 12 hours, how many times have you vomited?

7 or more	5–6	3–4	1–2	None
(5 points)	(4 points)	(3 points)	(2 points)	(1 point)

3. In the last 12 hours, how many times have you had retching or dry heaves without bringing anything up?

7 or more	5–6	3–4	1–2	None
(5 points)	(4 points)	(3 points)	(2 points)	(1 point)

Total score is the sum of replies to each of the three questions.

Nausea score:

Mild NVP = ≤ 6

Moderate NVP = 7–12

Severe NVP ≥ 13

Source: Koren et al., 2005.

Physical Examination: Components of the Physical Exam to Consider

- Vital signs
- Interval weight gain or loss
- Usual prenatal evaluation, including examination of the following factors:
  - Overall appearance
    - Weight loss
    - Skin turgor, heart rate, and other signs of dehydration
    - Self-care and hygiene
  - Abdominal examination

Clinical Impression: Differential Diagnoses to Consider

(ICD9data.com, 2012)

- Physiologic nausea and vomiting of pregnancy
- Also consider:
  - Hyperemesis gravidarum
  - Hydatidiform mole
  - Ectopic implantation
- Mental health conditions
  - Bulimia
  - Anxiety
  - Depression
- Other medical conditions
  - Gallbladder disease
  - Pyelonephritis
  - Gastroenteritis
  - Hyperthyroidism

Diagnostic Testing: Diagnostic Tests and Procedures to Consider

- Urine dipstick for ketones and glucose
- Urinalysis
- Blood urea nitrogen, creatinine, serum ketones, and electrolytes
- Thyroid evaluation: thyroid-stimulating hormone, T_3, and T_4
- Liver function testing
- CBC or white blood cell count
- Pelvic ultrasound
- Ultrasound of the gallbladder
- *H. pylori* testing

Providing Treatment: Therapeutic Measures to Consider

(King & Brucker, 2011)

- Treat conservatively, progressing as indicated by symptoms (Table 2-2)
- Vitamin B_6 (pyridoxine)
  - 10–25 mg PO TID
  - If no relief, add doxylamine succinate (Unisom) 12.5 mg (½ tablet) PO QID or after meals only
- Ginger
  - At least 1 g total daily, in divided doses
  - 250 mg QID in capsule form
  - 1 tsp grated fresh rhizome
  - 2 mL liquid extract
  - 2-in. piece of crystallized ginger, 0.25 mg thick
  - 8 oz ginger ale (real ginger)
- Initiate medications if relief not obtained from conservative measures or symptoms warrant
- IV hydration when indicated
  - Hydration alone may resolve symptoms
  - NS is the fluid of choice to correct hyponatremia
  - 500 mL bolus to start
  - Thiamine 100 mg to first liter of IV fluid (Cunningham, Levano, Bloom, Hauth, Rouse, & Spong, 2010)
  - Titrate to maintain urinary specific gravity within the normal range

Providing Treatment: Complementary and Alternative Measures to Consider

- Peppermint tea
- Foods rich in B vitamins
  - Wheat germ
  - Molasses
  - Brewer's yeast
- Acupressure at Neiguan P6 point via wristbands
- Acupuncture
- Hypnosis

Table 2-2 Common Medicinal Treatments for Nausea and Vomiting in Pregnancy

AGENT GENERIC (BRAND)	ORAL DOSE	SIDE EFFECTS	FDA PREGNANCY CATEGORY	COMMENTS
Pyridoxine (vitamin B$_6$)	10–25 mg q 8 h		A	Vitamin B$_6$ alone or B$_6$–antihistamine combination advised as first-line treatment.
Vitamin B6–doxylamine (Unisom SleepTabs) combination	Pyridoxine10–25 mg q 8 h, doxylamine 25 mg at bedtime, 12.5 mg in the A.M. PRN, and 12.5 mg in the afternoon PRN	Sedation	A	Available over the counter (OTC)
Ginger (considered a food supplement)	At least 1 g daily in divided doses	Reflux, heartburn		Wide variety of forms available. Generally recognized as safe in pregnancy. Available OTC.
Antihistamines				
Doxylamine (Unisom SleepTabs)	12.5–25 mg PO q 8 h or 25 mg in P.M. PO	Sedation	A	
Diphenhydramine (Benadryl)	25–50 mg q 8h	Sedation	B	
Diphenhydrinate (Dramamine)	50–100 mg PO q 4–6 h	Sedation	B	
Hydroyzibe (Atarax, Vistaril)	50 mg q 4–6 h	Sedation	B	
Meclazine (Antivert, Bonine)	25 mg q 6 h	Sedation	B	
Phenothiazines				
Prochlorperazine (Compazine)	5–10 mg q 4–6 h	Anticholinergic effects, dry mouth, dystonic reaction	C	Also available as buccal tablet.
Promethazine (Phenergan)	12.5–25 mg q 4–6 h	Sedation, anticholinergic effects, dry mouth, extrapyramidal symptoms	C	Severe tissue injury with IV use. Black box warning.
Benzamides				
Metoclopramide (Reglan)	5–10 mg q 8 h	Extrapyramidal symptoms, agitation, anxiety, acute dystonic reaction	B	Tardive dyskinesia. Black box warning.
Serotonin Antagonists				
Ondansetron (Zofran)	4–8 mg q 6 h	Headache, diarrhea, constipation, fatigue	B	Available in orally dissolving tablet.

(continues)

Table 2-2   Common Medicinal Treatments for Nausea and Vomiting in Pregnancy (continued)

AGENT GENERIC (BRAND)	ORAL DOSE	SIDE EFFECTS	FDA PREGNANCY CATEGORY	COMMENTS
Butyophenones				
Droperidol (Inapsine)	1.25–2.5 mg IM or IV only	Extrapyramidal symptoms, prolonged QT syndrome	C	Reserved for those patients who do not obtain relief with other regimens. To be used only following medical consultation and if other medications have failed to resolve symptoms, secondary to risk for prolonged QT syndrome. Black box warning.
Glucocorticoids				
Methylprednisolone (Medrol)	16 mg q 8 h for 3 days, then taper down over 2 weeks	Small increased risk of cleft lip if used prior to 10 weeks' gestation	C	Avoid use before 10 weeks' gestation.

Source: Adapted from King & Brucker, 2011; Niebyl, 2010.

Providing Support: Education and Support Measures to Consider

- All women with nausea and/or vomiting should be encouraged to to take the following steps:
  - Take prenatal vitamins at night or discontinue until symptoms resolve
  - Eat small amounts of bland, dry, high-protein foods every 2 hours
  - Increase intake of protein and complex carbohydrates
  - Limit dietary fat
  - Drink cold, clear, carbonated, flat, or sour fluids between meals
  - Avoid dehydration
  - Increase sleep, rest, and fresh air
  - Avoid brushing teeth soon after meals
  - Avoid triggers such as strong odors, fatigue, heat, and stuffy rooms

- Advise family of need for support
- Provide reassurance that symptoms resolve around 12 to 16 weeks' gestation for most women
- Review when to call
  - ADL become significantly affected
  - Unable to keep down food or fluids for more than 12 hours
  - Signs and symptoms of dehydration
  - Abdominal pain
  - Weakness, lethargy, or confusion

Follow-up Care: Follow-up Measures to Consider

- Document
- Return for care
  - As scheduled for gestation
  - As needed for worsening symptoms
  - Recommend hospital care for IV rehydration as needed

Multidisciplinary Practice: Consider Consultation or Referral

- Acupuncture therapy
- Hypnosis therapy
- OB/GYN services
  - Hyperemesis
  - Dehydration
- For diagnosis or treatment outside the midwife's scope of practice

CARE OF THE PREGNANT WOMAN WITH PICA

Key Clinical Information

Pica is defined as the craving and purposeful consumption of nonfood items for more than one month. Earth (geophagy), raw starches (amylophagy), and ice (pagophagy) are the most commonly reported pica substances in the United States (Young, 2010). Pica may be accepted in some cultures and subcultures; for example, clay eating and starch eating are seen in the United States in some southern, rural, African American communities, primarily among women and children (Ellis & Schnoes, 2006). The prevalence of this practice is not known because pica is often undisclosed, unrecognized, and underreported. The nature and amount of ingested substances determine the health consequences of this behavior.

Client History and Chart Review: Components of the History to Consider

(Ellis & Schnoes, 2006)

- Gestational age
- Identify
  - Nonfood substances craved or consumed
  - Cultural or ethnic expressions of pica
  - Social issues that may contribute to pica
    - Inadequate diet
    - Cultural expectations
- Evaluate
  - Client's diet and nutritional resources
  - Use of vitamin and mineral supplements
  - Previous hematocrit and hemoglobin
  - Prior history of anemia or nutritional deficiencies

Physical Examination: Components of the Physical Exam to Consider

- Vital signs
- Interval weight gain or loss
- Assess nutritional status
- Evaluate for symptoms of anemia
  - Color of mucous membranes
  - Capillary refill
  - Orthostatic hypotension
  - Elevated heart rate

Clinical Impression: Differential Diagnoses to Consider

(ICD9data.com, 2012)

- Pica
- Anemia
- Lead toxicity

Diagnostic Testing: Diagnostic Tests and Procedures to Consider

- Hematocrit and hemoglobin
- Lead screening
- Anemia workup (see the "Care of the Pregnant Woman with Anemia" section)

Providing Treatment: Therapeutic Measures to Consider

- Iron replacement therapy if anemia is present
- Multivitamin and mineral supplements

Providing Treatment: Complementary and Alternative Measures to Consider

- Iron-rich foods (see "A Nutritional Primer")
- Sea vegetables high in iron and trace minerals, such as kelp, nori, and wakame
- Red raspberry leaf tea
- Yellow dock

Providing Support: Education and Support Measures to Consider

- Explore concerns about pica with the client
  - Pica may interfere with good nutrition
  - Provide or arrange for nutritional education
  - Encourage client to avoid nonfood items
- Try offering substitute items
  - Laundry starch, ice: frozen fruit pops
  - Clay: food-grade seaweed
  - Other acceptable nutritional items

Follow-up Care: Follow-up Measures to Consider

- Document
- Return for care
  - As scheduled for gestation
  - Follow-up laboratory values as indicated
  - Inquire about continued pica practices

Multidisciplinary Practice: Consider Consultation or Referral

- Diet counseling
- Social services
  - Women, Infants, and Children (WIC) program
  - Food stamps
  - Food bank
- OB/GYN or medical services
  - For severe pica accompanied by anemia
  - For elevated lead levels
- For diagnosis or treatment outside the midwife's scope of practice

CARE OF THE PREGNANT WOMAN WITH ROUND LIGAMENT PAIN

Key Clinical Information

Round ligament pain is an unpleasant sensation that ranges from sharp knifelike pain to dull intermittent pain in the lower abdominal and inguinal areas of the pregnant woman. It is believed that virtually all pregnant women will experience this pain at some point in their pregnancy, so education and reassurance are important (Varney et al., 2004). Round ligament pain may be a frequent occurrence between 16 and 20 weeks' gestation. It may mimic, or mask, uncommon yet more serious conditions, such as appendicitis or ovarian torsion. Round ligament pain can cause significant distress, especially in the athletic woman who continues to jog or in women who have highly physical jobs. An objective pain scale is recommended to assess and document the client's pain level.

Client History and Chart Review: Components of the History to Consider

- Gestational age
- Evaluation of the pain
  - Onset, location, severity, and duration
  - Quality of the pain
    - Intermittent or constant
    - Sharp or dull
    - Exacerbating factors
  - Associated symptoms
    - Cramping
    - Backache
    - Nausea and vomiting
    - Change in bowel or bladder function
- Relief measures used and efficacy
- Activities of daily living
  - Employment activities
  - Lifestyle activities
  - Limitations secondary to pain

Physical Examination: Components of the Physical Exam to Consider

- Vital signs
- Verify location of pain; observe and palpate the area
- Note posture and overall appearance
- Abdominal examination
  - Palpate for tenderness
    - Guarding
    - Rebound pain
    - Referred pain
  - Uterine examination
    - Fundal height
    - Fetal heart rate

- ◆ Presence of contractions
- ◆ Consistency and position of uterus
- Pelvic examination as indicated
  - ▪ Cervical or vaginal discharge
  - ▪ Dilation and/or effacement
- Evaluate for CVA tenderness

Clinical Impression: Differential Diagnoses to Consider

(ICD9data.com, 2012)

- Round ligament pain
- Also consider:
  - ▪ Urinary tract infection
  - ▪ Ectopic pregnancy
  - ▪ Preterm labor
  - ▪ Placental abruption
  - ▪ Acute abdomen secondary to the following conditions:
    - ◆ Ovarian torsion
    - ◆ Renal calculi
    - ◆ Pyelonephritis
    - ◆ Appendicitis
    - ◆ Gallbladder disease
    - ◆ Pelvic inflammatory disease

Diagnostic Testing: Diagnostic Tests and Procedures to Consider

- Urinalysis
- CBC, with differential
- Ultrasound evaluation
  - ▪ Pelvis
    - ◆ Uterus, ovaries, and tubes
    - ◆ Appendix
  - ▪ Abdomen
    - ◆ Kidneys, ureters, and bladder
    - ◆ Gallbladder

Providing Treatment: Therapeutic Measures to Consider

- Maternity abdominal support or girdle
- Pain relief (King & Brucker, 2011): acetaminophen

Providing Treatment: Complementary and Alternative Measures to Consider

- Muscle strengthening and stretching
  - ▪ Yoga
  - ▪ Swimming
  - ▪ Prenatal exercise class
- Reflexology to waist and pelvic points
- Herbal remedies
  - ▪ Red raspberry leaf tea
  - ▪ Massage with arnica-infused massage oil

Providing Support: Education and Support Measures to Consider

- Reassurance of normalcy
- Provide information on cause of round ligament pain
- Self-help measures
  - ▪ Pelvic tilt
  - ▪ Arise slowly from bed
  - ▪ Warm baths
  - ▪ Applying gentle heat to area
  - ▪ Positioning
    - ◆ Knees to abdomen
    - ◆ Bending toward pain to ease ligament tension
    - ◆ Side-lying with pillow under abdomen
  - ▪ Limit lifting and twisting
  - ▪ Ask for help as needed
- Warning signs
  - ▪ Onset of contractions
  - ▪ Persistent abdominal pain
  - ▪ Fever
  - ▪ Onset of nausea and vomiting
  - ▪ Vaginal bleeding or discharge
  - ▪ Pain with intercourse or bowel movement

Follow-up Care: Follow-up Measures to Consider

- Document
- Return for care
  - ▪ As scheduled for gestation
  - ▪ As indicated by test results
  - ▪ With onset of warning signs

Multidisciplinary Practice: Consider Consultation or Referral

- Physical therapy for movement evaluation
- OB/GYN services
  - Abdominal pain inconsistent with round ligament pain
  - Abnormal test results
- For diagnosis or treatment outside the midwife's scope of practice

CARE OF THE PREGNANT WOMAN WITH VARICOSE VEINS

Key Clinical Information

Varicose veins are distended veins that experience abnormal collections of blood caused by weak venous walls or improperly functioning venous valves. Varicosities develop in approximately 40% of pregnant women (Blackburn, 2007). Itching, swelling, or pain can accompany varicose veins, and they generally worsen as the pregnancy progresses and with each subsequent pregnancy. Care must be taken to avoid trauma to these vessels, as it may result in hematoma formation, superficial phlebitis, or thrombophlebitis. Frequent rest periods with the feet elevated higher than the heart are essential for women with varicose veins. High-quality support hose are helpful in easing the discomfort of significant lower-limb varicosities. For women with vulvar varicosities, snug-fitting panties, bicycle shorts, or a girdle may be needed to provide counterpressure.

Client History and Chart Review: Components of the History to Consider

- Gestational age
- Onset and location of varicose veins
  - Changes with pregnancy
  - Associated symptoms
    - Pain
    - Edema
    - Redness or discoloration
    - Other symptoms
  - Current relief measures and their effects

- Use of medications
  - Aspirin
  - Nonsteroidal anti-inflammatory drugs
- Past medical history
  - Varicose veins
  - Superficial phlebitis
  - Thrombophlebitis
- Activities of daily living
  - Employment activities
  - Recent immobility

Physical Examination: Components of the Physical Exam to Consider

- Examination of varicosities
  - Location(s)
  - Number
  - Size
  - Severity
- Serial calf measurements
- Evaluate for symptoms of other conditions:
  - Superficial phlebitis
    - Heat
    - Redness or discoloration
    - Tenderness
  - Deep vein thrombosis
    - Pain
    - Positive Homans' sign (low specificity)
    - Leg edema

Clinical Impression: Differential Diagnoses to Consider

(ICD9data.com, 2012)

- Varicose veins
- Superficial phlebitis
- Deep vein thrombosis

Diagnostic Testing: Diagnostic Tests and Procedures to Consider

- Serial calf measurements
- Testing for bleeding or clotting disorders
  - Coagulations factors
  - Superficial phlebitis

- D-Dimer
- PTT, PTT
- Ulrasound as indicated to evaluate for deep vein thrombosis

Providing Treatment: Therapeutic Measures to Consider

- Support garments
  - Compression hosiery
    - Apply after elevating the legs for 10 minutes
    - Wear daily
  - Foam pad to support vulvar varicosities: use with close-fitting but nonconstricting undergarment
  - Maternity abdominal support to relieve pressure on pelvic veins
- Thromboprophylaxis: women with a history of thrombosis or thrombophilia may be candidates for prophylactic treatment with low-dose anticoagulants in pregnancy (ACOG, 2010b)
- For symptoms of early superficial phlebitis: consider use of a broad-spectrum antibiotic, such as Keflex

Providing Treatment: Complementary and Alternative Measures to Consider

- Increase intake of onions and garlic in the diet
- Herbal remedies (Romm, 2010)
  - Bilberry tablets or capsules TID
    - Strengthen capillaries
    - Reduce platelet aggregation
  - Horse chestnut tea, tincture, or capsule
- Positioning
  - Leg elevation above the heart
  - Leg inversion (right-angle position)

Providing Support: Education and Support Measures to Consider

- Provide information regarding the physiologic basis of varicose veins

- Encourage:
  - Use and application of support hose
  - Rest with legs elevated
  - Regular mild exercise, especially walking or swimming
- Avoidance of the following:
  - Constrictive clothing
  - Long periods of standing or sitting
  - Crossing legs while sitting
  - Leg massage
- Medication instructions
- Warning signs
  - Persistent or worsening pain
  - Unilateral edema of extremity
  - Localized redness, heat, or tenderness
  - Fever

Follow-up Care: Follow-up Measures to Consider

- Document
- Return for care
  - As scheduled for gestation
  - Onset of warning signs
  - Four to seven days for suspected early superficial phlebitis
  - Evaluate closely in the early postpartum period

Multidisciplinary Practice: Consider Consultation or Referral

- OB/GYN services
  - For candidates for thromboprophylaxis
  - Severe vulvar varicosities
  - Suspected or confirmed
    - Phlebitis
    - Thrombophlebitis
- For diagnosis or treatment outside the midwife's scope of practice

WEB RESOURCES FOR CLINICIANS

RESOURCE	URL
The rights of childbearing women	http://www.childbirthconnection.org/article.asp?ck=10084
Pregnant women who need a flu shot (CDC)	http://www.cdc.gov/flu/pdf/freeresources/pregnant/flushot_pregnant_Factsheet.pdf
Centering Pregnancy© group prenatal care	http://www.centeringhealthcare.org/pages/centering-model/pregnancy-overview.php
"Smoking Cessation During Pregnancy: A Clinician's Guide to Helping Women Quit Smoking" (ACOG)	http://www.acog.org/departments/healthIssues/scdp/files/scdp.pdf
"Motivational Interviewing: A Tool for Behavior Change" (ACOG)	http://mail.ny.acog.org/website/SMIPodcast/MotivationalInterview.pdf
"Preventing Preterm Birth: The Role of 17α-Hydroxyprogesterone Caproate" (ACOG)	http://mail.ny.acog.org/website/17PResourceGuide.pdf

REFERENCES

American College of Nurse–Midwives (ACNM). (2004). *Evidence-based home birth practice: Home birth practice handbook* (2nd ed.). Silver Springs, MD: Author.

American College of Obstetricians and Gynecologists (ACOG). (2008). Preventing preterm birth: The role of 17α hydroxyprogesterone caproate. Retrieved from http://mail.ny.acog.org/website/17PResourceGuide.pdf

American College of Obstetricians and Gynecologists (ACOG). (2010a). Committee opinion number 471: Smoking cessation during pregnancy. *Obstetrics & Gynecology, 166,* 1241–1244.

American College of Obstetricians and Gynecologists (ACOG). (2010b). Practice bulletin number 124: Inherited thrombophelias in pregnancy. *Obstetrics & Gynecology, 118*(3), 730–740.

Arnesen, S. (2006). Environmental health information resources: Healthy environments for healthy women and children. *Journal of Midwifery & Women's Health, 51,* 35–38.

Blackburn, S. (2007). *Maternal, fetal and neonatal physiology: A clinical perspective.* Philadelphia, PA: Saunders.

Bottomley, C., & Bourne, T. (2009). Management strategies for hyperemesis. *Best Practice & Research: Clinical Obstetrics & Gynaecology, 23*(4), 549–564.

Centers for Disease Control and Prevention (CDC). (2010a). 2010 guidelines for the prevention of perinatal group B streptococcal disease. Retrieved from http://www.cdc.gov/groupbstrep/guidelines/guidelines.html

Centers for Disease Control and Prevention (CDC). (2010b). Prevention and control of influenza with vaccines: Recommendations of the Advisory Committee on Influenza Practices, 2010. Retrieved from http://www.cdc.gov/mmwr/preview/mmwrhtml/rr5908a1.htm

Cunningham, C., Levano, K., Bloom, S., Hauth, J., Rouse, D., & Spong, C. (2010). *Williams obstetrics* (23rd ed.). New York, NY: McGraw-Hill.

Davis, E. (2004). *Hearts and hands: A midwife's guide to pregnancy and birth* (4th ed.). Berkeley, CA: Celestial Arts.

Dowswell, T., & Neilson, J. (2008). Interventions for heartburn in pregnancy. *Cochrane Database Systematic Review, 4,* CD007065.

Ellis, C. R., & Schnoes, C. J. (2006). Eating disorder: Pica. Retrieved from http://www.emedicine.com/PED/topic1798.htm

England, A. (1994). *Aromatherapy for mother and baby.* Rochester, VT: Healing Arts Press.

Facco, F., Kramer, J., Ho, K., Zee, P., & Groban, W. (2010). Sleep disturbances in pregnancy. *Obstetrics & Gynecology, 115*(1), 77–83.

Frye, A. (2007). *Understanding diagnostic tests in the childbearing year* (7th ed.). Portland, OR: Labrys Press.

Gojnic, M., Dugalic, V., Papic, M., Vidakovic, S., Milicevic, S., & Perulov, M. (2005). The significance of detailed examination of hemorrhoids during pregnancy. *Clinical Obstetrics & Gynecology, 32,* 183–184.

Hensley, J. G. (2009). Leg cramps and restless legs syndrome during pregnancy. *Journal of Midwifery & Women's Health, 54*(3), 211–218.

ICD9.com. (2012). The web's free 2012 medical coding reference. Retrieved from www.ICD9data.com.

Ickovics, J., Kershaw, T., Westdhal, C., Magriples, U., Massey, Z., Reynolds, H., & Schindler-Rising, S. (2007). Group prenatal care and perinatal outcomes. *Obstetrics & Gynecology, 110*, 330–339.

Institute for Clinical Systems Improvement (ICSI). (2006). *Routine prenatal care.* Bloomington, MN: Author. Retrieved from http://www.icsi.org/home/

Institute of Medicine (IOM). (2009). *Weight gain during pregnancy: Reexamining the guidelines.* Washington, DC: National Academies Press.

Janssen, P., Saxell, L., Page, L., Klein, M., Liston, R., & Lee, S. (2009). Outcomes of planned home birth with registered midwife versus planned hospital birth with midwife or physician. *Canadian Medical Association Journal, 181.* doi: 10.1503/cmaj.081869

Johnson, K., & Davis, B. A. (2005). Outcomes of planned home birth with certified professional midwives: Large prospective study in North America. *British Medical Journal, 330.* doi: 10.1136/bmj.3307575.1416

Jordan, R. (2010). Prenatal omega-3 fatty acids: Review and recommendations. *Journal of Midwifery & Women's Health, 55*(6), 520–528.

King, T., & Brucker, M. (2011). *Pharmacology for women's health.* Sudbury, MA: Jones & Bartlett Learning.

Koren, G., Piwko, C., Ahn, E., Boskovic, R., Maltepe, C., Einarson, A., . . . Unger, W. (2005). Validation studies of the Pregnancy–Unique Quantification of Emesis (PUQE) scores. *Journal of Obstetrics & Gynecology, 25*(3), 241–244.

March of Dimes (MOD). (2010). Caffeine in pregnancy. Retrieved from http://www.marchofdimes.com/pregnancy/nutrition_caffeine.html

Nakhai-Pour, H., Broy, P., Sheehy, O., & Berard, A. (2011). Use of nonaspirin nonsteroidal anti-inflammatory drugs during pregnancy and the risk of spontaneous abortion. *Canadian Medical Association Journal.* doi: 10.1503/cmaj.110454

Niebyl, J. (2010). Nausea and vomiting in pregnancy. *New England Journal of Medicine, 363*(16), 1544–1550.

Pennick, V. E., & Young, G. (2007). Interventions for preventing and treating pelvic and back pain in pregnancy. *Cochrane Database Systematic Review,* CD001139.

Romm, A. (2010). *Botanical medicine for women's health.* St. Louis, MO: Churchill Livingstone.

Rubak, S., Sandbaek, A., Lauritzen, T., & Christensen, B. (2005). Motivational interviewing: A systematic review and meta-analysis. *British Journal of General Practice, 55*, 305–312.

Sarris, J., & Byrne, G. (2011). A systematic review of insomnia and complementary medicine. *Sleep Medicine Reviews, 15*, 99–106. doi: 101016/j.smrv2010.04.001

Varney, H., Kriebs, J. M., & Gegor, C. L. (2004). *Varney's midwifery* (4th ed.). Sudbury, MA: Jones and Bartlett.

Walker, D., Day, S., Lirette, H., Mooney-Hescott, C., McCully, L., & Vest, V. (2002). Reduced frequency prenatal visit schedules in midwifery practice: Attitudes and use. *Journal of Midwifery & Women's Health, 47*(4), 269–277.

Walls, D. (2009). Herbs and natural therapies for pregnancy, birth and breastfeeding. *International Journal of Childbirth Education, 24*(2), 28–37.

Young, S. (2010). Pica in pregnancy: New ideas about an old condition. *Annual Review of Nutrition, 30*, 403–422.

CHAPTER 3

Care of the Pregnant Woman with Prenatal Variations

Midwives support women with pregnancy complications and variations through prompt identification and initiation of treatment for these concerns to ensure the best possible outcome for mother and baby. The ability to anticipate problems in pregnancy is an essential component of skilled midwifery practice. Midwives must be steadfast in their belief that pregnancy is a normal physiologic condition while retaining a healthy respect for problems and complications that can develop. During evaluation of potential or developing problems, the midwife actively engages the mother in decision making regarding the options for care of herself and her unborn baby.

Among the Hallmarks of Midwifery Care are advocacy for informed choice, shared decision making, and the right to self-determination (American College of Nurse–Midwives, 2007). Although the mother may have limited or no control over the development of problems during her pregnancy and may feel threatened when they arise, the midwife can enhance the mother's sense of control by presenting options in the areas where client choice is possible. Respect for each woman's needs is especially important when an unexpected problem develops.

Many women look to their midwife to present a balanced view of developing problems, the diagnostic evaluation process, and treatment options. Although many women choose to be active participants in all of their healthcare decisions, the expectation is that the midwife will clearly identify a recommended course of action. Recommendations are based on the midwife's judgment of what constitutes best care for the mother and the fetus in light of the presenting problem. Occasionally, the midwife's recommendations may run contrary to either the mother's preferences or standard hospital-based expectations for obstetric care. A clear, focused, and confidently presented midwifery plan of care, accompanied by a rationale backed by evidence-based resources, can be helpful in providing guidance to the client who hesitates at the indicated obstetric intervention, or in promoting understanding among providers in the medical setting where the midwife may feel pressured to intervene without a clear indication.

Midwifery care of problems during pregnancy forms a continuum from least intervention to most intervention. The skilled midwife can move along this continuum in either direction, understanding that appropriate medical or obstetric intervention in the presence of complication should always serve the mother's and baby's needs and is congruent with midwifery philosophy.

CARE OF THE PREGNANT WOMAN WITH ABDOMINAL PAIN

Key Clinical Information

Many women will experience self-limited periods of abdominal pain due to the normal physiologic changes during pregnancy. Normal etiologies of abdominal pain in pregnancy include round ligament pain, constipation, and heartburn. Medical complications such as appendicitis and cholecystitis can prove challenging to diagnose during pregnancy because symptoms of these conditions can mimic normal pregnancy discomforts. During pregnancy, the approximate incidences of appendicitis and cholecystitis are each 1 in 1000 women (Cunningham, Levano, Bloom, Hauth, Rouse, & Spong, 2010). Timing of abdominal pain in relation to gestational age provides key information to diagnose trimester-specific conditions such as ectopic pregnancy. A detailed history and exam are essential to narrow down the various differential diagnoses of abdominal pain in pregnancy. Abdominal pain associated with vaginal bleeding is addressed in a separate section later in this chapter.

Client History and Chart Review: Components of the History to Consider

- Age, GP TPAL
- Gestational age
- Review of prior ultrasound findings
- Location
  - Lower abdomen
  - Upper abdomen
  - Radiating to back: Cholecystitis
- Onset and duration

- Diet history
  - Timing of pain in relation to meals
  - Consider cholecystitis if pain occurs after fatty meals
- Characteristics
  - Sharp, dull
  - Constant, colicky
  - Severe, mild
- Associated symptoms
  - Nausea and vomiting
  - Constipation
  - Diarrhea
  - Syncope
  - Vaginal bleeding
  - Visual changes
  - Dysuria
  - Urinary urgency
  - Abdominal itching
  - Dark urine
  - Light-colored stools
  - Fatigue
- History of pica
- Bowel activity
- Relieving and exacerbating factors
- Recent trauma

Physical Examination: Components of the Physical Exam to Consider

- Vital signs, including pulse, temperature, and blood pressure (BP)
- Pain scale rating
- Diaphoresis
- Presence of jaundice
- Murphy's sign
  - Palpation of costal margin
  - RUQ pain with inhalation
  - Gasp or breath "catching": positive result
  - Indicative of gallbladder disease
- Abdominal exam
  - Presence of rigidity
  - Pain location
  - Assess rebound tenderness and muscle guarding
  - Bowel sounds

- McBurney's point assessment: Appendix moves progressively closer to gallbladder as gestation progresses
- Pelvic exam
  - Speculum exam
  - Look for products of conception in first trimester
- Suprapubic tenderness

Clinical Impression: Differential Diagnoses to Consider (ICD9Data.com, 2012)

- Abdominal pain
- Acute cholecystitis
- Cholecystitis: unspecified
- Cholelithiasis
- Appendicitis
- Peptic ulcer
- Acute cystitis
- Spontaneous abortion
- Ectopic pregnancy

Diagnostic Testing: Diagnostic Tests and Procedures to Consider

- 📞 Ultrasound
  - Uterus
  - Abdomen
  - Gallbladder
- Quantitative HCG
- Urinalysis and culture
- 24-hour urine collection if HELLP is suspected
- CBC: WBC elevation
- Liver enzyme panel
- Serum amylase and lipase
- Non-stress test (NST)
- Possible endoscopy or laparoscopy

Providing Treatment: Therapeutic Measures to Consider

- 📞 For pathologic diagnoses:
  - Analgesia
  - Intravenous fluids
  - Surgery

- See the following sections:
  - "Care of the Pregnant Woman with Vaginal Bleeding, First Trimester"
  - "Care of the Pregnant Woman with Vaginal Bleeding, Second and Third Trimesters"
  - "Care of the Pregnant Woman with Constipation"
  - "Care of the Pregnant Woman with Preterm Labor"
- For less severe or physiologically normal diagnoses, see the following sections:
  - "Care of the Pregnant Woman with Round Ligament Pain"
  - "Care of the Pregnant Woman with Heartburn"
  - "Care of the Pregnant Woman with Constipation"

Providing Treatment: Complementary and Alternative Measures to Consider

- According to diagnosis
- For mild cholelithiasis
  - Low-fat diet
  - Fiber-rich foods
  - Cleanse the gallbladder
    - Oatmeal, pears, beets, artichoke, dandelion greens, flax seed and meal
    - Milk thistle herb capsules
    - Olive oil and lemon juice flush

Providing Support: Education and Support Measures to Consider

- Reassurance of normalcy if physiologically-normal diagnoses
- As required for normal diagnosis
- Supportive presence if surgical intervention is needed
  - Surgery may be delayed until after pregnancy, such as in mild cholelithiasis
  - Surgery may be done regardless of pregnancy, such as in appendicitis

Follow-up Care: Follow-up Measures to Consider

- Document
- As required for normal diagnoses

Multidisciplinary Practice: Consider Consultation, Collaboration, or Referral

- Medical consult for the following conditions:
  - Significantly elevated WBC
  - Suspected problem requiring surgical intervention
  - Emergent situation
  - Diagnostic uncertainty
- For diagnosis or treatment outside the midwife's scope of practice

CARE OF THE PREGNANT WOMAN WITH ANEMIA

Key Clinical Information

Iron-deficiency anemia due to dietary deficiencies is the most common form of anemia in pregnant women. In developed countries, 20% of pregnant women have iron-deficiency anemia, whereas in developing countries more than half of pregnant women have this disorder (Rioux & LeBlanc, 2007). Anemia affects the oxygenation of both mother and fetus and can result in diminished fetal growth, maternal exhaustion, increased susceptibility to infection, and related complications, such as prematurity (Centers for Disease Control and Prevention [CDC], 2011b). Prompt diagnosis, treatment, and follow-up of anemia, along with attention to the overall nutritional status of the mother, are critically important for ensuring fetal well-being and for optimizing maternal health before the onset of labor.

Client History and Chart Review: Components of the History to Consider

- Age, GP TPAL
- Gestational age
- Interconceptional spacing
- Current hematocrit and hemoglobin
- Potential causes of anemia
  - Tobacco use
  - History of closely spaced pregnancies
  - Blood loss, heavy menses

- Chronic illness
- Malabsorption syndromes
  - Hookworms
  - Bariatric surgery
- Living in higher altitudes
- Malignancy
- Higher risk for thalassemia or sickle cell
  - African descent
  - Mediterranean descent
  - Asian descent
- Presence of anemia-related symptoms
  - Fatigue
  - Dizziness
  - Headache
  - Sore tongue
  - Pica (eating nonfood items such as starch or clay, or chewing ice)
  - Dyspnea
  - Palpitations or tachycardia
- Usual dietary patterns
  - General nutrition
  - Dietary iron sources
    - Prenatal vitamin use
    - Most have 30 mg elemental iron
    - Iron supplement use
- Use of over-the-counter (OTC) medications
  - Antacids and calcium supplements reduce iron absorption in the gut

Physical Examination: Components of the Physical Exam to Consider

- Vital signs, including pulse and blood pressure (BP)
- Affect and energy level
- Glossitis
- Pallor of skin and mucous membranes
  - Inspect oral mucosa
  - Inspect conjunctival mucosa
- Brittle nails
- Examination for potential causes of anemia
  - Bruising
  - Bleeding

Clinical Impression: Differential Diagnoses to Consider (ICD9Data.com, 2012)

- Physiologic anemia of pregnancy
- Iron-deficiency anemia
- Other anemia
  - Pernicious
  - Hemolytic
  - Sickle cell
  - Thalassemia

Diagnostic Testing: Diagnostic Tests and Procedures to Consider

- Complete blood count (CBC) with indices in simple iron-deficiency anemia:
  - Microcytic
  - Hypochromic
  - Serum ferritin: decreased
  - Total iron binding capacity: increased
- Stool for occult blood, ova, and parasites
- See Table 3-1 for criteria for diagnosing anemia in pregnancy.

Providing Treatment: Therapeutic Measures to Consider

- Iron replacement therapy for hemoglobin less than 11 g/dL or low serum ferritin (King & Brucker, 2011; Rioux & LeBlanc, 2007; University of Maryland Medical Center, 2007)
  - 60–120 mg elemental iron daily
  - Iron salts:
    - Ferrous sulfate (Feosol, Slow Fe)
      - 65 mg elemental iron
      - 1 PO TID
    - Ferrous gluconate (Fergon, Fertinic)
      - 27 mg elemental iron
      - 2 PO BID
    - Ferrous fumarate (Feostat, Chromagen)
      - 35 mg elemental iron in 325-mg tablet
      - 300–600 mg/day in divided doses
    - Polysaccharide iron complex (Niferex 150)
      - 150 mg elemental iron
      - 1–2 capsules PO daily
- Floradix iron liquid
  - 2 tsp BID
  - Vegetarian liquid formula
  - Causes less GI upset than iron salts
- Continue supplementation through 3 months postpartum
- IM or IV Imferon for severe or recalcitrant anemia
  - May cause anaphylactic reaction
  - Use with caution and following consult
- Increase high-iron food sources (see "A Nutritional Primer")

Providing Treatment: Complementary and Alternative Measures to Consider

(Romm, 2010; University of Maryland Medical Center, 2007)

- Chlorophyll: Liquid or capsule
  - May stimulate RBC production
  - Increases in hemoglobin and hematocrit are often seen in 2 weeks

Table 3-1 Criteria for Diagnosing Anemia in Pregnancy		
PREGNANT WOMEN	**HEMOGLOBIN**	**HEMATOCRIT**
First trimester	< 11.0 g/dL	< 33.0%
Second trimester	< 10.5 g/dL	< 32.0%
Third trimester	< 11.0 g/dL	< 33.0%

Source: CDC, 2011b.

- Blackstrap molasses
  - 1 Tbs daily
  - A good source of iron, B vitamins, and minerals, and a gentle bowel stimulant
- Spirulina (blue-green algae)
  - 1 tsp daily
- Gentian
  - Add 1 tsp powder to 3 cups water
  - Take 1 Tbs 30 minutes prior to meals
- Dried nettle leaf infusion
  - May stimulate RBC production
- Yellow dock and dandelion root syrup
  - May stimulate RBC production
  - ½ oz of each herb in 4 cups water simmered down to 1 cup, add ½ cup blackstrap molasses
  - 1–2 Tbs 1–2 times daily
- Alfalfa: Capsule or liquid
- Cast-iron cookware
  - Nonenamel surface
  - Adds elemental iron

Providing Support: Education and Support Measures to Consider

- Physiologic nature of anemia in pregnancy
- Pica decreases iron absorption
- Iron supplementation recommendations
  - Dosages
  - Separate supplement from the following sources:
    - ♦ Meals
    - ♦ Calcium intake
    - ♦ Fiber cereals and supplements
    - ♦ Other supplements (e.g., prenatal vitamins)
  - ⚠ Keep iron supplements away from children
- For best absorption, take the following steps:
  - Take with vitamin C or water
  - Take at bedtime
  - Avoid caffeine and black teas
- Common side effects
  - Gastrointestinal upset, constipation, or diarrhea
  - Nausea
  - Heartburn
  - Black stools
  - GI symptoms occur in 10–20% of those taking iron supplements (King & Brucker, 2011)
- Management of common side effects: Increase fluids, daily dietary fiber, and activity

Follow-up Care: Follow-up Measures to Consider

- Document
- List parameters for consultation
- Return for care
  - Repeat hematocrit and hemoglobin 4–6 weeks after initiating therapy
  - Add indices for persistent anemia if no improvement occurs

Multidisciplinary Practice: Consider Consultation, Collaboration, or Referral

- Nutritional consult
- Social services
  - WIC
  - Food stamps
  - Local food pantry
  - Smoking cessation programs
- Medical consult
  - For abnormal indices or elevated serum ferritin
  - For anemia resistant to conventional therapy
  - For concern regarding cause of anemia
- For diagnosis or treatment outside the midwife's scope of practice

CARE OF THE PREGNANT WOMAN EXPOSED TO CYTOMEGALOVIRUS

Key Clinical Information

Cytomegalovirus (CMV) is a herpes virus with the ability to remain dormant within the body for life, similar to Epstein-Barr virus and varicella zoster virus. Approximately 80% of adults in the United States have had CMV infection. CMV is the most common viral infection in newborns in the United States, with approximately 30,000 new cases occurring each year.

Most women who contract CMV during pregnancy do not transmit the infection to the fetus. While most newborns with prenatally acquired infection will not be affected by the disease, long-term effects such as hearing loss or mental and physical developmental disabilities occur in approximately 20% of infants born with congenital infection. Most women have had an asymptomatic CMV infection prior to childbearing; however, 4 in 10 childbearing women will not have had a CMV infection before becoming pregnant. Maternal immunity does not prevent reoccurrence, and maternal antibodies do not prevent fetal infection (Cunningham et al., 2010). The risk of CMV-related complications in infants born to women infected 6 months or more before conception is very low (CDC, 2010a). Approximately 50% to 80% of childbearing-age women have experienced a CMV infection prior to pregnancy (CDC, 2010a).

Primary transmission of CMV occurs through person-to-person contact such as kissing, or through mucosal absorption of CMV-infected urine or saliva, or through contact with fomites handled by infected individuals. Because infected infants and children can shed the virus in body fluids, CMV is more commonly found in daycare settings, where diaper changes and handling of children's toys can facilitate the pathogen's transmission.

Universal laboratory screening of pregnant women for CVM infection is not currently recommended. Instructing pregnant women on avoiding CMV infection by thorough hand washing techniques and avoiding potential contact is prudent. Although CMV can be passed through breastmilk, infections contracted through breastfeeding usually result in no clinical illness. Pregnant women with symptoms of mononucleosis should be evaluated for CMV infection.

Client History and Chart Review: Components of the History to Consider

- Current gestational age
- Employment history
- History of recent outbreak with close contact
  - Preschool teachers
  - Pediatric care workers

  - Woman with infants or preschool-age children in day care
- Presence of symptoms
  - Fever and chills
  - Malaise
  - Headache
- Most infected people are asymptomatic

Physical Examination: Components of the Physical Exam to Consider

- Vital signs, including temperature
- Routine prenatal surveillance
- Evaluate for the following:
  - Hepatosplenomegaly
  - Lymphadenopathy
  - Arthralgia

Clinical Impression: Differential Diagnoses to Consider (ICD9Data.com, 2012)

- Cytomeglovirus
- Other human herpes virus
- Other viral diseases complicating pregnancy

Diagnostic Testing: Diagnostic Tests and Procedures to Consider

- Viral culture or polymerase chain reaction (PCR) testing
  - Urine, saliva, or throat swab specimens
  - Testing is expensive and not widely used
- Serologic testing
  - IgM and IgG antibody linked to CMV (ELISA)
  - IgG avidity assay tests antibody maturity and provides for better detection of primary CMV infection
  - Compare acute-phase and convalescent-phase serum samples for diagnosis
  - Seroconversion of CMV-specific IgG is diagnostic for primary infection

Providing Treatment: Therapeutic Measures to Consider

- No treatment available for CMV infection is currently available.

Providing Treatment: Complementary and Alternative Measures to Consider

For possible exposure, consider the following measures:

- Herbs for immune system support
- Symptomatic treatment
- Stress reduction techniques: breathing techniques, yoga, guided imagery, journaling

Providing Support: Education and Support Measures to Consider

- Reassurance:
  - Few maternal infections result in fetal infection
  - Later-gestation infection typically does not result in any fetal problems
- Explanation of lab testing and diagnosis
- Potential for fetal compromise with infection
  - May have no effect
  - Possible developmental deficits

Follow-up Care: Follow-up Measures to Consider

- Document client discussions and testing plan
- Amniotic fluid testing offered to women positive for primary CMV infection
  - Negative testing does not always exclude fetal infection
- Ultrasound for fetal effects such as microcephaly, ascites, and oligohydramnios
- Other fetal surveillance done as clinically indicated
- Pediatric evaluation and follow-up after birth

Multidisciplinary Practice: Consider Consultation, Collaboration, or Referral

- OB/GYN services
  - Maternal infection with CMV
  - Fetus with evidence of fetal growth restriction or anomaly
- For diagnosis or treatment outside the midwife's scope of practice

CARE OF THE PREGNANT WOMAN WITH FEMALE GENITAL CUTTING

Key Clinical Information

Female genital cutting (FGC) is "the partial or total removal of the female external genitalia or other injury to the female genital organs for cultural or other nontherapeutic reasons" (World Health Organization, 2010). Conservative estimates state that FGC affects more than 200,000 women in the United States. Most of these women are refugees or immigrants from African nations where the practice of FGC is widespread. Women with FGC are more likely to have birth related complications than those who do not have FGC. There is a positive correlation between the more extensive FGC type and more adverse perinatal complications, including obstructed labor, fetal distress, perineal tears and wound infections, and postpartum hemorrhage and sepsis. Nonobstetric complications include urinary tract infections, dyspareunia, and dysmenorrhea.

FGC is typically performed on girls ranging in age from infancy to 13 years. Reasons given for the practice of FGC include ensuring virginity/monogamy, cleanliness (removal of unclean genitalia) and beauty, marriage eligibility, creating a shared experience, and religious associations, although FGC is not mandated by any known religious practice. In caring for a patient with FGC, it is very important that the midwife consider a woman's attitude toward her own body and the impact of her family and culture on her decision making regarding her FGC. Careful attention toward adequate open and sensitive communication regarding gynecologic and obstetric care and choices for the woman with FGC is essential.

Client History and Chart Review: Components of the History to Consider

- Age
- FGC history
  - Country of origin
  - Age at time of FGC
  - Perception/memory of personal FGC
  - Description of FGC (typing)

- Reproductive history
  - GP TPAL
  - Menstrual status
- Vaginal birth or cesarean delivery
  - Pelvic exam/Pap smear history
  - Prior history of defibulation
- Current sexual practices
  - Number of lifetime partners
  - Patient perception of sexual satisfaction
  - Acceptability of discussing sexuality
- History of the following conditions:
  - Urinary tract infections
  - Dysmenorrhea
  - Dyspareunia
  - Perinatal complications
- Cultural status
  - Personal attitude toward FGC and its effects on her body, life, and labor
  - Family and partner attitudes toward FGC
- Special considerations for the infibulated woman
  - Pregnancy/childbearing plans
  - Attitudes toward defibulation
  - Thoughts about re-infibulation

Physical Examination: Components of the Physical Exam to Consider (American Academy of Pediatrics, 1998)

It is important that the healthcare provider maintain a nonjudgmental attitude during the physical examination. The following factors should be taken into account while doing the pelvic examination:

- The appearance of FGC is widely variable.
- FGC is generally categorized by the types shown in Figure 3-1.
- Note the following:
  - Diameter of the vaginal introitus
  - Size of vaginal introitus
  - Character and degree of vulvar scar tissue
  - Perineal tissue elasticity

Clinical Impression: Differential Diagnoses to Consider (ICD9Data.com, 2012)

Female genital cutting status

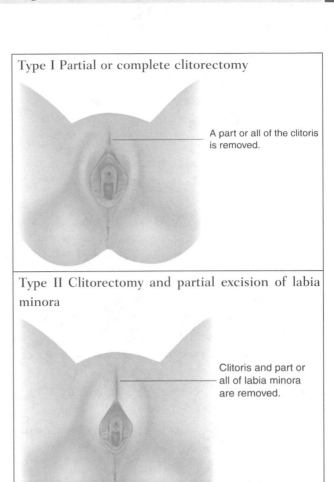

Type I Partial or complete clitorectomy

A part or all of the clitoris is removed.

Type II Clitorectomy and partial excision of labia minora

Clitoris and part or all of labia minora are removed.

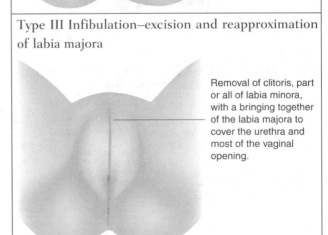

Type III Infibulation–excision and reapproximation of labia majora

Removal of clitoris, part or all of labia minora, with a bringing together of the labia majora to cover the urethra and most of the vaginal opening.

Type IV All other procedures not described here

Figure 3-1 Types of Female Genital Cutting
Source: Toubia, 1994.

Diagnostic Testing: Diagnostic Tests and Procedures to Consider

- Urinalysis to screen for asymptomatic UTI
- Limited vaginal exams in labor for descent of presenting part

Providing Treatment: Therapeutic Measures to Consider

- Care of the perineum of a pregnant/laboring woman with Type I or Type II FGC
  - Similar for women without FGC
  - Special consideration given to minimizing invasive exams
- Care of the perineum of a pregnant/laboring woman with Type III FGC
  - Offer defibulation in the second trimester of pregnancy
  - Consider an anterior episiotomy at the time of birth
  - Laceration or anterior episiotomy are repaired under local or epidural anesthesia

---

Anterior Episiotomy

A midline upward incision is made immediately prior to the birth of the baby to open the scar tissue, thereby allowing the birth to occur. The repair focuses on hemostasis of scar tissue and allowing for physiologic passage of urine and menstrual flow. If an anterior episiotomy is indicated, it is critical to engage in discussion with the woman about her anatomical and cultural goals of repair. For cultural reasons, some women prefer to have a portion of the incision re-infibulated.

Providing Treatment: Complementary and Alternative Measures to Consider

- Perineal massage (prenatal or intrapartum)
- Warm compresses
- Expectant "hands-off" management of second stage

Providing Support: Education and Support Measures to Consider

Provide information about the following issues:

- Defibulation prior to intercourse, pregnancy, or labor
- Management of FGC before and after birth
- Legal issues surrounding FGC in the United States

Follow-up Care: Follow-up Measures to Consider

- Document the type of FGC in the client's chart
- Document the client's preference for management of her FGC
- Note referrals for deinfibulation

Multidisciplinary Practice: Consider Consultation, Collaboration, or Referral

- OB/GYN services
  - For deinfibulation under anesthesia prior to pregnancy or in second trimester
  - For complex laceration repair
- Culturally appropriate mental health services or support groups for clients experiencing emotional repercussions of FGC
- For diagnosis or treatment outside the midwife's scope of practice

CARE OF THE PREGNANT WOMAN WITH FETAL DEMISE

Key Clinical Information

Early pregnancy loss before 20 weeks' gestation is considered a spontaneous or missed abortion, or miscarriage, whereas after 20 weeks' gestation it is considered a fetal death or stillbirth. In a majority of cases, the cause of fetal demise is unable to be determined (American College of Obstetricians and Gynecologists [ACOG], 2009). Some fetal or placental conditions are clearly incompatible with life, whereas other fetal loss may be related to maternal illness, heredity, medical conditions such as diabetes, and hypertension, or to unknown factors. Genetic investigation and counseling may be useful for exploring potential causes of fetal demise, particularly for the woman with a history of recurrent losses.

Fetal demise can occur at any stage of pregnancy. No matter when it occurs, a common response is for the mother to wonder what she did wrong. Emotional support and grief counseling are important components of care to parents.

Client History and Chart Review: Components of the History to Consider

- Gestational age
- Regression of signs of pregnancy
  - Absence of fetal activity
  - Absence of fetal heart tones
  - Other associated signs and symptoms such as decreased or absent breast tenderness
- Vaginal bleeding or discharge
- Back pain or cramping
- Previous human chorionic gonadotropin (HCG) results
- Precipitating event(s), if any
  - Idiopathic
  - Trauma/physical abuse
  - Substance abuse
- Medication and herb use
- Risk factors for stillbirth
  - Infection
  - Exposure to environmental toxins
  - Maternal age extremes
  - Multiple gestation
  - Body mass index (BMI) > 30
  - Race: African Americans' risk of stillbirth is twice that of Caucasian women
  - Maternal disorders, such as diabetes, hypertension, renal disease, and lupus
- Current emotions of self, partner, and significant others
- Current coping mechanisms
- Review birth and surgical history

Physical Examination: Components of the Physical Exam to Consider

- Maternal vital signs
- Abdominal exam
  - Fundal height for gestational age
  - Uterine tenderness
  - Absence of fetal heart tones
- Pelvic examination
  - Boggy feeling to uterus
  - Palpation of buckled fetal skull
  - Cervical status/Bishop's score

Clinical Impression: Differential Diagnoses to Consider (ICD9Data.com, 2012)

- Intrauterine fetal demise
  - Early, before 20 weeks' gestation
  - Late, after 20 weeks' gestation
- Missed abortion
- Ectopic pregnancy
- Blighted ovum
- Pseudocyesis
- Hydatidiform mole

Diagnostic Testing: Diagnostic Tests and Procedures to Consider

- Maternal blood work
  - CBC
  - Kleihauer-Betke test
  - Hemoglobin A_{1c}
  - Rapid plasma reagin/Venereal Disease Research Laboratory test
  - Serum/urine toxicology screen
- Weekly testing in expectant management
  - Prothrombin time (PT), partial thromboplastin time (PTT)
  - Fibrinogen, fibrin degradation products
  - Platelets
- Ultrasound
  - Absent fetal heart beat (verified by two examiners)
  - Overlapping of fetal cranial bones: Spalding's sign
  - Presence of gas in fetal abdomen: Robert's sign
- Fetal evaluation (ACOG, 2009)
  - Cord blood
  - Placenta to pathology for gross and microscopic examination
  - Placental cultures
  - Fetal x-rays and autopsy with consent of parents

- Genetic testing with consent and if indicated
  - Anomalies
  - Family history
  - Recurrent fetal losses

Providing Treatment: Therapeutic Measures to Consider

(Belkin & Wilder, 2007)

- Expectant management
  - May be emotionally difficult
  - Increased risk of disseminated intravascular coagulation (DIC) after 3 weeks
  - Observe for onset of the following conditions:
    - Fever
    - DIC
    - Rupture of membranes (ROM) or labor
- Surgical dilatation and evacuation (D & E) in early pregnancy
- Induction of labor
  - Laminaria or Foley catheter
  - Prostin E$_2$ suppositories
  - Misoprostol 50–100 mg per vagina or PO if no uterine scar
  - Oxytocin induction after 32 weeks' gestation

Providing Treatment: Complementary and Alternative Measures to Consider

Natural remedies may be used to stimulate labor:

- May not be effective before 32 weeks' gestation
- Blue/black cohosh infusion or tincture
- Castor oil
- Acupressure points spleen 6 or gallbladder 21

Providing Support: Education and Support Measures to Consider

(Belkin & Wilder, 2007)

- Discuss cause of death if known
- Options for birth
  - Discussion regarding labor initiation
    - Maternal preferences
    - Parameters for consultation
    - Therapeutic measures to initiate labor

- Location for birth
- Anticipated course of events
- Care of the body
  - May vary with gestational age
  - Family time
  - Autopsy or testing
  - Burial, cremation, or hospital disposal
- Funeral or memorial service
- Postpartum period
  - Lochia
  - Lactation suppression
  - RhIG if indicated
  - Rubella if non-immune
- Grief
  - Support groups and community resources
  - Review stages of grief

Follow-up Care: Follow-up Measures to Consider

- Document
  - Maternal response
  - Course of labor and birth
  - Anomalies, if any
  - Examination and testing of fetal remains
  - Care and arrangements for the fetus
  - Placental disposition
  - Planned follow-up
- Follow-up care
  - Weeks 1–6
    - Phone, home, or office visit
    - Results of any testing
    - Evaluation of emotional status
  - Weeks 2–6
    - Postpartum check
    - Initiation of birth control as needed
    - Support and referrals as needed

Multidisciplinary Practice: Consider Consultation, Collaboration, or Referral

- For social support
  - Grief counseling
  - Support groups
- Medical/obstetric care
  - Maternal preference

- Evidence of DIC or molar pregnancy
- Mother who prefers surgical D & E in early pregnancy
- Induction of labor as indicated by the following:
  - Midwifery practice parameters
  - Maternal preference or condition
- For diagnosis or treatment outside the midwife's scope of practice

CARE OF THE PREGNANT WOMAN WITH GESTATIONAL DIABETES

Key Clinical Information

Gestational diabetes mellitus (GDM) occurs in 4% to 10% of all pregnant women in the United States (U.S. Preventive Services Task Force [USPSTF], 2008). This condition is defined as carbohydrate intolerance and increased insulin resistance first recognized in pregnancy. Women with diabetes found at the first prenatal visit should receive a diagnosis of overt diabetes, not gestational diabetes (American Diabetes Association [ADA], 2011a). The carbohydrate intolerance of GDM presents on a continuum ranging from mild to severe, with maternal and fetal effects increasing with the degree of carbohydrate intolerance. Potential problems that may be seen in GDM are primarily related to the fetus/infant and include fetal macrosomia, secondary to elevated levels of circulating glucose resulting in increased fetal insulin and fat deposition, low blood sugar, and jaundice after birth.

There is no consensus among field experts on screening timing, methods, and populations; diagnostic criteria; and management, although some common practices are used. Some providers may screen, diagnose, or manage GDM outside these common practices yet still remain within the boundaries of evidence-based care.

Most women diagnosed with GDM can maintain euglycemia with appropriate diet therapy and moderate exercise. Other women may require oral hypoglycemics or insulin therapy. Daily attention to diet is imperative, with a variety of food sources providing excellent nutrition and a balance of proteins, fats, and complex carbohydrates. Keeping a food and blood glucose diary can be very helpful in making dietary recommendations that are culturally and financially reasonable. Exercise increases glucose uptake and insulin sensitivity and has been found to be as effective as insulin for some women, making exercise an important component of GDM management (Mottola, 2008).

Client History and Chart Review: Components of the History to Consider

- Age, GP TPAL
- Gestational age
- Risk factors for gestational diabetes
  - Maternal age > 25 years
  - BMI > 28 kg/m²
  - Previous fasting blood sugar (FBS) in the range of 110–125 mg/dL
  - Suspected or documented previous gestational diabetes
  - Previous infant weighing > 4100 g
  - Previous unexplained fetal demise
  - Polyhydramnios
  - Previous birth of a child with a congenital anomaly
  - Polycystic ovarian syndrome
- Family history of diabetes in a first-degree relative
- Ethnicity-related risk factors for type 2 diabetes (ADA, 2011b)
  - African American
  - Alaskan Native
  - Hispanic American
  - Native American
  - South or East Asian
  - Pacific Islander
- Symptoms of gestational diabetes
  - Glycosuria
  - Size larger than appropriate for dates
  - Polyuria
  - Polydipsia
  - Loss of energy

Physical Examination: Components of the Physical Exam to Consider

- Vital signs, including weight
- BMI
- Weight gain
- Serial fundal height
- Estimated fetal weight in third trimester

Clinical Impression: Differential Diagnoses to Consider (ICD9Data.com, 2012)

- Gestational diabetes
- Diabetes mellitus
- Fetal macrosomia secondary to the following:
  - Gestational diabetes
  - Constitutionally large fetus
- Polyhydramnios

Diagnostic Testing: Diagnostic Tests and Procedures to Consider

- Dip urinalysis for glucose
- First-visit or first-trimester serum screening for women at risk for type 2 diabetes/gestational diabetes
- Universal screening for gestational diabetes unless low risk: 24–28 weeks' gestation

- Serum screening may be omitted for low-risk women who meet all of the following criteria in Table 3-2 (Cunningham et al., 2010; Metzger et al., 2007)
  - One-hour glucose challenge test (50 mg glucose)
    - Value > 130–140 mg/dL is suspicious for gestational diabetes
    - Three-hour oral glucose tolerance test if 1-hour screen is elevated
    - Value > 200 mg/dL is diagnostic of gestational diabetes
  - One-step screening *and* diagnosis: Blood draws after fasting, as well as 1 hour and 2 hours after 75 mg oral glucose load
- Diagnosis: Two or more elevated blood levels in one-step testing (Table 3-3) or 3-hour glucose tolerance test (Table 3-4)
- Ongoing maternal laboratory assessment: Hemoglobin A_{1c}
  - Normal range: 4.0–8.2%
  - Less than 6% preferable in pregnancy
  - Self-monitored blood glucose
- Monitor for preeclampsia: Increased incidence in the presence of GDM
- Ultrasound for fetal anomalies and fetal growth

Table 3-2 Screening for Gestational Diabetes		
LOW RISK: SERUM TESTING NOT REQUIRED	**AVERAGE RISK: SCREEN AT 24–28 WEEKS' GESTATION**	**HIGH RISK: SCREEN AS SOON AS POSSIBLE**
Member of ethnic group of low prevalence*	Those women who are not at low or high risk	Obese (BMI > 30)
No known diabetes mellitus (DM) in a first-degree relative		Prior history of GDM
Age < 25 years		Glycosuria
Normal BMI		First-degree family history of DM
No history of abnormal glucose metabolism		
No history of prior poor obstetrical outcome		

*High-prevalence groups: African Americans, Hispanic Americans, East Asians (India, Middle East), Pacific Islanders, and Native Americans.

Table 3-3   One-Step Testing Diagnostic Criteria for Gestational Diabetes: 75-mg Two-Hour Screen and Diagnosis

TIME OF SAMPLE	CRITICAL LEVEL
Fasting	95 mg/dL
1 hour	180 mg/dL
2 hours	140 mg/dL

If two or more values meet or exceed the target level, GDM is diagnosed.

This method is recommended by the American Diabetes Association, though it is not yet widely used in the United States.

Providing Treatment: Therapeutic Measures to Consider

- Regular exercise
- Dietary therapy
  - Caloric intake by weight, ranging from 1800 to 2400 kcal/day
    - Underweight (BMI < 18.5): 40 kcal/kg/day
    - Average weight (BMI = 18.5–24.9): 30 kcal/kg/day
    - Overweight (BMI = 25–29.9): 24 kcal/kg/day
    - Obese (BMI > 30): 12–15 kcal/kg/day
  - Six small meals daily (Moore, 2010)
    - Three meals and three snacks
    - Complex carbohydrates: 35–40% of diet
    - Fat: 30% or less of diet
- Self-monitored blood glucose (Metzger et al., 2007)
  - Fasting glucose < 95 mg/dL

Table 3-4   Three-Hour Oral Glucose Tolerance Test (OGTT) Diagnostic Criteria for Gestational Diabetes

TIME OF SAMPLE	CRITICAL LEVEL
Fasting	105 mg/dL
1 hour	190 mg/dL
2 hours	165 mg/dL
3 hours	145 mg/dL

- 1 hour postprandial glucose
  - Postprandial monitoring superior to preprandial monitoring
  - Less than 140 mg/dL 1 hour after start of meal
  - Less than 120 mg/dL 2 hours after start of meal
- Oral hypoglycemics (Dhulkotia, Bolarinde, Fraser, & Farrell, 2010)
  - Are more convenient for women and require less intensive use instruction
  - Reduce risk of hypoglycemia compared to insulin
  - Glyburide (Pregnancy Category B)
    - Use after organogenesis
    - 📞 Consult for use and dosage
  - Metformin (Pregnancy Category B)
    - Limited to clinical trials (Ardilouze, Mahdavian, & Baillargeon, 2010)
    - 📞 Consult for use and dosage
- 📞 Insulin therapy
  - Initiate when more than 20% of the 2-hour postprandial glucose values exceed 120 mg/dL (ACOG, 2001b)
  - 📞 Consult for use, recommended types of insulin, and dosages
  - Titrate to maintain glycemic control

Providing Treatment: Complementary and Alternative Measures to Consider

- Cinnamon ¼ to ½ tsp daily (Hlebowicz, Darwiche, Bjorgell, & Almer, 2007)
- Herbs
  - Bilberry (Foster, 1996)
  - Chicory
  - Dandelion
  - Red raspberry tea

Providing Support: Education and Support Measures to Consider

(Metzger et al., 2007; Varney, Kriebs, & Gegor, 2004)

- Risks and benefits of options for care
- Diabetic education—the cornerstone of management

- Diabetic education
  - What GDM is
  - How GDM can affect pregnancy
  - Reassurance of likely normal pregnancy progression and outcome with stable euglycemia
  - Dietary control
    - Instruct in complex carbohydrate foods
    - Sample menus of three small meals and two to three snacks per day
    - Importance of not skipping meals
    - Dietary recommendations for glucose control
  - Physical activity recommendations
    - Benefits of aerobic exercise in blood glucose control
    - 30 minutes of walking, swimming, bike riding, or dancing on most days of the week
    - No exercise in fasting state
    - If exercising right after a meal, have a snack of one fruit serving after exercise
    - If exercising 2 hours or more after a meal, have a snack of one fruit serving before exercise
  - Medication instruction as needed
  - Daily home glucose monitoring
    - Ideal frequency not established
    - Glucometer with memory and log book to bring to each visit
    - Four to seven times per day until glycemic control is established
      - Fasting
      - 1 or 2 hours after start of meals
      - Bedtime
    - Daily self-monitoring may be reduced once glycemic control is established
    - Four times per day for 2 days per week— fasting and after meals
- ⚠ Warning signs and symptoms
  - Call with pattern of abnormal blood glucose values
  - Decreased fetal movement
  - Signs and symptoms of hypoglycemia

Follow-up Care: Follow-up Measures to Consider

- Document
- Review psychological adjustment to diabetes diagnosis
- Prenatal follow-up
  - Maternal and fetal evaluation
  - Blood glucose follow-up
    - Evaluate results at each visit
    - Periodic laboratory testing for validation of the following:
      - Home monitoring results
      - Glycemic control
    - Medication use
- Fetal assessment (Moore, 2010)
  - Method and initiation timing depend on the individual woman and her level of glycemic control
  - Fetal kick counts beginning approximately 34 weeks' gestation
  - Ultrasound for estimated fetal weight (EFW) and growth discrepancies
    - Ultrasound to detect anomalies for women diagnosed with GDM in the first trimester
  - Non-stress test (NST)
  - Biophysical profile (BPP)
- Labor and birth plan
  - If well-controlled blood sugars and no other problems, can wait until 40 weeks' gestation to consider induction of labor (ACOG, 2001b)
  - ◔ Consider induction before 40 weeks' gestation for the following circumstances:
    - Client on insulin therapy
    - Fetal macrosomia
    - Poor or marginal control
    - Nonreassuring fetal status
  - Plan to have the birth at a facility with newborn special care available: Anticipate respiratory distress syndrome (RDS)
  - If EFW > 4500 g, cesarean delivery may decrease the likelihood of brachial plexus injury in the infant (ACOG, 2001b)
  - Plan for pediatric care at birth

- Postpartum follow-up
  - Most women return to euglycemia quickly after birth
  - Self-monitor FBS and 2-hour postprandial blood sugar for 7 days
    - Evaluate as soon as possible for diabetes mellitus in the presence of either of the following conditions:
      - FBS > 120 mg/dL
      - Two-hour postprandial blood sugar > 160 mg/dL
  - FBS at 6 weeks postpartum
    - FBS > 126 mg/dL is diagnostic of diabetes mellitus
  - Interconceptional risk reduction
    - Weight loss
    - Diet improvements
  - Blood glucose checked every 1 to 3 years

Multidisciplinary Practice: Consider Consultation, Collaboration, or Referral

- Nutrition education and counseling: Referral to certified diabetic educator or registered dietician
- Social services, as indicated
- Medical, obstetric, or pediatric services
  - Referral to diabetic clinic for pregnant women
  - Gestational diabetes not controlled by diet
    - Initiation of insulin or glyburide
    - Ongoing medication dosage requirements
  - Fetal macrosomia, fetal growth restriction (FGR), or anomalies
  - Newborn care at birth
- For diagnosis or treatment outside the midwife's scope of practice

CARE OF THE PREGNANT WOMAN WITH HEPATITIS

Key Clinical Information

Hepatitis includes a range of viral illnesses that may be transmitted via blood or body fluids. Vertical transmission of hepatitis B, C, E, and G may occur to the fetus during pregnancy. Without treatment shortly after birth, as many as 90% of infants born to hepatitis B–infected mothers will become infected (ACOG, 2007b). Infected infants may become chronic carriers or may develop significant illness. Infected women may present with acute illness, or they may be chronic carriers—that is, asymptomatic but able to transmit infection (CDC, 2011a).

Client History and Chart Review: Components of the History to Consider

- Gestational age
- Immunization status—hepatitis A and B
- Potential exposure to hepatitis
  - Healthcare professional
  - IV drug use, shared needles
  - Sexual contacts
  - HIV-positive women
  - Presence of tattoos
  - Ingestion of raw shellfish
  - Hemodialysis patients
  - Blood or organ recipient before 1992
  - International travelers
  - Daycare workers
  - Immigrants from the following regions:
    - Asia
    - Africa
    - Pacific Islands
    - Haiti
    - Middle East
    - Eastern Europe
- Presence, onset and duration, and severity of symptoms
  - Malaise and lethargy
  - Fever and chills
  - Right upper quadrant pain
  - Jaundice
  - Nausea and vomiting
  - No symptoms: At least half of all initial hepatitis B virus (HBV) infections are asymptomatic

Physical Examination: Components of the Physical Exam to Consider

- Vital signs, including weight
- Examine for evidence of jaundice
  - Skin
  - Mucous membranes
  - Sclera
- Palpate and percuss the following:
  - Liver margins
  - Splenomegaly
  - Right upper quadrant pain

Clinical Impression: Differential Diagnoses to Consider (ICD9Data.com, 2012)

- Hepatitis A
- Hepatitis B
- Hepatitis C
- Cholestasis of pregnancy
- Cholelithiasis
- Other liver disorders in pregnancy

Diagnostic Testing: Diagnostic Tests and Procedures to Consider

- Hepatitis B profile, multiple antigen/antibody screen
- Hepatitis A screen for those at risk
  - Recent immigrants from or travelers to high-risk countries: Central and South America, rural Mexico
- Hepatitis C screen for those at risk
  - HIV-positive women
  - Current or former IV drug users
- Liver function tests
  - Elevation occurs during acute phase (CDC, 2011a)

Providing Treatment: Therapeutic Measures to Consider

- Illness must run its course
- Supportive therapy for woman
- Consider immunization series
  - For at-risk noninfected women
  - May be used during pregnancy

- Hepatitis B (Pregnancy Category C)
- Hepatitis A (Pregnancy Category C)

Providing Treatment: Complementary and Alternative Measures to Consider

- Herbs for immune support
  - Milk thistle tea (Foster, 1996)
  - Dandelion tea, tincture or capsule
  - Turmeric
  - Green tea
  - Reishi mushroom extract
- Adequate rest

Providing Support: Education and Support Measures to Consider

(CDC, 2011a)

- Provide information about hepatitis
  - Transmission, prevention, and self-care
    - Refrain from sharing household items such as toothbrushes and razors
    - Other family members should be tested for HBV
    - Cover cuts and skin lesions
    - Use condoms
    - Reaffirm no alcohol
    - Consult a healthcare provider before taking any OTC medications
    - Hepatitis B is *not* transmitted by kissing, hugging, coughing, food, water, or casual contact
  - Vaginal birth is recommended; cesarean delivery is recommended only for specific indications
  - Preterm birth risk is increased with acute HBV infection; education about warning signs should be given as needed
  - Medication recommendations for infant
    - Significant reduction in hepatitis B fetal transmission with immunoglobulin injection after birth
  - Breastfeeding: Not contraindicated for non-immunized infant

- Discussion regarding the following topics:
  - Options for care of self and infant
  - Location for birth
  - Parameters for referral

Follow-up Care: Follow-up Measures to Consider

- Document
- Return for care
  - Per routine for carrier
  - Weekly for acute phase of infection
    - Periodic liver function tests
    - Fetal evaluation with acute illness
- Administer to infant born to hepatitis B–positive mother
  - Hepatitis B immune globulin: 0.5 mL IM in anterior thigh within 12 hours of birth
  - Three-dose hepatitis B vaccine
    - Engerix-B 10 mg/0.5 mL
    - Recombivax HB 5 mg/0.5 mL
    - IM in anterior thigh shortly after birth
    - Repeat in 1 and 6 months

Multidisciplinary Practice: Consider Consultation, Collaboration, or Referral

- Epidemiologic support
- Medical services
  - Acute hepatitis, any type
  - Hepatitis C, to hepatitis specialist
- Pediatric care provider consultation
  - Before birth
  - Collaborative plan for newborn care
- For diagnosis or treatment outside the midwife's scope of practice

CARE OF THE PREGNANT WOMAN WITH HERPES SIMPLEX VIRUS

Key Clinical Information

The prevalence of herpes simplex virus (HSV) infection has risen in the last several decades, and this disease poses an important health problem in pregnancy. The risk of infection of the infant with HSV varies with the incidence of primary versus secondary infection in the mother (ACOG, 2007a). When primary genital HSV infection occurs during pregnancy, the perinatal transmission rate may be as high as 50%. This condition should be differentiated from a nonprimary genital infection with a first outbreak of lesions, which has a perinatal transmission rate of 33%. With secondary, or recurrent, genital HSV infection during pregnancy, the perinatal transmission rate diminishes to 0 to 3%.

Three categories of neonatal disease are distinguished: localized disease of the skin, eye, and mouth; central nervous system disease; and disseminated disease. The mother may be asymptomatic in as many as 80% of instances in which the infant is infected (ACOG, 2007a).

Client History and Chart Review: Components of the History to Consider

- Gestational age
- Sexual history
- Previous history
  - Genital or oral herpes
  - Other sexually transmitted infections (STIs)
- Duration and quality of present symptoms
  - Location and number of vesicular lesions
    - Oral
    - Genital
  - Symptoms
    - Pain
    - Tingling
    - Dysuria
- Primary infection associated with the following symptoms:
  - Fever
  - Headache and photophobia
  - Malaise
  - Aseptic meningitis

Physical Examination: Components of the Physical Exam to Consider

- Vital signs, including temperature
- Usual prenatal evaluation

- Physical evaluation with emphasis on the following:
  - Oral examination
  - Inguinal lymph nodes
    - Enlargement
    - Tenderness
  - External genitalia, buttocks, and pelvic region
  - Characteristic lesions
    - Vesicles
    - Shallow ulcers
- Speculum examination, as needed
  - Presence of other STI symptoms
  - Cervical discharge
  - Cervical or uterine motion tenderness

Clinical Impression: Differential Diagnoses to Consider (ICD9Data.com, 2012)

- HSV infection
- Other STIs
- Genital trauma

Diagnostic Testing: Diagnostic Tests and Procedures to Consider

(CDC, 2010b)

- Cell culture and polymerase chain reaction (PCR) for HSV
  - Negative culture or PCR does not indicate absence of HSV infection
- Type-specific serum testing for HSV antibody titer
  - Documents primary versus nonprimary first episode versus recurrent infection
  - Useful if the woman is asymptomatic and her sexual partner has a history of HSV
  - Repeat in 7–10 days
- Other STI testing
  - With symptoms
  - As indicated by history

Providing Treatment: Therapeutic Measures to Consider

(ACOG, 2007a)

- Valtrex (valacyclovir hydrochloride)
  - Pregnancy Category B

  - Pregnancy registry: 800-722-9292, extension 39437
  - Dose: 500 mg BID for 5 days
  - Begin medication within 24 hours of first symptoms
  - For suppressive therapy at 36 weeks' gestation until birth: 500 mg PO daily (for clients with more than 9 recurrences/year)
- Famvir (Famciclovir)
  - Pregnancy Category B
  - Dose: 125 mg BID for 5 days
  - Begin medication within 6 hours of first symptoms
  - For suppressive therapy at 36 weeks' gestation until birth: 250 mg PO BID
- Zovirax (Acyclovir)
  - Pregnancy Category C
  - Pregnancy registry: 800-722-9292, extension 58465
  - Topical ointment 5%
    - Apply three times per day for 7 days
  - Initial outbreak
    - 200 mg PO five times a day for 10 days
  - Recurrent outbreak
    - 200 mg PO five times per day for 7 days
    - Repeat treatment as needed
  - Suppression or severe recurrent outbreaks: 400 mg PO BID for 6–12 months
  - For suppressive therapy at 36 weeks' gestation until birth: 400 mg PO daily
- Acetaminophen (Tylenol) for pain relief

Providing Treatment: Complementary and Alternative Measures to Consider

(Romm, 2010)

- Lysine
  - 1000 mg PO BID for 3 months
  - Combine with vitamin C 500 mg
  - Begin with first sign of an outbreak
- Dietary recommendations
  - Include foods high in lysine
    - Chicken, turkey
    - Milk, yogurt, cheese

- ◆ Fish
- ◆ Cooked beans
- ◆ Eggs
- ◆ Soybeans
  - ▪ Avoid foods high in arginine
    - ◆ Chocolate, coffee, cola
    - ◆ Peanuts, cashews, pecans, almonds
    - ◆ Sunflower and sesame seeds
    - ◆ Oatmeal
    - ◆ Coconut
    - ◆ Gelatin
- Lemon balm and echinacea root tea, two to four cups daily
- Echinacea
  - ▪ Use to prevent outbreaks
  - ▪ Tincture up to 30 drops daily
  - ▪ Tablets/capsules 250–100 mg daily for 2 weeks
- Lemon balm cream: Reduces lesion pain
- Tea tree essential oil: *Topically only*

Providing Support: Education and Support Measures to Consider

- Information about HSV infection
  - ▪ CDC STI Hotline: 800-232-4636
  - ▪ Potential effects of infection on the following:
    - ◆ Pregnancy
    - ◆ Anticipated location for birth
    - ◆ Newborn
    - ◆ Labor and birth plans
    - ◆ Potential for cesarean delivery with prodromal symptoms or visible lesions in labor
- Discussion of the following topics:
  - ▪ Treatment options
  - ▪ Labor and birth options
  - ▪ Maternal preferences
  - ▪ Partner safety (CDC, 2010b)
    - ◆ Abstain from sexual activity when prodromal symptoms or lesions are present
    - ◆ HSV-2 transmission is reduced with daily valacyclovir
    - ◆ Transmission can occur in the absence of prodromal symptoms or lesions

- ◆ Male latex condoms may reduce genital herpes transmission
- Rest and comfort measures
  - ▪ With initial outbreak
  - ▪ To enhance immune response

Follow-up Care: Follow-up Measures to Consider

- Document
- Return for care
  - ▪ Per routine with history of herpes
  - ▪ For culture with active lesion
  - ▪ Primary herpes
    - ◆ If symptoms persist for more than 10 days
    - ◆ If symptoms worsen
      - ➤ Stiff neck
      - ➤ Unremitting fever
      - ➤ Inability to urinate
- Labor care
  - ▪ Vaginal birth if the mother does not have any active lesions or prodromal symptoms of vulvar pain or burning
    - ◆ Active lesion remote from genital region: Occlusive dressing applied
    - ◆ Limit cervical exams
    - ◆ Limit use of scalp electrode or intrauterine pressure catheter (IUPC)
  - ▪ Cesarean birth is recommended if the mother has active genital lesions or prodromal symptoms of vulvar pain or burning
    - ◆ Before ROM
    - ◆ As soon as possible with prelabor rupture of membranes (PROM)
    - ◆ May delay with preterm premature rupture of membranes (PPROM) for steroid therapy
- Breastfeeding is encouraged unless active lesions are present on the breast

Multidisciplinary Practice: Consider Consultation, Collaboration, or Referral

- ⚠ For symptoms of herpes meningitis
- For multidisciplinary labor plan
  - ▪ Presence of active lesions
  - ▪ Potential for cesarean delivery

- For pediatric follow-up after HSV exposure
- For diagnosis or treatment outside the midwife's scope of practice

CARE OF THE PREGNANT WOMAN WITH HUMAN IMMUNODEFICIENCY VIRUS

Key Clinical Information

Universal screening of pregnant women for human immunodeficiency virus (HIV) infection is recommended as early as possible during pregnancy. Some women may feel threatened by the thought of HIV testing; all women should be notified that HIV testing is included in the standard prenatal testing profile, and the woman's decision should be documented if she declines HIV testing (opt-out testing). Many states require HIV-specific pretest counseling and documentation of informed consent prior to screening. Early screening allows for prompt confirmation of the HIV diagnosis through follow-up testing and administration of antiretroviral medication, which can decrease the incidence of perinatal transmission of the infection from 13–25% to less than 2% (CDC, 2010b). Vertical transmission may be reduced in infants who reach term, are appropriate weight for the stage of gestation, and are born by elective cesarean section close to term. Women who test negative yet are at risk for HIV infection should be retested in the third trimester. Breastfeeding is contraindicated where access to safe breastmilk substitutes and clean water is assured (CDC, 2010b). Optimal care of the HIV-infected pregnant woman requires coordinated care between HIV specialists, maternity care providers, and supportive services (National Institutes of Health [NIH], 2010).

Client History and Chart Review: Components of the History to Consider

- Gestational age
- Gynecologic and sexual history
  - Previous HIV testing
  - Number of sexual partners
    - Self and/or partner(s)
      - Sexual practices
      - STIs
      - Substance abuse
        - IV drug use
        - Other substance use
      - Blood transfusions
    - Abnormal Pap smears
- History of opportunistic infections: Presence of current symptoms
  - Malaise
  - Fever
  - Cough
  - Skin lesions
- History of HIV infection
  - Prior medical care and medication regimens
  - Stability of disease
  - Presence of current symptoms

Physical Examination: Components of the Physical Exam to Consider

- Vital signs, including temperature
- Head, eyes, ears, nose, and throat (HEENT)
  - Fundoscopic exam
  - Oral examination for thrush or lesions
- Skin lesions
- Respiratory system
  - Cough
  - Adventitious breath sounds
  - Shortness of breath
  - Night sweats
- Liver margins
- Lymph nodes
  - Characteristics of enlarged nodes
  - Location(s) of enlarged nodes
- Pelvic examination
  - Internal or external lesions
  - Symptoms of STIs

Clinical Impression: Differential Diagnoses to Consider (ICD9Data.com, 2012)

- HIV disease/acquired immunodeficiency syndrome

- Asymptomatic HIV infection status
- Other STIs

Diagnostic Testing: Diagnostic Tests and Procedures to Consider

(NIH, 2010)

- Rapid HIV test
- HIV enzyme-linked immunosorbent assay (ELISA) test
- HIV Western blot test

Providing Treatment: Therapeutic Measures to Consider

(U.S. Public Health Service Task Force [USPHSTF], 2010)

- 📞 New-onset antiretroviral therapy
  - Consider delay of therapy onset until after first trimester unless needed for maternal health
    - Diminishes drug-related teratogenicity
    - Improves adherence once early nausea has passed
  - Use current facility guidelines for medication regimen
  - Management of side effects is important to maximize adherence
- Established antiretroviral therapy: Do not discontinue antiretroviral therapy upon pregnancy diagnosis
- Modified antiretroviral treatment for perinatal prophylaxis: Intrapartum therapy
- Initiation of other therapies based on diagnosis
- CD4 cell count and viral load every trimester or as noted in facility protocol
- First-trimester ultrasound to confirm gestational age: Scheduled operative birth at 38 weeks' gestation recommended
- Second-trimester ultrasound anatomy scan: Limited data are available on the effects of combined therapy on the fetus
- Screen for other STIs

- Scheduled cesarean section at 38 weeks' gestation for women with the following conditions:
  - HIV RNA copies > 1000/mL near time of delivery
  - Unknown HIV RNA copies near time of delivery

Providing Treatment: Complementary and Alternative Measures to Consider

- Supportive measures
- Most immune-stimulating herbs are not recommended
- Cautious use of herbals/homeopathic remedies for the following indications:
  - Appetite stimulation
  - Skin integrity
  - Emotional and spiritual balance

Providing Support: Education and Support Measures to Consider

- Provide information, listening, and discussion on the following topics:
  - HIV and acquired immunodeficiency syndrome (AIDS)
  - Prevention and transmission
  - Benefits of testing
  - Viral load evaluation and significance
    - Perinatal transmission
    - Potential effects on the baby
  - Medication and treatment options
    - Antiretroviral medication (for self and/or baby)
      - Benefits
      - Risks
      - Side effects
      - Alternatives
    - Scheduling operative birth near term
- Lifestyle issues
  - Encourage use of the following measures:
    - Abstinence or consistent condom use
    - No sharing of needles
  - Breastfeeding is contraindicated where safe breastmilk substitutes are available

Follow-up Care: Follow-up Measures to Consider

- Document
  - Informed consent for testing
  - Laboratory results
  - Maternal response to
    - Diagnosis
    - Treatment recommendations
- Discussions
  - Client preferences
  - Consultations and referrals
  - Anticipated location for birth
- Follow-up care
  - Review psychological adjustment to HIV diagnosis
  - Coordinate testing with primary care provider/site
  - Pediatric consult for newborn care and follow-up
  - Register with the CDC Antiretroviral Pregnancy Registry: 800-258-4263 or http://www.apregistry.com
  - Observe for side effects of medications
    - May cause hepatic toxicity
    - May mimic HELLP syndrome
  - Antiviral drug-resistance testing (NIH, 2010)
- Return visits
  - As indicated by prenatal course and gestation
  - For support

Multidisciplinary Practice: Consider Consultation, Collaboration, or Referral

- Social support services
  - Support groups
  - Mental health referrals
  - Victim advocacy groups
  - Clean needle programs
  - Substance abuse treatment options
- OB/GYN and medical services
  - For all newly diagnosed HIV-positive women
  - For coordination of antiretroviral regimen
  - For HIV-positive women with the following conditions:
    - Onset of infection

- Decrease in CD4 cell counts
- Significant medication side effects
- For diagnosis or treatment outside the midwife's scope of practice

CARE OF THE WOMAN WITH HYPERTENSIVE DISORDERS IN PREGNANCY

Key Clinical Information

In the United States, hypertensive disorders are the most common causes of medical complications in pregnancy, affecting 2% to 10% of all pregnancies (Cunningham et al., 2010). Hypertension in pregnancy can be chronic (occurring before 20 weeks' gestation and persisting beyond 42 days, postpartum), can arise during pregnancy (gestational hypertension or preeclampsia), or can represent preeclampsia superimposed on chronic hypertension. Of the various hypertensive disorders, preeclampsia—either alone or superimposed on chronic hypertension—is the most dangerous (Cunningham et al., 2010). It can lead to complications such as eclampsia and HELLP syndrome and is one of the leading causes of maternal mortality in both the developed and developing world. Differential diagnosis can be challenging because gestational hypertension can present with a wide array of symptoms. Onset of clinical signs and symptoms suggesting gestational hypertension and/or preeclampsia should prompt careful evaluation, thereby ensuring that there is ample opportunity to institute early treatment. Laboratory testing is the most reliable way to assess a woman's potential for development of gestational hypertension. Treatment improves the likelihood of the pregnancy resulting in a healthy mother and healthy baby and increases the potential for a vaginal birth.

Client History and Chart Review: Components of the History to Consider

- Gestational age
- Presence, onset, and durations of symptoms (Table 3-5)

Table 3-5   Hypertensive Disorders of Pregnancy

HYPERTENSIVE DISORDER	SIGNS AND SYMPTOMS	CRITERIA FOR DIAGNOSIS
Chronic hypertension May be mild, moderate, or severe	Predates 20th week of pregnancy or persists beyond usual postpartum period. May have cardiac enlargement, vascular changes, renal insufficiency.	BP ≥ 140/90 mild/mod BP ≥ 170/110 severe Two or more BP elevations > 4 hr apart
Preeclampsia PIH, mild	Gestational age of ≥ 20 weeks Onset of: Elevated BP Proteinuria Elevated reflexes Fundal heights small for dates Elevated hemoglobin secondary to hemoconcentration Elevated serum uric acid (normal range 1.2–4.5 mg/dL)	Hypertension after 20 weeks: 1. Systolic ≥ 140 mm Hg, *or* 2. Diastolic ≥ 90 mm Hg 3. On two occasions ≥ 6 hr apart New onset proteinuria: 1. 1–2+ dip, on 2. Two specimens, in 3. Absence of UTI, *or* 4. ≥ 300 mg in 24-hr urine
Preeclampsia PIH, severe	Signs of mild PIH, plus 1. Clonus 2. Diminished renal function (elevated BUN, diminished urinary output, serum creatinine > 1.2 mg/dL, decreased creatinine clearance) 3. Headache 4. Visual disturbances 5. Epigastric discomfort 6. IUGR and/or oligohydramnios by ultrasound May have onset of 1. HELLP syndrome 2. Eclampsia 3. Pulmonary edema	Hypertension: 1. Systolic ≥ 160 mm Hg 2. Diastolic ≥ 110 mm Hg 3. Two readings ≥ 6 hr apart Proteinuria: 1. New onset, *or* 2. 3–4+ dip 3. ≥ 5 g in 24-hr urine
Eclampsia	Grand mal seizure(s) Fetal distress Placental abruption	Gestational hypertension with seizure that is responsive to initiation of MgSO$_4$ therapy
HELLP Syndrome (HELLP = Hemolysis, Elevated Liver enzymes and Low Platelet count)	Epigastric pain General malaise Abnormal coagulation profile (low fibrinogen prolonged prothrombin time, prolonged partial prothrombin time)	Hemolysis of red blood cells Elevated liver enzymes (AST, ALT, LDH) Low platelets (< 100,000)

Sources: ACOG, 2001a, 2002; Varney, Kriebs, & Gegor, 2004.

- Evaluate for factors associated with preeclampsia
  - Nulliparity
  - African American or Asian race
  - Prior history of preeclampsia
  - Family history of hypertension or preeclampsia
  - Obesity
  - Maternal age < 18 years or > 35 years
  - Multi-fetal gestation
  - New partner
    - Exposure to partner's sperm for 6 months or more may protect against preeclampsia
    - Maternal immunologic recognition of partner's sperm
  - Hydatidiform mole
  - Fetal hydrops
  - Preexisting medical disorders
    - Essential hypertension
    - Diabetes mellitus
    - Collagen vascular disease
    - Renal vascular disease
    - Antiphospholipid disease
    - Cardiovascular disease
    - Thrombophilias
    - Sickle cell disease
    - Dyslipidemia
- Evaluate for chronic hypertension risk factors
  - Age > 35 years
  - Family history of chronic or gestational hypertension
- Social factors that may contribute to gestational hypertension
  - Poor nutrition
  - Tobacco use
  - Alcohol use
  - Excessive sodium intake
  - Current vasoactive drug use
    - Nasal decongestants
    - Cocaine
- Presence, onset, and durations of symptoms

Physical Examination: Components of the Physical Exam to Consider

- Vital signs, including BP and weight
- Weight: Patterns of gain

- BP evaluation
  - Two occasions, more than 6 hours apart
  - Allow a "rest" period after the following circumstances:
    - Anxiety
    - Pain
    - Smoking
    - Exercise
  - Equipment of correct size should be used
  - Sitting position used for each BP
  - Arm should be supported at the level of the heart
- Evaluation of extremities
  - Presence or absence of edema
  - Deep tendon reflexes
- Abdominal examination
  - Fundal height for evaluation of fetal growth
  - Liver margins
  - Epigastric pain
- Fundoscopic examination
  - Papilledema
  - Vessel narrowing
- Monitor pulmonary status

Clinical Impression: Differential Diagnoses to Consider (ICD9Data.com, 2012)

- Gestational hypertension
  - Preeclampsia, mild
  - Preeclampsia, severe
- Transient hypertension
- Essential hypertension
- Pregnancy-induced hypertension (PIH) superimposed on chronic hypertension
- HELLP syndrome
- Elevated BP without diagnosis of hypertension

Diagnostic Testing: Diagnostic Tests and Procedures to Consider

- Baseline preeclampsia laboratory testing for women with chronic hypertension and those at high risk
- Note: Normal ranges may vary by laboratory
  - Urine dipstick for protein

- Hematocrit (normal range: 10.5–14 g/dL)
- Platelet count (normal range: 130,000–400,000/mL)
- Liver function tests
  - Aspartate aminotransferase (AST/SGOT) (normal range: 0–35 IU/L)
  - Alanine aminotransferase (ALT/SGPT) (normal range: 5–35 IU/L)
  - Lactate dehydrogenase (LDH) (normal range: 0–250 IU/L)
- Coagulation studies
  - Fibrinogen
  - Prothrombin time (PT), partial thromboplastin time (PTT)
- Renal function tests
  - Serum uric acid (normal range: 1.2–4.5 mg/dL)
  - Serum albumin (normal range: 2.5–4.5 g/dL)
  - Serum creatinine (normal range: 1.0 mg/dL)
  - Blood urea nitrogen (BUN) (normal range: 7–25 mg/dL)
  - 24-hour urine for protein and creatinine
    - Initiate based on symptoms, clinical presentation, or when dip urinalysis indicates protein
    - Analysis of the first 4 hours for protein-to-creatinine ratio of a 24-hour collection
    - Reasonable rule-out test for proteinuria > 0.3g/day (Côté et al., 2008)
- Fetal evaluation
  - Fetal kick counts daily
  - NST and BPP: At diagnosis
  - Frequency determined by clinical condition and gestational age
    - Biweekly is the typical schedule
    - Amniotic fluid index (AFI) # (5 cm)
    - EFW: Should be within the 10th percentile for gestational age (GA)
  - Immediately with change in maternal condition (National Heart, Lung, and Blood Institute, 2000)
- Ultrasound
  - At diagnosis

- Schedule as indicated by maternal and fetal condition
  - Amniotic fluid index
  - Fetal growth evaluation

Providing Treatment: Therapeutic Measures to Consider

- For women at moderate to high risk for preeclampsia
  - Increase calcium intake (Sibai & Cunningham, 2009): 1500–2000 mg daily
  - Low-dose aspirin therapy (Bujold et al., 2010)
    - Start before 16 weeks' gestation
    - 50–150 mg daily
    - Reduces risk of FGR, preterm birth, and hypertension
    - Benefits of reducing preeclampsia outweigh risk in pregnancy
- Consider hospitalization
  - Upon initial diagnosis to determine severity and progression
  - If restricted activity is not possible at home
  - If the client shows progressive signs and symptoms
- Medications
  - Sustained BP > 160 mm Hg systolic
  - Sustained BP > 105 mm Hg diastolic
- Outpatient: Methyldopa (Aldomet) (King & Brucker, 2011)
  - Pregnancy Category B
  - Chronic hypertension
  - Longest safety record in pregnancy
- Inpatient
  - Hydralazine
    - 5 mg IV or 10 mg IM
    - Repeat at 20-minute intervals until BP is stable
    - Repeat as needed approximately every 3 hours
    - Change medication if no response occurs by dosing of 20–30 mg
  - Labetalol
    - ⚠ Do not use in women with asthma or congestive heart failure

- ◆ 20 mg IV bolus
- ◆ May give 40 mg IV in 10 minutes, followed by
  - ➤ 80 mg IV for two doses
  - ➤ Maximum dose 220 mg
- ◆ Pregnancy Category C
  - ■ Nifedipine
    - ◆ 10 mg PO
    - ◆ Repeat in 30 minutes
- MgSO₄ therapy (Leeman, Dresang, & Fontaine, 2006)
  - ■ 4 to 6 g bolus, slow IV
  - ■ Followed by 2 g/hr IV or 5 g 50% MgSO₄ IM every 4 hours
  - ■ Titrated to renal output and reflexes
  - ■ Monitor
    - ◆ BP
    - ◆ Therapeutic MgSO₄ level 5 4–7 mg/dL
    - ◆ Monitor reflexes
    - ◆ Intake and output
  - ■ Calcium gluconate at bedside
- Avoid
  - ■ Angiotensin-converting enzyme inhibitors
  - ■ Angiotensin II receptor agonists
  - ■ Atenolol (beta blocker)
  - ■ Thiazide diuretics
- Perform labor induction or cesarean section if no improvement occurs or the client's condition worsens

Providing Treatment: Complementary and Alternative Measures to Consider

(Romm, 2010)

- Garlic
  - ■ Inhibits platelet aggregation and inflammation
  - ■ 800 mg daily
  - ■ Discontinue 3 weeks before due date
- Cramp bark tincture
- Hawthorn berry tincture
  - ■ Best for chronic hypertension
  - ■ Infusion: one cup daily
  - ■ Tincture: 15 drops TID

- Chlorophyll liquid or capsules
- Stress reduction techniques: Breathing techniques, yoga, guided imagery, journaling

Providing Support: Education and Support Measures to Consider

- Discussion with client and family regarding the following topics:
  - ■ Diagnosis
  - ■ Treatment options and recommendations
- Home care: preeclampsia
  - ■ Adequate diet
  - ■ Rest periods throughout the day
  - ■ Daily fetal movement counting
  - ■ Home BP monitoring
  - ■ Home urine protein by dipstick
  - ■ Daily weights
  - ■ Call the healthcare provider in the event of elevating BP, proteinuria, significant weight increase, or decreased fetal movement
  - ■ Return to the provider's office every 2 to 3 days
  - ■ Hospitalization or induction if symptoms worsen
- Potential need for the following measures:
  - ■ Hospitalization or more frequent prenatal visits
  - ■ OB/GYN consultation/referral
  - ■ Change in planned location for birth
  - ■ Pediatric care at birth
  - ■ Newborn special care after birth
- ⚠ Indications for immediate care
  - ■ Epigastric pain
  - ■ Visual disturbance
  - ■ Severe headache unrelieved by acetaminophen

Follow-up Care: Follow-up Measures to Consider

- Document
  - ■ List parameters for consultation and referral
  - ■ Update the plan of care weekly or as indicated
- Continued assessment for preeclampsia in women with the following conditions:
  - ■ Gestational hypertension
  - ■ Chronic hypertension

- Increased frequency of office visits (biweekly)
  - Fetal surveillance testing
  - Maternal evaluation/laboratory values
  - Consider hospitalization in the following circumstances:
    - Inability of the mother to follow the provider's recommendations
    - Signs and symptoms indicating a worsening condition
- Indications for delivery
  - Persistent or severe headache
  - Persistent or severe abdominal pain
  - Abnormal liver function tests
  - Rising serum creatinine
  - Thrombocytopenia
  - Pulmonary edema
  - Eclampsia
  - Abruptio placentae
  - Oligohydramnios
  - Nonreassuring NST
  - FGR noted by ultrasound
  - Abnormal biophysical profile

Multidisciplinary Practice: Consider Consultation, Collaboration, or Referral

- OB/GYN services
  - For chronic hypertension in pregnancy
  - With diagnosis or suspicion of preeclampsia or gestational hypertension
  - Signs and symptoms of worsening condition
  - For any indications for delivery (see the preceding section)
- For diagnosis or treatment outside the midwife's scope of practice

CARE OF THE PREGNANT WOMAN WITH INADEQUATE WEIGHT GAIN

Key Clinical Information

Optimal weight gain during pregnancy is based on the woman's prepregnant BMI and age (see "A Nutritional Primer"). Inadequate weight gain may indicate a number of medical problems. More commonly, however, inadequate nutrition is due to psychosocial issues, such as poverty, substance abuse, mental illness, or simply poor food choices. Women with a history of anorexia or bulimia may have difficulty maintaining adequate intake to support growth of a healthy baby. Overweight women may require fewer calories during pregnancy while still demonstrating an adequate fundal growth pattern. Weight gain is a gross marker for the nutritional status of the mother, and it is a factor in body image issues for many women. A woman's body undergoes remarkable changes during pregnancy; she should be helped to appreciate the beauty of such changes. The focus of diet counseling should be on healthy food choices from a variety of whole foods in appropriate portions. In most cases, appropriate weight gain follows from a nutritious diet.

Client History and Chart Review: Components of the History to Consider

- Age of client
- Gestational age
- Review of gestational dating parameters
- Review of BMI and weight gain pattern to date
- Nutritional assessment; see "A Nutritional Primer"
  - 24-hour diet recall
  - Appetite, taste for food
  - Preferred diet and portion size
  - Food sources available
- Assessment for eating disorders
  - Use of enemas and laxatives
  - Eating in secret
  - Binge eating
  - Self-induced vomiting after eating
- Assessment for depression
- Physical health issues
  - Activity level and general metabolic rate
  - Involvement in athletics and exercise frequency
  - Presence of symptoms
    - Nausea and vomiting
    - Constipation, diarrhea

- ◆ Abdominal pain
- ◆ Pica
- Prior health history
  - Presence of maternal illness or infection
  - Gastrointestinal and malabsorption disorders
  - Bariatric surgery
  - Hyperthyroidism
  - Hepatitis
  - Anemia
  - Malnutrition
  - Anorexia or bulimia
- Emotional and spiritual health issues
  - Family and personal support for pregnancy
    - ◆ Education level
    - ◆ Social living conditions and financial resources
    - ◆ Physical abuse
  - Stress levels and coping skills: Physical response to stress
  - Other mental health issues
- Substance abuse

Physical Examination: Components of the Physical Exam to Consider

- Vital signs, including height and weight
- BMI and weight distribution
  - Adult BMI charts for women > 18 years
  - Adolescent BMI-for-age charts for women < 18 years (Groth, 2007)
- Abdominal examination
  - Fundal height
    - ◆ For gestation
    - ◆ Fundal height growth curve
  - Bowel sounds
  - Palpation of abdomen
- Dental/oral evaluation
  - Caries
  - Abscess
- Evaluation of other symptoms

Clinical Impression: Differential Diagnoses to Consider (ICD9Data.com, 2012)

- Short maternal stature, constitutional
- Small-for-gestational-age baby

- Intrauterine fetal growth restriction
- Malnutrition, secondary to conditions such as the following:
  - Homelessness
  - Poverty
  - Substance abuse
  - Physical abuse
    - ◆ Anorexia nervosa
    - ◆ Bulimia
  - Mental illness

Diagnostic Testing: Diagnostic Tests and Procedures to Consider

- Calculate the BMI-specific recommended weight gain (see "A Nutritional Primer")
- Laboratory testing
  - Toxicology if drug use suspected
  - Thyroid-stimulating hormone
  - Serum albumin
  - Hepatitis screen
- Fetal kick counts
- Ultrasound for evaluation of the following:
  - Gestational age
  - Interval fetal growth
  - Evidence of FGR
  - Amniotic fluid index

Providing Treatment: Therapeutic Measures to Consider

- Prenatal vitamin and mineral supplement PO once daily
- Diet and nutrition counseling
  - Normal-weight women need 300 extra calories per day while pregnant
  - Daily calorie intake may range from 1800 cal/day to 2400 cal/day, depending on the woman's BMI
  - Explore suitable food choices
    - ◆ Adequate protein, fat, and carbohydrates
    - ◆ 🌐 Culturally acceptable foods
    - ◆ Use of additional dietary supplements as needed

- Consider hospitalization in the following circumstances:
  - Malnutrition
  - Anorexia or bulimia
  - Significant mental illness

Providing Treatment: Complementary and Alternative Measures to Consider

- Dietary supplements
  - Smoothies
  - Energy bars
- Herbal appetite stimulants
  - May be combined for flavor and effectiveness
  - Alfalfa, 500 mg daily (avoid with lupus or allergies to pollen)
  - Dandelion root tea, one cup BID (avoid with history of gallstones)
  - Hops tea, one to two cups daily
  - Chamomile tea, one to two cups daily

Providing Support: Education and Support Measures to Consider

- Provide information about the following topics:
  - Weight gain and fetal growth pattern
  - Maternal and fetal nutrient needs from the maternal diet
  - Examples of high-calorie, nutrient-dense foods
  - Anticipated weight gain for gestation
    - FGR infants
    - Constitutionally small infants
- Fetal kick counts
- Warning signs
  - ⚠ Decreased fetal motion
  - PIH signs and symptoms
- Potential effect on the following issues:
  - Planned location for birth
  - Need for pediatric care at birth
- Importance of the following considerations:
  - Fundal/fetal growth over weight gain
  - Maternal and fetal well-being
  - Dietary needs during pregnancy
    - Small frequent meals

- Balanced selection of food choices
- Adequate caloric intake
- Excessive or rapid weight gain risks
  - Increased maternal insulin resistance
  - Postpartum or future obesity
- Provide support
  - Develop the plan of care with the client
  - Address client and family concerns

Follow-up Care: Follow-up Measures to Consider

- Document
- Reevaluate weekly or biweekly
  - Diet review
  - Interval fetal growth
  - Signs and symptoms of PIH
- Address client concerns and preferences
  - Nutritional counseling
  - Emotional issues
- Parameters for consultation or referral

Multidisciplinary Practice: Consider Consultation, Collaboration, or Referral

- Nutritional counseling: Refer to a dietician as needed
- Social services referral
  - Enroll the family in a supplemental nutrition program, such as the WIC program
  - Refer to local food assistance programs
- Obstetric/pediatric services
  - For persistent poor weight gain accompanied by the following:
    - Delayed fetal growth
    - PIH
  - For transfer of care or change planned location of birth
- Medical services
  - Evidence of malnutrition
  - Suspected or documented mental health issues
  - Suspected or documented medical illness
- For diagnosis or treatment outside the midwife's scope of practice

CARE OF THE PREGNANT WOMAN WHO IS OBESE

Key Clinical Information

Obesity is defined as a body mass index (BMI) measurement of 30 or greater. Approximately one in four reproductive-age women in the United States currently meets the BMI criterion for obesity. There is an ethnic disparity in obesity rates, however, with this condition having a prevalence of 49% in non-Hispanic black women, 39% in Mexican American women, and 31% in non-Hispanic white women (March of Dimes, 2010).

Obesity contributes to reproductive health problems such as infertility, miscarriage, preeclampsia, gestational diabetes, thromboembolic disorders, perinatal depression, large-for-gestational-age fetus, excessive pregnancy weight, labor induction, and operative birth. Maternal obesity also increases the risk of preterm birth due to medical complications, stillbirth, neural tube defects, and birth injury. Weight gain during pregnancy is important, even in obese women (ACOG, 2005). In fact, assisting obese women achieve a healthy amount of weight gain through diet and lifestyle modification is an important goal during prenatal care to reduce the risk of complications during delivery and postpartum. Babies born to obese women have an increased risk of childhood obesity (March of Dimes, 2010). Postpartum, obese women have a higher risk for postpartum hemorrhage and delayed lactogenesis.

Client History and Chart Review: Components of the History to Consider

- Current gestational age
- GP TPAL
- Prior maternity history
  - Weight gain pattern in prior pregnancies and their outcomes
  - Newborn weight
  - Gestational diabetes
  - Preeclampsia or hypertension

- Health history
  - Hypertension
  - Heart disease
  - Lipid disorders
  - Depression
- Family members and obesity
- Diet assessment
- Food resources assessment
- Activity assessment
- Screening for depression: The Edinburgh Depression Scale is valid for use in pregnancy
- Additional risk factors for gestational diabetes (see "Care of the Pregnant Woman with Gestational Diabetes")

Physical Examination: Components of the Physical Exam to Consider

- Blood pressure with appropriate-size cuff
- Weight and height: Make an accurate BMI determination
- Maternal skin and adipose tissue
  - Abdominal pannus
  - Skin fold disorders
    - ◆ Intertrigo
    - ◆ Candidosis
- Uterine size
- Routine prenatal visit exam per gestational age

Clinical Impression: Differential Diagnoses to Consider (ICD9Data.com, 2012)

- BMI between 30 and 39
- BMI of 40 or higher

Diagnostic Testing: Diagnostic Tests and Procedures to Consider

- Ultrasound for verification of uterine size and gestational age: Periodic ultrasound may be needed to monitor serial uterine growth
- One-hour OGTT at first visit; repeat at 24 to 28 weeks' gestation if normal on the first visit
- Assess urine dip for glucose and protein at every visit due to the increased risk for gestational diabetes and preeclampsia in the women who is obese

Providing Treatment: Therapeutic Measures to Consider

- Nutritional counseling and support
  - Gain 11–20 lb in pregnancy
  - Increase intake of fruits, vegetables, and complex carbohydrates
  - Reduce intake of refined carbohydrates and processed foods
  - Reduce intake of fats, sugar, and high-glycemic-index foods such as peas, potatoes, corn, and rice
  - Advise the woman not to lose weight in pregnancy
- Provide prescription for increased activity
  - Walking 30 minutes per day and increasing the amount of time devoted to this activity; can be divided into segments each day
  - Low-impact aerobics
  - Water aerobics
  - Yoga
- Offer anomaly screening by ultrasound and serum screening
- Teach signs and symptoms of deep venous thrombosis (DVT)
- Birth place discussion: The increased risks associated with obesity should be considered when determining environment for birth
- Anesthesia consult in labor for vaginal birth after cesarean (VBAC) or induction

Providing Treatment: Complementary and Alternative Measures to Consider

Take the focus off the number on the scale:

- Validate the woman as a beautiful person
- Reinforce her healthy lifestyle choices
- Acknowledge the difficulty of making change

Providing Support: Education and Support Measures to Consider

- Use appropriate language such as the actual BMI number instead of broader terms such as "morbid obesity"

- Be sensitive to providing respectful and honest care, as obese women often encounter judgmental attitudes from healthcare providers (Nyman, Prebensen, & Flensner, 2010)
- Instruct the client about the benefits of increased activity
- Provide logs in which she can record her daily activity
- Provide positive feedback for diet and activity changes
- Encourage family involvement and social support

Follow-up Care: Follow-up Measures to Consider

- Document (Jevitt, 2009)
  - BMI and serial weight and fundal heights
  - Weight gain advised
  - Glucose screening results
  - Anomaly serum screening offered
  - Anomaly screening by ultrasound offered
  - Nutritional counseling and referrals
  - Teaching done on signs and symptoms of DVT
- Plan for postpartum weight loss
- Return for care
  - Per routine for prenatal care
  - More frequently for support as needed
  - Individualized based on clinical presentation

Multidisciplinary Practice: Consider Consultation, Collaboration, or Referral

- Nutritional services for ongoing nutritional assessment and counseling
- Lactation consultant for instruction and support
- Consult with obstetrical/perinatal services
  - Abnormal uterine growth
  - Elevated blood pressure
  - Elevated glucose testing results
  - Abnormal genetic screening
- For diagnosis or treatment outside the midwife's scope of practice

CARE OF THE PREGNANT WOMAN EXPOSED TO PARVOVIRUS (FIFTH DISEASE)

Key Clinical Information

Human parvovirus B19 causes erythema infectiosum, also known as fifth disease. It is spread by hand-to-mouth contact and by respiratory secretions, most often in the springtime. Viremia occurs 4 to 14 days after inoculation and may last several days (Cunningham et al., 2010). Symptoms may include a lacy rash on the face, trunk, and extremities. In addition, the hand, wrist, and knee joints may swell. Elementary teachers and women with elementary school–aged children are more prone to exposure. Fortunately, most women contract parvovirus as children and are not at risk for primary infection during pregnancy. Parvovirus infection during pregnancy is considered to pose a low risk for fetal morbidity; however, it may result in fetal hydrops, aplastic anemia, or fetal growth restriction (FGR), especially if infection occurs in the first half of pregnancy (CDC, 2005).

Client History and Chart Review: Components of the History to Consider

- Current gestational age
- Blood type and Rh
- Rubella and rubeola titers
- Employment history
- History of recent outbreak with close contact
  - School teachers
  - Healthcare workers
  - Woman with school-aged child
- Symptoms of parvovirus infection
  - Rash
  - Fever
  - Malaise
  - Myalgia, arthralgia

Physical Examination: Components of the Physical Exam to Consider

- Vital signs, including temperature
- Routine prenatal surveillance

- Evaluate for the following conditions:
  - Flulike symptoms
    - Fever
    - Headache
  - Rash
    - Diffuse maculopapular rash
    - May appear on the face, trunk, and extremities
    - Occurs several days after fever
    - Resolves in 7–10 days
  - Joint and muscle pain, especially in the hands, wrists, and knees
- Some patients may be asymptomatic

Clinical Impression: Differential Diagnoses to Consider (ICD9Data.com, 2012)

- Fifth disease, erythema infectiosum, parvovirus B19
- Other viral exanthema
- Allergic rash

Diagnostic Testing: Diagnostic Tests and Procedures to Consider

- Serologic testing for parvovirus B19
  - Indications
    - Post-exposure
    - Positive clinical signs and symptoms
    - Fetal nonimmune hydrops
  - Parvovirus B19 IgM and IgG
    - Positive IgM indicates recent infection
    - Positive IgG indicates current immunity; if the woman is not immune, repeat the test in 3–4 weeks
- Ultrasound every 2 weeks for those individuals who test positive for parvovirus infection
  - Fetal cardiac, spleen, and liver evaluation
  - Fetal hydrops

Providing Treatment: Therapeutic Measures to Consider

No treatment for parvovirus B19 infection is available. However, heightened fetal surveillance is recommended if seroconversion occurs.

Providing Treatment: Complementary and Alternative Measures to Consider

In women with possible exposure to parvovirus B19, consider the following measures:

- Herbs for immune support: Astragalus
- Stress reduction techniques: Breathing techniques, yoga, guided imagery, journaling

Providing Support: Education and Support Measures to Consider

- Provide reassurance: Most adults are immune to the virus
- Explain the screening and management plan
- Identify the warning signs to report
  - Rash
  - Decreased fetal movement
- Note the potential for fetal compromise with infection
  - May have no effect
  - Spontaneous abortion (SAB) in first trimester
  - Fetal death in second trimester (3–6 weeks post maternal infection)
  - Nonimmune hydrops
  - Severe anemia
  - Viral-induced cardiomyopathy
- Parvovirus B19 is not associated with birth defects

Follow-up Care: Follow-up Measures to Consider

(Hunt & Hunt, 2010)

- Document
- Testing
  - Positive IgG: Immune, no further testing is necessary
  - Negative IgG: Past or current infection; repeat testing in 3–4 weeks
- Return for care
  - In 2–3 weeks post-exposure
  - At the onset of signs or symptoms
- Mother with acute illness
  - Follow for hydrops: Biweekly ultrasound for 12 weeks
  - Provide emotional support

Multidisciplinary Practice: Consider Consultation, Collaboration, or Referral

- OB/GYN services
  - Maternal infection with parvovirus B19
  - Fetus with evidence of the following conditions:
    - Cardiomyopathy
    - Hydrops
    - Anemia
- For diagnosis or treatment outside the midwife's scope of practice

CARE OF THE PREGNANT WOMAN WITH PRURITIC URTICARIAL PAPULES AND PLAQUES OF PREGNANCY

Key Clinical Information

Pruritic urticarial papules and plaques of pregnancy (PUPPP) is a form of urticaria that most commonly appears in the third trimester. These pruritic dermatoses typically erupt on the abdomen but may extend to the torso and extremities (Brzoza, Kasperska-Zajac, Oles, & Rogala, 2007). The condition generally resolves within 6 weeks after the birth of the infant. There are no systemic disorders associated with PUPPP; therefore treatment is aimed at relieving the symptoms, which can range from mild to severe in nature.

Client History and Chart Review: Components of the History to Consider

- Gestational age
  - Most often primipara
  - Third trimester
- Onset, duration, and severity of symptoms
  - Pruritic papules often begin in striae (Brzoza et al., 2007)
    - May have small vesicles
    - Surrounded by narrow, pale halo
    - Severe itching
  - Pattern of spread
    - Abdomen and striae
    - Periumbilical area not involved
    - Trunk and limbs
    - Face, palms, and soles spared

- Other associated signs and symptoms
- Presence of allergies
  - Medications
  - Exposure to topical irritants
- Exposure to viral infections: Provide immune titers as indicated
- Self-help remedies and their effects

Physical Examination: Components of the Physical Exam to Consider

- Vital signs, including temperature
- Abdominal distention: Striae gravidarum
- Location and appearance of lesions
  - Erythematous, edematous papules
  - Urticarial plaques
  - Papulovesicular lesions
- Evaluate as needed for signs related to other differential diagnoses

Clinical Impression: Differential Diagnoses to Consider (ICD9Data.com, 2012)

- PUPPP
- Scabies
- Allergic dermatitis
  - Drug or food reaction
  - Poison ivy
- Impetigo
- Viral exanthema
- Herpes gestationis
- Erythema multiform
- Cholestasis of pregnancy

Diagnostic Testing: Diagnostic Tests and Procedures to Consider

- Culture of vesicular lesions
  - Herpes
  - Impetigo
  - Scabies skin prep
- Immune titers as needed
  - Rubella
  - Rubeola
  - Varicella

- Liver function tests to evaluate for cholestasis
  - Alkaline phosphatase
  - Gamma-glutamyl transferase

Providing Treatment: Therapeutic Measures to Consider

- Topical antipruritic lotions
  - Calamine or Caladryl (over-the-counter preparations)
  - Doxepin HCl 5% cream (Pregnancy Category B)
- Oral antihistamines
  - Diphenhydramine HCl (Benadryl)
    - 25–50 mg every 4–6 hours
    - Pregnancy Category B in third trimester
  - Loratadine (Claritin)
    - 10 mg daily
    - Pregnancy Category B in third trimester
  - Cetirizine HCl (Zyrtec)
    - 5–10 mg daily
    - Pregnancy Category B in third trimester
  - Hydroxyzine (Atarax)
    - 25–100 mg PO daily
    - Pregnancy Category C
- Topical corticosteroids
  - Pregnancy Category C
  - Rule out viral cause before using the following medications:
    - Alclometasone dipropionate 0.05%
    - Aclovate cream or ointment
    - Hydrocortisone 1%
    - Cortisporin cream
    - Hytone cream, lotion, or ointment
    - Triamcinolone acetonide 0.025%, 0.1%, or 0.5%
    - Aristocort cream
    - Kenalog cream, lotion, or ointment
- Oral steroid therapy
  - Prednisone 0.5–1 mg/kg/day PO
    - Use the minimum effective dose
    - Taper off doses when symptoms abate
  - Pregnancy Category B

- Use with caution in women with the following conditions:
  - Gestational diabetes
  - Hypertension
- Topical relief of itching
  - Colloidal oatmeal baths
  - Calendula cream or calendula-infused oil
  - Olive oil
  - Aloe gel

Providing Treatment: Complementary and Alternative Measures to Consider

(Romm, 2010)

- Topical relief of itching
  - Chamomile cream
  - Gotu kola ointment
  - Chinese skullcap
  - St. John's wort extract
- Internal use
  - Yellow dock root tea
  - Dried nettle leaf tea

Providing Support: Education and Support Measures to Consider

- PUPPP not associated with fetal jeopardy
- Instructions to call the healthcare provider if symptoms persist or worsen
- Address client concerns
- Treatment options
- Medication instructions
  - Topical steroids
    - Apply a thin film only
    - Do not cover or occlude
    - May be systemically absorbed
  - Oral steroids
    - Take as directed
    - Do not stop suddenly

Follow-up Care: Follow-up Measures to Consider

- Document
- Return for care

- Per routine for prenatal care
- If symptoms worsen or additional symptoms develop

Multidisciplinary Practice: Consider Consultation, Collaboration, or Referral

- Dermatology services
- For diagnosis or treatment outside the midwife's scope of practice

CARE OF THE PREGNANT WOMAN WHO IS RH NEGATIVE

Key Clinical Information

Rh alloimmunization or ABO incompatibility can have devastating effects on both mother and baby. Infants are at risk when fetomaternal bleeding initiates the process of Rh or ABO incompatibility or if the mother became sensitized previously after blood transfusion. This outcome can result when an Rh-positive infant is born to an Rh-negative mother, an infant with type A or B blood is born to a mother with type O blood, an infant with type B or AB blood is born to a mother with type A blood, or an infant with type A or AB blood is born to a mother with type B blood. ABO incompatibility can lead to hemolytic disease in the newborn accompanied by jaundice; the latter condition is usually successfully treated with phototherapy.

Often, the baby who is being carried when the fetomaternal bleeding occurs does not have a problem, but instead the mother becomes sensitized. This problem then manifests itself in a subsequent pregnancy when maternal antibodies attack the fetal blood. Alloimmunization can result in fetal hydrops, congestive heart failure, and fetal anemia. Adherence to established guidelines in the treatment of the Rh-negative mother significantly decreases the incidence of fetal hemolytic disease and its sequelae (ACOG, 1999).

Client History and Chart Review: Components of the History to Consider

- Gestational age
- Previous blood transfusions

- Prior pregnancy history
  - Unexplained fetal losses
  - Stillbirth
  - Miscarriage
- Ectopic pregnancy
- Termination of pregnancy at more than 8 weeks since last menstrual period
- Previous Rh immune globulin injection
- Knowledge of own blood type and the pathophysiology of the incompatibility

Physical Examination: Components of the Physical Exam to Consider

Routine prenatal surveillance

Clinical Impression: Differential Diagnoses to Consider (ICD9Data.com, 2012)

- Rh-negative mother
- Rh-sensitized mother
- ABO-sensitized mother

Diagnostic Testing: Diagnostic Tests and Procedures to Consider

- Maternal: test at the first prenatal visit, and repeat at 24–28 weeks for Rh-negative mothers
  - Type and Rh factor
  - Antibody screen (indirect Coombs test)
  - Antibody identification for positive antibody screen
  - Early Rh immune globulin (RhIG) testing after amniocentesis or threatened SAB may give a positive titer at the 24- to 28-week screen
- Maternal test results
  - Titer < 1:8 anti-D suggests passive immunity from RhIG
  - Titer > 1:8 suggests active immunization due to Rh incompatibility
  - Rh(D)-negative or type O mother
    - ◆ Plan to obtain cord blood at birth for analysis
    - ◆ Maternal/newborn follow-up postpartum

Providing Treatment: Therapeutic Measures to Consider

(ACOG, 1999)

- RhIG is indicated for an unsensitized Rh-negative client in the following circumstances:
  - Amniocentesis
  - Chorionic villus sampling
  - External version
  - Trauma, such as a car accident
  - Placenta previa
  - Abruptio placentae
  - Fetal death
  - Multiple gestation
  - 28 weeks' gestation prophylaxis if the father of the baby is Rh positive or his Rh status is unknown
  - Accidental transfusion of Rh-positive blood to an Rh-negative person
- Give RhIG (Pregnancy Category C) in the following circumstances (Moise & Brecher, 2004):
  - Threatened or spontaneous miscarriage at later than 12 weeks' gestation: 50 or 300 mg IM
  - Procedures or trauma: 300 mg IM
  - 28- to 36-week prophylaxis: 300 mg IM with negative 28-week antibody screen
    - ◆ Consider redosing if pregnancy continues for longer than 12 weeks from the first dose
    - ◆ If paternity is certain and the father is Rh negative, antepartum prophylaxis is not needed (ACOG, 1999)
  - Postpartum: 300 mg IM or IV
    - ◆ Provide to an unsensitized Rh-negative mother with an Rh-positive infant
    - ◆ Give as soon as possible after birth, preferably within 72 hours postpartum
    - ◆ Can be given up to 28 days postpartum for some benefit
    - ◆ Adjust dose for large fetomaternal transfusion based on laboratory results
  - Intravenous RhIG is available as Rhophylac

- For women who refuse antenatal RhIG, perform an antibody screen (indirect Coombs test) every 4 weeks prenatally

Providing Treatment: Complementary and Alternative Measures to Consider

- Maintain a healthy pregnancy and placenta
  - Consume a well-balanced diet
  - Ensure adequate trace mineral intake
- Limit invasive procedures
- Avoid traumatic placental delivery

Providing Support: Education and Support Measures to Consider

Provide information about the following topics:

- Rh and blood type status
- Rh immune globulin
  - Prophylaxis and desired result
  - Potential risks with RhIG
    - Transfusion-type adverse reactions
    - Mercury sensitivity or reaction with RhoGAM
  - Potential risks without RhIG
    - Maternal sensitization
    - Fetal hydrops or other complications with future pregnancy
    - Difficulty of cross-matching blood for the woman in the future (e.g., after an accident or surgery)
    - Potential for jaundice in the infant due to Rh or ABO incompatibility

Follow-up Care: Follow-up Measures to Consider

- Document
  - Indication for RhIG
  - Rh-negative and antibody status
  - Client education, discussion, and preferences
- Observe for potential blood transfusion–type reactions
  - Warmth at injection site
  - Low-grade fever
  - Flushing

- Chest or lumbar pain
- Poor clotting
- If mother is Rh(D) negative or type O
  - Newborn
    - Type and Rh
    - Direct Coombs test
    - Bilirubin levels
  - Maternal testing postpartum
    - Type and Rh
    - Antibody screen (indirect Coombs test)
    - Antibody ID for positive antibody screen
    - Fetal red cell screen
- Kleihauer-Betke quantitative testing
  - Determine the volume of fetal blood in the maternal system and the dosage of RhIG to give to the mother
  - Performed when a high risk of fetomaternal hemorrhage exists
    - Previa
    - Abruption
    - Abdominal trauma
    - Hydrops
    - Sinusoidal fetal heart patterns
    - Unexplained fetal demise

Multidisciplinary Practice: Consider Consultation, Collaboration, or Referral

- OB/GYN or perinatology services
  - For Rh-negative mother with a positive antibody screen
  - Evidence of large fetomaternal bleed
  - Transfusion-type reactions
- For diagnosis or treatment outside the midwife's scope of practice

CARE OF THE PREGNANT WOMAN WITH SIZE–DATE DISCREPANCY

Key Clinical Information

Serial fundal height measurements during pregnancy provide a clinical estimation that, along with other parameters, is used to form a broad assessment of fetal growth. Discrepancies in uterine size and gestational age can be physiologic: Many infants are simply constitutionally small or large. Overweight and obese women may measure consistently larger for dates, which can reflect maternal adipose tissue rather than fetal weight. For other women, size–date discrepancy may signal a problem, with the most common causes including fetal growth restriction (FGR) and gestational diabetes mellitus (GDM). Increased fetal surveillance and attention to maternal health help to prevent over- or under-intervention when fetal size–date discrepancy is noted.

Client History and Chart Review: Components of the History to Consider

(Cunningham et al., 2010)

- GP TPAL
- Review accuracy of last menstrual period and estimated date of confinement (EDC—the "due date")
- Verify gestational age
  - Estimated date of conception
  - Uterine size at first visit
  - Date of quickening
  - Early ultrasound report
- Pregnancy history
  - Review past and current fundal growth curve
  - Hypertension
  - Preeclampsia
  - Gestational diabetes
  - Birth weights of prior infants
- Social history
  - Diet and weight gain pattern
  - Maternal activity patterns
  - Tobacco, alcohol, or drug use
  - Poverty
  - Psychosocial factors
    - Stress
    - Mental illness
    - Abuse
- Family history
  - Personal or family history of diabetes
  - Hypertension
  - Other preexisting disease
  - Ethnic norm for fetal weight

- Review of systems
  - Shortness of breath, palpitations
  - Signs or symptoms of illness
  - Fetal activity

Physical Examination: Components of the Physical Exam to Consider

- Vital signs, including BP and BMI
- Weight gain/loss and pattern
- General appearance and well-being
- Palpation of thyroid
- Cardiopulmonary evaluation
- Abdominal examination
  - Fundal height
  - Interval growth
  - Fetal lie
  - Fetal heart rate (FHR)
- Extremities
  - Reflexes
  - Edema
  - Physical evidence of substance abuse
- Pelvic examination
  - Station of presenting part
  - Evidence of ROM

Clinical Impression: Differential Diagnoses to Consider (ICD9Data.com, 2012)

- Poor fetal growth affecting management of the mother
- Excessive fetal growth affecting management of the mother
- Small-for-dates fetus
  - Fetal growth restriction
  - Small for gestational age (SGA)
  - Constitutionally small infant
  - Oligohydramnios
- Congenital malformations
- Large-for-dates fetus
  - Large for gestational age (LGA)
  - Gestational or maternal diabetes
  - Multiple pregnancy
  - Polyhydramnios
  - Constitutionally large infant
  - Fibroid uterus

- Symmetric versus asymmetric FGR secondary to the following conditions:
  - Hypertension
  - Underlying maternal disease or infection
  - Poor nutrition

Diagnostic Testing: Diagnostic Tests and Procedures to Consider

- Dip urinalysis
- Urine toxicology
- Diabetes screen
- Maternal antiphospholipid antibody testing
- Maternal drug screen
- Symmetric FGR
- Fetal karyotype
- Titers for the following infections:
  - Toxoplasmosis
  - Cytomegalovirus
  - Herpes virus
- Preeclampsia laboratory profile
- Ultrasound evaluation
  - Verify singleton versus multiple pregnancy
  - Confirm estimated date of birth (EDB) by ultrasound parameters
  - Fetal anomaly study
  - Fetal growth: May be done serially
    - Schedule at least 3 weeks apart
    - Abdominal circumference: Decreased in asymmetric FGR
  - Amniotic fluid index (AFI) for oligohydramnios or polyhydramnios
  - Placenta previa
  - Chronic placental abruption
  - Presence of uterine fibroids
- 🕿 Ultrasound evaluation for FGR
  - Confirm EDB by ultrasound parameters
  - Fetal anomaly study
  - Fetal growth: May be done serially
    - Schedule at 2–3 weeks apart
    - Abdominal circumference: Decreased in asymmetric FGR
  - AFI for oligodydramnios or polyhydramnios
  - Placenta previa

- Chronic placental abruption
- Presence of uterine fibroids
- Fetal surveillance begins as early as FGR is suspected
  - Weekly or biweekly non-stress test (NST), biophysical profile (BPP)
  - Consider oxytocin challenge test (OCT) or contraction stress test (CST) if NST is nonreactive
- Weekly or biweekly AFI: normal range > 6
- LGA/macrosomia
  - Ultrasound evaluation
    - Poor diagnostic power for estimated fetal weight (EFW) and macrosomia
    - Accurate approximately one-third of the time (Wagner, 2011)
  - Clinician palpation of EFW is more accurate than ultrasound
  - A multiparous woman's perception of fetal size is more accurate than ultrasound (Campaigne & Conway, 2007)
- LGA/polyhydramnios
  - Ultrasound evaluation

Providing Treatment: Therapeutic Measures to Consider

- Treat underlying medical condition(s)
  - Preeclampsia
  - Gestational diabetes
  - Infection
  - Anemia
- Substance abuse treatment
- 🕿 FGR
  - Decrease maternal activity
  - Consume a high-quality diet
  - Avoid substances that may affect placental efficiency, such as smoking or illegal drug use
  - Encourage the left lateral position to enhance uteroplacental blood flow
  - Ensure adequate nutrition and oxygenation
  - ⚠ Consider delivery if fetal compromise is evident

- LGA/macrosomia
  - Not an indication for induction (ACOG, 2000b; Suneet et al., 2005)
  - Not a contraindication for vaginal birth after cesarean (VBAC)
  - ⚠ Both ultrasound and clinical estimates of fetal weight are imprecise
  - 🔧 Cesarean may be considered in the following circumstances:
    - EFW > 5000 g in a nondiabetic mother
    - EFW > 4500 g in a diabetic mother
- LGA/polyhydramnios
  - Consider amnio-reduction of fluid (therapeutic amniocentesis)
  - Antacids for increased heartburn

Providing Treatment: Complementary and Alternative Measures to Consider

Alternative measures vary with condition causing the size/date discrepancy.

Providing Support: Education and Support Measures to Consider

- Provide information about the following topics:
  - Implications for continued care
  - Options for treatment
  - Parameters for intervention
- Nutritional counseling and surveillance as needed
- Potential for serial evaluation of fetal well-being
- Potential for change in location or providers for birth
- Provide support and reassurance
- Address client and family concerns

Follow-up Care: Follow-up Measures to Consider

- Document
  - Results of diagnostic testing
  - Discussions with client and family
  - Note findings with indications for consultation or referral
- Anticipated follow-up
  - Serial fetal assessment: Weekly or biweekly
  - Update plan weekly or as indicated by findings

- Assess nutritional intervention understanding and adherence
- Anticipate the need for birth before term in the presence of the following conditions:
  - Positive CST
  - Oligohydramnios
  - Ultrasound documentation of limited cranial growth
- LGA infant: Anticipate potential for shoulder dystocia
- Anticipate need for fetal/neonatal resuscitation

Multidisciplinary Practice: Consider Consultation, Collaboration, or Referral

- OB/GYN services
  - Prenatal consultation based on maternal and fetal condition
  - Documented FGR
  - Potential referral to high-risk obstetrics service
  - With induction
  - With anticipated LGA infant
  - As indicated or needed during labor and birth
- Pediatric services
  - Anticipated preterm infant
  - FGR
  - Maternal diabetes
  - Chronic maternal malnutrition
  - Anticipated newborn resuscitation
- Social services as indicated
  - Tobacco, drug, or alcohol use
  - Poor social support systems
  - WIC, food stamps, local food assistance
- For diagnosis or treatment outside the midwife's scope of practice

CARE OF THE PREGNANT WOMAN WITH TOXOPLASMOSIS INFECTION

Key Clinical Information

Acute primary maternal infection with toxoplasmosis puts the unborn baby at increased risk for congenital toxoplasmosis infection. Infection in pregnancy is more likely to be transmitted to the fetus as the pregnancy progresses toward term. The risk of congenital fetal toxoplasmosis infection rises from 15% in women who contract toxoplasmosis in the first trimester to 30% in women who develop this infection during the second trimester, and peaks at 60% during the last trimester (CDC, 2011c). Complications of maternal toxoplasmosis infection can include spontaneous abortion or miscarriage, fetal demise, fetal microcephaly, chorioretinitis, cerebral calcifications, and abnormalities of the cerebrospinal fluid. Because prevalence of this disease is low in the United States, however, routine screening for toxoplasmosis during pregnancy is not currently recommended (ACOG, 2000a). Preventive measures for pregnant women to employ are essential to protecting them and their children from infection.

Client History and Chart Review: Components of the History to Consider

- Gestational age
- Fetal activity
- Query regarding possible source of exposure
  - Cat feces, fur, and bedding
  - Raw or rare meat (primary source)
  - Soil or sand
  - Unwashed fruit or vegetables
  - Contaminated water or milk
- Onset, duration, and severity of symptoms
  - Fever
  - Exhaustion
  - Sore throat
  - Swollen lymph nodes
  - Other associated symptoms
- Most people infected are symptomatic

Physical Examination: Components of the Physical Exam to Consider

- Vital signs, including temperature
- Evaluation for lymphadenopathy
- Evaluation for liver margins
- Fundal height growth

Clinical Impression: Differential Diagnoses to Consider (ICD9Data.com, 2012)

- Toxoplasmosis
- Mononucleosis
- Influenza
- Other viral illnesses

Diagnostic Testing: Diagnostic Tests and Procedures to Consider

- Toxoplasmosis testing
  - Preconception as needed
  - Retest every trimester as needed
- Types of tests
  - IgG-Sabin-Feldman dye test
  - IgM-immunofluorescent antibody (IFA): If titers exceed 1:512, recent acute infection is likely
  - Possible exposure
    - IgG and IgM negative: no infection or previous exposure
    - IgG positive and IgM negative: previous infection/immunity
    - Both IgG and IgM positive: possible acute infection, repeat for rising titers
- Recheck IgM in 3 weeks: If titers are rising, acute infection is likely

Providing Treatment: Therapeutic Measures to Consider

Provide maternal therapy per the perinatologist's or obstetrician's orders

- Spiramycin
- Pyrimethamine, sulfadiazine, and folic acid

Providing Treatment: Complementary and Alternative Measures to Consider

- Immune support
  - Maintain a high-quality diet
  - Rest
  - Echinacea
- Astragalus tea, tincture, or capsule
- Emotional support and reassurance

Providing Support: Education and Support Measures to Consider

- Prevention measures (CDC, 2011c): Avoid the following:
  - Contact with cats, cat feces, and cat bedding
  - Travel during pregnancy to areas with endemic toxoplasmosis
  - Drinking untreated water
  - Handling raw meat whenever possible
  - Eating rare-cooked meat
    - Cook whole cuts of meat to 145 degrees
    - Cook ground meat to 160 degrees
    - Cook poultry to 165 degrees
  - Eating unwashed fruits and vegetables
- Recommended practices
  - Careful hand washing with soap and water
  - Use of gloves in the following situations:
    - Gardening
    - Cleaning litter or sandbox
    - Preparing raw meat
  - Clean surfaces after handling raw meat
- Information and discussion about the following topics:
  - Test results and diagnosis
  - Options for care
  - Recommendations for continued care
  - Optimal location for birth
  - Pediatric care for birth
  - Breastfeeding recommended

Follow-up Care: Follow-up Measures to Consider

- Document
- Positive maternal titer
  - Ultrasound at 20–22 weeks' gestation for fetal anomalies
  - Serial ultrasounds as indicated
  - Percutaneous umbilical blood sampling (PUBS) for fetal IgM and culture
  - Evaluation of the newborn for congenital infection
- Return for care
  - Per prenatal routine
  - Provide ongoing support

Multidisciplinary Practice: Consider Consultation, Collaboration, or Referral

- Diagnosis of acute toxoplasmosis—referral
  - Perinatology
  - Genetic counseling
  - Counseling or support group
- For diagnosis or treatment outside the midwife's scope of practice

CARE OF THE PREGNANT WOMAN WITH URINARY TRACT INFECTION

Key Clinical Information

The physiologic changes experienced by pregnancy enhance the risk of ascending urinary tract infection (UTI). Urinary tract infection during pregnancy can have a variety of presentations. Asymptomatic bacteriuria is common in pregnancy, and acute pyelonephritis occurs in as many as 30% of women with previously untreated asymptomatic bacteriuria (Johnson & Kim, 2011). Pyelonephritis is a serious complication for both the woman and her fetus, as it is associated with premature delivery and low-birth-weight infants. Simple cystitis can also occur during pregnancy and can be extremely painful. Renal calculi typically present with flank pain, accompanied by blood or leukocytes in the urine. UTIs can lead to renal damage, severe pain, and increased risk of preterm labor. The economic costs and impact on quality of life related to UTIs may be considerable.

Client History and Chart Review: Components of the History to Consider

- Gestational age
- Current symptoms
  - Onset, duration, and severity
  - Dysuria, urgency, frequency, and burning
  - Fever, chills
  - Nausea, vomiting
  - Flank pain, back pain, suprapubic pain or heaviness
  - Colicky pain
  - Hematuria

- Self-diagnosis in women with history of UTI
- Symptoms of preterm labor
- Other associated symptoms
- Review history related to the following issues:
  - UTIs
  - Renal calculi
  - Recent urinary catheterization
  - Frequency of intercourse, new partner
  - Voiding and fluid intake habits
  - Recent antibiotic therapy
  - Structural or functional abnormalities of the urinary tract
  - Intimate-partner violence
  - Chronic conditions, such as sickle cell trait/ disease and diabetes

Physical Examination: Components of the Physical Exam to Consider

- Vital signs, including temperature
- Evaluation of hygiene
- Abdominal evaluation
  - Fetal heart tone
  - Presence of contractions
  - Suprapubic tenderness
  - Guarding or rebound tenderness
  - Distended bladder
- Signs of renal involvement
  - Fever
  - Costovertebral angle (CVA) tenderness
- Pelvic examination
  - External genitalia and ureters
  - Vaginal discharge or odor
  - Evaluate cervical length, consistency, and dilation
  - Station of presenting part

Clinical Impression: Differential Diagnoses to Consider (ICD9Data.com, 2012)

- Urinary tract
  - Asymptomatic bacteriuria
  - Cystitis
  - Pyelonephritis
  - Renal calculi

- Pregnancy-related diagnoses
  - Preterm labor
  - Preeclampsia
  - Concealed abruption
  - Ectopic pregnancy
- Appendicitis
- STI

Diagnostic Testing: Diagnostic Tests and Procedures to Consider

- Urinalysis
  - Dip
    - Positive nitrites: First-morning urine collection is more accurate
    - Positive leukocytes: Frequent false positives
    - Positive nitrites with positive leukocytes is predictive of UTI
  - Microscopy
    - Blood (red blood cells)
    - Pyuria (white blood cells)
    - Bacteria
    - Casts
- Gram stain: Positive result correlates with positive culture
- Urine culture and sensitivity testing from a clean-catch sample are indicated for the following conditions:
  - Symptoms of UTI
  - Positive urinalysis
  - History of UTI
  - Sickle trait
  - Diabetes
  - Chronic renal disease
  - Hypertension
  - Test of cure after treatment
  - Repeat every 6–12 weeks for remainder of pregnancy
- Urine culture findings
  - Less than 10,000 colonies
    - No infection
    - Treatment not indicated
  - Colonies of 25,000–100,000
    - Asymptomatic bacteriuria
    - Treatment indicated

- More than 100,000 colonies
  - UTI if pathogenic bacteria are present
  - Contamination if mixed bacteria are present
  - Treat when UTI is present
  - Check for sensitivity of the identified bacteria to the prescribed drug
- Presence of Group B *Streptococcus* (GBS) in urine
  - Treatment indicated with any colony count of GBS
  - Additional vaginal/rectal screening is not needed, as the urine test is considered GBS positive
- For complicated UTI (pyelonephritis, calculi)
  - CBC
  - Electrolytes
  - Blood urea nitrogen, creatinine
  - Renal ultrasound
  - Strain all urine
- Ultrasound to evaluate for the following conditions:
  - Maternal hydronephrosis
  - Calculi
  - Fetal status
- Screening for recurrent UTI
  - Group B *Streptococcus*
  - Sickle cell
  - Glucose-6-phosphate dehydrogenase (G6PD)
  - Diabetes
  - Kidney function
    - Blood urea nitrogen
    - Creatinine, 24-hour creatinine clearance
    - Total protein

Providing Treatment: Therapeutic Measures to Consider

(ACOG, 2011; King & Brucker, 2011)

- Keflex
  - Pregnancy Category B
  - 250 mg PO QID or 500 mg BID for 7–14 days
  - First choice for GBS in urine

- Ampicillin
  - Pregnancy Category B
  - 250–500 mg PO QID for 7–10 days
  - High rates of bacterial resistance
- Augmentin
  - Pregnancy Category B
  - 250 mg PO QID for 7–10 days
  - High rates of bacterial resistance
- Macrobid
  - Pregnancy Category B
  - Simple cystitis: 100 mg PO BID for 3 days
  - Simple or recurrent UTI: 100 mg PO BID for 7–10 days
  - First choice for suppressive therapy: 50–100 mg daily
  - ⚠ Avoid before 13 weeks' gestation unless it is the best choice: May be associated with increased risk of birth defects
  - ⚠ Do not use after 36 weeks' gestation: Can cause newborn anemia
  - ⚠ Do not use with G6PD anemia
- Sulfatrimethoprim DS
  - Pregnancy Category C
  - 1 (400/80 mg) PO BID for 7–10 days
  - ⚠ Avoid before 13 weeks' gestation unless it is the best choice: May be associated with increased risk of birth defects
  - ⚠ Do not use after 36 weeks' gestation: Can cause newborn anemia
  - ⚠ Do not use with G6PD anemia
- Pyridium for dysuria
  - Pregnancy Category B
  - 200 mg TID after meals
  - Maximum six doses
- Consider a prescription for *Candida* treatment PRN for women who frequently get UTIs with antibiotic therapy
- Pyelonephritis
  - Hospitalization
  - IV hydration
    - 200 mL/hr
    - Balanced electrolyte solution

- Antibiotics
  - IV Cefoxitin 1–2 g every 6 hours or other cephalosporins
  - Change to PO when the patient has been afebrile for 24 hours
- Provide for adequate pain control

Providing Treatment: Complementary and Alternative Measures to Consider

(Romm, 2010)

- Live culture probiotics
- Vitamin C 500 mg up to 200 mg daily during acute infection
- Herbals
  - Cranberry juice
  - Concentrated cranberry tablets, 1–2 tablets every 4–6 hours with fluid
  - Oregano tincture or capsules

Providing Support: Education and Support Measures to Consider

- Medication instructions: Take full antibiotic course
- Review warning signs of progression
  - Fever and chills
  - Flank pain
  - Urinary urgency or burning
  - Hematuria
  - Generalized abdominal pain
  - Nausea, vomiting, loss of appetite, inability to maintain hydration
- Review perineal hygiene
  - Void immediately after intercourse
  - Blot after voiding
  - Wipe front to back after bowel movement
- When to call or come in for care
  - Symptoms do not resolve within 24 hours
  - Symptoms worsen
  - Symptoms recur
- Indications for hospitalization
- Indications for a consult or referral

- Encourage the following practices:
  - Increased frequency of voiding: Every 1–2 hours while awake
  - Increased fluid intake
    - Water preferable
    - Cranberry juice or tea
    - One cup of fluid per hour while awake
  - Avoid the following:
    - Caffeine
    - Excess vitamin C
    - Sugars

Follow-up Care: Follow-up Measures to Consider

- Document
- Maternal surveillance
  - Observe for improvement
  - Change antibiotics based on sensitivities
  - Culture for test of cure
  - Perform urinalysis on each visit to assess for blood, nitrites, and leukocytes
  - Culture each trimester
  - Suppressive therapy after two positive cultures
  - Observe for signs and symptoms of preterm labor
- Fetal surveillance: Monitor FHR and activity
- Hospital discharge is appropriate in the following circumstances:
  - 24 hours on PO antibiotics
  - Afebrile
  - Calculi passed
  - No signs or symptoms of preterm labor

Multidisciplinary Practice: Consider Consultation, Collaboration, or Referral

- OB/GYN services
  - Pyelonephritis
  - Renal calculi
  - Threatened preterm labor
- For diagnosis or treatment outside the midwife's scope of practice

CARE OF THE PREGNANT WOMAN WITH VAGINAL BLEEDING, FIRST TRIMESTER

Key Clinical Information

Although vaginal bleeding in the first trimester is a relatively common occurrence, affecting as many as 15% to 25% of pregnant women (Snell, 2009), it must be considered serious until all potential abnormal causes have been effectively ruled out. The precipitating cause may not readily present itself and can take some investigation to identify. Serial evaluation with quantitative β-HCG levels and ultrasound can assist in evaluation. Ectopic pregnancy should always be considered. This emotionally difficult time is made more so by uncertainty and lack of effective treatments. The midwife must present a cautious prognosis while maintaining hope when such a stance is warranted.

Client History and Chart Review: Components of the History to Consider

- Onset, duration, and severity of bleeding
  - Color, amount, and characteristics of discharge
  - Precipitating events, if any
  - Presence of cramping or abdominal pain
  - Fever or flu-like symptoms
  - Presence or regression of pregnancy symptoms
  - Other associated symptoms
- Estimated gestational age
  - Last menstrual period
  - Date of conception, if known
  - Ultrasound report, if done
- Pregnancy/gynecologic history
  - GP TPAL
  - Blood type and Rh
  - Risk factors for ectopic pregnancy
    - Pelvic inflammatory disease
    - Intrauterine device
    - Gynecologic surgery
    - STIs
  - Previous pregnancy losses

- History
  - Abnormal Pap smears
  - STIs
  - Vaginal infections
  - Infertility
  - Cesarean birth
- Potential exposure
  - STIs
  - Viral infections
  - Physical abuse or trauma

Physical Examination: Components of the Physical Exam to Consider

(Snell, 2009)

- Vital signs
- FHR as appropriate for gestation
- External genitalia
  - Trauma
  - Lesions
  - Varicosities, hemorrhoids
  - Blood or discharge at introitus
- Speculum examination
  - Blood or discharge
    - From vaginal vault
    - From cervix
  - Visual cervical dilation
  - Presence of products of conception (POC) at os or in vaginal vault
  - Presence of erosion, polyps, or other cervical cause of bleeding
- Bimanual examination
  - Cervical dilation
  - Uterine size for dates
  - Uterine tenderness or pain
  - Presence of adnexal mass or pain
  - Presence of cervical motion tenderness

Clinical Impression: Differential Diagnoses to Consider (ICD9Data.com, 2012)

- Implantation bleeding
- Spontaneous abortion
  - Threatened SAB
  - Inevitable SAB

- Incomplete SAB
- Complete SAB
- Missed SAB
- Ectopic pregnancy
- Molar pregnancy
- Cervical bleeding
  - Cervicitis
  - Cervical polyps
  - Cervical trauma
  - Cervical cancer
- STIs

Diagnostic Testing: Diagnostic Tests and Procedures to Consider

- Serial quantitative β-HCG 48 hours apart (Table 3-6)
- CBC
- Type and Rh status
- Infection screening if indicated
- Coagulation studies if missed abortion is suspected
  - Prothrombin time
  - Partial prothrombin time
  - Fibrinogen level
  - Platelets
- Ultrasound
  - Fetal heart motion
  - Dating
  - Placenta previa or abruptio
  - Ectopic

Table 3-6 Anticipated HCG Level	
WEEKS POST-LMP	**LEVEL (MIU/ML)**
4	5–425
5	18–7350
6	1080–56,500
7–8	7650–230,000
9–12	25,700–288,000
13–16	13,500–253,000
17–24	4060–65,500

Source: Frye, 2007.

Providing Treatment: Therapeutic Measures to Consider

- Expectant management
  - Pelvic rest, await spontaneous resolution to SAB
  - Bleeding can be significant
  - Clear parameters and reassurance
- Medical management: Methotrexate for ectopic pregnancy
- Surgical management: D & C or D & E
- Discussion of risk/benefits of each option
- Rh immune globulin for Rh-negative mother (see "Care of the Pregnant Woman Who Is Rh Negative")
- Iron replacement therapy for anemia (see "Care of the Pregnant Woman with Anemia")
- Misoprostol for incomplete SAB < 13 weeks' gestation
  - 600–800 mg PO or vaginally
  - Repeat dose if POC are not passed within 8–24 hours

Providing Treatment: Complementary and Alternative Measures to Consider

- For early pregnancy loss: Encourage expulsion of products of conception with blue or black cohosh tincture
- Herbal treatment for missed abortion (Romm, 2010)
  - Evening primrose oil capsules 1000 mg BID for 2 days
  - Tincture of cotton root, black cohosh, or blue cohosh
  - Take 2.5 mL every 4 hours; repeat daily up to 5 days
- Promote healing after SAB
  - Rescue remedy
  - Herbal combinations that may include the following herbs:
    - Red raspberry leaf
    - Vitex berries
    - Black haw root

- Bleeding during pregnancy with rising HCG levels (Frye, 1998)
  - Red raspberry leaf
  - False unicorn root
  - Wild yam root
  - Black haw

Providing Support: Education and Support Measures to Consider

- For threatened SAB: Provide emotional support
- Discuss the following topics:
  - Potential for miscarriage
  - Options for care
  - Expectant care
  - Tests available
  - Potential findings
  - RhIG for Rh-negative mother
- For SAB:
  - Pelvic rest
  - Avoid heavy lifting
  - Call if bleeding increases or is accompanied by pain
  - If awaiting spontaneous resolution of SAB at home, call or seek care immediately in the following circumstances:
    - Heavy bleeding with pain for more than 1 hour
    - Faintness or weakness
    - Adnexal pain
    - Fever
- After SAB:
  - Abstain from intercourse for 2 weeks
  - Bleeding may last 7–10 days
  - Discuss birth control if desired
- In case of incomplete SAB: Provide information on options for care
- For ectopic pregnancy, discuss the following options:
    - Surgical treatment
    - Medical treatment
- For bleeding of unknown etiology:
  - Reassurance that 50% of women with bleeding go on to have a healthy pregnancy

- Warning signs given, with indications when to call the healthcare provider
- Plan for follow-up
- Before next pregnancy:
  - Take a multivitamin with folic acid daily
  - Improve nutrition if indicated
  - Avoid cigarettes, drugs, and alcohol

Follow-up Care: Follow-up Measures to Consider

- Document
- ⚠ Rule out
  - Molar pregnancy
  - Choriocarcinoma
  - Ectopic pregnancy
  - Incomplete SAB
- Follow β-HCG levels
  - 48 to 96 hours in case of threatened SAB
  - Repeat every 3–5 days until either of the following occurs:
    - Clear regression
    - Appropriate increase
  - 4–6 weeks post-SAB
- Ultrasound follow-up
  - No intrauterine pregnancy (IUP) seen on ultrasound
    - Serial HCG levels
    - Continued positive or elevated HCG
      - ⚠ Suspect ectopic pregnancy
      - Repeat ultrasound in 2–7 days
  - Subchorionic bleeding on ultrasound
    - Follow-up ultrasound for anomalies
    - Follow β-HCG levels
- After SAB
  - Examination in 2–4 weeks
  - Evaluate return to nonpregnant state
  - Assess emotional status
  - Initiate birth control if desired

Multidisciplinary Practice: Consider Consultation, Collaboration, or Referral

- OB/GYN services
  - Ectopic pregnancy
  - No IUP seen on ultrasound

- Molar pregnancy
- Excessive bleeding
- Dilatation and curettage as indicated or desired
- Cervical lesion or suspected cervical cancer
- Genetic counseling for recurrent losses
- Other referrals as needed
  - Pathology or genetic evaluation of products of conception
  - Evaluation for problems that can lead to SAB
    - Maternal disease (e.g., lupus, *Listeria* infection, syphilis)
    - Congenital anomalies of the genital tract
    - Previous cervical surgery
    - Hormonal imbalances
    - Fibroids
- Social services
  - Mental health services
  - Grief counseling
- For diagnosis or treatment outside the midwife's scope of practice

CARE OF THE PREGNANT WOMAN WITH VAGINAL BLEEDING, SECOND AND THIRD TRIMESTERS

Key Clinical Information

When a woman presents with vaginal bleeding in the latter part of the second trimester or in the third trimester, evaluation and stabilization of the mother and fetus are the immediate goals. There are benign causes for spotting or bleeding in this time frame, such as postcoital or postexamination spotting, vaginal or cervical infection or inflammation, and labor with bloody show. However, the midwife must be vigilant for signs and symptoms of placenta previa and placental abruption. Bleeding is a frightening experience for the woman; the midwife's prompt attention and action are reassuring.

Client History and Chart Review: Components of the History to Consider

- Onset, duration, and severity of bleeding
  - Color, amount, and characteristics of discharge

- Precipitating events, if any
- Presence of contractions, abdominal pain, or no pain
- Other associated symptoms
- Recent examination or intercourse
- Recent trauma or strain
- Gestational age: Location of placenta on prior ultrasound, if done
- Fetal activity
- Pregnancy and gynecologic history (Cunningham et al., 2010)
  - GP TPAL
  - Blood type and Rh
  - Risk factors for placenta previa
    - Multiparity
    - Maternal age > 35 years
    - Previous placenta previa
    - Previous uterine surgery, including cesarean section
    - Multiple pregnancy
    - Smoking
  - Risk factors for abruptio placentae
    - Maternal hypertensive disorders
    - Advanced maternal age or parity
    - Poor nutritional status
    - Previous abruptio placentae
    - Chorioamnionitis
    - Smoking
    - External cephalic version
    - Preterm rupture of membranes
    - Uterine leiomyoma
    - History of Factor V Leiden thrombophelia
    - Sudden decrease in uterine volume (e.g., with spontaneous or artificial rupture of membranes [SROM or AROM])
    - Blunt abdominal trauma
    - Cocaine use, especially crack cocaine

Physical Examination: Components of the Physical Exam to Consider

- Vital signs
- Pain rating or assessment
- FHR pattern

- Abdominal evaluation
  - Uterine enlargement
  - Uterine pain
  - Board-like abdomen
- ⚠ No vaginal examination until placenta location is known
- External genitalia evaluation
  - Trauma
  - Lesions
  - Varicosities, hemorrhoids
  - Blood or discharge at introitus
- Speculum examination if no placenta previa
  - Blood or discharge
    - From vaginal vault
    - From cervix
  - Visual cervical dilation
  - Presence of erosion, polyps, or other cervical cause of bleeding
- Bimanual examination if no placenta previa
  - Cervical dilation, effacement, and station
  - Presenting part
  - Status of membranes

Clinical Impression: Differential Diagnoses to Consider (ICD9Data.com, 2012)

- Abruptio placentae
- Placenta previa
- Early labor
- Premature labor
- Bleeding, secondary to the following conditions:
  - Postcoital spotting
  - Postexamination spotting
  - Trauma
  - Cervicitis
- STIs

Diagnostic Testing: Diagnostic Tests and Procedures to Consider

- Ultrasound evaluation for previa, abruption, and fetal status
- NST, BPP
- Type and Rh status
- CBC, hematocrit, and hemoglobin

- Type and cross-match
- Coagulation studies
  - Prothrombin time
  - Partial prothrombin time
  - Fibrinogen level
  - Platelets

Providing Treatment: Therapeutic Measures to Consider

- For benign spotting
  - Pelvic rest until spotting resolves
  - Treatment of underlying cause, if known (e.g., bacterial vaginosis)
  - Reassurance and review of danger signs
- For labor at term or preterm: See "Care of the Woman During Labor and Birth"
- 🕐 For placenta previa
  - If bleeding stops and fetal response is reassuring:
    - May go home on bed rest
    - Strict pelvic rest, avoiding the following:
      - Intercourse, orgasm
      - Douching
      - Placement of anything in the vagina
    - Plan for cesarean section at term
    - Plan for emergency transport as needed
  - If bleeding continues and fetal response is nonreassuring:
    - Assemble surgical team and neonatal resuscitation team
    - Plan for emergency cesarean section
  - Marginal previa
    - Plan for vaginal birth if bleeding is minimal or stops and fetal response is reassuring
    - May cautiously support, induce, or augment labor with consultation
- 🕐 For abruptio placentae
  - If bleeding is minimal or stops and fetal response is reassuring:
    - May cautiously support, induce or augment labor per consultant
    - Hospital birth with physician available

- If bleeding is significant or continues and fetal response is nonreassuring:
  - Assemble surgical team and neonatal resuscitation team
  - Plan for emergency cesarean section
- Rh immune globulin for Rh-negative mother (see "Care of the Pregnant Woman Who Is Rh Negative")
- Iron replacement therapy for anemia (see "Care of the Pregnant Woman with Anemia")
- Fluid and blood replacement as indicated

Providing Treatment: Complementary and Alternative Measures to Consider

There are no alternative treatments for placenta previa or abruptio placentae.

Providing Support: Education and Support Measures to Consider

- Nonemergent bleeding
  - Provide support and reassurance
  - Review cause, treatment, and warning signs
  - Provide clear indications for when to call the healthcare provider
- During an emergency
  - Briefly explain the nature of the emergency
  - Keep the client and family apprised of what is happening
  - Provide emotional support

- After an emergency
  - Provide information about the emergency
  - Employ compassionate listening
- Education
  - Potential for recurrence in future pregnancies
  - Status and prognosis of the infant

Follow-up Care: Follow-up Measures to Consider

- Document
  - Findings, client response, and plan of care
  - Parameters for immediate care
- Rh immune globulin for Rh-negative mother
- Iron replacement therapy for anemia
- Postpartum
  - Examination in 1–4 weeks
  - Evaluate return to nonpregnant state
  - Assess emotional status
  - Initiate birth control if desired

Multidisciplinary Practice: Consider Consultation, Collaboration, or Referral

- OB/GYN services
  - Placenta previa
  - Abruptio placentae
- For diagnosis or treatment outside the midwife's scope of practice

WEB RESOURCES FOR CLINICIANS

RESOURCE	URL
Patient Information	
Dietary sources of iron and of vitamin C (CDC)	http://www.cdc.gov/nutrition/everyone/basics/vitamins/iron.html
"What Do I Need to Know About Gestational Diabetes" (National Diabetes Clearing House, 2006)	http://diabetes.niddk.nih.gov/dm/pubs/gestational/
"A Patient's Guide to Managing Gestational Diabetes" (NIH, 2004)	http://www.nichd.nih.gov/publications/pubs/upload/Managing_Gestational_Diabetes_rev.pdf
Clinician Information	

Female genital mutilation (World Health Organization, 2011)	http://www.who.int/mediacentre/factsheets/fs241/en/
Recommendations for antiretroviral therapy in pregnancy (NIH, 2011).	http://aidsinfo.nih.gov/contentfiles/PerinatalGL.pdf
March of Dimes	http://www.marchofdimes.com/professionals/patients.html

REFERENCES

American Academy of Pediatrics. (1998). Female Genital Mutilation. *Pediatrics, 102,* 153-156.

American College of Nurse–Midwives. (2007). Hallmarks of midwifery care: Core competencies for basic midwifery practice. Retrieved from http://www.acnm.org/siteFiles/descriptive/Core_Competencies_6_07.pdf

American College of Obstetricians and Gynecologists (ACOG). (1999; reaffirmed 2010). *Practice bulletin no. 147: Prevention of RhD alloimmunization.* Washington, DC: Author.

American College of Obstetricians and Gynecologists (ACOG). (2000a; reaffirmed 2009). Practice bulletin no. 20: Perinatal viral and parasitic infections. *Obstetrics & Gynecology, 96*(3), 1–13.

American College of Obstetricians and Gynecologists (ACOG). (2000b; reaffirmed 2010). *Practice bulletin no. 22: Fetal macrosomia.* Washington, DC: Author.

American College of Obstetricians and Gynecologists (ACOG). (2001a). *Clinical management guidelines, no. 29: Chronic hypertension in pregnancy.* Washington, DC: Author.

American College of Obstetricians and Gynecologists (ACOG). (2001b; reaffirmed 2010). Practice bulletin no. 30: Gestational diabetes. *Obstetrics & Gynecology, 98,* 525–538.

American College of Obstetricians and Gynecologists (ACOG). (2002). *Clinical management guidelines, no. 33: Diagnosis and management of preeclampsia and eclampsia.* Washington, DC: Author.

American College of Obstetricians and Gynecologists (ACOG). (2005). Obesity in pregnancy: ACOG committee opinion no. 315. *Obstetrics & Gynecology, 106*(3), 671–675.

American College of Obstetricians and Gynecologists (ACOG). (2007a). Practice bulletin no. 82: Management of herpes in pregnancy. *Obstetrics & Gynecology, 109,* 1489–1498.

American College of Obstetricians and Gynecologists (ACOG). (2007b). Practice bulletin no. 86: Viral hepatitis in pregnancy. *Obstetrics & Gynecology, 110,* 941–956.

American College of Obstetricians and Gynecologists (ACOG). (2009). *Practice bulletin no. 102: Management of stillbirth.* Washington, DC: Author.

American College of Obstetricians and Gynecologists (ACOG). (2011). Committee opinion no. 494: Sulfonamides, nitrofurantoin and risk of birth defects. *Obstetrics & Gynecology, 117*(6), 1483–1485.

American Diabetes Association (ADA). (2011a). Diagnosis and classification of diabetes mellitus. Retrieved from http://care.diabetesjournals.org/content/34/Supplement_1/S62.full.pdf+html

American Diabetes Association (ADA). (2011b). Standards of medical care in diabetes—2011. Retrieved from http://care.diabetesjournals.org/content/34/Supplement_1/S11.full.pdf+html

Ardilouze, J., Mahdavian, M., & Baillargeon, J. (2010). Brick by brick: Metformin for gestational diabetes? *Expert Review of Endocrinology & Metabolism, 5*(3), 353–357.

Belkin, T., & Wilder, J. (2007). Management option for women with midtrimester fetal loss: A case report. *Journal of Midwifery & Women's Health, 52*(2), 164–167.

Brzoza, Z., Kasperska-Zajac, A., Oles, E., & Rogala, B. (2007). Pruritic urticarial papules and plaques of pregnancy. *Journal of Midwifery & Women's Health, 52*(1), 44–48.

Bujold, E., Roberge, S., Lacasse, Y., Bureau, M., Audibert, F., Marcoux, S., Giguere, Y. (2010). Prevention of preeclampsia and intrauterine growth restriction with aspirin started in early pregnancy: A meta-analysis. *Obstetrics & Gynecology, 116*(2), 402–414.

Campaigne, A., & Conway, D. (2007). Detection and prevention of macrosomia. *Obstetrics and Gynecology Clinics of North America, 34*(2), 309–322.

Centers for Disease Control and Prevention (CDC). (2005). Parvovirus B19 infection and pregnancy. Retrieved from http://www.cdc.gov/ncidod/dvrd/revb/respiratory/B19&preg.htm

Centers for Disease Control and Prevention (CDC). (2010a). Cytomegalovirus and congenital CMV. Retrieved from http://www.cdc.gov/cmv/clinical/index.html

Centers for Disease Control and Prevention (CDC). (2010b). Sexually transmitted diseases treatment guidelines. Retrieved from http://www.cdc.gov/std/treatment/2010/

Centers for Disease Control and Prevention (CDC). (2011a). Hepatitis B information for health professionals. Retrieved from http://www.cdc.gov/hepatitis/HBV/PerinatalXmtn.htm#section1

Centers for Disease Control and Prevention (CDC). (2011b). Iron and iron deficiency anemia. Retrieved from http://www.cdc.gov/nutrition/everyone/basics/vitamins/iron.html

Centers for Disease Control and Prevention (CDC). (2011c). Toxoplasmosis prevention and control. Retrieved from http://www.cdc.gov/parasites/toxoplasmosis/prevent.html

Côté, A. M., Brown, M., Lam, E., von Dadelszen, P., Firoz, T., Liston, R., & Magee, L. (2008). Diagnostic accuracy of urinary spot protein:creatinine ratio for proteinuria in hypertensive pregnant women: Systematic review. *British Medical Journal, 336,* 1003. doi: 10.1136/bmj.3952.543947.BE

Cunningham, C., Levano, K., Bloom, S., Hauth, J., Rouse, D., & Spong, C. (2010). *Williams obstetrics* (23rd ed.). New York, NY: McGraw-Hill.

Dhulkotia, J., Bolarinde, O., Fraser, R., & Farrell, T. (2010). Oral hypoglycemic agents vs insulin in management of gestational diabetes: A systematic review. *American Journal of Obstetrics & Gynecology, 203,* 457e1–457e9.

Foster, S. (1996). *Herbs for your health.* Loveland, CO: Interweave Press.

Frye, A. (1998). *Holistic midwifery: A comprehensive textbook for midwives in homebirth practice. Vol. 1: Care during pregnancy.* Portland, OR: Labrys Press.

Frye, A. (2007). *Understanding diagnostic tests in the childbearing year* (7th ed.). Portland, OR: Labrys Press.

Groth, S. (2007). Are the Institute of Medicine recommendations for gestational weight gain appropriate for adolescents? *Journal of Obstetric, Gynecologic, & Neonatal Nursing, 36,* 21–27.

Hlebowicz, J., Darwiche, G., Bjorgell, O., & Almer, L. (2007). Effect of cinnamon on post-prandial blood glucose, gastric emptying and satiety in healthy subjects. *American Journal of Clinical Nutrition, 85,* 1552–1556.

Hunt, M., & Hunt, R. (2010). Parvovirus and fifth disease. *Microbiology and Immunology On-line, University of South Carolina School of Medicine.* Retrieved from http://pathmicro.med.sc.edu/mhunt/parvo.htm

ICD9Data.com. (2012). The web's 2012 free medical coding source. Retrieved from http://www.icd9data.com/

Jevitt, C. (2009). Pregnancy complicated by obesity: Midwifery management. *Journal of Midwifery & Women's Health, 54*(6), 445–451.

Johnson, E., & Kim, E. (2011). Urinary tract infections in pregnancy. *Medscape.* Retrieved from http://emedicine.medscape.com/article/452604-overview

King, T., & Brucker, M. (2011). *Pharmacology for women's health.* Sudbury, MA: Jones & Bartlett Learning.

Leeman, L., Dresang, L., & Fontaine, P. (2006). Medical complications in pregnancy: Advanced life support in obstetrics (update). Retrieved from http://www.aafp.org/online/etc/medialib/aafp_org/documents/cme/courses/clin/also/chapterb.Par.0001.File.tmp/Chapter%20B.pdf

March of Dimes. (2010). Obesity in pregnancy. Retrieved from http://www.marchofdimes.com/professionals/medicalresources_obesity.html

Metzger, B., Buchanan, T., Coustan, D., de Leiva, A., Dunger, D., Hadden, D., Zoupas, C. (2007). Summary and recommendations of the Fifth International Workshop–Conference on Gestational Diabetes Mellitus. *Diabetes Care, 30,* S251–S260.

Moise, K. J., & Brecher, M. E. (2004). Package insert for rhesus immune globulin. *Obstetrics & Gynecology, 103,* 998–999.

Moore, T. (2010). Diabetes mellitus and pregnancy. Retrieved from http://emedicine.medscape.com/article/127547-overview#aw2aab6c20

Mottola, M. (2008). The role of exercise in the prevention and treatment of gestational diabetes mellitus. *Current Diabetes Reports, 8*(4), 299–304.

National Heart, Lung, and Blood Institute. (2000). Working group on high blood pressure in pregnancy. Retrieved from http://www.nhlbi.nih.gov/guidelines/archives/hbp_preg/

National Institutes of Health (NIH). (2010). Recommendations for use of anti-retroviral drugs in pregnant HIV infected women for maternal health and interventions to reduce prenatal transmission in the United States. Retrieved from http://aidsinfo.nih.gov/contentfiles/PerinatalGL.pdfb

Nyman, V., Prebensen, A., & Flensner, G. (2010). Obese women's experiences of encounters with midwives and physicians during pregnancy and childbirth. *Midwifery, 26,* 424–429.

Rioux, F. M., & LeBlanc, C. P. (2007). Iron supplementation during pregnancy: What are the risks and benefits of current practice? *Applied Physiology, Nutrition, and Metabolism, 32,* 282–288.

Romm, A. (2010). *Botanical medicine for women's health.* St. Louis, MO: Churchill Livingstone.

Sibai, B., & Cunningham, G. (2009). Prevention of preeclampsia. In M. Lindheimer, J. Robert, & F. Cunningham (Eds.), *Chesley's hypertensive disorders of pregnancy* (3rd ed., p. 215). New York, NY: Elsevier.

Snell, B. (2009). Assessment and management of bleeding in the first trimester of pregnancy. *Journal of Midwifery & Women's Health, 54*(6), 483–491.

Suneet, P., Grobman, W., Gherman, R., Chauhan, V., Chang, G., Magann, E., & Hendrix, N. (2005). Suspicion and treatment of the macrosomic fetus: A review. *American Journal of Obstetrics & Gynecology, 193*(2), 332–346.

Toubia, N. (1994). Female circumcision as a public health issue. *New England Journal of Medicine, 331*(11), 712–716.

University of Maryland Medical Center. (2007). Anemia. Retrieved from http://www.umm.edu/altmed/articles/anemia-000009.htm

U.S. Preventive Services Task Force (USPSTF). (2008). Screening for gestational diabetes mellitus: U.S. Preventive Services Task Force recommendation statement. *Annals of Internal Medicine, 148*(10), 759–765.

U.S. Public Health Service Task Force (USPHSTF), Panel on Treatment of HIV-Infected Pregnant Women and Prevention of Perinatal Transmission. (2010). *Recommendations for use of antiretroviral drugs in pregnant HIV-1–infected women for maternal health and interventions to reduce perinatal HIV-1 transmission in the United States.* Rockville, MD: Author. Retrieved from http://www.guideline.gov/content.aspx?id=16305&search=antiretroviral+pregnancy

Varney, H., Kriebs, J. M., & Gegor, C. L. (2004). *Varney's midwifery* (4th ed.). Sudbury, MA: Jones and Bartlett.

Wagner, A. (2011). Ultrasound diagnosis of fetal macrosomia found to be inaccurate. Retrieved from http://www.familypracticenews.com/news/more-top-news/single-view/ultrasound-diagnosis-of-fetal-macrosomia-found-inaccurate/36fa34152d.html

World Health Organization (WHO). (2010). Female genital mutilation. Retrieved from http://www.who.int/mediacentre/factsheets/fs241/en/

Care of the Woman During Labor and Birth

Continuous therapeutic presence at the side of women in active labor is a hallmark of midwifery care and remains the essence of being "with woman." It is common wisdom among those who are "with woman" during labor and birth that confidence is a vital asset to the birthing process. A confident woman is one who has faith in her ability to prevail no matter which circumstances she is given and can call forth the emotional stamina, positive attitude, and coping behaviors necessary to ensure an optimal outcome. Midwives are privileged to support women in developing this belief in themselves and offer support through being present, wiping a brow, squeezing a hand, rubbing a back, or whispering "You are strong; you can do it."

Women in labor are women who are experiencing some of their most vulnerable, creative, and powerful moments. Birth is a transformational process that brings forth new life while irrevocably altering the mother's life in a myriad of ways. Labor and birth collectively represent a major life event, one that is recognized as a significant psychophysiologic event embedded in social processes. For many of the 4 million women who give birth in the United States every year, this event is normal, healthy, and a cause for celebration.

Giving birth is an important developmental milestone in a woman's life, with influences on mother, child, and family that extend beyond the birth itself. The birth of a child is a singular and significant marker event in a woman's life history. For many women, time is designated as "life before children" and "life after children." Women carry vivid memories of their birth experiences throughout their lives.

Women from many cultures and all walks of life come to midwives for birth care. These women look to midwives for safe, compassionate, maternity care. One reason many women choose midwifery care is to have a natural ally in their attempts to achieve the birth experience they desire during this formative and transitional time. Women expend an incredible amount of energy in the process of laboring and bringing forth their children, while remaining vigilant in protecting their birth experience, including the possible need to navigate the complexities of the healthcare system. Few women have the resources to attend to all these tasks at once, and the supportive midwife acts on behalf of the mother as both an advocate and a guide.

Midwives remain underutilized as care providers in many U.S. hospitals and birth settings despite evidence that these caregivers provide high-quality maternity and women's health care in a humane and cost-effective manner. Integration of midwives into every maternity and women's healthcare setting will make midwifery care accessible to all women across America.

Midwifery care is distinguished from obstetric care by the belief that pregnancy and birth are fundamentally healthy physiologic functions, as opposed to pathologic processes. This perspective assists midwives in evaluating women's needs during this time, while remaining vigilant for conditions that hold the potential to be problematic. An inherent dynamic tension exists between the two views of birth—normal versus pathologic—which can be harnessed for the woman's benefit.

National standards for midwifery care are expressed as local expectations and practices for midwifery care. Such practices can vary geographically throughout the United States as well as by birth location. Familiarity with state, regional, and local standards for birth care eases the way for negotiation when adopting an innovative or uncommon practice. Use of scientific resources is useful in developing midwifery policy, but it should not supersede the hallmarks and traditions of sound midwifery care that have served women so well. Nowhere in the life of a woman is individualized care more important than during labor and birth.

ASSESSMENT OF THE WOMAN IN LABOR

Key Clinical Information

Assessment of the woman in labor encompasses not only physical evaluation of both mother and baby, but also meticulous assessment of the woman's coping skills and strengths that she brings to the task of bringing forth her child. A comprehensive and accurate labor assessment forms the foundation for development of the midwifery plan of care and may provide critical information that influences the mother's care as labor progresses. Sorting out false from true labor and ascertaining onset of progressive labor are important judgments that influence later clinical decision making.

Client History and Chart Review: Components of the History to Consider

- Verify last menstrual period (LMP), estimated date of conception (EDC), and anticipated gestational age
- Determine
  - Onset of labor
  - Frequency, length, and duration of contractions
    - Pain level
    - Coping skills
  - Status of membranes
    - Presence of meconium
  - Presence of bloody show
  - Recent nutritional intake
  - Hydration status
- Perform labor risk assessment
  - Current pregnancy course
  - Prenatal laboratory review
  - Group B *Streptococcus* (GBS) status
  - Other risk factors
- Previous pregnancy and birth history
  - Length of previous labors
  - Size of previous infants
  - Previous use of anesthesia in labor
  - Previous problems in labor and birth
- Review past medical and surgical history
  - Allergies
  - Medication and herb use
  - Previous anesthesia
  - Surgical procedures
  - Chronic and acute illnesses
  - Injuries

- Social history
- Maternal well-being
  - Coping mechanisms for labor
    - Emotional status
    - Developmental status
    - Support people
  - Preferences for labor and birth
    - 🌐 Cultural practices
    - Support for labor
    - Birth plan
- Fetal well-being: Fetal activity patterns
- Review of systems (ROS)
  - Genitourinary system
  - Respiratory system
  - Circulatory system
  - Gastrointestinal system
  - Nervous system
  - Musculoskeletal system

Physical Examination: Components of the Physical Exam to Consider

- Maternal and fetal vital signs
- Abdominal examination
  - Contraction pattern: frequency, duration, and strength
  - Fetal evaluation
    - Fetal lie, presentation, position, and variety
    - Fetal heart rate (FHR) (ACNM, 2006b; Macones, et al., 2008)
      - ➤ Auscultation or electronic fetal monitoring (EFM)
      - ➤ Fetal heart rate patterns
      - ➤ Baseline variability
      - ➤ Baseline, periodic and episodic changes
  - Estimated fetal weight (EFW)
- Pelvic examination
  - Determine presenting part
  - Dilation and effacement
  - Verify status of membranes
  - Station
  - Presence of bleeding or show

- Assess external genitalia, perineum, and pelvic floor
  - Presence of any lesions
  - Presence of female genital cutting
- Presence of amniotic fluid
  - Pooling
  - Nitrazine testing
  - Ferning
  - Meconium staining
- Extremities
  - Reflexes
  - Edema
- Pre-anesthesia considerations
  - Dentition
  - Airway
  - Cardiopulmonary status
  - Spine
- Evaluate additional body systems as indicated by the following factors:
  - History
  - Client presentation
  - Physical examination findings
  - Diagnostic test results

Clinical Impression: Differential Diagnoses to Consider

(ICD9data.com, 2012)

- Threatened labor
- Onset of labor at term
  - Prolonged first stage of labor
  - Early or threatened labor
  - Normal birth
  - Premature rupture of membranes (PROM) unspecified as to episode of care

Diagnostic Testing: Diagnostic Tests and Procedures to Consider

- Testing is performed as indicated by the following factors:
  - Client history
  - Active risk factors
  - Facility or practice standards

- Urinalysis
  - Dip for protein and glucose
  - Microscopic evaluation as needed
- Complete blood count (CBC)
- Type and screen/cross-match
- Other screening as indicated by history and physical exam
- Ultrasound
  - Fetal presentation
  - Amniotic fluid index (AFI)
  - Biophysical profile
  - Placental location and integrity

Providing Treatment: Therapeutic Measures to Consider

- Expectant management
  - Watchful waiting
  - Oral hydration and nutrition
  - Ambulation and position changes
  - Support people present
- As indicated by the mother's history or by the facility's protocol
  - Saline lock for venous access
  - IV fluids for hydration, or venous access
    - GBS antibiotic prophylaxis (see "Care of the Woman with Group B *Streptococcus* Colonization")
    - Magnesium sulfate for pregnancy-induced hypertension (PIH) (see "Care of the Woman with Hypertensive Disorders of Pregnancy in Labor")
    - Gestational diabetes on insulin (see "Care of the Pregnant Woman with Gestational Diabetes")
- Medications
  - As indicated by maternal history
  - As indicated by fetal status

Providing Treatment: Complementary and Alternative Measures to Consider

- Hydrotherapy
- Doula

Providing Support: Education and Support Measures to Consider

- Provide information
  - Role of birth professionals
    - Labor evaluation process
    - Expected care during labor and birth
  - Hydration options
  - Activity options
  - Pain relief or comfort options
    - Nonpharmaceutical
    - Pharmaceutical
- Positions for birth
- Indications for the following measures:
  - Artificial rupture of membranes
  - Internal examinations
  - Medications
- Provide progress updates
- Provide encouragement and support
- Provide information for shared decision making/informed consent

Follow-up Care: Follow-up Measures to Consider

- Document admission history and physical exam
- Reevaluate for presence of progress
  - As indicated by maternal and fetal status
  - Every 2–4 hours
  - Document in progress notes
- Monitor client responses
  - To support people
  - To unfamiliar care providers
  - To labor progress and information
- Note
  - Anticipated progression
  - Anticipatory thinking
  - Consultations or referrals

Multidisciplinary Practice: Consider Consultation, Collaboration, or Referral

- For diagnosis or treatment outside the midwife's scope of practice

CARE OF THE WOMAN IN FIRST-STAGE LABOR

Key Clinical Information

The first stage begins with the onset of labor as indicated by regular uterine contractions together with progressive cervical change, commonly accepted to begin at 4 cm dilation, and ends with complete dilation of the cervix. Ongoing evaluation of the woman in labor provides the midwife with necessary information for determining maternal and fetal well-being during labor. The range of progress during labor considered "normal" varies widely. The midwife plays a critical role in providing maternal support and reassurance while at the same time remaining vigilant for subtle variations in maternal or fetal condition that may indicate the presence of or potential for developing problems. Early identification of actual or potential problems allows problem-solving measures and treatments to be initiated promptly and proactively, with a goal of the best outcome possible for mother and baby in the given circumstances.

Client History and Chart Review: Components of the History to Consider

- Chart review or verbal report
- Prior labor and birth history
  - GP TPAL
  - LMP, EDC, gestational age
  - Prenatal course
  - Birth plan or preferences
- Interval history since admission, at least every 2–4 hours
  - Frequency, length, and duration of contractions
  - Pain level
  - Pattern of labor
  - Status of membranes
  - Presence of bloody show
  - Recent fetal and maternal vital signs
  - Maternal coping ability
- Internal examination
  - When last assessed

- Cervical dilation, effacement
- Presenting part and station
- Presence of pelvic pressure
- Deviations from anticipated labor course
- Initial midwifery plan of care

Physical Examination: Components of the Physical Exam to Consider

- Maternal and fetal vital signs
  - Maternal blood pressure, pulse, respirations, and temperature
  - FHR pattern and variability
- Evaluation of fetal response to labor
  - Methods
    - Auscultation
      - Fetoscope
      - Doppler
    - Evaluate for 60 seconds
    - Evaluate during and after contraction
    - Electronic fetal monitoring (ACNM, 2006b)
      - External fetal monitoring
        - Intermittent
        - Continuous
      - Internal scalp electrode
        - Not indicated for low-risk pregnancy
        - Direct electrocardiogram
        - For continuous assessment and evaluation of abnormal FHR patterns
    - Observation of fetal activity
  - Note fetal heart tone (FHT)
    - At least every 30 minutes
    - Immediately after ROM
    - After pain medication
      - At medication peak
    - With change in contraction pattern
    - As indicated by the following:
      - Course of labor
      - Stage of labor
      - Previous FHR patterns

> **Minimum Frequency for Intermittent Auscultation of Fetal Heart Rate in Labor**
>
> - Without risk factors
>   - Every 30 minutes in active labor
>   - Every 15 minutes in second stage
> - With risk factors
>   - Every 15 minutes in active labor after a contraction
>   - Every 5 minutes in second stage
>
> *Sources:* ACOG, 2005; Varney, Kriebs, & Gegor, 2004.

- Evaluation of maternal response to labor
  - Methods
    - Observation
    - Palpation of uterus
    - External tocotransducer
    - Intrauterine pressure catheter (IUPC)
  - Coping ability
    - Effectiveness of support people
    - Maternal behavior during labor
      - ➤ Cultural responses to labor
      - ➤ Maternal attitude and approach
      - ➤ Pain relief techniques and needs
      - ➤ Emotional coping ability
  - Contraction pattern
    - Duration
    - Frequency
    - Strength
    - Maternal behavior during contraction
- Pelvic examination
  - Cervical dilation, effacement
  - Status of membranes
  - Presenting part
  - Station
  - Position
  - Reevaluate pelvimetry
  - Assess soft tissues
    - Distensibility
    - Anatomic configuration and landmarks
- Urinary system
  - Bladder distention
  - Urine: protein and ketones
  - Output
- Hydration and nutrition
  - Fluid intake
  - Nutritive intake
  - Nausea and vomiting
  - Energy level
- Evaluate for signs of labor progress
  - Change in maternal behavior
    - Decreased coping
    - Agitation or expressed concerns
    - Urge to push
  - Vaginal examination when indicated: Fewer than four examinations decreases risk of maternal infection
  - Before administration of pain medication
  - Ongoing evaluation while providing supportive care and comfort measures
- Additional assessments as indicated

Clinical Impression: Differential Diagnoses to Consider

(ICD9data.com, 2012)

- Normal birth
- Long labor
- Other threatened labor unspecified as to episode of care
- Also consider
  - Fetal–maternal hemorrhage antepartum condition or complication
  - Maternal conditions, such as PIH
- Labor dystocia, secondary to the following conditions:
  - Fetopelvic disproportion unspecified as to episode of care
  - Dysfunctional labor
    - Other and unspecified uterine inertia
    - Hypertonic incoordinate or prolonged uterine contractions unspecified as to episode of care
    - Obstructed labor

- Fetal position
    - Malposition and malpresentation of fetus
    - Breech presentation without mention of version
    - Face or brow presentation unspecified as to episode of care

Diagnostic Testing: Diagnostic Tests and Procedures to Consider

- Dip urine for protein and ketones
- Testing as indicated by the following:
    - Labor progression and status
    - Developing maternal or fetal risk factors
        - Preeclampsia
        - Suspected breech
        - Labor dystocia
    - Fetopelvic disproportion
        - Placental abruption

Providing Treatment: Therapeutic Measures to Consider

- (Gabbe, Niebyl, & Simpson, 2007; Greulich & Tarrant, 2007; King & Brucker, 2011)
- [www] Physiologic management of labor (Albers, 2007)
    - Watchful waiting
    - Onset of active labor at 4 cm: Send home for early labor; do not admit to hospital if low risk and less than 4 cm
    - Allow broad time frame for progressive labor
    - Encourage
        - Gentle activity
        - Food and drink
        - Rest times
        - Music
        - Relaxation
        - Visualization
- False or prodromal labor
    - Reassurance
    - Medications (see "Care of the Woman with Prolonged Latent-Phase Labor")

- Morphine 15–20 mg SC or IM: May consider giving an additional 10 mg 20 minutes later if no relief is noted
        - Vistaril 50–100 mg IM
- Uterine hyperstimulation (spontaneous or induced)
    - Reassurance
    - Hydration, PO or IV
    - Terbutaline 0.25 mg SC
    - Therapeutic rest: Morphine 15–20 mg IM as above
- Active management of labor
    - Augmentation of labor with oxytocin infusion (see "Care of the Woman Undergoing Induction or Augmentation of Labor")
    - Amniotomy
- IV access as indicated
    - Client history
    - Facility standard
    - Consider saline lock versus continuous IV
    - Maintain an IV start kit on hand for use as needed
- Sedatives, anxiolytics, and antiemetics
    - Vistaril 50 mg IM
        - Early or active labor
        - Causes sedation
        - Reduces anxiety
        - May combine with analgesic to potentiate effects
    - Phenergan 50 mg PO, IM, or IV
        - Use in early or active labor
        - Causes sedation
        - Reduces anxiety
        - Treats nausea and vomiting
        - May combine with analgesic to potentiate effects
        - Preferred route of administration is deep IM (see black box warning)
- Analgesic medications (King & Brucker, 2011)
    - May decrease newborn respiratory drive
    - May be reversed as needed with naloxone
        - ⚠ Use naloxone with caution in clients with suspected narcotic addiction

- Newborn dose: 0.1 mg/kg IM, SQ, or IV
- Watch for rebound effect
  - Fentanyl
    - 50–100 mcg IM or IV every 1–2 hours
  - Stadol (butorphanol)
    - 1–2 mg IM every 3–4 hours
    - 1–2 mg IV every 2–4 hours
  - Nubain (nalbuphine)
    - 10–20 mg SQ or IM or IV every 1–2 hours
  - Demerol: Active labor
    - 75 mg IM every 2–4 hours
    - 75–80 mg IV every 2–4 hours
  - Nitrous oxide inhalation analgesia (American College of Nurse–Midwives [ACNM], 2009)
    - Nitronox: 50% oxygen/50% nitrous oxide
    - Self-administered by the woman
    - Rapid onset and reversal
    - Few adverse effects to mother or baby
    - Limited availability in the United States
- Regional anesthetic
  - Requires IV hydration
  - May decrease placental perfusion secondary to hypotension
  - Epidural
    - Continuous infusion possible
    - May diminish urge to push
  - Intrathecal
    - Generally one-time dose
    - Lasts 2–12 hours depending on the medications used
- Hydration
  - Oral fluid intake
  - IV fluids
- Consider IV access for the following conditions:
  - Grand multiparity
  - Overdistended uterus (e.g., twins, polyhydramnios)
  - Oxytocin administration
  - History of postpartum hemorrhage
  - Maternal dehydration or exhaustion
  - Fetal distress with fatigued mother

- Any condition requiring quick intravenous access (e.g., preeclampsia)
- Lactated Ringer's or similar balanced electrolyte solution
  - Fluid bolus of 300–1000 mL
    - Before regional anesthesia
    - To correct dehydration or volume depletion
  - Maintenance dose of 100–200 mL/hr
  - Titrate to urinary output
- Labor dystocia
  - IV oxytocin (see "Care of the Woman Undergoing Induction or Augmentation of Labor")
  - Nipple stimulation
  - Artificial ROM if vertex is well applied and station is 0 or below
- Catheterize as needed for a distended bladder if the woman is unable to void (DeSevo & Semeraro, 2010): Intermittent catheterization is preferred over an indwelling catheter
  - Prevents UTIs
  - Minimizes urethral damage
  - Maintains independence and psychological well-being

Providing Treatment: Complementary and Alternative Measures to Consider

(Romm, 2010)

- Pain relief
  - Hydrotherapy
    - Shower
    - Tub
  - Acupressure/acupuncture
  - Hypnobirthing
  - Massage
    - Effleurage
    - Lower back
    - Neck and shoulders
  - Ice packs
  - Hot packs
  - Sterile water papules for back pain

- Transcutaneous electrical nerve stimulation unit
- Frequent voiding
- Position changes
  - Encourage upright positions
  - Birth ball
  - Rocking chair
  - Hands and knees
  - Squatting
  - Side-lying
  - Walking
- Doula or support person
- Induction of endogenous oxytocin release
  - Nipple stimulation
  - Sex/orgasm
- Plant-based labor stimulants
  - Castor oil
  - Cotton root
  - Black haw/crampbark
  - Motherwort
  - Red raspberry
  - Evening primrose oil
  - Black or blue cohosh
    - Traditional use
    - Mixed reports regarding safety

Providing Support: Education and Support Measures to Consider

- Active listening to maternal concerns
- Information and discussion
  - Fetal and maternal well-being
  - The progress of labor
  - The process of labor
  - Any imposed limits, or medical therapies, with rationale
- Informed consent process for anticipated procedures
- Emotional support
  - Continuous presence of support people
  - Continuous presence of the midwife while the client is in active labor or for problems
  - Familiar environment or objects

- Reassurance that labor is a normal physiologic process
- Encourage maternal control
  - Food and fluid as desired
  - Position changes as desired
  - Frequent voiding
  - Timing of maternal and fetal evaluation

Follow-up Care: Follow-up Measures to Consider

- Document (see "Office Visit or Progress Note")
- Reevaluate every 1–4 hours in active labor
  - Anticipate labor progress
  - Notify additional personnel as indicated

Multidisciplinary Practice: Consider Consultation, Collaboration, or Referral

- As indicated by collaborative practice agreements
- For diagnosis or treatment outside the midwife's scope of practice

CARE OF THE WOMAN IN SECOND-STAGE LABOR

Key Clinical Information

The second stage of labor begins with complete dilation of the cervix and ends with the birth of the baby. During this stage, the fetus must traverse the bony confines of the pelvis and the soft tissues of the birth canal before emerging from the womb. Fetal position at entry to the pelvis contributes to the duration and difficulty of second-stage labor. Prenatal evaluation of the internal pelvic diameters, known as pelvimetry, can be very useful in anticipating the course of second-stage labor and in offering suggestions for maternal positioning to facilitate fetal descent.

The second stage of labor includes three phases (Roberts, 2002): (1) the latent phase—a lull in uterine activity; (2) the active expulsive phase—forceful bearing-down efforts; and (3) the final transition phase—the head emerges. "Laboring down" is a term used to describe ongoing support during passive fetal descent secondary to uterine forces, in a woman who is completely dilated and not actively pushing due an absence of the urge to push from physiologic or anesthetic conditions. This physiologic process allows the fetal head to mold and reposition to fit the maternal pelvis as it descends. Encouraging the woman to listen to her body during second-stage labor is a hallmark of midwifery care and promotes a quiet, calm, yet focused, woman-centered atmosphere in the birth environment.

Client History and Chart Review: Components of the History to Consider

- Documented pelvimetry
- EFW
- Review the progress of first-stage labor
  - Labor curve
  - Fetal presentation and position
  - Maternal positioning
  - Maternal attitude and coping
  - Analgesia or anesthesia
- Review the progress of second-stage labor
  - The length of the second stage varies and can last more than 5 hours
  - A 2-hour second stage is not an independent indication for assisted delivery (Gabbe et al., 2007; Rouse et al., 2009)
  - Progressive second-stage labor includes the following considerations:
    - Presence of effective contractions
    - Steady descent
    - Maternal and fetal well-being
- Previous labor and birth history
  - Previous infants' weights
  - Second-stage length
  - Shoulder dystocia
  - Assisted or operative births
    - Forceps
    - Vacuum extractor
    - Cesarean delivery

Physical Examination: Components of the Physical Exam to Consider

- Abdominal examination: Evidence of fetal descent
  - Abdominal contour changes
  - Fetal position changes
  - Descent in location of FHT

- Pelvic examination
  - Verify complete dilation
  - Assess
    - Location of sutures
    - Flexion of fetal head
    - Fetal molding
    - Effectiveness of bearing down
    - Rate of descent
    - Caput formation
  - Bulging of perineum
- Fetal well-being
  - Frequent FHT assessment
  - FHR may decelerate in midpelvis
  - ⚠ Head compression may cause FHR decelerations
    - FHR should return to greater than 100 between contractions
    - FHR less than 90: Anticipate resuscitation
- Determine maternal well-being
  - Vital signs
  - Assess hydration
  - Evaluate energy level
  - Determine the woman's coping ability
  - Assess for bladder distention: May cause second-stage obstruction or third-stage hemorrhage
  - Perineal tissue elasticity and anatomic configuration
- Evaluate for signs or symptoms of the following conditions:
  - Arrested descent
  - Slow descent
  - Caput formation
  - Fetal distress
  - Maternal exhaustion
  - Perineal edema or blanching

Clinical Impression: Differential Diagnoses to Consider

(ICD9data.com, 2012)

- Spontaneous vaginal birth
- Perineal injury
  - First-degree laceration

- Second-degree laceration
- Third-degree laceration
- Fourth-degree laceration
- Episiotomy
- Also consider these conditions:
  - Fetal distress affecting management of the mother
  - Precipitate labor, unspecified as to episode of care
  - Other specified fetal and placental problems affecting management of the mother, unspecified as to episode of care
  - Cord around the neck with compression complicating labor and delivery, unspecified as to episode of care
  - Other and unspecified cord entanglement with compression complicating labor and delivery
- Slowly progressive second stage, with the following:
  - Other malposition or malpresentation, unspecified as to episode of care
  - Persistent posterior presentation
  - Shoulder dystocia during labor and delivery
- Failure of descent during second stage
  - Obstructed labor
  - Fetopelvic disproportion, unspecified as to episode of care

Diagnostic Testing: Diagnostic Tests and Procedures to Consider

- A limited number of vaginal examinations may be performed to assess descent of the presenting part.

Providing Treatment: Therapeutic Measures to Consider

- Physiologic management of labor (Albers, 2007)
  - Continuous labor support
  - Avoid a rigid interpretation of the Friedman curve
  - Intermittent auscultation of fetal heart tones
  - Nonpharmacologic methods of pain relief
    - Breathing and relaxation techniques

- Remaining upright and mobile as desired
- Hydrotherapy
- Touch/massage
- Acupuncture
  - Onset of pushing with maternal urge (Roberts, 2002)
    - Delayed pushing
    - Open glottis pushing
    - Avoid arbitrary time limits
    - Supporting upright positioning
- Active management of labor (Brown, Paranjothy, Dowswell, & Thomas, 2009)
  - Accurate diagnosis of active labor
  - Amniotomy
  - Augmentation with oxytocin
    - Slight reduction in cesarean section rate
    - Highly interventional
    - Unclear which elements are responsible for the reduction in cesarean section rates
- Nitrous oxide inhalation analgesia (ACNM, 2009)
  - Nitronox: 50% oxygen/50% nitrous oxide
  - Self-administered by the woman
  - Well suited to use in second-stage labor due to its rapid onset and reversal
  - Few adverse effects to mother or baby
  - Limited availability in the United States
- Local or other anesthesia for the following procedures:
  - Episiotomy
  - Laceration repair as needed
- Catheterization if the woman's bladder is distended and she is unable to void
- Positioning for second stage and birth
  - Semi-sitting
  - Left lateral
  - Squatting
  - Standing
  - Hands and knees
  - Birthing stool
  - Birthing tub
- Lithotomy position with feet braced
  - Flattens sacral spine
  - Opens midpelvis

- Rotates symphysis anteriorly
- Assists with persistent posterior
- Assists with slow descent
- Water birth
- Perineal management
  - Hot packs to perineum
  - Perineal lubrication
  - Perineal massage
  - Perineal support
    - Hands on
    - Hand poised
  - EMLA cream before birth for local anesthesia (Franchi et al., 2009)

Recipe for Perineal Massage Oil

- Used for prenatal or birth perineal massage
- Place dried calendula petals and arnica leaves in a slow cooker
- Cover completely with cold-pressed oil; use wheat germ, apricot kernel, sweet almond, or olive oil
- Simmer on low for 6 hours
- Strain out herbs
- Allow to cool
- Add contents of one to two vitamin E capsules
- Store in a dark glass jar out of direct sunlight
- Use at room temperature or warmed in a hot pack

Source: Walls, 2007.

- Family participation in birth
- Management of nuchal cord
  - Birth maneuvers for an infant with a nuchal cord
    - Reduce cord and slip it over the infant's head
    - Deliver the infant's shoulders through the loop of the cord
    - Somersault maneuver (see "Somersault Maneuver" box)

- Clamp, cut, and unwind the cord after birth of the infant's head

Somersault Maneuver

- Consider this maneuver for a nuchal cord with a bit of give to it.
- As the shoulders are delivered, gently push the infant's head toward the mother's thighs.
- Keep the infant's head next to the mother's perineum as the rest of the body emerges.
- The infant "somersaults" out and the cord is untangled from his or her neck.

Source: Varney et al., 2004.

- Timing of clamping and cutting (Eichenbaum-Pikser & Zasloff, 2009; McDonald & Middleton, 2009)
  - Immediate
  - Delayed: Generally considered 2–3 minutes or longer
  - After cessation of pulsation
  - Lotus birth
    - Umbilical nonseverance
    - Umbilical cord and placenta detach several days after birth
  - Family member cuts the cord
- Assisted birth
  - Manual assistance (see "Care of the Woman with Shoulder Dystocia")
  - Vacuum extraction (see "Care of the Woman Undergoing Vacuum-Assisted Birth")
- Collect a cord blood sample
  - For an Rh-negative mother
  - Per facility or practice standard
  - As indicated by history
  - If sending a specimen to a cord blood bank
  - Consider cord blood gases in nonvigorous infants
- Cord blood banking
  - Private
  - Public

Phases of the Second Stage of Labor

- Latent phase: a lull in uterine activity
- Active expulsive phase: forceful bearing-down efforts
- Final transition phase: the head emerges

Source: Roberts, 2002.

Providing Treatment: Complementary and Alternative Measures to Consider

(Romm, 2010)

- Induction of endogenous oxytocin release
  - Nipple stimulation
  - Sex/orgasm
- Plant-based labor stimulants
  - Castor oil
  - Cotton root
  - Black haw/crampbark
  - Motherwort
  - Red raspberry
  - Evening primrose oil
  - Black and blue cohosh
    - Traditional use
    - Mixed reports regarding safety
- Acupressure/acupuncture
- Sterile water papules for back pain
- Hypnobirthing methods

Providing Support: Education and Support Measures to Consider

- Second stage of labor
  - Allow for natural expulsive efforts
  - Direct pushing efforts when needed
  - Review range of normal sensations during this stage
  - Reassure the client regarding normal expulsion of excrement and bodily fluids
  - Instruct when not to push
- Immediate care after birth
  - Discuss the plan for newborn handling
    - Skin to skin

- Reasons for separation
- Initial evaluation process for baby
- Cord cutting
  - Review warning signs and symptoms
    - Hemorrhage
    - Infection
  - Prepare for third-stage sensations and procedures
  - Give positive, supportive feedback to the mother and family
  - Take a moment to honor this event

Follow-up Care: Follow-up Measures to Consider

- Document (see "Birth Note")
- Provide newborn resuscitation as indicated
- Evaluate perineal integrity
  - Note any episiotomy or lacerations
    - Extent and location(s)
  - Consider no repair in the following circumstances:
    - Laceration is first or second degree *and*
    - Approximates well *and*
    - Is not bleeding
  - Repair, if necessary
    - Dermabond
    - Suture
    - Medications
  - Provide local anesthesia, as needed via infiltration or EMLA cream
  - Provide analgesia, as needed
- IV fluids
- Observe mother and newborn after birth
  - Bonding
  - Breastfeeding
  - Maternal stability
  - Signs of third-stage labor
- Provide for ongoing care postpartum

Multidisciplinary Practice: Consider Consultation, Collaboration, or Referral

- OB/GYN on unit or on standby
  - Arrest of descent
  - Anticipated shoulder dystocia

- - Fetal distress
  - Repair of third- or fourth-degree lacerations
- Pediatrician or neonatologist, on unit or on standby
  - Fetal distress
  - Newborn resuscitation
  - Shoulder dystocia
- For diagnosis or treatment outside the midwife's scope of practice

CARE OF THE WOMAN IN THIRD-STAGE LABOR

Key Clinical Information

The third stage of labor begins with the birth of the baby and ends with the delivery of the placenta. Significant blood loss can occur before or after the birth of the placenta. Active management of the third stage is promoted in a joint statement by the International Confederation of Midwives and the International Federation of Gynecology and Obstetrics (International Confederation of Midwives, 2006). Active management strategies typically include administration of a uterotonic drug within 2 minutes after the infant's shoulders are delivered and controlled traction of the umbilical cord in conjunction with uterine contractions, accompanied by counter traction on the uterus to prevent uterine inversion. Delayed cord clamping is compatible with active management of third-stage labor. Current available evidence suggests that the key strategy in reducing hemorrhage is the prophylactic administration of a uterotonic drug, with synthetic oxytocin being the preferred medication (McDonald, 2007).

The evidence for active management of third-stage labor is being questioned, however (Fahy, 2009). Support for physiologic management of the third stage in women at low risk for postpartum hemorrhage is consistent with the midwifery tenet of supporting normal processes with minimal intervention. American midwives have been reluctant to embrace the active management of third-stage labor and generally have the luxury of practicing in resource-rich

settings, with personnel and medications to treat hemorrhage readily available.

Complete evaluation of the placenta includes manual palpation of the maternal surface and visual inspection of both sides of the placenta for areas of fragmentation, divots, or torn blood vessels that may indicate retained placental parts.

Client History and Chart Review: Components of the History to Consider

- Previous birth history
  - Previous postpartum hemorrhage
- Risk factors for postpartum hemorrhage
  - Overdistended uterus
  - Large infant
  - Precipitous labor and birth
  - Prolonged first or second stage
  - Cervical manipulation
  - Anemia
- Course of labor and birth

Physical Examination: Components of the Physical Exam to Consider

- Vital signs
- Evaluate for tears or lacerations
  - Vagina
  - Periurethral area
  - Rectum
  - Cervix
- Expectant management: Observe for placental separation
  - Lengthening cord
  - Globular fundus
  - Gush of blood
- Verify that placenta is intact (Gabbe et al., 2007)
  - Visual examination of maternal and fetal surfaces
  - Tactile examination of the maternal surface
  - Cord insertion and vessel pattern
  - Look for gross pathologic changes
  - Examine for the number of cord vessels (two arteries, one vein)

Clinical Impression: Differential Diagnoses to Consider

(ICD9data.com, 2012)

- Normal spontaneous vaginal birth
- Third-stage labor with the following conditions:
  - Postpartum hemorrhage
    - High vaginal laceration during and after labor
    - Laceration of cervix
    - Other immediate postpartum hemorrhage, unspecified as to episode of care
    - Delayed and secondary postpartum hemorrhage
  - Retained placenta without hemorrhage
    - Accreta
    - Percreta
    - Increta

Diagnostic Testing: Diagnostic Tests and Procedures to Consider

- Send placenta to pathology for evaluation (Hargitaib, Marton, & Cox, 2004)
  - Maternal indications
    - Retained placenta
    - Abnormal gross placental examination
    - Placental abruption
    - Diabetes
    - Chronic hypertension or PIH
    - Preterm birth (less than 35 weeks, gestation)
    - Post-term birth (more than 42 weeks, gestation)
    - Unexplained fever
    - Previous poor pregnancy outcome
    - No or minimal prenatal care
    - Substance abuse
    - Unexplained elevation of α-fetoprotein
  - Fetal indications
    - Stillbirth
    - Neonatal death
    - Multi-fetal gestation
    - Intrauterine fetal growth restriction
    - Congenital anomalies

- Hydrops fetalis
- Admission to neonatal intensive care
- Low 5-minute Apgar score (less than 6)
- Umbilical artery pH (less than 7.20)
- Meconium-stained fluid
- Polyhydramnios or oligohydramnios
- Fetal cord blood testing
  - Cord blood type and Rh
  - Cord blood gases

Providing Treatment: Therapeutic Measures to Consider

- Cord care
  - Clamp and cut cord
  - Collect a cord blood sample
- Physiologic management of the third stage (Fahy, 2009)
  - Encourage the infant to nurse at breast
  - Observe for signs of placental separation: May take up to 30 minutes
  - Once separation has been observed:
    - Gentle expulsion with maternal effort
    - Place one hand on the symphysis to guard the uterus
    - Use gentle traction on the cord to guide the placenta
    - Avoid excessive force on the cord
  - After birth of the placenta:
    - Evaluate firmness of the uterus
    - Massage to firmness as needed
    - Provide nipple stimulation or breastfeeding for oxytocin release
    - Give oxytocin as needed for uterine atony
      - 10 units IM
      - 10–20 units in IV fluids
- Active management of the third stage
  - Verify the presence of a singleton infant
  - Early cord clamping is not required (Fahy, 2009)
  - Drain placental blood and reapply the clamp
    - Provides for a small reduction in the length of the third stage (Soltani, Poulose, & Hutchon, 2011)
    - Reduces the amount of blood loss

- Uterotonic medication
  - With birth of anterior shoulder *or*
  - After birth of entire infant
    - No prenatal ultrasound
    - Palpation of fundus to verify presence of a singleton fetus
- Assess for placental separation
- When the placenta appears separated (Gabbe et al., 2007):
  - Provide controlled cord traction
  - Guard the uterus with one cupped hand
  - Apply gentle, steady pressure on the uterus toward the maternal chest
  - Guide the placenta down into the vagina
- When the placenta is visible, guide to expel it:
  - Use ring forceps to twist trailing membranes into a "rope"
  - Tease membranes out as necessary
  - Carefully examine the placenta for integrity
- Repair of episiotomy or lacerations as needed
- Excessive bleeding (see "Care of the Woman with Postpartum Hemorrhage")
  - Ensure IV access
  - Uterine atony
    - Fundal massage
    - Bimanual compression
    - Administer uterotonic medication
  - Lacerations
    - Locate source of bleeding
    - Clamp the vessel
    - Pack as needed
    - Ensure prompt repair
  - Retained placenta or fragments
    - Perform manual exploration of the uterus
    - Perform or arrange for manual removal of the placenta or endometrial curettage
- Analgesic, as needed
  - For after pains
  - To facilitate laceration repair
- If there are no signs of placental separation after more than 30 minutes:
  - No bleeding is evident
  - Assume abnormal implantation

- Prepare for potential surgical removal of the placenta

Providing Treatment: Complementary and Alternative Measures to Consider

- Leave the cord intact until the placenta is delivered
- Allow the placenta to come naturally
- Induce endogenous oxytocin release through
  - Nipple stimulation
  - Sex/orgasm
- Plant-based labor stimulants
  - Castor oil
  - Cotton root
  - Black haw/crampbark
  - Motherwort
  - Red raspberry
  - Evening primrose oil
  - Black and blue cohosh
    - Traditional use
    - Mixed reports regarding safety
- Perineal swelling
  - Comfrey compresses
  - Arnica oil
  - Ice to the perineum after birth

Providing Support: Education and Support Measures to Consider

- Encourage skin-to-skin mother–baby contact
- Encourage breastfeeding of the baby
- Be gentle
- Provide information
  - Third-stage labor
  - Need for repair, if any
  - Interventions, if indicated
- Offer to show the placenta, and respect the client's request: Inquire if the placenta is desired by the family
- Show the client a firm fundus
- Advise the woman to notify the midwife or support staff in the following circumstances:
  - Fundus is "boggy"
  - Flow is excessive
  - Concerns about the baby arise

Follow-up Care: Follow-up Measures to Consider

- Document (see "Birth Note")
- Postpartum evaluation: 1 to 2 hours after birth or until the client is stable
- Documentation
  - Every 15 minutes for the first hour
    - Vital signs
    - Fundal/flow checks
  - Evaluate maternal–infant bonding
- Follow-up evaluation within 12–24 hours

Multidisciplinary Practice: Consider Consultation, Collaboration, or Referral

- Obstetric service for excessive bleeding uncontrolled by the following methods:
  - Oxytocin, methylergonovine maleate (Methergine), or misoprostol (Cytotec)
  - Bimanual compression
- As needed for the following indications:
  - Vaginal lacerations beyond the midwife's scope of practice
  - Rectal lacerations
  - Cervical lacerations
  - Suspected retained placental parts
    - Placenta that is undelivered 30–60 minutes after birth of the infant
    - Significant vaginal bleeding
- For diagnosis or treatment outside the midwife's scope of practice

CARE OF THE WOMAN UNDERGOING AMNIOINFUSION

Key Clinical Information

During amnioinfusion, sterile fluid such as Ringer's lactate or normal saline is instilled into the uterine cavity via intrauterine catheter to replace or expand amniotic fluid volume. Amnioinfusion is recognized as an effective way to reduce fetal risks associated with cord compression (Hofmeyr, 2010a, 2010b, 2010c), and it may increase the rate of vaginal birth in the presence of fetal distress by decreasing the frequency and severity of variable decelerations and by improving umbilical cord pH.

Amnioinfusion is not without risk. It has been associated with overdistention of the uterus, resulting in increased basal uterine tone and sudden deterioration of the FHR pattern. Amnioinfusion is not recommended for dilution of meconium-stained amniotic fluid, as it does not alter the rate of meconium aspiration syndrome or other respiratory disorders in the neonate (American College of Obstetricians and Gynecologists [ACOG], 2006; Hofmeyr, 2010a, 2010b, 2010c).

Client History and Chart Review: Components of the History to Consider

- LMP, EDC, gestational age
- Maternal vital signs, including temperature
- Cervical status
- Fetal presentation
- Status of membranes
- Indications for amnioinfusion: Presence of variable decelerations associated with cord compression
- Contraindications to amnioinfusion
  - Presence of amnionitis
  - Polyhydramnios
  - Uterine hypertonus
  - Multi-fetal gestation
  - Known uterine anomaly
  - Severe fetal distress
  - Nonvertex presentation
  - Fetal scalp pH less than 7.20
  - Placental abruption or placenta previa

Physical Examination: Components of the Physical Exam to Consider

- Maternal vital signs, including temperature
- Vaginal examination
  - Check status of membranes: Amniotomy must be performed if SROM has not occurred
  - Check dilation, effacement, and station: Birth should not be imminent
  - Verify presenting part

- Place intrauterine pressure catheter
- Place fetal scalp electrode if indicated
- Abdominal examination
  - Verify there is a singleton fetus in vertex lie
  - Evaluate FHR: Variable decelerations presenting before 8–9 cm
  - Evaluate for signs of amnionitis

Clinical Impression: Differential Diagnoses to Consider

(ICD9data.com, 2012)

- Amnioinfusion is appropriate for treatment of variable decelerations, secondary to cord compression.

Diagnostic Testing: Diagnostic Tests and Procedures to Consider

- Preoperative laboratory tests
- Evaluation of effectiveness of amnioinfusion through fetal heart rate patterns

Providing Treatment: Therapeutic Measures to Consider

- Insert an intrauterine pressure catheter, if one is not already in place: Use a double-lumen IUPC if available
- Internal fetal scalp lead or external Doppler
- Procedure
  - Infuse sterile saline or Ringer's lactate into the intra-amniotic space
  - Warmed solution is not required
  - Give a bolus infusion
    - For treatment of variable decelerations
    - 250–600 mL at a rate of 10–15 mL/min
    - Usual bolus: 500 mL in 30 minutes
    - May follow with a bolus of 250 mL after deceleration resolves
  - Provide a continuous infusion
    - May begin with a 250-mL bolus
    - 10 mL/min for 1 hour
    - Maintenance rate of 3 mL/min
    - May take 20–30 minutes to see an effect

- Intrauterine fetal resuscitation measures
  - Maternal position changes
  - Oxygen therapy
  - Terbutaline therapy
  - Emergency cesarean section
- ⚠ Do not delay preparations for cesarean delivery while performing amnioinfusion
- Assess uterine resting tone and FHT continuously

Providing Treatment: Complementary and Alternative Measures to Consider

- Watchful waiting
- Variable decelerations
  - Maternal positioning to optimize FHR
  - Avoid stimulation of labor
  - Maternal hydration
- Prepare for resuscitation of infant

Providing Support: Education and Support Measures to Consider

- Address concerns about the infant
- Provide information to allow informed consent
- Address client and family concerns
- Identify risks, benefits, and alternatives
  - When used for indications for amnioinfusion, the benefits often outweigh the risks
  - Elevated risk of endometritis/ chorioamnionitis
- Educate regarding client requirements
  - Positioning for procedure
  - The woman is confined to bed post procedure
- Continuous fetal and maternal monitoring

Follow-up Care: Follow-up Measures to Consider

- Document (see "Procedure Notes")
- Observe for complications
  - Deterioration of FHR
  - Uterine hypertonus
  - Cord prolapse
  - Uterine scar separation
  - Amniotic fluid embolism

- Placental abruption
- Signs or symptoms of infection
- Monitor and document
  - Maternal and fetal response
  - Progress of labor

Multidisciplinary Practice: Consider Consultation, Collaboration, or Referral

- OB/GYN services
  - With indication for amnioinfusion
  - For potential surgical consult
  - For complications related to amnioinfusion
- Pediatric services
  - Fetal distress
  - Meconium aspiration syndrome
  - Newborn resuscitation
- For diagnosis or treatment outside the midwife's scope of practice

CARE OF THE WOMAN UNDERGOING CESAREAN BIRTH

Key Clinical Information

In many settings, the midwife cares for the woman whose newborn is born via cesarean section. Scheduled cesarean section may be due to previous cesarean birth, nonvertex presentation, or placenta previa. Unplanned cesarean birth may be due to failure to progress, significant fetal distress, or placental abruption. Midwives discuss with all women the possibility of cesarean section, the benefits when this procedure is done for clear indications, and the risks inherent in the surgery. Additionally, the midwife quotes her or his personal and practice statistics for primary cesarean section and overall cesarean section rates so that women have a sense of how likely it is that this event will occur under the care of this particular midwife or practice.

The choice of elective cesarean section as a substitute for vaginal birth is typically a fear-based response to perceptions of exaggerated danger of labor and vaginal birth combined with pressure from the provider (ACNM, 2005; National Institutes of Health

[NIH], 2010; Sakala & Corry, 2007). Vaginal birth remains the optimal route for birth except in clearly defined circumstances.

The mother who is anticipating an unmedicated birth or a planned birth center or home birth may need additional assistance in coping with the disappointment of the unexpected change in birth plans and in assimilating the events surrounding the procedure and its outcome. Any mother who undergoes cesarean birth can have conflicting feelings about her labor and birth experience and will benefit from the midwife's gentle care.

Client History and Chart Review: Components of the History to Consider

- See "Care of the Woman Undergoing Cesarean Birth as First Assist"
- Indication for cesarean birth
- Client response to the need for cesarean birth
- Complete maternity admission history
  - Pregnancy/gynecologic history
  - Medical and surgical history
  - Review of systems
  - Laboratory values
  - Social history
- Interval labor history as applicable

Physical Examination: Components of the Physical Exam to Consider

- Complete maternity admission physical examination
- Physical examination related to indication for cesarean birth

Clinical Impression: Differential Diagnoses to Consider

(ICD9data.com, 2012)

- Primary cesarean section
- Repeat cesarean section
  - After vaginal birth after cesarean (VBAC) attempt
  - Additional codes to document indication for cesarean section

Diagnostic Testing: Diagnostic Tests and Procedures to Consider

- Preoperative laboratory tests
  - Urinalysis
  - CBC with differential
  - Type and screen or type and cross-match
- Other necessary laboratory tests as indicated by maternal/fetal status
  - Fetal lung maturity assessment
  - Preeclampsia laboratory panel
  - Clotting studies
  - Antibody identification

Providing Treatment: Therapeutic Measures to Consider

- NPO (6-hour minimum preferred)
- IV access and fluids
  - Lactated Ringer's, D_5 lactated Ringer's, normal saline, or similar balanced electrolyte solution
  - 14- to 20-gauge IV catheter
  - Bolus of 500–1000 mL if regional anesthesia is anticipated
  - Maintenance rate 100–150 mL/hr
- Foley catheter
  - Inserted in labor and delivery/admission unit
  - Inserted in holding area
  - Inserted after regional anesthesia (preferred)
- Notify appropriate personnel of pending surgery
  - OB/GYN services
  - Anesthesia
  - Nursing or operating room supervisor
  - Pediatrics
- Medications per anesthesia
- Maternal and fetal monitoring as indicated

Providing Treatment: Complementary and Alternative Measures to Consider

- Failure to progress is a common indication for primary cesarean section (Lowe, 2007)
- Based on the indication for cesarean section, consider the following:
  - Watchful waiting

- Pain management
- Rest and nutrition
- Augmentation of labor
- VBAC
- Provide emotional support
  - Allow/encourage family or support person(s) in the operating room
  - Engage the mother in decision making where possible

Providing Support: Education and Support Measures to Consider

- Obtain informed consent
  - Discuss indication(s) for cesarean birth
  - Provide an interpreter as necessary
  - Explain risks and possible harms
    - Infection
    - Bleeding
    - Injury
      - Bowel or bladder
      - Fetus
      - Uterus
      - Blood loss
      - Long-term sequelae
  - Explain benefits
    - Birth in a controlled environment
    - Expedited birth
    - Cesarean section may decrease risk to mother or baby, based on the indication for cesarean birth
      - Breech/transverse lie
      - Cephalopelvic disproportion (CPD)
      - Severe PIH
      - Preterm fetus
  - Explain alternatives to the procedure
    - Continued labor
    - Vaginal birth, based on indication(s)
- Discuss recommendations and process with the family: Maternal participation in decision making may affect the following issues:
  - Feelings about surgical birth
  - Bonding with the baby
  - Self-image as a woman

- Considerations for client and family education
  - Time in the operating room and postanesthesia unit
  - If the support person(s) may stay with the mother
  - Expected care for the baby after birth
- Anticipated postoperative care
- Provide emotional support related to the following issues:
  - Indication for cesarean birth
  - Changes in birth circumstances
    - Birth plans
    - Birth attendant
    - Birth location

Follow-up Care: Follow-up Measures to Consider

- Document
- Assist at surgery if qualified (see "Care of the Woman Undergoing Cesarean Birth as First Assistant")
- Remain with the client if possible during surgery
- Review the experience with the client postpartum
- Provide postoperative care as applicable
- Obtain an operative note for the midwife's records
- Discuss future childbirth choices of VBAC or repeat cesarean
  - Based on type of uterine incision
  - Based on probability of recurrence of cesarean indication
  - Based on maternal preference and access to care

Multidisciplinary Practice: Consider Consultation, Collaboration, or Referral

- OB/GYN services
  - Confirmed or suspected indication for cesarean birth as indicated by the following considerations:
    - Midwife scope of practice
    - Practice setting
    - Client preference
    - Collaborative practice agreement
  - Development of complications postoperatively

- Pediatric services: Newborn care or resuscitation at birth
- Anesthesia service
  - Preoperative evaluation
  - Postoperative pain control, as needed
  - Postanesthesia complications
- For diagnosis or treatment outside the midwife's scope of practice

CARE OF THE WOMAN UNDERGOING CESAREAN BIRTH AS FIRST ASSISTANT

Key Clinical Information

Many midwives have expanded their clinical practice to include assisting with cesarean section and/or gynecologic surgery (ACNM, 2006a, 2008b). By first assisting, the midwife provides greater continuity of care to women and greater versatility within her or his clinical practice (Tharpe, 2007). First-assisting skills enhance the midwife's ability to perform perineal repairs when needed and lead to a greater appreciation of the complexities of the female body. Working with the surgeon provides an opportunity to develop another facet of the multidisciplinary collaborative relationship.

Client History and Chart Review: Components of the History to Consider

- Review the current pregnancy history
  - Prenatal laboratory values
  - Admission laboratory values
  - Course of labor/interval history
  - Indication for cesarean birth
    - Maternal
    - Fetal
    - Urgent versus scheduled
- Review the past pregnancy and birth history
  - Previous cesarean birth
  - History of postpartum hemorrhage
- Medical history
  - Allergies
  - Medication or herb use
  - Medical conditions
    - Asthma

- ◆ Cardiac dysfunction
- ◆ Respiratory disorders
- ◆ Scoliosis or spinal surgery
  - ■ Previous surgeries
    - ◆ Response to anesthesia
      - ➤ General
      - ➤ Regional
- • Social history
  - ■ Support systems
  - ■ Smoking
  - ■ Alcohol or drug use
- • Client concerns
- • Review of systems

Physical Examination: Components of the Physical Exam to Consider

- • Maternal and fetal vital signs
- • Admission physical, with focus on the following:
  - ■ Cardiopulmonary system
  - ■ Gastrointestinal system
  - ■ Fetal presentation and EFW
- • Preoperative considerations
  - ■ Maternal body mass index
  - ■ Mobility of the following structures:
    - ◆ Jaw
    - ◆ Neck
    - ◆ Back
  - ■ Positioning limitations

Clinical Impression: Differential Diagnoses to Consider

(ICD9data.com, 2012)

- • Primary cesarean section
- • Repeat cesarean section
  - ■ After attempting VBAC
  - ■ Additional codes to document indication for cesarean section

Diagnostic Testing: Diagnostic Tests and Procedures to Consider

- • Preoperative laboratory tests (see "Care of the Woman Undergoing Cesarean Birth")

- • Additional testing as indicated
  - ■ Ultrasound localization of the placenta
  - ■ Coagulation studies

Providing Treatment: Therapeutic Measures to Consider

- • Ensure IV access and patency
- • Ensure airway patency
- • Assist with induction of general or regional anesthesia as needed
- • Actively assist the surgeon and surgical team (Tharpe, 2007)
  - ■ Preoperative patient preparation
  - ■ Regional or general anesthesia
  - ■ Positioning and draping
  - ■ Retraction
  - ■ Dissection
  - ■ Suctioning
  - ■ Extraction of the infant and the placenta
  - ■ Clamping and cutting the umbilical cord
  - ■ Suctioning of the infant as needed
  - ■ Obtaining cord blood for laboratory tests
  - ■ Hemostasis
  - ■ Closures
- • Procedure
  - ■ Pre-briefing
    - ◆ Planned procedure
    - ◆ Anticipated variations
    - ◆ Expected role of the first assistant
  - ■ ⚠ Surgical "time-out"
    - ◆ Correct patient
    - ◆ Correct procedure (tubal)
    - ◆ Antibiotic prophylaxis
    - ◆ Antithromobolytic device
    - ◆ Allergies or risk factors
  - ■ Verification of adequate anesthesia
  - ■ Abdomen opened in layers using sharp and blunt dissection
    - ◆ Skin
    - ◆ Subcutaneous fat
    - ◆ Fascia
    - ◆ Muscle
    - ◆ Peritoneum

- Bladder flap (optional)
- Uterine incision
    - Follow scalpel with suction
    - Position bladder blade to provide exposure
    - Incision extended with scissors or bluntly with traction
- Rupture of membranes
- Removal of bladder blade
- Head/buttocks delivery
    - Manual
    - Vacuum extractor
    - Piper forceps for after-coming head with breech
- Fundal pressure on request for birth of body
- Wiping or suctioning the infant's mouth and nares
- Clamp and cut the cord, delay or milk the cord when possible
- Cord blood collection
- Administration of medications by anesthesia
    - Medications given after cord is clamped
    - Oxytocin
    - Anxiolytics
    - Narcotics
    - Antiemetics
- Placenta
    - Spontaneous expulsion with controlled cord traction
        - ➤ Associated with decreased risk of infection
        - ➤ Associated with decreased blood loss
    - Manual removal of the placenta
        - ➤ Identification of attachment location: Shear the placenta off the endometrium with cupped fingers
        - ➤ Opportunity to learn this skill in a controlled environment
    - Surgeon preference
- Uterus inspected and cleared of debris
- Uterus closed in layers
    - Assistant "follows" suture
    - Uterus exteriorized or left in situ

Decreasing Risk for Women Desiring Future VBAC

Double-layer uterine closure is recommended for women who are future VBAC candidates (Bujold, Bujold, Hamilton, Harel, & Gauthier, 2002; NIH Consensus Panel, 2010).

- Inspection of other organs
    - Examine the ovaries, fallopian tubes, and appendix
    - Tubal ligation is done at this point as indicated
- Closure of layers per surgeon preference (Ethicon, 2004): Assistant "follows" or sutures
- Sterile dressing applied
- Postprocedure debriefing
    - Review procedure
    - Identify what went well
    - Identify areas for improvement or change
    - Goal is quality integrated family-centered care

Providing Treatment: Complementary and Alternative Measures to Consider

- Provide for maternal autonomy and involvement
    - Allow the mother to walk to the operating room
    - Allow maternal choice of music
    - Provide information about the procedure as desired by the patient
- Allow/encourage the presence of support person(s)
    - Preoperative area
    - Holding area
    - Operating room
    - Postanesthesia care unit (PACU)
- Encourage the mother to hold the baby as soon as possible
    - Can put the baby in a skin-to-skin position on the mother's chest during closure
    - Needs assistance with securing the baby

- Allow the support person(s) to care for the infant until the mother is able to do so

Providing Support: Education and Support Measures to Consider

- Provide emotional support
- 🌐 Provide a respectful environment
  - Mother/baby care
  - Advise family of delays
  - Address concerns regarding the indication for cesarean birth
- Advise the client of related routines
  - Anesthesia
  - Cesarean section procedure
  - Newborn care
  - Recovery room
  - Postoperative course
- Provide active listening to client and family concerns

Follow-up Care: Follow-up Measures to Consider

(Tharpe, 2004)

- Document postoperative care provided
  - Discussions regarding the labor or birth
  - Maternal feelings regarding the birth events
  - Baby care or feeding
  - Self-care instructions
  - Postoperative surgical rounds
- Ensure adequate pain control
  - Long-acting spinal or epidural medications
  - Patient-controlled analgesia
  - IM narcotics
  - PO narcotics
  - PO nonsteroidal anti-inflammatory drugs
- Postoperative laboratory tests: CBC or hematocrit and hemoglobin
- Physical examination
  - Vital signs
  - Reproductive system
  - Cardiopulmonary system
    - ◆ Assess for signs or symptoms
      - ➤ Anemia

- ➤ Hypovolemia
  - ◆ Incentive spirometry
- Gastrointestinal system
  - ◆ Auscultate for bowel sounds
  - ◆ Note passage of flatus
  - ◆ Note passage of stool
- Urinary system
  - ◆ Ensure voiding after catheter removal
  - ◆ Assessment
    - ➤ Urinary retention
    - ➤ Post void residual
    - ➤ Urinary tract infection
    - ➤ Bladder injury
    - ➤ Bladder spasm
- ☎ Assess for signs and symptoms of postoperative complications
  - Thrombus or embolism
  - Atelectasis
  - Infection
  - Ileus
  - Emotional difficulties
- Evaluate client's emotional response
  - To the events and procedure
  - To the newborn
  - To the parenting demands
- Evaluate for postpartum depression risk
- Other postoperative follow-up
  - Advance diet as tolerated
  - Ambulate when full sensation is restored
  - Discontinue use of the Foley catheter when the client is able to ambulate
  - Discontinue the IV/saline lock when the client is taking PO fluid well

Multidisciplinary Practice: Consider Consultation, Collaboration, or Referral

- OB/GYN services
  - Presence of intraoperative or postoperative complications
  - For postoperative care per collaborative practice agreement
- For diagnosis or treatment outside the midwife's scope of practice

CARE OF THE WOMAN WITH CORD PROLAPSE

Key Clinical Information

Cord prolapse is the descent of the umbilical cord along the side of (occult) or in front of (overt) the presenting part. Funic presentation refers to the umbilical cord as the presenting part between the fetus and the cervix when membranes are intact. Cord prolapse is a true clinical emergency. Unless compression of the cord is relieved, the fetus will be deprived of oxygen and can suffer brain and organ damage or death. In this situation, the midwife must elevate the presenting part off the umbilical cord while calling for immediate assistance (Varney et al., 2004). Emergency cesarean delivery is performed to save the infant's life unless birth can be accomplished vaginally within minutes. Placing the mother into the knee–chest position or Trendelenburg position can diminish cord compression.

Cord prolapse is a rare but catastrophic event with an incidence of 0.1% to 0.6%. This incidence rises in transverse and breech presentations and varies with type of breech. The infant mortality rate is 9% with cord prolapse. Practice drills for cord prolapse management prepare birth providers for management of this rare event where timely interventions are essential.

Client History and Chart Review: Components of the History to Consider

- LMP, EDC, gestational age
- ⚠ Identify risk factors for cord prolapse
  - Polyhydramnios
  - Multi-fetal gestation
  - Prematurity
  - High/ill-fitting presenting part
  - Nonvertex presentation
  - Compound presentation
  - Recent intrapartum interventions
  - Status of membranes
    - ◆ Artificial ROM
    - ◆ Spontaneous ROM
- Fetal heart rate

- Previously documented FHR
  - FHR changes
  - Maternal medical or pregnancy problems

Always Be Prepared

Cord prolapse can occur in the absence of risk factors.

Physical Examination: Components of the Physical Exam to Consider

- Diagnosis and prevention
  - Avoid ROM unless the presenting part is engaged
  - Evaluate the FHR after ROM
    - ◆ Severe bradycardia suggests cord prolapse
    - ◆ Severe FHR drop with resolution suggests an occult cord or a true knot in the cord
- Abdominal examination
  - Evaluation of fluid volume
  - Determination of fetal lie and presentation
  - Estimation of fetal weight
- Vaginal examination
  - Determine the presenting part(s)
  - Feel for a frank or occult cord (Varney et al., 2004)
    - ◆ In vaginal fornices
    - ◆ At cervical edge
    - ◆ Through lower uterine segment
  - Identify the station and cervical dilation
- Assess for factors contributing to cord prolapse
  - Floating presenting part
  - Bulging bag of waters
  - Ballooning or hourglass membranes

Clinical Impression: Differential Diagnoses to Consider

(ICD9data.com, 2012)

- Cord prolapse
  - Occult
  - Frank
- Fetal distress due to cord compression

Diagnostic Testing: Diagnostic Tests and Procedures to Consider

- Preoperative laboratory testing STAT if not obtained previously
- CBC
- Type and screen/cross-match

Providing Treatment: Therapeutic Measures to Consider

- Manually lift the presenting part off the cord
  - Place the mother in left lateral, Trendelenburg, or knee–chest position
  - Place the entire hand in the vagina
  - Lift the presenting part out of the pelvis
  - Evaluate for fetal response: Monitor FHR closely
  - Keep the cord warm and moist
  - Maintain the mother in knee–chest or Trendelenburg position
  - Arrange for STAT surgical delivery, including transport if necessary
- In the presence of suspected occult cord prolapse:
  - Discontinue any oxytocin if running
  - Give O_2 by mask at 6–8 L/min
  - Positioning
    - Knee–chest position *or*
    - Trendelenburg position with left lateral tilt
  - Elevation of the presenting part off of the cord
    - Manually
    - Insert Foley catheter
      - Instill 500 mL sterile saline into the mother's bladder to lift the presenting part off the cord
      - Clamp off the catheter
      - Release the clamp when the mother is prepped for a cesarean section
  - Cord care
    - Cover the cord with warm saline–soaked gauze
    - Minimize manipulation to prevent cord spasm

- Maintain elevation of the presenting part off the cord until birth
  - Maintain continuous evaluation of FHR
- Terbutaline
  - To decrease contractions and uterine tone
  - 0.25 mg SQ or 0.125–0.25 mg IV
- Prep for STAT cesarean section
- ⚠ Consider vaginal birth in the following circumstances:
  - Complete dilation and low station
  - Anticipated rapid second-stage labor
  - Operative birth: Use of forceps or vacuum

Providing Treatment: Complementary and Alternative Measures to Consider

There is no alternative to timely intervention in this situation.

Providing Support: Education and Support Measures to Consider

- Education: Include cord prolapse as a risk factor in the following situations:
  - Vaginal breech birth
  - Multi-fetal gestation
  - Polyhydramnios
- During the emergency:
  - Briefly explain the nature of the emergency
  - Keep the client and family advised of what is happening
  - Provide emotional support
- After the emergency:
  - Compassionate listening
  - Information about the emergency

Follow-up Care: Follow-up Measures to Consider

- After birth:
  - ⚠ Document, as soon as possible after birth
  - Provide the client with information about the events as applicable
  - Encourage the client to verbalize feelings and understanding

- Consider peer review and HIPAA compliance
  - Overall case review
  - Learning experience
  - Maternal and fetal outcomes

Multidisciplinary Practice: Consider Consultation, Collaboration, or Referral

- OB/GYN services
  - Funic presentation
  - Suspected or confirmed cord prolapse
  - Fetal distress unresponsive to therapy
- Pediatric services
  - Fetal distress unresponsive to therapy
  - Newborn resuscitation
  - Newborn evaluation after emergency
- Social services
  - Counseling
  - Support group
- For diagnosis or treatment outside the midwife's scope of practice

CARE OF THE WOMAN WITH GROUP B *STREPTOCOCCUS* COLONIZATION

Key Clinical Information

On average, 10% to 30% of women are colonized, either vaginally or rectally, with group B *Streptococcus* (GBS) (Centers for Disease Control and Prevention [CDC], 2010). GBS may cause maternal urinary tract infection, chorioamnionitis, postpartum endometritis, or wound infection. Approximately half of the infants born to colonized mothers may themselves become colonized with GBS. In turn, approximately 1% of colonized infants develop significant complications related to GBS infection (CDC, 2010).

Early-onset GBS disease occurs in the presence of maternal colonization accompanied by additional risk factors associated with GBS disease. The rate of early-onset GBS disease has diminished significantly since the institution of antibiotic prophylaxis in the early 1990s. The associated newborn mortality rate for early-onset GBS disease in full-term infants is 2% to 3% (CDC, 2010). Late-onset GBS disease is defined as that which occurs between 1 week

and several months of age. Late-onset GBS disease occurs in as many as 20% of infants with GBS sepsis. Complications of neonatal GBS infection include meningitis, pneumonia, and sepsis.

Client History and Chart Review: Components of the History to Consider

- GP TPAL, EDC
- Review prenatal course, including GBS cultures
  - Performed at 35–37 weeks
  - Rectovaginal
  - Urine
- Note documented discussions
  - GBS status
  - Antibiotic prophylaxis in labor
- GBS status unknown: Evaluate risk factors for risk-based management
- Identify risk factors associated with neonatal sepsis (CDC, 2010)
  - African American ethnicity
  - Positive GBS culture
  - GBS bacteriuria in pregnancy
  - Previous infant with GBS sepsis
  - Previous chorioamnionitis
  - Preterm PROM
  - ROM greater than 18 hours
  - Maternal fever (greater than 38°C [100.4°F]) in labor
  - Preterm birth/low birth weight
- Review labor course
  - Onset and progression of labor
  - Fetal and maternal vital signs
  - ROM
    - Odor and color
    - Anticipated time from ROM to birth

Physical Examination: Components of the Physical Exam to Consider

- Vital signs
- Usual maternal and fetal labor evaluation
- Evaluate for symptoms of chorioamnionitis
  - Febrile mother
  - Significant and persistent fetal tachycardia

- Odor to amniotic fluid
  - Uterine tenderness (late sign)
- Observe newborn immediately after birth for symptoms of sepsis
  - Pallor and poor tone
  - Respiratory distress
  - Slow irregular pulse

Clinical Impression: Differential Diagnoses to Consider

(ICD9data.com, 2012)

- GBS screening

Diagnostic Testing: Diagnostic Tests and Procedures to Consider

- Obtain GBS culture at 35–37 weeks, gestation
  - Distal vagina to rectum, through anal sphincter
  - Note the patient's allergies on the laboratory slip requesting culture and sensitivities
    - ⚠ If allergic to penicillin (PCN) and at high risk for anaphylaxis
    - History of anaphylaxis
    - Angioedema, respiratory distress, or urticaria following use of PCN or cephalosporin (CDC, 2010)
  - Self-collection is an option for women (Tora & Dunn, 2000)
  - Use selective broth medium for GBS
  - Urine culture
- GBS culture is not required and prophylaxis in labor is recommended in the following circumstances:
  - Positive GBS in urine culture this pregnancy
  - Previous infant with GBS disease
- CBC with differential
- Cultures at birth if no GBS results are available
  - Amnion/placenta
  - Infant's axilla, groin, or ear fold

Providing Treatment: Therapeutic Measures to Consider

- Follow current CDC recommendations (CDC, 2010)

- GBS negative: No treatment
- GBS unavailable
  - Use risk-based strategy
  - Offer antibiotics in the following situations:
    - Anticipated birth at less than 37 weeks, gestation
    - Intrapartum fever (greater than 38°C [100.4°F])
    - ROM greater than 18 hours
- GBS positive: Prophylaxis treatment recommended at labor onset or rupture of membranes
  - Positive culture during this pregnancy
  - Previous infant with GBS disease
  - GBS bacteriuria in current pregnancy
  - Local standards for risk factors
- Intrapartum prophylaxis is *not* indicated in the following cases:
  - Negative culture during this pregnancy
  - Client opts out
- Allow time for two doses of antibiotics before birth if possible
- Note antibiotic allergies
  - PCN allergy, but not at risk for anaphylaxis:
    - Cefazolin 2 g IV followed by 1 g IV every 8 hours until birth
  - PCN allergy, at high risk for anaphylaxis:
    - Clindamycin 900 mg IV every 8 hours until birth *or*
    - Vancomycin 1 g IV every 12 hours until birth
- Penicillin G: 5 million units IV followed by 2.5–3 million units every 4 hours until birth
- Ampicillin: 2 g IV followed by 1 g every 4 hours until birth

Providing Treatment: Complementary and Alternative Measures to Consider

- Expectant management
- Herbal remedies as prophylaxis
  - Astragalus root tea, tincture, or capsule to build immunity
  - Echinacea for 2–3 weeks only, just before birth

- Tea of lemon balm and oregano, 2 to 3 cups daily for several weeks
- Raw garlic, no more than 1 clove per week, 2–3 weeks before birth
- Chlorhexidine vaginal wash (see "Chlorhexidine Vaginal Wash" box)
- For clients on antibiotic prophylaxis, replace bacteria in gut
  - Acidophilus capsules
  - Live culture yogurt
- Immediate evaluation and treatment of symptomatic newborn

Chlorhexidine Vaginal Wash

Chlorhexidine gluconate 4% (Hibiclens) is available over the counter.

- Place 1 Tbs Hibiclens in a measuring cup
- Fill with water to 1 cup mark to yield a 0.25% solution
- Vaginal flush:
  - Use 200 cc in a douche bottle
  - Insert into vagina
  - Avoid inadvertent cervical insertion
  - Gently expel solution
- Vaginal wipe:
  - Soak cotton gauze in the solution
  - Wrap around exam fingers
  - Wipe vaginal walls, labia, and perineum
  - Repeat every 6 hours, making new solution each time

Source: Ross, 2007.

Providing Support: Education and Support Measures to Consider

- Discuss the following topics:
  - Practice routine regarding GBS screening
  - Treatment options if the woman is GBS positive

- Provide information to allow informed decision making
  - Current CDC recommendations
  - Risks and benefits of antibiotics
  - Individual risk for GBS disease in the infant
  - Alternatives to current recommendations
- Provide information regarding neonatal sepsis
  - May occur from birth through 3 months
  - Seek care immediately if any symptoms develop
    - Lethargy
    - Pallor
    - Nonvigorous suck
    - Fever

Follow-up Care: Follow-up Measures to Consider

- Document all discussions
  - GBS culture results
  - Treatment plan options
  - Client preferences for care
  - Risk factors for GBS infection
- Schedule regular newborn assessment

Multidisciplinary Practice: Consider Consultation, Collaboration, or Referral

- OB/GYN services
  - Women with intrapartum fever (greater than 38°C [100.4°F])
  - Women with positive GBS tests and preterm labor or PROM
  - Signs or symptoms of chorioamnionitis
  - Transfer of care or birth location due to GBS status or symptoms
- Pediatric services
  - GBS-positive client with abnormal FHR pattern
  - Infant whose mother has received antibiotics
  - Newborn conditions
  - Symptomatic infant
- For diagnosis or treatment outside the midwife's scope of practice

CARE OF THE WOMAN USING HYDROTHERAPY IN LABOR

Key Clinical Information

Hydrotherapy during labor typically involves maternal immersion in a tub of warm water covering the abdomen, although showers are also used during labor. Hydrotherapy provides therapeutic effects to the laboring woman, such as decreased pain, blood pressure, and edema; increased relaxation and satisfaction; and enhanced maternal movement, positioning, and fetal descent. Use of hydrotherapy in labor is as safe as labor in bed for selected women and improves women's satisfaction with their birth experience (Da Silva, De Oliveira, & Nobre, 2009; Eckert, Turnbull, & MacLennan, 2001). Additionally, water immersion during labor can have health-promoting benefits beyond maternal preferences for the conduct of labor and birth, such as a treatment option for certain kinds of labor dystocias (Cluett, Pickering, Getliffe, & Saunders, 2004). Women deserve the option and support to use hydrotherapy during labor and the opportunity to achieve the birth experience they desire.

Client History and Chart Review: Components of the History to Consider

- ⬦ The woman's stated preference for hydrotherapy
- Availability of hydrotherapy at the birth site with the following recommendations:
  - Water temperature recorded hourly while using the tub: Maintain between 95°F and 100°F
  - Debris seen in water removed with a net and discarded
  - Tub thoroughly cleaned and scrubbed between each use with infection control–approved disinfectant and process
  - Cultures of tub surface and water supply collected and recorded monthly
  - Single-use liners for birth tubs, if available
- Prior labor and birth history
  - GP TPAL
  - LMP, EDC, gestational age

- Prenatal course
- Birth plan or preferences
- Prior use of hydrotherapy in labor or birth
- Interval history since admission, at least every 2–4 hours
  - Frequency, length, and duration of contractions
  - Pattern of labor
  - Status of membranes
  - Presence of bloody show
  - Recent fetal and maternal vital signs
  - Maternal coping ability
  - Use of hydrotherapy: pattern and length of time
- Deviations from anticipated labor course
- Contraindications to use of tub hydrotherapy
  - Gestational age less than 37 weeks
  - Nonreassuring FHR pattern
  - Fetal malpresentation
  - Presence of thick, particulate meconium
  - IUGR
  - Multi-fetal gestation
  - Evidence of chorioamnionitis
  - Maternal or fetal tachycardia
  - Maternal fever greater than 100.4°F
  - Narcotic analgesia or epidural anesthesia
  - Oligohydramnios/polyhydramnios
  - Active infection with HSV, HBV, or HIV
  - Any fetal condition requiring continuous electronic fetal monitoring
  - Any medical or pregnancy condition that the midwife feels precludes use of the tub

Physical Examination: Components of the Physical Exam to Consider

- Maternal and fetal vital signs
  - Maternal blood pressure, pulse, and respirations
  - Maternal temperature hourly while using the hydrotherapy tub
  - FHR pattern and variability
- Labor progress
  - Contraction pattern
  - Cervical dilation, effacement

- Presenting part and station
- Presence of pelvic pressure
- Evaluation of fetal response to labor and hydrotherapy
  - Auscultation using waterproof Doppler for 60 seconds
  - Evaluate during and after contraction
  - Observation of fetal activity
  - Note FHTs according to ACOG standard for intermittent auscultation
    - Immediately after ROM
    - With change in contraction pattern
    - As indicated by course of labor and FHR pattern
- Evaluation of maternal response to labor and hydrotherapy
  - Observation of coping ability
    - Maternal attitude and approach
    - Cultural responses to labor
    - Pain relief techniques and needs, positions, and movement
    - Effectiveness of support people
  - Palpation of uterus and observation of contraction pattern
    - Duration
    - Frequency
    - Strength
    - Maternal behavior
- Urinary system
  - Bladder distention
  - Output
- Hydration and nutrition
  - Fluid intake
  - Nutritive intake
  - Nausea and vomiting
  - Energy level
- Evaluate for changes in cervical status or fetal descent
  - With change in maternal behavior
  - Before administration of pain medication
  - With urge to push
  - As needed for ongoing evaluation of labor progress

Clinical Impression: Differential Diagnoses to Consider

(ICD9data.com, 2012)

- Whirlpool, nonportable
- Application of a modality to one or more areas, whirlpool
- Progressive labor, with delivery

Diagnostic Testing: Diagnostic Tests and Procedures to Consider

- Dip urine for protein and ketones
- Testing as indicated
  - Based on labor progression and status
  - In case of developing maternal or fetal risk factors

Providing Treatment: Therapeutic Measures to Consider

(Stark, Rudell, & Haus, 2008)

- Latent-phase labor
  - Use for relaxation; may decrease contraction rate
  - See "Care of the Woman with Prolonged Latent-Phase Labor"
- www Active labor
  - Offer tub or shower in the absence of contraindications
  - Ensure that a competent support person is in attendance
  - The client and the midwife should agree on criteria regarding use of the tub or shower
  - Beneficial effects occur after 20–30 minutes in the tub
  - Assist the mother with periodic position changes
  - Enter and exit from the tub as determined by maternal preference
  - Discontinue use of the tub or shower in the following circumstances:
    - Persistent maternal or fetal tachycardia
    - Maternal temperature elevation greater than 100.4°F

◆ Complications that preclude use of a tub or shower
- A 30-minute break from hydrotherapy is recommended after 2 hours

- Hydration
  - Encourage oral fluid intake with cool liquids
  - Adequate hydration prevents maternal hyperthermia and dehydration
- If IV access is indicated, it is compatible with use of hydrotherapy
- Uterine hyperstimulation (spontaneous)
  - Reassurance
  - Hydration, PO or IV
  - Discontinue use of tub until resolution
  - May enter tub again, if desired, 30 minutes after resolution
- Labor dystocia (Cluett et al., 2004)
  - Discontinue use of the tub or shower if using hydrotherapy
  - Consider hydrotherapy if not in use
  - See "Care of the Woman with Labor Dystocia"

Providing Treatment: Complementary and Alternative Measures to Consider

- Position changes, especially upright positions
- Ambulation
- Frequent voiding
- Doula or support person
- Pain relief
  - Acupressure
  - Hypnobirthing
  - Massage
  - Ice packs
  - Hot packs
- Birth in the tub
  - Bring the newborn's head to the surface air immediately
  - Leave the infant's body immersed; observe and enjoy the newborn/maternal response
  - Provide newborn resuscitation and care as indicated by the status of the infant

- If needed, newborn resuscitation can occur on the mother's chest or on a water-resistant table placed in the tub
- Delivery of the placenta: Blood colors the waters; frequently a time of exit from the tub
- Complications during water birth
  - The woman is mobile; she may need to exit the tub quickly with assistance
  - The woman may need to change her position in the water, such as to her hands and knees, or to a squat
  - Observe the baby's face; ensure it does not reenter the water after coming to the air
  - A short cord may need to be clamped and cut immediately

Providing Support: Education and Support Measures to Consider

- Active listening to maternal concerns
- Information and discussion
  - Benefits and risks of hydrotherapy
    ◆ Fetal and maternal well-being
    ◆ Process and progress of labor
  - Guidelines for use of hydrotherapy tub, including contraindications, with their rationale
- Informed consent process for hydrotherapy
- Emotional support
  - Continuous presence of support people and midwife
  - Guidance and reassurance regarding hydrotherapy tub or shower use
- Encourage maternal control
  - Use/discontinuation of use of the hydrotherapy tub or shower as desired
  - Position changes as desired

Follow-up Care: Follow-up Measures to Consider

- Document
- Reevaluate the client every 1–4 hours in active labor
  - Anticipate labor progress
  - Notify additional personnel as indicated

Multidisciplinary Practice: Consider Consultation, Collaboration, or Referral

- OB/GYN services: For complications of labor
- Pediatric services: For fetal distress or neonatal concerns
- For diagnosis or treatment outside the midwife's scope of practice

CARE OF THE WOMAN WITH HYPERTENSIVE DISORDERS OF PREGNANCY IN LABOR

Key Clinical Information

Approximately 5% to 7% of pregnant women develop gestational hypertension, preeclampsia, or pregnancy-induced hypertensive (PIH) disorders (see "Care of the Pregnant Woman with Hypertensive Disorders in Pregnancy"). Prompt identification of PIH offers the opportunity for enhanced surveillance, which may increase the likelihood of vaginal birth and decrease the potential for maternal or fetal harm (Livingston, Livingston, Ramsey, Mabie, & Sibai, 2003). Women with mild preeclampsia are managed expectantly; treatment of moderate to severe PIH is geared toward preventing progression of the disorder. Hypertensive disorders in pregnancy remain among the top causes of maternal mortality. The goal in the care of PIH is to ensure the safety of the mother and the birth of a mature, healthy infant (Sibai, 2007).

PIH frequently causes elevations in maternal blood pressure, urinary protein, serum uric acid, and liver function tests. The maternal circulating blood volume is diminished, resulting in hypovolemia despite the presence of generalized peripheral edema. Placental and renal blood flow is frequently diminished. Platelets may fall well below the normal range. HELLP syndrome may occur without prior symptoms and is associated with an increased incidence of maternal morbidity, including a greater incidence of seizures, epigastric pain, nausea and vomiting, significant proteinuria, and stillbirth (Sibai, 2007).

Seizures may be the first sign of PIH and may occur as long as 24–48 hours postpartum.

Client History and Chart Review: Components of the History to Consider

- Prenatal history
  - EDC, LMP
  - Review of preeclampsia laboratory values if previously obtained
  - Vasoactive drug use (e.g., nasal decongestants, cocaine)
- Labor history, as applicable, or for the following purposes:
  - Cervical ripening
  - Induction
- Maternal blood pressure
  - During pregnancy
  - During evaluation
- Presence and onset of symptoms, including those indicating end-organ involvement:
  - Persistent severe headache
  - Epigastric pain or "heartburn"
  - Visual disturbance
  - Vague complaints of feeling unwell
- Evaluate for PIH risk factors
  - History of essential hypertension
  - Hydatidiform mole (10 times the risk)
  - Fetal hydrops (10 times the risk)
  - Primigravida (6–8 times the risk)
  - Hypertension in previous pregnancy, other than first pregnancy
  - Diabetes
  - Collagen vascular disease
  - Persistent nausea and vomiting
  - Renal vascular disease
  - Renal parenchymal disease
  - Multi-fetal gestation (5 times the risk)
  - African American and other ethnic minority status
  - Maternal age less than 20 years or greater than 35 years
- Other complicating medical factors
- Family history

Physical Examination: Components of the Physical Exam to Consider

- Serial blood pressure readings
  - Use a cuff of the correct size
  - Use the same maternal position for each blood pressure reading
  - Support the mother's arm at the level of the heart
- Evaluation for pitting edema
  - Face
  - Hands
  - Feet and lower legs
- Deep tendon reflexes
  - Patellar, Achilles tendon
  - 3+ or clonus indicates central nervous system irritability
- Optic fundi for evidence of edema or hemorrhage
- Pulmonary status evaluation
- Fetal status evaluation
- Pelvic examination, as indicated
  - Bishop's scope before induction
  - Labor progress

Clinical Impression: Differential Diagnoses to Consider

(ICD9data.com, 2012)

- Gestational hypertension (PIH)
  - Preeclampsia, mild
  - Preeclampsia, severe
  - Eclampsia
- Transient hypertension
- Essential hypertension
- PIH superimposed on chronic hypertension
- HELLP syndrome
- Elevated blood pressure without diagnosis of hypertension

Mild Preeclampsia

- Blood pressure of 140/90 mm Hg to 159/109 mm Hg
- Proteinuria of 0.3 g or higher in a 24-hour urine specimen

Source: ACOG, 2002a.

Severe Preeclampsia

- Blood pressure of 160/110 mm Hg or higher
- Proteinuria of 5 g or higher in a 24-hour urine specimen
- Oliguria
- Cerebral or visual disturbances
- Pulmonary edema or cyanosis
- Epigastric or right upper quadrant pain
- Impaired liver function
- Thrombocytopenia
- Fetal growth restriction

Source: ACOG, 2002a.

Diagnostic Testing: Diagnostic Tests and Procedures to Consider

- Baseline preeclampsia/preoperative laboratory panel
  - Urinalysis
  - CBC with differential
    - Platelet count (normal range: 130,000–400,000/mL)
    - Elevated hematocrit may indicate severity of hypovolemia
  - Serum uric acid (normal range: 1.2–4.5 mg/dL)
  - Type and screen or cross-match
  - Renal function testing
    - Blood urea nitrogen
    - Creatinine (normal range: less than 1.0 mg/dL)
  - Liver function testing
  - Coagulation studies, in the presence of the following:
    - Abnormal liver function tests
    - Abruptio placentae
- Fetal surveillance
  - Biophysical profile
  - Amniotic fluid index
- Fetal monitoring
  - Decreased variability
  - Pattern of late decelerations

Providing Treatment: Therapeutic Measures to Consider

(Sibai, 2007)

- [www] Expectant management
  - Preferred for gestation less than 37 weeks
  - Increased bed rest
  - Monitoring of blood pressure, weight, and reflexes
  - Serial fetal surveillance
  - Serial preeclampsia laboratory tests
  - Medications as indicated below: Not typically used for mild preeclampsia
- Active management
  - Expedited delivery
  - Steroids to promote fetal lung maturity as needed
  - IV access and fluids
  - Route of birth dictated by the following factors:
    - Maternal and fetal condition
      - A preterm fetus may do best with cesarean delivery
      - Prompt delivery is indicated for an eclamptic mother
      - $MgSO_4$ may slow labor/induction (ACOG, 2002a)
    - Anesthesia concerns
      - Prompt cesarean section may be preferred
      - Labile blood pressure may be a contraindication to regional anesthesia
      - Edema may make endotracheal intubation more difficult
- Medications
  - $MgSO_4$ (anticonvulsant)
    - 4–6 g IV bolus followed by 2 g/hr
    - Titrate based on renal output and reflexes (ACOG, 2002a)
    - Have calcium gluconate immediately available at the bedside
  - Oxytocin induction or augmentation of labor as necessary

- Antihypertensive medications
  - Of only limited benefit
  - [🕿] Hydralazine, nifedipine, or labetolol is commonly used
  - Used to regulate labile blood pressure
    - From 170/110 mm Hg down to 130/90 mm Hg (optimal)
    - Monitor intake and output
      - Hourly intake and output
      - NPO
      - Foley catheter
      - IV fluids on pump

Providing Treatment: Complementary and Alternative Measures to Consider

Supportive care is provided in addition to medical therapies:

- Quiet dark room
- Rest in left lateral position
- Support people present or available
- A calm atmosphere of caring and safety

Providing Support: Education and Support Measures to Consider

- Provide information about the following topics:
  - Diagnosis
  - Options for care
  - Symptom recognition
  - Anticipated course of events: Need for calm and quiet
- Discussion regarding potential for the following events:
  - Change in birth plans
  - Medical interventions
  - Initiation of labor
  - Newborn special care
- Address client and family concerns
- Instruct the client/family to notify the provider if additional symptoms develop
  - Epigastric pain
  - Scotomata
  - Visual disturbance
  - Severe headache unrelieved by acetaminophen

Follow-up Care: Follow-up Measures to Consider

- Follow vital signs, reflexes, and symptoms
  - At least every 2–4 hours
  - For 24–48 hours postpartum
- Repeat preeclampsia or HELLP laboratory tests
- Document

Multidisciplinary Practice: Consider Consultation, Collaboration, or Referral

- OB/GYN services
  - Suspected or confirmed preeclampsia
  - For women requiring transport due to PIH
  - For women with labile PIH
- Pediatric services
  - For presence at birth in case of maternal PIH
  - When fetal status concerns arise
    - Preterm birth
    - Nonreassuring FHR patterns
- For diagnosis or treatment outside the midwife's scope of practice

CARE OF THE WOMAN UNDERGOING INDUCTION OR AUGMENTATION OF LABOR

Key Clinical Information

Induction is the stimulation of the uterus by an external agent with the intent to start labor before the onset of spontaneous labor. Augmentation is the use of similar techniques to enhance uterine contractions after labor has started. Induction or augmentation of labor may be initiated for a wide variety of clinical indications. Induction is recommended in cases when the fetus is believed to be safer outside the uterus than inside it, for maternal indications, or for both. Rates of induction are increasing in the United States, with the 1990 rate of 9.5% rising to 22.8% in 2007—a 140% increase (Simpson, 2011). Avoidance of elective induction of labor is recommended because spontaneous labor offers substantial benefits to both mother and baby (ACNM, 2010). Induction-associated risks, such as late-term prematurity and increased rates of operative birth, are not warranted in the absence of evidence-based maternal or fetal indications for the induction.

Practices vary tremendously in terms of the approach to induction and augmentation. Maternal involvement in the decision-making process is essential, because stimulation of labor can contribute to maternal feelings of success or failure based on maternal motivation and attitude toward the induction or augmentation process. Midwives can best support women and foster vaginal birth through purposeful nonintervention in the absence of complications in the current milieu of rising elective induction rates.

Client History and Chart Review: Components of the History to Consider

(Simpson, 2011)

- Prenatal record review
  - LMP, EDC, gestational age
  - EFW
- Identification of indication for induction
  - Maternal indications
    - Absolute indications: Chorioamnionitis
    - Relative indications
      - Preeclampsia/eclampsia
      - Chronic hypertension
      - Gestational diabetes
      - Maternal medical complications, such as diabetes or renal disease
  - Fetal indications
    - Absolute indications
      - Chorioamnionitis
      - Fetal compromise
      - Intrauterine growth restriction
      - Isoimmunization
    - Relative indications
      - Post dates (greater than 41–42 weeks, gestation)
      - PROM
      - Fetal macrosomia
      - Fetal demise
      - Fetus with major congenital anomaly
      - Prolonged ROM
      - Other fetal risk in utero

- Uteroplacental indications
  - Absolute indications: Placental abruption, partial and stable
  - Relative indications
    - Unexplained oligohydramnios
    - Placental insufficiency
- Identification of indication for augmentation
  - Maternal indications
    - Nonprogressive labor
    - Insufficient contraction pattern
    - Maternal fever
    - Prolonged ROM
  - Fetal indications: Nonreassuring FHT
- Contraindications to induction or augmentation
  - Maternal contraindications
    - Absolute contraindications
      - Classical uterine incision
      - Active genital herpes
      - Serious chronic medical conditions
      - Pelvic structure abnormality
      - Invasive cervical cancer
    - Relative contraindications
      - Cervical carcinoma
      - Grand multiparity
      - Heart disease
      - Severe maternal hypertension
      - Uterine overdistention (secondary to polyhydramnios or multi-fetal gestation)
  - Fetal contraindications
    - Absolute contraindications
      - Transverse/oblique lie
      - Extreme fetal compromise
    - Relative contraindications
      - Nonengaged presenting part
      - CPD
      - Malpresentation
      - Fetal macrosomia
  - Uteroplacental contraindications
    - Absolute contraindications
      - Cord prolapse
      - Placenta previa
      - Vasa previa

- Relative contraindications
  - Low-lying placenta
  - Unexplained vaginal bleeding
  - Cord presentation
  - Myomectomy involving the uterine cavity
- Misoprostol contraindications: Previous uterine scar
- Obtain labor admission history or review interval labor history

Physical Examination: Components of the Physical Exam to Consider

- Maternal and fetal vital signs
- Assess fetal and maternal well-being
  - Contraction status
  - Frequency, duration, strength
  - Palpation
  - External or internal monitoring
- Pelvic examination
  - Bishop's score
    - 6 or greater is considered favorable for induction for multiparous women
    - 8 or greater is considered favorable for induction for nulliparous women (see Table 4-1)
  - Pelvimetry to rule out CPD
  - Cervical status
    - Effacement
    - Dilation
    - Consistency
  - Status of membranes
  - Descent of presenting part

Clinical Impression: Differential Diagnoses to Consider

(ICD9data.com, 2012)

- Induction of labor, secondary to:
  - PROM
  - Preeclampsia
  - Post-term pregnancy (42 weeks, gestation or later)

Table 4-1 Bishop's Score				
	0	**1**	**2**	**3**
Dilation	0	1–2 cm	3–4 cm	5–6 cm
Effacement	0–30%	40–50%	60–70%	80+%
Station	−3	−2	−1/0	+1/+2
Consistency	Firm	Medium	Soft	N/A
Position	Posterior	Mid-position	Anterior	N/A

N/A: not applicable.
Source: Bishop, 1964.

- Maternal diabetes mellitus
- Maternal medical problems
- Intrauterine fetal growth restriction
- Fetal demise
- Augmentation of labor, secondary to:
  - Dysfunctional labor
  - Uterine inertia

Diagnostic Testing: Diagnostic Tests and Procedures to Consider

- Fetal evaluation
  - Non-stress test (NST)/contraction stress test (CST)
  - Biophysical profile
  - Amniotic fluid index
  - Fetal kick counts
- Fetal surveillance
  - Intermittent auscultation for FHR
  - Continuous fetal monitoring
- Preoperative laboratory tests
  - CBC
  - Urinalysis
  - Type and screen (or red-topped tube to hold)
  - Other laboratory tests as indicated

Providing Treatment: Therapeutic Measures to Consider

- Cervical-ripening agents (King & Brucker, 2011)
  - Prostin E_2
    - Prepidil
    - Cervidil

- Hospital-compounded Prostin E_2 gel 2–6 mg
- Misoprostol (may result in induction)
  - Off-label use
  - Informed consent recommended
  - 100 mcg tablet divided into four 25 mcg pieces
  - PO or in posterior vaginal fornix (25–50 mcg)
  - Repeat doses
    - Oral: every 2 hours
    - Vaginal: every 3–6 hours
- Laminaria
- Foley catheter balloon
  - Place inside internal os
  - Fill with 30 mL fluid
  - Tape to the client's thigh
- Induction/augmentation
  - Amniotomy
  - Oxytocin infusion
    - 10 units oxytocin/1000 mL IV solution such as lactated Ringer's
    - Titrate until a contraction pattern of every 3 minutes is achieved
    - Rates vary
      - Examples include 0.5–2 mU/min
      - Increase 1–2 mU/min every 15–60 minutes
    - Maximum dose: 20–40 mU/min
    - Conservative physiologic rate based on oxytocin half-life and receptor response (Simpson, 2011)

➤ Initiate at 1 mU/min
➤ Increase 1–2 mU/min every 30–40 minutes
➤ Discontinue oxytocin once active labor is achieved
➤ Prolonged high-dose infusions increase the risk of postpartum atony

- Potential complications
  - Overstimulation of the uterus
    - More common with 50 mcg dosing of misoprostol
    - With category 1 FHR:
      ➤ Maternal repositioning
      ➤ IV fluid bolus of 500 mL
      ➤ If uterine activity not normal by 10 minutes, decrease rate by half or discontinue oxytocin
    - With category 2 FHR:
      ➤ Discontinue oxytocin
      ➤ Maternal repositioning
      ➤ Consider O_2 at 10 L/min
      ➤ IV fluid bolus of 500 mL
    - If no response, consider 0.25 terbutaline sub-Q
  - Fetal distress
  - Under-dosing and maternal exhaustion
  - Water intoxication, a form of hyponatremia (oxytocin)

Providing Treatment: Complementary and Alternative Measures to Consider

- Repeated antepartum fetal surveillance
- Encourage patience and watchful waiting for the woman, family, and provider
- Cervical ripening/initiation of labor
  - Nipple stimulation
  - Sexual intercourse
  - Castor oil 2–4 oz PO
  - Stripping of membranes
  - Herbs
    - Evening primrose oil: Apply to cervix or take orally
    - Red raspberry tea every 1–2 hours in labor

Providing Support: Education and Support Measures to Consider

- Outline recommendations for care
  - Indication for induction or augmentation
  - Obtain informed consent
  - Client/family preferences
- Note potential for the following measures:
  - Transport if out-of-hospital
  - IV access
  - Fetal monitoring
- Potential restrictions with induction/augmentation
  - NPO
  - Clear liquids
  - IV oxytocin
  - Electronic fetal monitoring
  - Limited mobility
  - Operative assistance at birth
    - Vacuum extraction
    - Forceps
    - Cesarean section
- Provide support

Follow-up Care: Follow-up Measures to Consider

- Document
- Address client preferences
- Evaluate maternal/fetal status at regular intervals
  - Evaluate for progress
  - Evaluate based on the indication for induction/augmentation
  - Update plan after each evaluation
- Ensure access to emergency services as needed
- Encourage the client to express her feelings and concerns

Multidisciplinary Practice: Consider Consultation, Collaboration, or Referral

- OB/GYN services
  - Before induction or ripening per collaborative practice agreement
  - Women requiring cesarean section or other assisted birth

- As needed for transport or evaluation of maternal compromise
- Pediatric services: For evidence or suspicion of fetal compromise
- For diagnosis or treatment outside the midwife's scope of practice

CARE OF THE WOMAN WITH LABOR DYSTOCIA

Key Clinical Information

There is no consensus on how to define nonprogressive labor. Current evidence does not support strict interpretation and application of the Friedman criteria (Albers, Schiff, & Gorwoda, 1996; Lowe, 2007). When labor does not progress, the suspected mechanism(s) should be clearly identified so that the healthcare provider can systematically select appropriate treatment. In some instances, fetal size or positioning can slow the progression of labor, while the uterus works hard to literally push past the difficulty. Failure to progress is a common diagnosis that can have multiple components (Lowe, 2007). Delay in progression can be related to the effectiveness of uterine contractions, the size of the mother's pelvis in relation to the size of the fetus, fetal position (Hart & Walker, 2007) or anatomy, or psychosocial factors that inhibit labor progress. The challenge to the midwife is to identify and treat the specific component(s) causing the delay. Time and patience are often rewarded with slow and steady progress. When the uterus is not working efficiently, augmentation of labor via oxytocin can help prevent prolonged labor and avoid unnecessary cesarean birth. Patience is essential because the pattern of labor for many women does not follow the average labor curve. These women need time and support for their own pace for labor and birth (Albers et al., 1996).

Client History and Chart Review: Components of the History to Consider

- GP TPAL
- LMP, EDC, gestational age

- Review of labor
  - Onset of labor
  - Progress of labor
  - Fetal response to labor
  - Maternal response to labor
  - Status of membranes
    - Color of fluid
    - Length of rupture
  - Oral intake of food or fluids
  - Positions used and results
  - Use of analgesia/anesthesia
  - Estimated fetal weight
  - Previous clinical evaluation of fetal lie
- Previous labor and birth history
- Inquiry into potential barriers to labor progress
  - Cultural
  - Developmental
  - Emotional or social
  - Physical
    - Positioning
    - Hydration
    - Nutrition
    - Voiding

Physical Examination: Components of the Physical Exam to Consider

- Maternal and fetal vital signs
- Evaluate for signs of maternal exhaustion
  - Tachycardia
  - Ketonuria
  - Trembling
  - Lethargy
- Maternal attitude
  - Positive and persistent
  - Discouraged
  - Fear or anxiety
  - Tension
- Abdominal examination
  - Fetal lie, presentation, and position
  - Estimated fetal weight
  - Signs of engagement
  - Uterine contractions: Frequency, duration, and intensity
  - Bladder distention

- Pelvic examination
  - Cervix
    - Dilation and effacement
    - Position
    - Edema or asymmetry of cervix
  - Presenting part
    - Verification of presenting part
    - Application to the cervix
    - Station
    - Asyncliticism
    - Caput formation
    - Molding
  - Pelvimetry
- Fetal vital signs
  - FHR variability
  - Fetal activity
  - Fetal response to stimulation

Clinical Impression: Differential Diagnoses to Consider

(ICD9data.com, 2012)

- Slowly progressive labor
- Presence of a protraction disorder
  - Dilation
- Presence of an arrest disorder
  - Arrest of dilation
  - Prolonged second stage
- Secondary to the following:
  - Dysfunctional labor
  - Fetopelvic disproportion
  - Fetal presentation or position
  - Additional codes to document associated conditions

Diagnostic Testing: Diagnostic Tests and Procedures to Consider

- Urine for ketones
- Uterine pressure catheter to evaluate uterine contractions
- Preoperative laboratory tests with consideration for potential cesarean section

Providing Treatment: Therapeutic Measures to Consider

- Watchful waiting
- Assess maternal environment for stress factors
  - Fear and pain
  - Light and noise
  - Dysfunctional family or staff members
- Hydration
  - PO clear liquids
  - IV bolus of 500 mL of solution suitable for labor: Maintain at 125–200 mL/hr
- Rest, if maternal and fetal statuses are stable
  - Consider morphine sulfate 10–20 mg IM in early labor: ⚠ Have Narcan immediately available
  - Pain relief to facilitate rest/relaxation
- Clinical repositioning techniques
  - Manual flexion of vertex
  - Massage and stretch cervical lip over presenting part
  - Hip press to open midpelvis
- Active management of labor (Institute for Clinical Systems Improvement, 2004)
  - Oxytocin (see "Care of the Woman Undergoing Induction or Augmentation of Labor")
  - Amniotomy
- Empty bladder
- Antibiotic prophylaxis
  - Not indicated with negative GBS status
  - With ROM greater than 18 hours if GBS status is unknown or per facility guidelines
  - With maternal fever or elevated WBC

Providing Treatment: Complementary and Alternative Measures to Consider

(Simkin & Ancheta, 2011)

- Watchful waiting
- Explore emotional issues that may interfere with labor
  - Fear
  - Previous trauma, such as rape or abortion

- Family issues (e.g., gender of infant, history of abuse)
- Imposed deadlines related to the following considerations:
  - Labor management
  - Interventions
- Encourage position changes
  - Hands and knees
  - Side-lying
  - Walking
  - Rocking chair
  - Semi-sitting
  - Stair stepping or other asymmetrical positions
- Empty bladder and bowels
- Hydrotherapy
  - Tub
  - Whirlpool
  - Shower
- Lying flat on the back with knees flexed can encourage descent
  - Opens pelvic inlet
  - Flattens sacrum
  - The woman can move upright once the fetus's vertex descends
- Use upright positions once the head enters the pelvis
  - Squatting
  - Squatting bar
  - Birth stool
  - Standing
  - Sitting
    - Birth ball
    - Birth tub
    - Bed
    - Chair
    - Toilet
- If contractions slow secondary to fatigue and the mother and fetus are both stable:
  - Sleep
  - Provide nutrition and hydration
  - Allow more time
  - Close monitoring of maternal and fetal well-being

- Stimulate contractions
  - Nipple stimulation
  - Herbal remedies (see "Care of the Woman Undergoing Induction or Augmentation of Labor")

Providing Support: Education and Support Measures to Consider

- Discuss findings with the client and family
  - Describe the options available
  - Address client and family concerns
  - Formulate a plan with the patient
    - Potential need to transport if out-of-hospital
    - Recommendations for midwifery care
- Increased potential for augmentation in the following scenarios:
  - Prolonged ROM
  - Dysfunctional labor
- Increased potential for cesarean section in the following scenarios:
  - Protracted active labor
  - Failure to descend
  - Maternal or fetal exhaustion

Follow-up Care: Follow-up Measures to Consider

- Reassess
  - Every 1–3 hours
  - After initiation of treatments
  - With maternal or fetal indication
- Update the plan of care after each assessment
  - Maternal and fetal response
  - Interval change
  - Clinical impression
  - Discussions with client and family
  - Planned course of action

Multidisciplinary Practice: Consider Consultation, Collaboration, or Referral

- OB/GYN services
  - For persistently nonprogressive labor
  - Suspected fetopelvic disproportion
  - Fetal malposition

- For fetal or maternal distress
- For transport
- Pediatric services:
  - Nonreassuring FHR pattern
- For diagnosis or treatment outside the midwife's scope of practice

CARE OF THE WOMAN WITH MECONIUM-STAINED AMNIOTIC FLUID

Key Clinical Information

Meconium-stained amniotic fluid occurs in approximately 7% to 22% of all pregnancies (Fraser, Hofmeyr, Lede, & Faron, 2005), with increasing frequency in advancing gestational age. Although it is more common in the post-term pregnancy, it can also occur before term. Meconium-stained amniotic fluid is theorized to be the result of either an acute or chronic hypoxic event leading to relaxation of the fetal anal sphincter, allowing meconium to be released into the amniotic fluid.

Meconium aspiration syndrome affects 1.7% to 35.8% of infants born with meconium staining of the amniotic fluid (Fraser et al., 2005). Meconium aspiration syndrome can occur when the fetus born through meconium-stained fluid breathes meconium into the lungs, but it occurs more often in utero in an already-compromised fetus with preexisting pulmonary abnormality or compromise. Thick meconium-stained amniotic fluid is an indication to step up fetal surveillance for signs of fetal distress and to prepare for intrauterine and extrauterine resuscitation.

Client History and Chart Review: Components of the History to Consider

- Verify EDC, gestational age
- Assess fetal well-being
  - Reassuring FHR pattern
  - Patterns of fetal activity
- Characteristics of meconium in fluid
  - Thin
  - Moderate
  - Thick

- Risk factors for meconium aspiration syndrome
  - Maternal factors
    - Fewer than five prenatal visits
    - Oligohydramnios
    - Term or post-term pregnancy
  - Labor risk factors
    - Consistency of meconium
    - Abnormal FHR patterns
    - Precipitous birth
    - Cesarean birth
  - Fetal factors
    - Advancing gestational age (greater than 42 weeks)
    - Apgar score less than 7 (1 or 5 minutes)

Physical Examination: Components of the Physical Exam to Consider

- Abdominal examination
  - FHT in relation to contractions
  - Fetal movement
  - Fluid adequacy (thick meconium may be present in conjunction with oligohydramnios)
  - Frequency, duration, and strength of contractions
  - Fetal lie and presentation (meconium aspiration is common with breech presentations)
- Pelvic examination
  - Cervical status
  - Confirmation of presentation
  - Station of presenting part

Clinical Impression: Differential Diagnoses to Consider

(ICD9data.com, 2012)

- Meconium-stained amniotic fluid
- Meconium noted at birth, affecting infant
- Fetal distress

Diagnostic Testing: Diagnostic Tests and Procedures to Consider

- Evaluation of fetal well-being

- Intermittent auscultation: Follow ACOG "with risk factors" guidelines (ACOG, 2005)
  - Every 15 minutes in active labor after a contraction
  - Every 5 minutes in second stage
- Electronic fetal monitor
  - External
  - Internal
- Ultrasound
  - AFI
  - Fetal presentation
- Preoperative laboratory tests
  - Nonreassuring FHR pattern
  - Arrest of dilation or descent
  - Per facility standard

Providing Treatment: Therapeutic Measures to Consider

- ⚠ Amnioinfusion is recommended for meconium-stained fluid only with the presence of variable decelerations associated with cord compression (see "Care of the Woman Undergoing Amnioinfusion")
- Prepare for potential outcomes
  - Vigorous newborn: Routine care
  - Suctioning for newborns
    - Suction newborns who are not vigorous
    - Suction newborns who are initially vigorous but develop respiratory distress
    - Use intubation and suction with an endotracheal tube (American Academy of Pediatrics/American Heart Association, 2010)
  - Neonatal resuscitation
  - Neonatal transport

Providing Treatment: Complementary and Alternative Measures to Consider

- Expectant management
- Gentle birth
- Suctioning method determined by the midwife's scope of practice, such as DeLee or Res-Q-Vac

Providing Support: Education and Support Measures to Consider

- Most healthy term infants with meconium-stained fluid do not develop meconium aspiration syndrome
- Advise the client of the potential risks associated with meconium
  - Meconium aspiration syndrome
  - Trauma potential with intubation
- ▽ Advise the client of the potential for interventions
  - Transport if an out-of-hospital birth is planned
  - Immediate clamping and cutting of the cord for hand-off of the newborn to the pediatric team
  - Intubation of the newborn
  - Oxygen for the newborn
  - Newborn special care
  - Antibiotic therapy for the infant
- Prompt treatment of an infant with meconium aspiration syndrome decreases the following risks:
  - Severe respiratory disorders
  - Newborn death
- Provide ongoing information
  - In labor
  - At birth
  - If the newborn needs special care

Follow-up Care: Follow-up Measures to Consider

- Have all resuscitation equipment on hand and tested
- Anticipate the newborn's condition at birth
  - A professional who is skilled in intubation should be present if possible
  - Additional personnel for newborn resuscitation should be present, as needed
- Document infant assessment and care

Multidisciplinary Practice: Consider Consultation, Collaboration, or Referral

- OB/GYN services
  - Abnormal FHR patterns
  - Thick or particulate meconium

- ▪ Documented or suspected oligohydramnios
- ▪ For change in planned location of birth
- Consider hospital birth with the following conditions:
  - ▪ Meconium-stained amniotic fluid
  - ▪ Postdates pregnancy
  - ▪ Abnormal FHR pattern
- Pediatric services
  - ▪ Presence of meconium
  - ▪ Anticipation of a compromised newborn
  - ▪ Newborn resuscitation
  - ▪ Respiratory distress in the neonate
- For diagnosis or treatment outside the midwife's scope of practice

CARE OF THE WOMAN WITH MULTI-FETAL GESTATION

Key Clinical Information

Midwives will occasionally diagnose multi-fetal gestation in women in every setting where they provide prenatal care. Incidence of multi-fetal gestation has increased by 65% in the case of twin pregnancies and by 400% in triplet and higher-order pregnancies largely due to more widespread use of assisted reproductive technologies (Gabbe et al., 2007). Early identification of the multi-fetal gestation provides an opportunity to assess for and address potential complications before they arise.

Midwives provide prenatal care and labor and birth care to women with twin gestation in some settings. In the home birth setting, the midwife assumes the responsibility for advising parents of the increased risk of adverse outcomes with multi-fetal pregnancy when birth occurs in the home. Regardless of the planned birth location, the midwife must have a means to provide access to obstetric or pediatric care if it is indicated. Multi-fetal pregnancy is associated with increased risks for preterm labor, preeclampsia, preterm ROM, intrauterine fetal growth restriction, twin-to-twin transfusion, and perinatal death. Vertex–vertex presentation is the most common presentation of twins, however, and vaginal birth is recommended for these women

in the absence of the same indications for cesarean delivery as for singleton births (Gabbe et al., 2007).

Client History and Chart Review: Components of the History to Consider

- LMP, EDC, gestational age
- Contributing factors for multi-fetal gestation
  - ▪ Family history of multi-fetal gestations
  - ▪ Personal history of multi-fetal gestations
  - ▪ Use of fertility drugs
  - ▪ Use of in vitro fertilization or other assisted reproductive technologies (Gabbe et al., 2007)
- History suggestive of multi-fetal gestation
  - ▪ Fundal growth pattern
  - ▪ Size larger than dates by examination
  - ▪ Fetal motion not detected by 18–20 week size
  - ▪ Elevated α-fetoprotein results
- ⚠ Multi-fetal pregnancy complications include increased incidence of the following conditions:
  - ▪ Fetal anomalies
  - ▪ Spontaneous abortion
  - ▪ Maternal anemia
  - ▪ Preeclampsia
  - ▪ Preterm labor
    - ◆ Uterine irritability
    - ◆ Cervical changes
    - ◆ Preterm PROM
  - ▪ Polyhydramnios
  - ▪ Placental abruption
- Other pregnancy considerations
  - ▪ Rh status
  - ▪ Medical conditions
- Social support
  - ▪ Nutrition status
  - ▪ Working or living conditions
  - ▪ Response to multi-fetal gestation

Physical Examination: Components of the Physical Exam to Consider

- Interval weight gain
- Abdominal examination
  - ▪ Interval fundal growth pattern
  - ▪ Size larger than dates on two or more occasions

- ▪ Multiple small parts felt on palpation
- ▪ Two fetal hearts heard simultaneously at different rates via Doppler or fetoscope
- Pelvic examination: Cervical length and dilation

Clinical Impression: Differential Diagnoses to Consider

(ICD9data.com, 2012)

- Multi-fetal gestation
  - ▪ Twins
  - ▪ Triplets
  - ▪ Quadruplets
  - ▪ Other multi-fetal pregnancy

Diagnostic Testing: Diagnostic Tests and Procedures to Consider

- Maternal serum α-fetoprotein
- Amniocentesis
- Ultrasound evaluation
  - ▪ Gestational age
  - ▪ Presence of multi-fetal gestation
  - ▪ Presence of anomalies
  - ▪ Placenta(s) and membranes
    - ◆ Monochorionic
    - ◆ Dichorionic, diamniotic
  - ▪ Fetal gender(s)
  - ▪ Interval growth
  - ▪ Cervical evaluation
    - ◆ Width
    - ◆ Length
    - ◆ Funneling
- Antepartum surveillance
  - ▪ Serial ultrasounds every 3–4 weeks after 20 weeks (Gabbe et al., 2007)
  - ▪ For complications of multi-fetal gestation
    - ◆ Intrauterine growth restriction
    - ◆ Abnormal AFI
    - ◆ Discordant fetal growth
    - ◆ PIH
    - ◆ Fetal anomalies
    - ◆ Monoamniotic twins
  - ▪ Non-stress testing
  - ▪ Biophysical profile

Providing Treatment: Therapeutic Measures to Consider

- There is no evidence to support the use of the following modalities (Gabbe et al., 2007):
  - ▪ Cervical cerclage
  - ▪ Bed rest
  - ▪ Hospitalization
  - ▪ Home uterine activity monitoring
- Selective fetal termination
  - ▪ Common consideration with high-order multi-fetal gestation and in vitro fertilization
  - ▪ Poses ethical dilemmas
- Specialized multi-fetal clinics for prenatal care
- Treat
  - ▪ Preterm labor (see "Care of the Woman with Preterm Labor")
  - ▪ Preterm ROM (see "Care of the Woman with Prelabor Rupture of Membranes")
  - ▪ Preeclampsia (see "Care of the Pregnant Woman with Hypertensive Disorders in Pregnancy")
- Vertex–vertex twins
  - ▪ Anticipate vaginal birth
  - ▪ Second twin may require time to be born
  - ▪ Cesarean birth for same indications with singleton birth (Gabbe et al., 2007)
- Vertex–nonvertex twins
  - ▪ Consider vaginal birth for second twin weighing more than 1500 g
  - ▪ Consider cesarean birth based on the following considerations:
    - ◆ Fetal weight less than 1500 g
    - ◆ Maternal preference
    - ◆ Clinician skill and experience
- Nonvertex first twin
  - ▪ Cesarean delivery is recommended
  - ▪ Vaginal birth of nonvertex first twin has not been studied
  - ▪ Potential for locked twins with breech–vertex twins
- Ongoing evaluation of second fetus after first birth
  - ▪ Ultrasound

- Electronic fetal monitoring
- Close observation for complications
  - Cord prolapse
  - Placental abruption
  - Abnormal FHR pattern
- Stimulation or augmentation of labor, as needed
  - Oxytocin
  - Amniotomy
- For deteriorating fetal status
  - Internal podalic version as needed
  - Breech extraction
  - Cesarean birth of second twin

Providing Treatment: Complementary and Alternative Measures to Consider

- Diagnosis of twins via clinical examination
- Out-of-hospital birth
  - Uncomplicated multi-fetal gestation
  - Maternal preference
  - Informed choice considerations
  - Risk factors for individual
  - Midwife skill and experience
  - Distance/time to emergency care
- ⚠ Multi-fetal birth holds increased risk in every birth location
  - Vertex–vertex presentation has the highest likelihood of vaginal birth with minimal intervention and excellent outcome
  - Parental willingness to transfer for indications is an important consideration in plans for out-of-hospital birth
  - Emergency transport plans and communication with the receiving hospital are essential elements of plans for out-of-hospital birth of twins
- In-hospital birth
  - Vaginal birth
  - Birth room
  - Minimum of people
  - Opportunity to meet staff beforehand
  - Negotiation of preferences
  - Ability to see and touch babies immediately

- Care provided in the family's presence
- Rooming-in and breastfeeding fostered
- Cesarean birth
  - Support people present
  - Ability to see and touch babies immediately, if stable
  - Care provided in the family's presence
  - Rooming-in and breastfeeding fostered

Providing Support: Education and Support Measures to Consider

- Discussion and education regarding multi-fetal gestation
  - Anticipated care during pregnancy
  - Information on testing or surveillance
    - Procedures
    - Results
    - Implications
    - Options and recommendations
- Active listening to the client
  - Individual needs
  - Preferences
  - Collaborative planning of care
  - Options for high-risk care as indicated

Follow-up Care: Follow-up Measures to Consider

- Document
- Increased frequency of prenatal visits
  - By gestational age
  - As indicated by results of testing
  - In the presence of any complicating factors
  - As term approaches (third trimester)
- Identification of risk factors
  - Problem list
  - Update the plan as changes occur
- Labor: Anticipate potential complications
  - Preterm labor (see "Care of the Woman with Preterm Labor")
  - Prelabor ROM (see "Care of the Woman with Prelabor Rupture of Membranes")
  - Uterine inertia
  - Placental abruption
  - Postpartum hemorrhage

Multidisciplinary Practice: Consider Consultation, Collaboration, or Referral

- OB/GYN services
  - For all multi-fetal pregnancies per the midwife's scope of practice
  - For the multi-fetal gestation with complications
    - Maternal complications
    - Fetal complications
  - Triplet or greater multiple pregnancy
  - Maternal preference
- Pediatric services
  - Presence of prenatal complications
  - Immediate newborn care at birth
- Social services
  - Mothers of twins support group
  - Grief support group for pregnancy losses
  - Other support services
- For diagnosis or treatment outside the midwife's scope of practice

CARE OF THE WOMAN WITH A NONVERTEX PRESENTATION

Key Clinical Information

Breech presentation is the most common nonvertex presentation, occurring in 3% to 4% of term single-ton pregnancies. Compared to a vertex presentation, breech and other nonvertex presentations carry an increased risk of complications, such as cord prolapse and fetal injury. Specific prenatal techniques, such as postural management, moxibustion, Webster chiropractic technique, and hypnosis, when used during the prenatal period have demonstrated some benefit in turning breech to vertex presentation with no evidence of harmful effects (Pistolese, 2002; Romm, 2010).

ACOG (2000a) recommends external version to convert a breech or transverse lie to vertex presentation to decrease the risks associated with nonvertex presentations and avoid unnecessary cesarean delivery. Decisions about the mode of birth for term breech fetuses should be based on the experience of the provider; vaginal breech birth may be reasonable with careful selection criteria and labor management guidelines (ACOG, 2006). Planned cesarean section for nonvertex presentation does not apply to women who refuse surgical delivery, women whose birth is imminent at the time of diagnosis, or women whose second twin is a nonvertex presentation.

Client History and Chart Review: Components of the History to Consider

- LMP, EDC
- Previous maternity history
  - Previous breech births
  - Previous birth weights of children
  - Presence of uterine scars
- Contraindications for vaginal breech birth
  - Inexperienced birth attendant
  - Maternal preference for Cesarean birth
  - Birth attendant preference for Cesarean birth
  - Suspected CPD
  - Macrosomic fetus
  - Nonreassuring FHR patterns
  - Maternal or fetal complications
  - Previous history
    - Shoulder dystocia
    - Dysfunctional labor
    - Protracted labor
- Current pregnancy history
  - Methods of dating pregnancy
  - Current gestation
  - Rh status
  - Placental location
  - Presence of labor
- Contributing factors to nonvertex presentation
  - Maternal pelvic type and dimensions
  - Polyhydramnios
  - Lax abdominal muscle tone
  - Multiparity
  - Prematurity
  - Multi-fetal gestation
  - Placenta previa
  - Hydrocephalus
  - Fetal or uterine anomalies (Varney et al., 2004)

Physical Examination: Components of the Physical Exam to Consider

- Diagnosis of nonvertex presentation: Abdominal examination
  - Leopold's maneuvers
  - Determine fetal presentation, lie, and variety
  - Estimate fetal weight
  - Note abdominal muscle tone
  - Uterine tone
  - FHR and location
- Pelvic examination
  - Clinical pelvimetry
  - Cervical status
    - Palpation of presenting part through cervix or lower uterine segment
    - Determine fetal presentation, lie, and variety
    - Estimate fetal weight

Clinical Impression: Differential Diagnoses to Consider

(ICD9data.com, 2012)

- Pregnancy, nonvertex presentation
  - Breech
  - Transverse
  - Face or brow

Diagnostic Testing: Diagnostic Tests and Procedures to Consider

- Ultrasound
  - Confirmation of fetal position
  - Evaluation of placental position
  - Version may be performed under ultrasound guidance
- External cephalic version
  - Fetal evaluation
    - Preprocedure
    - During and post procedure
    - Continuous fetal monitoring
    - NST and/or biophysical profile (BPP)
  - Maternal
    - IV access
    - Preoperative laboratory tests

Providing Treatment: Therapeutic Measures to Consider

- External cephalic version (ACOG, 2000a)
  - Success rates of 35% to 86%
  - More successful in the following scenarios:
    - Multiparous women
    - Transverse or oblique lie
  - Use of tocolytics
    - For nulliparous women
    - For all women
  - Consider use of sedative, analgesia, or anesthesia
  - Rh immune globulin for Rh-negative women
  - Ready access to emergency cesarean delivery
- External cephalic version method, after fetal evaluation
  - Have the client empty her bladder
  - The client relaxes with knees bent and supported
  - Abdominal muscles must be relaxed
  - Attempt a forward roll using gentle, steady pressure
  - Lift the breech from the pelvis
  - Encourage the head toward the pelvis with gentle pressure and flexion
  - Attempt a backward roll if the forward roll is not successful
  - Two practitioners may work together to encourage the fetus to turn
  - ⚠ Stop the version with the following conditions:
    - Fetal bradycardia
    - Maternal pain
    - Vaginal bleeding
    - Rupture of membranes
    - Unsuccessful version
    - Successful version
- Vaginal breech birth may be considered (Gabbe et al., 2007)
  - EFW = 2000–3800 g
  - Frank breech
  - Adequate pelvis

- Flexed fetal head
- Fetal evaluation in labor
- Access to rapid cesarean birth
- Good progress is maintained in labor
- Experienced practitioner is available
- Informed consent and maternal desire for vaginal birth
- Cesarean birth may be prudent (Gabbe et al., 2007)
  - EFW is less than 1500 g or greater than 4000 g
  - Footling presentation
  - Small pelvis
  - Hyperextended fetal head
  - Absence of practitioner expertise
  - Nonreassuring fetal heart rate pattern
  - Arrest of progress
- Conduct of vaginal breech birth (Varney et al., 2004)
  - Hands off until birth to the umbilicus
    - Maintain flexion of the head
    - Pinard maneuver for extended legs
  - Gently pull down a loop of cord
  - Place a warm towel around the baby's body
  - Holding the baby's hips, provide gentle, steady, downward and outward traction
  - When axillae are in view, deliver one arm and shoulder, then other
  - Maintain cephalic flexion through pressure on the fetal maxilla
  - Provide upward traction of the body to facilitate slow birth of the head

Providing Treatment: Complementary and Alternative Measures to Consider

- Breech tilt position
  - Perform for 5 minutes, three to four times daily
  - Hips higher than head on tilt board
  - Music at maternal feet to encourage fetus to turn
- Hands and knees with or without pelvic rocking (Andrews & Andrews, 2004)

- Moxibustion (Romm, 2010)
  - Burn moxa cone 15 minutes daily
  - Place at outer corner of the little toe nailbed
- Acupuncture (Habek, Habek, & Jagust, 2003)

Providing Support: Education and Support Measures to Consider

- Provide information on risks, benefits, and availability
  - Vaginal breech birth
  - External cephalic version
  - Planned cesarean delivery
- Obtain informed consent for planned birth or procedure
  - Perinatal risk may be higher with vaginal birth—5% versus 1.6% (ACOG, 2006)
    - Short-term neonatal morbidity
    - Fetal injury or death
    - Neonatal injury or death
  - Maternal risk increased for cesarean section versus vaginal breech (Hofmeyr & Hannah, 2007)
- Encourage questions regarding options
- Consider maternal preferences in jointly determining the plan for care

Follow-up Care: Follow-up Measures to Consider

- Document
- Reconfirm
  - Fetal position before birth
  - Maternal preference for planned birth or procedure
- Persistent breech
  - Repeat version attempt
  - Reconsider vaginal breech or planned cesarean section
- Document
  - All discussions
  - Informed consent/informed choice
  - Maternal preferences for care
- For planned vaginal breech birth
  - Plan access to emergency care
  - Estimate fetal weight

- Plan for birth
  - Number, type, and skill of birth attendants
  - Presence of resuscitation team for newborn
  - Plan for emergency care

Multidisciplinary Practice: Consider Consultation, Collaboration, or Referral

- Chiropractic care: Webster technique for turning breech (Pistolese, 2002)
- OB/GYN services
  - For persistent nonvertex presentation
  - For cesarean delivery
  - For failed version
  - Maternal preference
  - Contraindications to vaginal breech birth
- Pediatric service: For newborn care after vaginal breech birth
- For diagnosis or treatment outside the midwife's scope of practice

CARE OF THE WOMAN WITH POSTPARTUM HEMORRHAGE

Key Clinical Information

Postpartum hemorrhage is defined as a blood loss of greater than 500 mL at delivery or within the first 24 hours after vaginal birth; it affects 1% to 3% of women in the first 24 hours after birth (Gregory, Main, & Lyndon, 2009). Postpartum hemorrhage is a leading cause of maternal mortality and morbidity in both developed and developing countries. The anemia that results from hemorrhage can be a significant contributor to delayed postpartum healing and predispose the woman to infection. Hemorrhage can be the primary indicator of retained placental tissue, uterine fatigue, significant lacerations, or disorders of coagulation. The primary cause of postpartum hemorrhage is uterine atony. Greater length of time to placental delivery increases the risk of postpartum hemorrhage; at more than 30 minutes, the risk of postpartum hemorrhage triples. Active management

of the third stage of labor is an evidence-based strategy that can reduce the risk of postpartum hemorrhage (Simpson, 2007).

Client History and Chart Review: Components of the History to Consider

- Past pregnancy history
  - Prior history of postpartum hemorrhage
  - Parity
    - Nulliparous
    - Grand multiparity
  - Cesarean section
  - Prior history of retained placenta
- Course of labor
  - Gestational age
  - Hematocrit and hemoglobin at onset of labor
  - Effectiveness of uterine contractions
  - Length of each stage
  - Oxytocin administration
  - Placental delivery and status
  - Genital tract laceration
- Risk factors for hemorrhage
  - Ethnic history
    - Asian
    - Hispanic
  - Preterm delivery
  - Precipitous labor and birth
  - Overdistention of the uterus
    - Fetal macrosomia
    - Polyhydramnios
    - Multi-fetal gestation
  - Prolonged third stage (Simpson, 2007)
  - PIH or HELLP syndrome
    - $MgSO_4$ use
    - Low platelets
  - Operative delivery
    - Vacuum extraction
    - Forceps
    - Uterine manipulation (i.e., version)
  - Placenta previa or abruption
  - Chorioamnionitis
  - Fetal demise
  - Disseminated intravascular coagulation (DIC)

- Medical history
  - Bleeding disorders
  - Asthma (avoid Prostin)
  - Hypertension (avoid Methergine)
- [www] Assessment for hemorrhage risk for women in labor (CMQCC Hemorrhage Task Force, 2010)
  - Low risk
    - No previous uterine incision
    - Singleton pregnancy
    - Fewer than or equal to four prior vaginal births
    - No known bleeding disorder
    - No history of postpartum hemorrhage
  - Moderate risk
    - Prior cesarean births or uterine surgery
    - More than four births
    - Chorioamnionitis
    - History of postpartum hemorrhage
    - Large uterine fibroids
    - Estimated fetal weight more than 4 kg
    - Morbid obesity (BMI greater than 35)
  - High risk
    - Placenta previa or low-lying placenta
    - Suspected placenta accreta or percreta
    - Hematocrit less than 30
    - Platelets less than 100,000
    - Active bleeding greater than show in labor
    - Known coagulopathy

Physical Examination: Components of the Physical Exam to Consider

- Evaluate the cause of bleeding
  - Uterine atony
  - Lacerations
  - Retained placental fragments
  - Partially separated placenta
  - Coagulopathy
- Evaluate bladder, empty as needed
- Evaluate for shock (estimated blood loss greater than 500 mL)
  - Rapid, thready pulse
  - Rapid, shallow respirations
  - Pale, clammy skin and mucous membranes
  - Anxiety or lack of affect

- Placenta undelivered
  - Evaluate the uterus for placental separation
    - Uterus globular, firm
    - Fundus rises and is mobile
    - Cord lengthens
    - Brandt-Andrews maneuver (see "Modified Brandt-Andrews Maneuver" box)
  - Assess for lacerations

Modified Brandt-Andrews Maneuver

- Hold the umbilical cord taut with a clamp in one hand
- Press downward just above the maternal symphysis with the other hand
- If the cord retracts, the placenta is not yet separated
- If the cord lengthens, the placenta has separated

Source: Varney et al., 2004.

- Placenta delivered
  - Examine placenta for completeness
  - Evaluate the uterus for atony
    - If atony present
      - Massage fundus
      - Bimanual compression
      - Consider retained placental or membrane fragments
    - If no atony, evaluate for a traumatic source of bleeding
      - Cervical lacerations
      - Vaginal lacerations
      - Uterine rupture

Clinical Impression: Differential Diagnoses to Consider

(ICD9data.com, 2012)

Postpartum hemorrhage, secondary to the following:

- Uterine atony
- Genital tract laceration(s)
- Retained placental tissue
- Clotting disorders

Diagnostic Testing: Diagnostic Tests and Procedures to Consider

- CBC
- Hematocrit and hemoglobin
- Platelets
- Type and cross-match
- Preeclampsia laboratory panel (see "Care of the Woman with Hypertensive Disorders of Pregnancy in Labor")
- Coagulation studies
  - Prothrombin time, partial thromboplastin time
  - Fibrinogen
- Ultrasound evaluation
  - Retained placental tissue
  - Hematoma formation

Estimating Blood Loss Through Hemoglobin Levels

Each 500 mL of blood lost roughly translates to a drop of 1 g in the hemoglobin level (Blackburn, 2007).

Providing Treatment: Therapeutic Measures to Consider

- **www.** Preventive measures
  - Controlled birth of infant to minimize tissue trauma
  - Physiologic management of third-stage labor (see "Care of the Woman in Third-Stage Labor"): For clients without risk factors for postpartum hemorrhage
  - Active management of third-stage labor (see "Care of the Woman in Third-Stage Labor")
    - Clients with risk factors for postpartum hemorrhage
    - All clients
  - Massage the uterus until it is firm once the placenta is born
  - Encourage breastfeeding and skin-to-skin contact with the infant

- Postpartum hemorrhage placenta in situ
  - Bleeding indicates partial separation
  - Manual exploration and removal may be necessary
    - Do not pull on the cord
    - Procedure for manual removal
      - Insert a sterile gloved hand into the vagina
      - Follow the cord to the placenta
      - Move the hand laterally to find the edge
      - Wedge the fingertips under the leading edge of the placenta
      - Shear the placenta off the uterine wall using short strokes
      - Remove the placenta
      - Treat the client for postpartum hemorrhage with the placenta delivered
      - Potential need for follow-up dilation and curettage (D & C)
- Postpartum hemorrhage with placenta delivered
  - Assess the placenta for completeness
  - Examine the vagina and cervix for lacerations
  - Assess maternal vital signs
- Perform bimanual compression
  - If the uterus fails to contract well
  - Decreases the blood supply to large uterine vessels
  - Will not diminish bleeding due to lacerations
  - Technique
    - One hand in the vagina against the lower uterine segment: Form into a fist in the anterior fornix
    - Second hand on the abdomen: Cup the posterior wall of the uterus
    - Bring hands firmly together
      - Uterus will be compressed between the hands
      - Maintain steady pressure until bleeding is controlled
      - Order uterotonic medications (Varney et al., 2004)

- Medications
  - Pitocin 10 units IM or 20–40 units/1000 mL normal saline or lactated Ringer's IV fluids
    - Rapid infusion
    - Preferred first-line therapy
  - Misoprostol (Cytotec) (King & Brucker, 2011)
    - 800 mcg rectally or sublingually in one dose: Range of dosing 400–1000 mcg
    - Thermostable uterotonic agent
    - Low incidence of side effects (abdominal pain and diarrhea)
    - Rapid onset of action
    - Half-life (oral): 20–40 min (Rx Med, n.d.)
  - Methergine 0.2 mg IM
    - May be repeated in intervals of 2-4 hours, for up to 7 days
    - Indicated for persistent boggy uterus
    - Avoid in a client with hypertension
  - Prostaglandin F_2 alpha (Hemabate) 250 mg IM or intramyometrial
    - Repeat every 20–90 minutes up to 8 doses
    - Significant side effects
    - Not the preferred first-line therapy
  - Prostaglandin E_2 alpha (Prostin E_2) 15 M, 0.25 mg IM
- IV therapy
  - Large-bore (16-gauge) catheter(s)
  - Lactated Ringer's, Normosol, or other similar solution
  - 10 units oxytocin/500 mL IV fluids
  - Run rapidly until atony subsides
  - Use second IV as needed for fluid replacement
- Uterine exploration for retained placental tissue: May need D & C under anesthesia
- Replacement blood transfusion
  - For estimated blood loss of greater than 1000 mL or signs of shock
  - Blood products, warmed to prevent hypothermia
    - Volume expanders (albumin, hetastarch, dextran)
    - Whole blood
    - Packed red blood cells
    - Other blood components as indicated
- For shock
  - Additional IV access
  - O_2 by mask
  - Trendelenburg or shock position
  - Foley catheter
  - Monitor intake and output closely
- Extreme bleeding
  - Packing
    - Deep vaginal or cervical lacerations
    - While awaiting surgical repair
  - Uterine tamponade balloon
    - Aortic compression
    - Emergency measure while awaiting surgical care
  - Surgical control of bleeding
    - Repair of lacerations
    - Suture ligature of bleeding vessels
    - Dilation and evacuation of retained placenta fragments
    - Hysterectomy or uterine artery ligation in extreme cases

Providing Treatment: Complementary and Alternative Measures to Consider

- Preventives
  - Nettle or alfalfa leaf infusion
    - Given during pregnancy
    - Given immediately after birth of the baby
  - Motherwort tincture
- Treatment of hemorrhage due to atony
  - Shepherd's purse tincture (Soule & Szwed, 2000)
  - Tincture made of blue cohosh and shepherd's purse
  - Breast stimulation

Providing Support: Education and Support Measures to Consider

- Discuss and arrange transport if out-of-hospital
- After resolution of hemorrhage
  - Discuss occurrence of hemorrhage

- If symptomatic, call for help before arising
- Take iron replacement therapy as directed
  - Dietary sources
  - Supplements
- Rest and adequate nutrition are essential for healing
- Reinforce knowledge of signs and symptoms of infection
  - How to recognize
  - When and how to call
- Active listening

Follow-up Care: Follow-up Measures to Consider

- Document findings, treatment, and client response
- Observe
  - Persistent bleeding
  - Signs of hypovolemia or anemia
    - Weakness
    - Dyspnea
    - Syncope
- CBC/hematocrit and hemoglobin
  - First postpartum day
  - Repeat if bleeding continues
  - 4- to 6-week check

Multidisciplinary Practice: Consider Consultation, Collaboration, or Referral

- OB/GYN services
  - Hemorrhage that does not respond
    - Immediately to treatment
    - As expected with appropriate treatment
  - Signs and symptoms of shock
  - For transport from out-of-hospital
  - For suspicion of the following conditions:
    - Retained placental fragments
    - Severe vaginal lacerations or hematomas
    - Cervical lacerations
    - Uterine rupture
- For diagnosis or treatment outside the midwife's scope of practice

CARE OF THE WOMAN WITH POST-TERM PREGNANCY

Key Clinical Information

Post-term pregnancy is defined as pregnancy that extends to or beyond 42 completed weeks. Approximately 4% to 7% of women have post-term pregnancies (Hermus, Verhoeven, Mol, Wolf, & Fiedeldeij, 2009). Accurate dating of the pregnancy is essential to making this diagnosis. Perinatal morbidity and mortality increase as gestational age advances beyond term as a function of placental aging. Additional fetal surveillance is typically initiated between 41 and 42 weeks, gestation in the form of biweekly non-stress tests. Post-term pregnancy is widely considered an indication for recommending induction. Women with a post-term pregnancy and an unfavorable cervix can be managed expectantly. Induction compared to expectant management yields a lower cesarean section rate and less meconium-stained fluid and its sequelae (Sanchez-Ramos, Olivier, Delke, & Kaunitz, 2003). The absolute difference in perinatal mortality is low, however, so women should be educated on both options.

Client History and Chart Review: Components of the History to Consider

- Assess EDC using multiple parameters
  - LMP
  - Conception date if known
  - First positive pregnancy test
  - Uterine size at first visit
  - Initial FHR
    - Fetoscope or stethoscope: 18–20 weeks
    - Doppler: 10–14 weeks
  - Quickening
  - Fundal height at umbilicus at 20 weeks
  - Early or mid-pregnancy ultrasound
- Post-term risk assessment
  - Fetal macrosomia
  - Fetal postmaturity syndrome
  - Oligohydramnios
  - Meconium aspiration syndrome

- Review history for additional factors that may prolong pregnancy
  - Adrenal hyperplasia
  - Maternal psychosocial stresses
  - Certain fetal anomalies
- Assess
  - Ongoing nutrition
  - Fetal activity and changes
  - Contraction patterns
  - Maternal concerns and state of mind

Physical Examination: Components of the Physical Exam to Consider

- Vital signs
- Weight
- Abdominal examination
  - Fetal presentation, position, lie, and variety
  - Fetal flexion and engagement
  - EFW
  - Palpate for the following conditions:
    - Fluid adequacy
    - Presence of contractions
- Pelvic examination
  - Calculate Bishop's score
  - Verify presenting part
  - Reassess pelvimetry

Clinical Impression: Differential Diagnoses to Consider

(ICD9data.com, 2012)

- Prolonged pregnancy: More than or equal to 42 weeks
- Term pregnancy: More than 37 weeks but less than 42 weeks

Diagnostic Testing: Diagnostic Tests and Procedures to Consider

Fetal surveillance

- Daily fetal kick counts
- Non-stress test
  - Weekly
  - Biweekly

- Biophysical profile
  - Weekly
  - Biweekly
- AFI as a separate indicator
- Contraction stress testing (ACOG, 2004)

Providing Treatment: Therapeutic Measures to Consider

- Watchful waiting—requirements:
  - Close observation of maternal and fetal well-being
  - Informed choice
  - Willingness to accept intervention as needed
- Cervical ripening (see "Care of the Woman Undergoing Induction or Augmentation of Labor")
  - No demonstrated benefit over expectant care for a healthy mother and fetus (ACOG, 2004)
  - As indicated by maternal or fetal status
    - Preeclampsia
    - Gestational diabetes
    - Nonreassuring fetal surveillance
  - Generally followed by induction of labor
- Induction (see "Care of the Woman Undergoing Induction or Augmentation of Labor")
  - Offered at or close to 42 completed weeks, gestation
  - As indicated by maternal or fetal status

Providing Treatment: Complementary and Alternative Measures to Consider

- Watchful waiting (see previous section)
- Alternative measures for cervical ripening/induction (see "Care of the Woman Undergoing Induction or Augmentation of Labor")

Providing Support: Education and Support Measures to Consider

- Discuss potential risks and benefits
  - Expectant management
  - Induction of labor
  - Interventions

- Review or teach
  - Post-term is after 42 weeks, gestation
  - Fetal kick count technique
  - Process of labor
  - Indications to call
- Discuss labor options
  - Obtain informed consent
  - Expectant care
  - Elective intervention
  - Indicated intervention
  - Any potential change in location or anticipated care for labor and birth
- Listen to and note the client's and family's preferences and concerns

Follow-up Care: Follow-up Measures to Consider

- Fetal surveillance
  - Evaluate fetal status every 3–7 days
  - Review results promptly
- Document the ongoing plan
- Anticipate the potential for complications (ACOG, 2004)
  - Meconium-stained amniotic fluid
  - Shoulder dystocia
  - Postpartum hemorrhage
  - Increased chance of cesarean
  - Newborn respiratory distress

Multidisciplinary Practice: Consider Consultation, Collaboration, or Referral

- OB/GYN services
  - Pregnancy after 42 weeks
  - Nonreassuring fetal testing
  - Concerns regarding reasons for post-term status
  - Change in location of birth due to fetal status/postdates
- Pediatric services
  - Anticipatory for post-term infant
  - As indicated by the following conditions:
    - Nonreassuring fetal surveillance
    - Meconium-stained amniotic fluid

- Shoulder dystocia
- Cesarean delivery
- Newborn respiratory distress
- For diagnosis or treatment outside the midwife's scope of practice

CARE OF THE WOMAN WITH PRELABOR RUPTURE OF MEMBRANES

Key Clinical Information

Prelabor rupture of membranes (PROM) is defined as the rupture of membranes before the onset of labor; it occurs in approximately 8% of term pregnancies (Marowitz & Jordan, 2007). Ninety percent of women with PROM enter labor by 24 hours post ROM. Management options for term PROM include induction and expectant management. Expectant management is a reasonable option to offer to selected women with PROM (ACOG, 2007; ACNM, 2008a). Preterm PROM is ROM that occurs before the pregnancy has reached the term mark.

Complications of PROM include complications related to preterm birth after PROM, fetal distress related to cord compression, and fetal infection. Maternal complications include maternal intraamniotic infection, increased risk of cesarean delivery, and postpartum endometritis (Gabbe et al., 2007).

Client History and Chart Review: Components of the History to Consider

- LMP, EDC, gestational age
- Relevant prenatal and maternity history
  - GBS status
  - Complications of current or previous pregnancy
  - Previous PROM
  - Sexually transmitted infection test results
- Current signs and symptoms
  - Onset of symptoms
  - Duration of symptoms
  - Amount, color, and consistency of vaginal leakage
  - Last sexual activity

- Presence of warning signs
  - Fever or chills
  - Palpitations
  - Uterine tenderness
  - Flank tenderness
- Presence of risk factors for PROM (Varney et al., 2004)
  - Nonvertex presentation
  - Previous pregnancy with PROM
  - Chorioamnionitis
  - Polyhydramnios
  - Multi-fetal gestation
  - Vaginal GBS or other pathogenic vaginal flora
  - Smoking more than ½ pack of cigarettes per day
  - Nutritional deficiencies
  - Family history of PROM
  - Cervical procedure
    - Loop electrocautery excision procedure (LEEP)
    - Conization
    - Cryosurgery
  - Occupational fatigue in nulliparas

Physical Examination: Components of the Physical Exam to Consider

- Vital signs with temperature every 1–2 hours
  - Maternal fever (temperature greater than 32.2°C [100.4°F])
  - Maternal or fetal tachycardia (maternal heart rate greater than 100, FHR greater than 160)
- Abdominal examination
  - Amniotic fluid volume/ballottement
  - Presence of contractions
  - EFW
  - Determine fetal presentation and lie
  - Frequent evaluation of FHR
  - Palpation for uterine tenderness
- Sterile speculum examination
  - Visualization of leakage of amniotic fluid
  - Visualization of cervix
  - Collection of specimen(s) for examination
    - Ferning

- Nitrazine
- GBS culture or screen
- Sterile digital vaginal examination (defer until labor begins)
  - Cervical dilation
  - Effacement
  - Station
  - Confirm presentation
  - Rule out cord prolapse

Clinical Impression: Differential Diagnoses to Consider

(ICD9data.com, 2012)

- Premature rupture of membranes
- Urinary incontinence
- Urinary tract infection
- Increased vaginal secretions
  - Due to pregnancy
  - Vaginitis
  - Sexually transmitted infection

Diagnostic Testing: Diagnostic Tests and Procedures to Consider

- Vaginal fluid evaluation
  - Nitrazine or pH testing (pH 7.0–7.7)
  - Ferning
  - Pooling
  - Wet prep and KOH
- Cultures as indicated, if expectant management is planned
  - GBS culture of vagina and rectum
  - Chlamydia/gonorrhea status
- Ultrasound evaluation
  - Oligohydramnios/AFI
  - Biophysical profile
  - Guidance for amniocentesis
- Amniocentesis for fetal pulmonary maturity testing
- CBC with differential: Maternal leukocytosis (WBCs greater than 16,000 in absence of labor)
- Urine for urinalysis and culture and sensitivity (C & S)
  - Clean catch
  - Straight catheter specimen

- Fetal surveillance
  - NST if greater than 32 weeks, gestation
  - Daily fetal movement counts
  - Biophysical profile/AFI

Providing Treatment: Therapeutic Measures to Consider

- Bed rest
  - Nonvertex presentation
  - Preterm PROM
- Expectant management based on gestational age (ACNM, 2008a)
  - Term pregnancy
    - Labor and birth occur within 28 hours in 95% of cases (Gabbe, 2007)
    - Observation of 24–72 hours is acceptable
    - Avoid digital examinations until labor is well established
    - Induction of labor (see "Care of the Woman Undergoing Induction or Augmentation of Labor")
  - Preterm pregnancy with no additional complications
    - Conservative management is preferred
    - Birth generally occurs within 7 days
    - Glucocorticoids to enhance fetal lung maturity
    - Tocolysis (rarely)
    - Transport to center with newborn special care
- Antibiotic treatment and induction for signs and symptoms of chorioamnionitis

Providing Treatment: Complementary and Alternative Measures to Consider

- Watchful waiting
  - No internal examinations
  - Temperature every 2 hours
  - Daily CBC
  - Adequate hydration and nutrition
  - Await onset of labor
- Stimulation of labor with natural remedies (see "Care of the Woman Undergoing Induction or Augmentation of Labor")

Providing Support: Education and Support Measures to Consider

- Discuss the significance of PROM
  - Anticipated fetal outcome for gestational age
  - Anticipated newborn care
  - Risks and benefits of options for care
  - Maternal risks with PROM
    - Ascending intrauterine infection
    - Increased incidence of intervention
  - Fetal risks with PROM
    - Umbilical cord compression
    - Ascending or preexisting infection
  - Potential need for medical care
  - Potential for change in plans
    - Birth plan
    - Location of birth
    - Birth attendant
- Provide education on signs and symptoms
  - Chorioamnionitis
  - Neonatal sepsis
  - Postpartum endometritis

Follow-up Care: Follow-up Measures to Consider

- Review and document results
  - Maternal testing
  - Fetal surveillance
    - Fetal kick counts
    - NST
    - Biophysical profile
    - Serial AFI
    - FHR
      - Intermittent auscultation of FHT
      - Continuous fetal monitoring
      - Cervical ripening or induction of labor (see "Care of the Woman Undergoing Induction or Augmentation of Labor")
  - Time lapsed since ROM
- Reassess for signs or symptoms of complications
  - Maternal fever
  - Abdominal tenderness
  - Nonreassuring FHT patterns
    - Tachycardia
    - Bradycardia

♦ Late or severe variable decelerations

♦ Decreased variability

- Update plan as changes occur
- ⚠ Expedite birth in the following circumstances:
  - Symptoms of infection develop
  - Fetal compromise occurs
  - Maternal preference
- Evaluate the mother and newborn postpartum
  - Endometritis
  - Other infection
  - Newborn sepsis
- Offer time for discussion and processing information
  - Labor and birth events
  - Outcomes
  - Potential effect on future pregnancies

Multidisciplinary Practice: Consider Consultation, Collaboration, or Referral

- OB/GYN services: Confirmed PROM
  - With delay in onset of labor
  - With signs or symptoms
    - ♦ Infection
    - ♦ Cord prolapse
    - ♦ Fetal compromise
- Pediatric services
  - Onset of labor with fetal or maternal infection
  - For birth as indicated by fetal status
  - Newborn evaluation after prolonged ROM
- For diagnosis or treatment outside the midwife's scope of practice

CARE OF THE WOMAN WITH PRETERM LABOR

Key Clinical Information

Preterm labor is defined as the onset of regular uterine contractions in a woman who is between 20 and 37 weeks, gestation, who in addition has either spontaneous ROM or progressive cervical change (ACOG, 2003). It is the second leading cause of neonatal mortality in the United States, occurring in approximately 10% of pregnancies (Reedy, 2007). Many women who have preterm contractions do not progress to preterm labor. Differentiation of preterm labor from preterm contractions can be challenging, especially for the midwife practicing in a rural area where perinatal services are limited or require substantial travel time. The combination of positive fetal fibronectin (fFN) testing and cervical length less than 25 mm is a strong predictor of impending preterm birth (ACOG, 2003; Reedy, 2007).

Client History and Chart Review: Components of the History to Consider

- EDC confirmation
  - LMP, menstrual cycles
  - Ultrasound dating
  - Beta-HCG results
  - Assisted reproductive technologies
- Prenatal treatment or monitoring for preterm labor prevention
- Determination of labor status
  - Signs and symptoms of preterm labor
    - ♦ Onset and duration of symptoms
    - ♦ May be vague
    - ♦ Mild or severe cramping
    - ♦ Dull backache
    - ♦ Suprapubic or pelvic pressure
    - ♦ Loose stools
    - ♦ Increased or "different" vaginal discharge
  - Precipitating factors
    - ♦ Sexual activity within 96 hours (see the discussion of fFN)
    - ♦ Prolonged standing or heavy lifting
    - ♦ Stress or trauma
    - ♦ Vaginal bleeding
- History or symptoms of infection
  - Urinary tract infections or asymptomatic bacteriuria
  - Vaginal infections or sexually transmitted infections
  - GBS

- ⬜ Risk factors for preterm birth
  - Adolescent pregnancy
  - Advanced maternal age
  - Prepregnant body mass index less than 19.8
  - Cervical cone biopsy
  - Poverty
  - Multi-fetal gestation
  - Tobacco use
  - Prior history of preterm birth
  - Intrauterine growth restriction
  - Uterine anomalies
- Previous determinations of cervical status
  - Length
  - Consistency
  - Funneling

Physical Examination: Components of the Physical Exam to Consider

- Maternal and fetal vital signs
- Abdominal examination
  - Presence of contractions
  - Uterine tenderness
  - Fetal heart rate
  - Estimated fetal weight for gestational age
  - Fetal presentation, position, and lie
  - Costovertebral angle (CVA) tenderness
- Pelvic examination
  - Sterile speculum exam for specimen collection
    - Fetal fibronectin fFN
    - GBS culture
    - Wet prep
    - Chlamydia/gonorrhea
    - Specimen for ferning
  - Cervical change from baseline
  - Status of membranes
  - Vaginal discharge
- Evaluation for complications of pregnancy that would favor delivery over tocolysis

Clinical Impression: Differential Diagnoses to Consider

(ICD9data.com, 2012)

- Preterm labor
- False preterm labor

- Multi-fetal gestation
- Pyelonephritis
- Renal calculi
- Abruptio placentae
- Gastritis
- Appendicitis
- Urinary tract infection
- Intrauterine fetal growth restriction

Diagnostic Testing: Diagnostic Tests and Procedures to Consider

- Laboratory tests
  - fFN
    - Collect before digital examination
    - Recent sexual activity or blood can affect results
  - GBS
  - Chlamydia
  - Gonorrhea
  - Wet prep
  - Ferning, nitrazine testing if spontaneous ROM suspected
  - STAT urinalysis, C & S
  - CBC with differential smear
  - Additional laboratory tests as indicated by client history and presentation
- Ultrasound—based on symptoms and gestational age
  - Cervical length and funneling
    - Length greater than 40 mm: Low risk
    - Length 40–26 mm: Moderate risk
    - Length less than 26 mm: High risk
  - Determination of approximate gestational age
  - Verification of number of fetuses
  - Placental location and status
  - AFI, biophysical profile
  - Guidance for amniocentesis
- ⬤ Amniocentesis for fetal surfactant and lecithin/sphingomyelin (L/S) ratio

Providing Treatment: Therapeutic Measures to Consider

- Rest
  - Stop work; avoid lifting

- Refrain from sexual arousal and intercourse
- Stop breastfeeding or other breast stimulation
- Hydration—IV or PO
- Tocolytic medications
  - Use before 34 weeks, gestation
  - Dilation less than 4 cm
  - Can prolong pregnancy 2–7 days or more
  - Allows antenatal transport and corticosteroids (Riley, Boozer, & King, 2011)
  - Calcium-channel blockers (Gabbe et al., 2007)
    - Less severe side-effect profile than β-agonists
    - May cause hypotension
    - Avoid in a client with liver disease
  - Nifedipine: 10–20 mg PO as initial dose
    - May repeat every 3–6 hours until contractions are rare
    - Maintenance with long-acting formulation, 30 or 60 mg PO every 8–12 hours
- Beta Agonists
  - Significant side-effect profile
  - Decrease dose for maternal heart rate greater than 130 beats/min
  - Begin with IV dosing
  - Change to PO dosing:
    - Labor stopped for 12–24 hours
    - 30 minutes before stopping IV dosing
  - Terbutaline
    - IV 2.5 mg/min; increase in 2.5-mg increments
    - Increase every 20 minutes based on effect
    - Maximum dose: 20 mg/min
    - SQ dose: 0.25 mg every 3 hours
    - PO dose: 2.5–5.0 mg every 4–6 hours
  - Ritodrine
    - IV dose: 0.05–0.35 mg/min
    - PO dose: 20 mg every 2–4 hours (ACOG, 2003)
- Magnesium sulfate
  - Loading dose: 4–6 g
  - Maintenance: 2–4 g/hr
  - $MgSO_4$ is typically stopped 12 hours after contractions cease
  - Tapering dose is not required

- Indomethacin (Moses, 2004)
  - Only used before 32 weeks, gestation: May cause premature closure of ductus arteriosis
  - Loading dose: 50 mg PO
  - Maintenance dose: 25 mg PO every 4 hours
  - Maximum dosing period: 48 hours
- Corticosteroid use (Riley et al., 2011)
  - Use between 24 and 34 weeks, gestation
  - Maximum benefit: 1–7 days postdosing
  - Betamethasone—two doses: 12 mg IM every 24 hours
  - Dexamethasone—four doses: 6 mg IM every 12 hours
- Selective cesarean for very preterm infant(s)

Providing Treatment: Complementary and Alternative Measures to Consider

- Observe for preterm contractions versus preterm labor
- Plant-based therapies
  - Black haw tea, tincture, or capsule
  - Valerian root tincture
  - Skullcap tincture
  - Cramp bark and wild yam tincture (1:1): ½ dropperful TID
- Assess overall nutritional status and provide supplements
  - Calcium citrate 1000 mg daily
  - Magnesium 500 mg daily

Providing Support: Education and Support Measures to Consider

- Threatened preterm labor
  - Avoid sexual arousal or activity
  - Call if symptoms resume or increase
  - Perform daily fetal kick counts
  - Encourage smoking cessation and improvement of nutrition as applicable
- Progressive preterm labor: topics of discussion
  - Best care in circumstances
  - Anticipated events for preterm birth
  - Neonatal care for gestational age
  - Need for family and social support and involvement

Follow-up Care: Follow-up Measures to Consider

- Document
  - Symptoms
  - Cervical changes
  - Fetal well-being
  - Treatment and education
  - Client response
- Threatened preterm labor
  - Negative cervical change and negative fFN (Reedy, 2007)
    - Standard prenatal care
    - Reassurance
    - fFN every 2 weeks; sooner if symptoms persist or increase
    - Consider serial ultrasound evaluation based on findings
      - Fetal surveillance
      - Cervical length
    - Follow as at high risk for preterm birth
  - Negative cervical change and positive fFN (Reedy, 2007)
    - Comfort measures
    - Education of woman and family
    - Weekly office visits
    - fFN every 2 weeks; sooner if symptoms persist or increase
    - Consider home monitoring
    - Consider antenatal corticosteroids (Riley et al., 2011)
    - Consider serial ultrasound evaluation based on findings
      - Fetal surveillance
      - Cervical length
    - Follow as at high risk for preterm birth
  - Positive cervical change and positive fFN (Reedy, 2007)
    - Consult OB/GYN or perinatologist
    - Antenatal corticosteroids (Riley et al., 2011)
    - Tocolysis in hospital
    - Activity restriction
    - Consider home monitoring
- Preterm labor and birth
  - Preterm infant care options locally or regionally
  - Consider transfer of care to perinatal specialist
- Provide support and reassurance
- Connect with community resources for assistance as indicated
  - Breastfeeding support
  - "Preemie" clothing
  - Rides to neonatal special care unit

Multidisciplinary Practice: Consider Consultation, Collaboration, or Referral

- OB/GYN or perinatal services
  - Suspected preterm labor
  - Confirmed preterm labor
- Consider transfer, as applicable
  - To hospital care
  - To a regional perinatal care center
- Pediatric services
  - For presence at birth
  - For follow-up of premature newborn
- Social services
  - Social support services
  - Parents of "preemies" support groups
  - Grief counseling as needed
- For diagnosis or treatment outside the midwife's scope of practice

CARE OF THE WOMAN WITH PROLONGED LATENT-PHASE LABOR

Key Clinical Information

The latent phase of labor is considered by some authorities to be prolonged when it exceeds approximately 20 hours in nullipara or 14 hours in multipara from the onset of regular contractions to the onset of active labor (4 cm dilation). However, labor frequently does not have a discrete beginning (Greulich & Tarrant, 2007), and the recall of the laboring woman can get lost in her excitement or anticipation of the baby's birth. Progressive cervical change is the hallmark of labor; persistent uterine contractions in the absence of cervical change should not be considered labor and should be treated as preparation for labor. Maternal fatigue caused by persistent irregular contractions can have a profound impact on the woman's labor energy levels and can influence the clinician to intervene when labor has not yet begun in earnest. Expectant management, therapeutic rest, and awaiting active labor are recommended for most women.

Client History and Chart Review: Components of the History to Consider

- LMP, EDC
- GP TPAL, gestational age
- Previous labor patterns in multipara
- Current contraction pattern
  - Onset of contractions
    - Intermittent contractions
    - Presence of regular contractions
    - Associated cervical change
  - Maternal response to contractions
  - Status of membranes
  - Associated factors and symptoms
    - Increase in vaginal discharge
    - Mucous plug
    - Spotting
    - Recent intercourse or orgasm
    - Use of alternative uterotonics
- Maternal and fetal well-being
  - Sleep, rest, and activity
  - Emotional response to situation
  - Nutrition and fluid intake
  - Fetal activity

Physical Examination: Components of the Physical Exam to Consider

- Fetal vital signs and well-being
  - FHT
  - Fetal movement
- Maternal well-being
  - Vital signs, including temperature
  - Abdominal examination
    - EFW
    - Fetal presentation and position
  - Pelvic examination for progressive changes
    - Cervical effacement

- Cervical dilation
- Descent of presenting part
- Status of membranes
- Pelvimetry
  - Assess hydration
    - Urine output, color, and specific gravity
    - Skin turgor
  - Signs of decreased coping ability
    - Excessive anxiety
    - Fear
    - Tension
  - Evaluate for signs of exhaustion

Clinical Impression: Differential Diagnoses to Consider

(ICD9data.com, 2012)

- Prolonged prodromal labor: False labor
- Dysfunctional labor
  - Uterine inertia
  - Malpresentation or malposition of the fetus
  - Obstructed labor

Diagnostic Testing: Diagnostic Tests and Procedures to Consider

- Fetal evaluation
  - NST
  - Fetal kick counts
  - Biophysical profile/amniotic fluid index as indicated
- Maternal evaluation
  - Urine—specific gravity
  - Evaluation of contractions
    - Palpation
    - External electronic monitoring
- Preoperative laboratory tests if concerned about labor progress

Providing Treatment: Therapeutic Measures to Consider

- Discharge to home (Greulich & Tarrant, 2007)
  - Instructions for rest, hydration, and nourishment

- Contact in presence of active labor
- Otherwise, keep next prenatal appointment
- Therapeutic rest
  - May stop contractions that occur from uterine irritability
  - Allows rest and restoration
    - Benadryl 50 mg PO
    - Ambien 10 mg PO
    - Morphine sulfate 10–20 mg IM or SQ (with or without Vistaril 50 mg IM)
    - Vistaril 50–75 mg IM
    - Demerol 25–50 mg IM (with or without Phenergan 25 mg)
- Hydration, oral or IV
- Stimulation of labor in women who are rested
  - Oxytocin stimulation
  - Artificial ROM

Providing Treatment: Complementary and Alternative Measures to Consider

- Watchful waiting (Greulich & Tarrant, 2007)
- Provide safe environment to allow for the following:
  - Rest, including intermittent naps
  - Hydration and adequate nutrition
- Warm bath/hydrotherapy
- Massage
- Strong chamomile or hops tea to facilitate rest
- Position changes to facilitate optimal fetal positioning
- Labor stimulation in women who are rested
  - Membrane sweeping
  - Sexual intercourse or orgasm
  - Nipple stimulation
  - Evening primrose oil: Apply directly to the cervix or take orally

Providing Support: Education and Support Measures to Consider

- Listen to maternal concerns
  - Explore fears related to labor, birth, and parenting
  - Provide reassurance

- Work to provide a safe-feeling birth environment
- Discuss options with woman and her significant other(s)
  - Review stages of labor
  - Rest
  - Stimulation of contractions
  - Potential change in birth plans
    - Location
    - Provider(s)

Follow-up Care: Follow-up Measures to Consider

- Document
- Update documentation after each evaluation
- Reevaluate every 1–2 hours
  - Response to therapy
  - Progressive labor signs
    - Strength and duration of contractions
    - Application of presenting part to cervix
    - Dilation and descent
    - Positioning of fetal vertex
    - Status of membranes
  - Developing maternal and fetal complications
    - Maternal exhaustion
    - Fetal distress
- If therapeutic rest is not successful
  - Consider stimulation of labor
  - Reevaluate potential causes of the labor dysfunction
- If progress does not occur, evaluate for evidence of the following:
  - Ineffective uterine contractions
  - Suboptimal fetal presentation or position
  - Fetopelvic disproportion

Multidisciplinary Practice: Consider Consultation, Collaboration, or Referral

- OB/GYN services
  - Diagnosis of arrest of latent phase
  - Lack of successful response to therapy
  - As needed for change of birth location
- For diagnosis or treatment outside the midwife's scope of practice

CARE OF THE WOMAN WITH SHOULDER DYSTOCIA

Key Clinical Information

Midwives and other maternity care providers consider shoulder dystocia to be one of the most frightening complications they encounter (Ramirez & Frye, 2004). Shoulder dystocia is defined as occurring when the fetal shoulders fail to deliver despite routine maneuvers. It is associated with significant fetal and maternal morbidity, perinatal mortality, and costly litigation. The incidence of shoulder dystocia is reported to be less than 0.6% to 1.4% (ACOG, 2002b; Jevitt, 2005). The potentially profound adverse effects of shoulder dystocia require all maternity care providers to be confident in diagnosing and responding to this condition. In the presence of shoulder dystocia, severe acidosis, fetal injury such as brachial plexus injury or fractured clavicle, or death can occur with a 4- to 5-minute delay between birth of the head to birth of the shoulders.

This uncommon obstetric emergency requires the midwife to be skilled in rapid identification of shoulder dystocia and specific interventions to remediate this situation. Mental preparedness includes knowing when to notify additional members of the care team, which can include midwives, OB/GYN physicians, maternity and pediatric nurses, pediatricians, and anesthesia personnel for immediate action. Nearly half of all shoulder dystocia cases occur in infants who weigh less than 4000 grams, indicating that it is not the infant's size alone that creates the difficulty, but rather the fit of this particular infant through the pelvis of this particular mother. Studies have been unable to reliably predict which mothers and infants will be at risk for shoulder dystocia (ACOG, 2002b).

Shoulder dystocia can be anticipated with a long second stage and the presence of the "turtle sign" after the head emerges. The head extends with difficulty, and the chin remains snug against the perineum. Restitution does not occur. The shoulders may be wedged in the pelvis—referred to as "tight shoulders"—or they may be impacted above the pelvic brim. Prompt identification of shoulder dystocia should result in the rapid initiation of systematic maneuvers to deliver the infant. Excessive traction on the infant's head has been associated with increased risk of newborn injury (Varney et al., 2004).

Shoulder dystocia is an event with a high incidence of allegations of malpractice and professional liability claims, so the midwife should be aware of strategies for liability risk reduction (ACNM, 2003a). Periodic drills of the birth team in managing this and other rare emergency events are an important part of preparedness to deal with this situation.

Client History and Chart Review: Components of the History to Consider

- LMP, EDC, gestational age
- Maternal height/weight
- Documented clinical pelvimetry
- ⚠ Potential risk factors for shoulder dystocia
  - Maternal diabetes
  - History of large infants
  - Maternal obesity
  - Postdate pregnancy
  - Large fetus, by palpation or ultrasound
  - History of prior difficult birth
  - History of prior shoulder dystocia
  - Cephalopelvic disproportion (ACOG, 2002b)
  - Dysfunctional labor
  - Prolonged second stage

Constant Vigilance!

Shoulder dystocia can occur in the absence of risk factors.

Physical Examination: Components of the Physical Exam to Consider

- Abdominal examination in labor
  - Fetal presentation and position
  - Flexion of the head at the pelvic brim
  - Estimate fetal weight with onset of labor
- Pelvic examination(s) during labor
  - Progression of cervical dilation

- Rate of descent
- Maternal tissue elasticity
- Pelvimetry
- At birth
  - Slow progression of extension
  - Retraction of the infant's head ("turtle sign")
  - Failure to restitute
  - Suffusion, discoloration of the infant's face
  - Need for one or more maneuvers to deliver the infant

Clinical Impression: Differential Diagnoses to Consider

(ICD9data.com, 2012)

- Shoulder dystocia
- Short cord
- Fetal anomaly

Diagnostic Testing: Diagnostic Tests and Procedures to Consider

- Ultrasound for EFW
  - Can be inaccurate by more than 1–2 lb
  - Size is often not the issue
- Preoperative laboratory tests

Providing Treatment: Therapeutic Measures to Consider

- Engage the mother in cooperating
- With the mother who is on her back
  - Perform the McRoberts maneuver (knees to shoulders and wide apart)
    - Advantages
      - Alters the angle of inclination of symphysis
      - Flattens the sacrum
      - Opens up the posterior pelvis
      - Reduces the amount of traction required to effect birth
      - May decrease traction-related fetal injury
    - Disadvantages: Requires two assistants
  - Request firm suprapubic pressure

- Encourage maternal pushing efforts
- Attempt birth
  - With *gentle* traction on the infant's head
  - If descent occurs, assist with birth
    - Place fingers on both of the infant's shoulders
    - Maintain the arms in close contact with the trunk
- If birth does not occur
  - Stop maternal pushing efforts
  - Insert the dominant hand in the vagina to check the position of the infant's shoulders
    - Place the hand on the infant's back
    - Palpate the anterior axillary crease
      - ⚠ *Do not* place fingers in the axilla
      - Apply firm traction toward the pubis to shift the suprascapular structures
        - Decreases the bisacromial diameter
        - Attempt rotation of the anterior shoulder into the pelvis
          - Use firm, gentle digital pressure
          - Rotate the infant's back toward the symphysis
          - Rotate the shoulders into the oblique
        - As anterior shoulder rotates, move the client to her hands and knees as needed
        - Maintain the infant's position
        - Use gentle outward traction, which should bring the posterior shoulder into the pelvis: Deliver the posterior arm
        - Encourage maternal pushing efforts
          - "Walk" the shoulders out using both hands
          - Place traction on the suprascapular bones
          - Keep the infant's arms close to the body
          - Use gentle, firm outward traction

> Rotate the infant manually from side to side
  - ★ The back should always be rotated toward the mother's symphysis
  - ★ "Corkscrew" the body out (Woods screw maneuver)
- With the mother on hands and knees for birth
  - Flex the legs so the belly rests on the legs
  - Knees to shoulders
  - Deliver the posterior arm first
- Water birth
  - Have the mother stand and lean over the tub: This may release the impaction
  - Assist as you would for a mother on hands and knees
  - Alternatively, have the mother exit the tub with assistance
    - ◆ Have her move to a hands and knees position, or on her back
    - ◆ Continue as described previously
- For severe unrelieved shoulder dystocia, consider the following:
  - Alternative positioning
  - Call for STAT obstetric and pediatric assistance
  - Fracture of the clavicle
  - Empty the mother's bladder with a straight catheter
  - Enlarge or cut an episiotomy if tissue dystocia is suspected
  - Rule out other causes of dystocia through direct palpation of pelvic contents
    - ◆ Fetal anomalies
    - ◆ Extremely short cord
  - Zavenelli maneuver (ACOG, 2002b; Varney et al., 2004)
    - ◆ Replacement of head in vagina
    - ◆ Reverse process of extension
    - ◆ Follow with immediate cesarean section
- Prepare for the following:
  - Full neonatal resuscitation (American Academy of Pediatrics/American Heart Association, 2010)

- Immediate postpartum hemorrhage
- Cesarean birth for documented macrosomia
- Consider cesarean birth with large EFW (Gabbe et al., 2007)
  - EFW > 4500 g in normoglycemic mothers
  - EFW > 4000 g in diabetic mothers
  - ⚠ All methods of estimating fetal weights are imprecise

Providing Treatment: Complementary and Alternative Measures to Consider

- Gaskin maneuver (Bruner, Drummond, Meenan, & Gaskin, 1998)
  - Rotate the mother to her hands and knees
  - Rotate the mother in the direction in which the infant is facing
  - This maneuver alters the pelvic geometry
  - Advantages
    - ◆ The position change may resolve the impaction
    - ◆ Gravity may facilitate birth
  - Disadvantages
    - ◆ Cannot use suprapubic pressure
    - ◆ May exaggerate the impaction
- Squatting
  - Advantages
    - ◆ The position change may resolve the impaction
    - ◆ Results in a wider pubic (outlet) angle
  - Disadvantages
    - ◆ Cannot use suprapubic pressure
    - ◆ May decrease the inlet dimensions
    - ◆ Offers limited access to the infant

Providing Support: Education and Support Measures to Consider

- Discuss the potential for difficult birth with a mother who has:
  - Documented macrosomia
  - EFW more than 1 lb larger than largest previous infant
  - History of shoulder dystocia

- 📋 Follow up after the birth with discussion of the following topics:
  - The care given
  - Infant well-being
  - Maternal feelings about the event:
    - ◆ Complications
    - ◆ Interventions
    - ◆ Outcomes
    - ◆ Labor and birth
- Review signs to be heeded for:
  - Postpartum endometritis
  - Postpartum depression

Follow-up Care: Follow-up Measures to Consider

- Immediately after birth:
  - Provide newborn resuscitation as necessary
  - Evaluate the infant for birth injury
  - Observe for postpartum hemorrhage after birth
  - Evaluate for maternal injury
- Document
  - ⚠️ Details in the birth note
    - ◆ Physical findings at birth
    - ◆ Identification of shoulder dystocia
    - ◆ Maneuvers used and their effects
    - ◆ Note any injury to the mother or the infant
    - ◆ Note the movement of the infant's arms
  - Consultations requested during birth
- ⚠️ Seek opportunities for peer support
  - Peer review (nondiscoverable)
  - Sentinel event reviews
  - Colleague support, HIPAA compliant

Multidisciplinary Practice: Consider Consultation, Collaboration, or Referral

- OB/GYN services
  - Potential for shoulder dystocia anticipated
  - Diagnosis of shoulder dystocia
- Pediatric services
  - In anticipation of neonatal resuscitation
  - For newborn evaluation after a difficult birth
- For diagnosis or treatment outside the midwife's scope of practice

CARE OF THE WOMAN UNDERGOING VACUUM-ASSISTED BIRTH

Key Clinical Information

Vacuum-assisted birth carries with it significant risks to mother and baby and increases liability for the midwife (ACOG, 2000b; Clark, 2005). The benefits of using the vacuum extractor to aid in the birth of the infant should clearly outweigh the potential risks associated with this procedure. Because using a vacuum at birth is not a basic midwifery skill, midwives who assist with birth using outlet vacuum extraction should be educated and trained in indications and contraindications, techniques, and complications associated with the use of the device. The most common indications for use of vacuum-assisted birth by midwives are nonreassuring fetal heart rate in second-stage labor and maternal exhaustion in second-stage labor (Clark, 2005).

Client History and Chart Review: Components of the History to Consider

- Verify LMP, EDC, and term gestation
- Relevant prenatal and labor history
  - Progress of labor, including second stage
  - Fetal and maternal response to labor
  - Pelvimetry
- ⚠️ Presence of contraindications to vacuum-assisted birth (ACNM, 2003b)
  - Weak or infrequent uterine contraction
  - Vertex not well engaged
  - Cephalopelvic disproportion
  - Preterm pregnancy (less than 37 weeks)
  - Suspected macrosomia
  - Nonvertex presentation
  - Uncooperative client
  - Poor maternal expulsive effort
- Indications for outlet vacuum-assisted birth (ACOG, 2000b)
  - Prolonged second stage
    - ◆ More than 3 hours for nullipara
    - ◆ More than 2 hours for multipara
  - Nonreassuring FHR pattern
  - Maternal exhaustion

- Outlet vacuum-assisted birth is not indicated for midwife exhaustion (Clark, 2005)

Physical Examination: Components of the Physical Exam to Consider

- Abdominal examination
  - Fetal lie, presentation, and position
  - EFW
  - Presence of adequate, effective, regular contractions
- Pelvic examination
  - Dilation must be complete
  - Station
    - Vertex visible at introitus: Outlet delivery
    - +2 station: Midforceps delivery; Physician management is recommended
  - Make a determination of vacuum extraction versus forceps versus cesarean section
  - Presence of caput or marked molding
  - Vacuum extraction increases the risk of fetal trauma
  - Assess fetal presentation and position

Clinical Impression: Differential Diagnoses to Consider

(ICD9data.com, 2012)

- Vacuum-assisted birth may be performed in the following circumstances:
  - Prolonged second-stage labor
  - Fetal distress
  - ▽ Maternal exhaustion

Diagnostic Testing: Diagnostic Tests and Procedures to Consider

- Preoperative laboratory tests
- Evaluation of the effectiveness of uterine contractions
  - Palpation
  - Electronic fetal monitoring
- Evaluation of the fetal response via FHR
  - Auscultation
  - Electronic fetal monitoring

Providing Treatment: Therapeutic Measures to Consider

- Oxytocin stimulation to improve contractions
- Vacuum-assisted birth procedure
  - Empty the mother's bladder and rectum
  - Consider local anesthesia
  - Consider episiotomy
    - May increase the risk of third- or fourth-degree laceration
    - A mediolateral episiotomy may give more room
  - Verify the position of vertex
  - Apply the vacuum cup to the "flexion point"—the area of the fetal head needed to achieve flexion without asynclitism
  - Verify that no maternal tissues are under the cup rim: Request suction
  - Use pressure of 4 in. Hg (100 mm Hg) between contractions
  - Use pressure of 15–23 in. Hg (500 mm Hg) with contractions
  - Apply gentle, steady traction
    - With contractions only
    - Follow curve of Carus
  - ⚠ Discontinue attempts to assist the birth with vacuum in the following circumstances:
    - The cup disengages three times
    - Scalp trauma is visible after the cup disengages
    - No progress is noted after three attempts at traction
    - Attempts for birth are met with no success after 15–30 minutes
    - Birth has not occurred within 10 accrued minutes of maximum suction

Risk Management Issues with Vacuum-Assisted Birth

- Do not allow the vacuum to remain at maximum levels for more than 10 accrued minutes.
- Do not follow a failed vacuum effort with a forceps attempt: The success rate is low, and the morbidity rate is high.

Providing Treatment: Complementary and Alternative Measures to Consider

- Assess for maternal and fetal well-being
  - Be patient
  - Allow a rest period
  - Provide for adequate hydration and nutrition
- Continue maternal pushing efforts
  - Encourage voiding
  - Push only with urge
- Vigilant assessment of maternal and fetal status
  - Vital signs
  - Fetal descent
- Position changes
  - Side-lying
  - McRoberts position
  - Lithotomy with leg support
    - Feet should push against a fixed object
    - Arms should pull
    - The back should be as flat as possible
    - Use of a squatting bar is helpful
  - Squatting
  - Birthing stool
  - Hands and knees
  - Floating in birthing tub

Providing Support: Education and Support Measures to Consider

- Discuss the issues with the client and family
  - Concerns related to slow progress
  - Options for care
  - Recommendations and indications
- Vacuum-assisted birth procedure: Discuss its risks and benefits with the client
  - Risk of fetal trauma
    - Cephalohematoma
    - Intracranial trauma
    - Shoulder dystocia
    - Ecchymosis, abrasions (ACOG, 2000b)
  - Risk of maternal trauma
    - Third- or fourth-degree laceration
    - Sulcus tears
    - Possible need for cesarean birth

- Benefits
  - Vaginal birth of infant
  - Faster than forceps or cesarean section
  - Less risk of fetal trauma than forceps
  - May decrease the need for cesarean birth

Follow-up Care: Follow-up Measures to Consider

- Prepare for potential postbirth care
  - Shoulder dystocia
  - Postpartum hemorrhage
  - Third- or fourth-degree laceration
  - Newborn injury
  - Newborn resuscitation
- Document (see "Procedure Note" or "Birth Note")
- Evaluate for maternal or neonatal injury
  - Examine the vagina carefully for lacerations
  - Examine the infant carefully for injury
- Discuss the birth with the mother and family
  - Allow exploration of feelings
  - Review indications for assisted birth

Multidisciplinary Practice: Consider Consultation, Collaboration, or Referral

- OB/GYN services
  - Indications for vacuum extraction
  - Maternal indications; cesarean section may be necessary
- Pediatric services
  - Fetal distress
  - Fetal injury
  - Evaluation of delayed signs of injury
- For diagnosis or treatment outside the midwife's scope of practice

CARE OF THE WOMAN DURING VAGINAL BIRTH AFTER CESAREAN SECTION

Key Clinical Information

Vaginal birth after cesarean (VBAC) provides carefully selected women with an alternative to a surgical birth of their infant. Successful VBAC results in significant benefits and fewer risks for women and infants than repeat cesarean birth. Midwives are qualified to care for women planning VBAC with appropriate arrangements for medical consultation and emergency care in place (ACNM, 2011). Application of the midwifery model of care increases successful VBAC rates and decreases primary cesarean section rates and the need for subsequent VBAC.

Uterine ruptures following cesarean section occur at a documented rate of approximately 0.5% to 1%. This rate is increased to 3.7% in women with more than one previous cesarean birth (ACOG, 2010). It is also increased in women with a single-layer uterine closure, two or more previous cesarean births, an interdelivery interval of 18 months or less, and labor augmented or induced with oxytocin (NIH, 2010). When uterine rupture does occur, outcomes are improved with the immediate availability of skilled surgical services.

In 2010, the National Institutes of Health issued a statement encouraging increased access to VBAC. In response, ACOG (2010) updated its guidelines, thereby broadening the categories of women who are candidates for VBAC while still encouraging VBAC only in hospitals equipped for rapid emergency surgical delivery. This edict tends to be interpreted conservatively and, therefore, continues to limit VBAC as an option for many women and providers.

Limited availability of the VBAC option in hospitals has led some women seeking this service to choose out-of-hospital birth sites—a choice steeped in controversy. Nevertheless, the noninterventive style of care provided in out-of-hospital settings and by midwives in the hospital setting is well suited to the needs of the woman choosing VBAC. The highest VBAC success rates are achieved when labor begins spontaneously and progresses normally. Women should be counseled as to their options, risks and benefits, and alterations in care if complications should develop. Most women seeking VBAC can safely be cared for by midwives (ACNM, 2011).

Client History and Chart Review: Components of the History to Consider

- Obtain operative records for previous cesarean section(s)
  - Indication for primary cesarean section
  - Gestational age with prior cesarean section
  - Length of labor
  - Cervical dilation at time of cesarean
  - Type of uterine incision
  - Type of uterine closure
  - Postoperative course
  - Wound infection
  - Endometritis
- Review medical history for the following factors, which are associated with less chance of VBAC success:
  - Renal disease
  - Seizure disorders
  - Heart disease
- Review current pregnancy course
- Identify positive predictors for the VBAC candidate (NIH, 2010)
  - Nonrepeating indication for previous cesarean section
  - Client motivated for vaginal birth
  - Previous vaginal birth
  - Vertex presentation
  - Bishop's score > 4
  - Two-layer uterine closure
  - No history of postoperative fever or infection
  - Maternal age less than or equal to 30 years
  - 24 or more months since previous cesarean section
  - Spontaneous onset of labor
  - Progressive labor
  - Non-Hispanic white ethnicity
  - Greater maternal height
  - BMI < 30
  - Previous VBAC
  - Previous baby weighing less than 4000 g
  - Lower gestational age at delivery
  - Cervical dilation on admission or with ROM
  - Cervical effacement reaching 75% to 90%

- Fetal head engagement or at a lower station
- Additional candidates for VBAC (ACOG, 2010)
  - Two prior low transverse incision cesarean births
  - Twin gestation with one prior low transverse incision cesarean birth
  - Gestation beyond 40 weeks
  - Suspected macrosomia
  - Prior low vertical incision
  - Unknown type of previous uterine incision, unless there is high suspicion of classical incision
- Women who are not generally candidates for VBAC (ACOG, 2010)
  - Classical uterine incision
  - Extensive transfundal uterine surgery
  - Previous uterine rupture
- Negative predictors for the VBAC candidate (ACOG, 2010; NIH, 2010)
  - Nonvertex presentation of infant
  - Single-layer uterine closure
  - Maternal age greater than 30 years
  - Less than 18 months since previous cesarean section
  - Nonprogressive labor
  - Hispanic or African American ethnicity
  - Single marital status
  - Less than 12 years of education
  - Maternal disease
  - Gestational age greater than 40 weeks
  - Labor induction or augmentation
    - 54% chance success with mechanical methods
    - 69% with pharmacologic means
  - Lower uterine segment (LUS) thickness < 2.3 mm
  - Recurrent indication for initial cesarean delivery
  - Maternal obesity
  - Preeclampsia
  - Increased neonatal birth weight (ACOG, 2010)

Physical Examination: Components of the Physical Exam to Consider

- Abdominal exam
  - Scar
  - Contractions
  - Leopold's maneuvers
  - Note pain or tenderness
- Comprehensive labor evaluation
  - Clinical pelvimetry with history of cephalopelvic disproportion (CPD) or failure to progress (FTP)
  - Estimated fetal weight
  - Presentation, position, engagement
  - Cervical status
  - Maternal and fetal vital signs
- Reevaluate progress at frequent intervals
- Maternal and fetal response to labor
  - Contraction pattern
  - Cervical change
    - Greater than 4 cm: approximately 86% success rate for VBAC
    - Greater than 75% effaced: approximately 81% success rate for VBAC (King, 2004)
  - Fetal descent
- Signs of uterine rupture
  - Fetal bradycardia or nonreassuring FHR
  - Maternal tachycardia
  - Abdominal pain: May or may not be present

Clinical Impression: Differential Diagnoses to Consider

(ICD9data.com, 2012)

- VBAC candidate
- Repeat cesarean section

Diagnostic Testing: Diagnostic Tests and Procedures to Consider

- Prenatal ultrasound for LUS thickness (Bujold, Jastrow, Simoneau, Brunet, & Gauthier, 2009)
- Preoperative laboratory tests
  - CBC with platelets
  - Type and screen

- Continuous observation of maternal and fetal status
  - 1:1 nurse or midwife care with auscultation
  - External fetal monitor
  - Internal fetal monitor

Providing Treatment: Therapeutic Measures to Consider

- Evaluate for onset of progressive labor
- Provide a supportive labor and birthing environment
- Limit invasive examinations or procedures
- Oral intake
  - NPO
  - Ice chips
  - Clear liquids
- IV access
  - Saline lock
  - Lactated Ringer's at 125 cc/hr
- Maternal and fetal evaluation of well-being
- Medications
  - ⚠️ Misoprostol and other prostaglandins are contraindicated for use with a scarred uterus
  - Oxytocin as indicated
    - Can be used to facilitate vaginal birth due to uterine inertia
    - Uterine overstimulation can increase risk of rupture (ACOG, 2004)
  - Pain relief as needed (see "Care of the Woman in First-Stage Labor")
- Careful management of third-stage labor: Increased risk of placenta accreta

Providing Treatment: Complementary and Alternative Measures to Consider

- Facilitate physiologic labor
  - Ambulation
  - Hydrotherapy
  - Positioning
  - Doula support
  - Adequate hydration and nutrition
- Foster maternal autonomy: Provide a supportive labor environment

Providing Support: Education and Support Measures to Consider

- 📋 Discuss options with the client and family
  - VBAC versus repeat cesarean section
  - Surgical coverage options
  - Location(s) for birth
  - Options for labor care and support
  - 🌐 Chance of blood product use
- Obtain signed informed consent
  - Success rate: 60% to 80% (NIH, 2010)
  - Incidence of catastrophic uterine rupture
    - Low transverse uterine incision: 0.19% to 0.8%
    - Other types of incision: Higher incidence
  - No increased risk with the following:
    - Oxytocin augmentation less than 5 mU/min
    - Infant weighing more than 4000 g
  - Increased risk with the following:
    - Induction of labor
    - Gestational age greater than 40 weeks
    - Single-layer closure at previous cesarean section
    - Increasing numbers of prior cesarean sections
    - Giving birth in a low-birth-volume hospital
    - Unfavorable cervix on admission
    - Obesity
    - Interbirth interval less than 18 months
  - Risk of maternal or fetal death with catastrophic rupture
  - Risks, benefits, and alternatives to VBAC
    - Risks of cesarean
      - Increased maternal mortality/morbidity
      - Significant adhesions
      - Bladder, ureter, and bowel injury
  - Discussion regarding facility/practice parameters for VBAC
- Anticipated care of VBAC women in labor
  - Labor procedures (e.g., IV, laboratory tests)
  - Average length of time for urgent cesarean section
    - At the facility
    - If transport is required

Follow-up Care: Follow-up Measures to Consider

- Consult OB/GYN of client choice prenatally
- ⚠ Uterine scar dehiscence or rupture
  - May result in fetal and/or maternal death
  - Can occur in labor or during birth
  - Can occur regardless of mode of birth
  - Access surgical services immediately
  - Ensure IV access
    - ◆ Provide fluid replacement
    - ◆ Order blood
  - Treat shock
- ▽ Document
  - Review of previous cesarean section operative notes
  - Discussions with the client and family
  - Client preference
  - Informed choice and consent
  - Treatment of complications
  - Consultations
- Update notes frequently, especially in labor

Multidisciplinary Practice: Consider Consultation, Collaboration, or Referral

- OB/GYN services
  - Previous incision that is not low transverse
  - Planned repeat cesarean section
  - Planned VBAC
  - STAT for client in labor with the following signs and symptoms:

- ◆ Symptoms of dramatic uterine rupture (ACOG, 2010)
    - ➤ Nonreassuring fetal status is the most common indication of uterine rupture (70%)
    - ➤ Increased uterine contractions
    - ➤ Vaginal bleeding, loss of fetal station
    - ➤ New onset of intense uterine pain
    - ➤ Sharp, shooting pain in lower abdomen
    - ➤ Feeling that something has torn
    - ➤ Fetal parts more easily palpated
    - ➤ Violent fetal movements followed by cessation of movements
    - ➤ Signs of shock
    - ➤ Referred pain to chest
  - ◆ Symptoms of quiet uterine rupture
    - ➤ Vomiting
    - ➤ Increased tenderness above abdomen
    - ➤ Severe suprapubic pain
    - ➤ Hypotonic uterine contractions
    - ➤ Lack of progress
    - ➤ Faintness
  - Evidence of developing dystocia or obstruction
  - Demand for repeat cesarean section
  - Retained placenta
- Pediatric services: Anticipated need for neonatal resuscitation
- For diagnosis or treatment outside the midwife's scope of practice

🌐 WEB RESOURCES FOR CLINICIANS

RESOURCE	URL
Changing Posterior Fetal Positions	Spinning Babies: http://spinningbabies.com/
Evidence-Based Practice	Childbirth Connection: http://www.childbirthconnection.org/
Hypertensive Disorders of Pregnancy	Diagnosis, Evaluation, and Management of the Hypertensive Disorders of Pregnancy: http://www.preeclampsia.org/pdf/gui206CPG0803_001.pdf
Obstetric Hemorrhage Toolbox	California Maternal Quality Care Collaborative: http://www.cmqcc.org/
Patient and Professional Resources	March of Dimes: http://www.marchofdimes.com/professionals/medicalresources.html
Waterbirth	Waterbirth International: http://www.waterbirth.org/

REFERENCES

Albers, L. (2007). The evidence for physiologic management of the active phase of the first stage of labor. *Journal of Midwifery & Women's Health, 52,* 207–215.

Albers, L., Schiff, M., & Gorwoda, J. G. (1996). The length of active labor in normal pregnancies. *Obstetrics & Gynecology, 87,* 355–359.

American Academy of Pediatrics/American Heart Association. (2010). *Textbook of neonatal resuscitation* (6th ed.). Elk Grove, IL: American Academy of Pediatrics.

American College of Nurse–Midwives (ACNM). (2003a). *Midwifery strategies for liability risk reduction: Shoulder dystocia.* Washington, DC: Author.

American College of Nurse–Midwives (ACNM). (2003b). *Vacuum assisted birth in midwifery practice* (2nd ed.). Washington, DC: Author.

American College of Nurse–Midwives (ACNM). (2005). *Position statement: Elective primary cesarean section.* Washington, DC: Author.

American College of Nurse–Midwives (ACNM). (2006a). *The midwife as surgical first assistant handbook.* Washington, DC: Author.

American College of Nurse–Midwives. (2006b). Position statement: Standardized nomenclature for electronic fetal monitoring. Retrieved from http://www.midwife.org/siteFiles/position/Standardized_Nomenclature_for_Electronic_Fetal_Monitoring.pdf

American College of Nurse–Midwives (ACNM). (2008a). *Position statement: Premature rupture of labor at term.* Washington, DC: Author.

American College of Nurse–Midwives (ACNM). (2008b). *Position statement: The certified nurse-midwife/certified midwife as first assistant at surgery.* Washington, DC: Author.

American College of Nurse–Midwives (ACNM). (2009). *Position statement: Nitrous oxide for labor anesthesia.* Washington, DC: Author.

American College of Nurse–Midwives (ACNM). (2010). *Position statement: Induction of labor.* Washington, DC: Author.

American College of Nurse–Midwives (ACNM). (2011). Clinical bulletin: Care for women desiring vaginal birth after cesarean. Washington, DC: Author.

American College of Obstetricians and Gynecologists (ACOG). (2000a). Practice bulletin #13: External cephalic version. In *2006 compendium of selected publications.* Washington, DC: Author.

American College of Obstetricians and Gynecologists (ACOG). (2000b). Practice bulletin #17: Operative vaginal delivery. In *2006 compendium of selected publications.* Washington, DC: Author.

American College of Obstetricians and Gynecologists (ACOG). (2002a). Practice bulletin #33: Diagnosis and management of pre-eclampsia and eclampsia. In *2006 compendium of selected publications.* Washington, DC: Author.

American College of Obstetricians and Gynecologists (ACOG). (2002b). Practice bulletin #40: Shoulder dystocia. In *2006 compendium of selected publications.* Washington, DC: Author.

American College of Obstetricians and Gynecologists (ACOG). (2003). Practice bulletin #43: Management of preterm labor. In *2006 compendium of selected publications.* Washington, DC: Author.

American College of Obstetricians and Gynecologists (ACOG). (2004). Practice Bulletin #55: Management of post-term pregnancy. In *2006 compendium of selected publications.* Washington, DC: Author.

American College of Obstetricians and Gynecologists (ACOG). (2005). Practice bulletin #70: Intrapartum fetal heart rate monitoring. In *2006 compendium of selected publications.* Washington, DC: Author.

American College of Obstetricians and Gynecologists (ACOG). (2006). *Committee opinion #340: Mode of term singleton breech delivery.* Washington, DC: Author.

American College of Obstetricians and Gynecologists (ACOG). (2007). *Practice bulletin #80: Premature rupture of membranes.* Washington, DC: Author.

American College of Obstetricians and Gynecologists (ACOG). (2010). *Practice bulletin #115: Vaginal birth after previous cesarean delivery.* Washington, DC: Author.

Andrews, C., & Andrews, E. (2004). Physical theory as a basis for successful rotation of fetal malpositions and conversion of fetal malpresentations. *Biological Research for Nursing, 6*(2), 126–140. doi: 10.1177/1099800404268318

Bishop, E. H. (1964). Pelvic scoring for elective induction. *Obstetrics & Gynecology, 24,* 267.

Blackburn, S. T. (2007). *Maternal, fetal and neonatal physiology: A clinical perspective* (3rd ed.). Philadelphia, PA: Saunders.

Brown, H. C., Paranjothy, S., Dowswell, T., & Thomas, J. (2009). Package of care for active management of labour for reducing cesarean section rates in low-risk women

[Review]. Cochrane Library, 3. doi: 10.1002/14651858. CD004907.pub2

Bruner, J., Drummond, S., Meenan, A. L., & Gaskin, I. M. (1998). The all fours maneuver for reducing shoulder dystocia. *Journal of Reproductive Medicine, 43*, 439–443.

Bujold, E., Bujold, C., Hamilton, E. F., Harel, F., & Gauthier, R. J. (2002). The impact of single-layer or double-layer closure on uterine rupture. American *Journal of Obstetrics & Gynecology, 186*, 1326–1330.

Bujold, E., Jastrow, N., Simoneau, J., Brunet, S., & Gauthier, R. J. (2009). Prediction of complete uterine rupture by sonographic evaluation of the lower uterine segment. *American Journal of Obstetrics & Gynecology, 201*, 320.e1–320.e6.

Centers for Disease Control and Prevention (CDC). (2010). Prevention of perinatal group B streptococcal disease: Revised guidelines from CDC, 2010. Retrieved from http://www.cdc.gov/groupbstrep/clinicians/obstetric-providers.html#guidelines

Clark, P. A. (2005). Use of the vacuum extractor by midwives: What has changed in the last decade? *Journal of Midwifery & Women's Health, 50*, 517–524.

Cluett, E. R., Pickering, R. M., Getliffe, K., & Saunders, N. J. S. G. (2004). Randomised controlled trial of labouring in water compared with standard of augmentation for management of dystocia in first stage of labour. *British Medical Journal, 328*(7435), 314–320.

CMQCC Hemorrhage Task Force. (2010). OB hemorrhage protocol. OB hemorrhage care guidelines: Checklist format V.1.4. Retrieved from http://www.cmqcc.org/resources/ob_hemorrhage/ob_hemorrhage_care_guidelines_checklist_flowchart_tablechart_v1_4

Da Silva, F. M. B., De Oliveira, S. M. J. V., & Nobre, M. R. C. (2009). A randomised controlled trial evaluating the effect of immersion bath on labour pain. *Midwifery, 25*(3), 286–294.

DeSevo, M. R., & Semeraro, P. (2010). Urinary Catheterization during epidural anesthesia. *Nursing for Women's Health, 14*(1), 11–13.

Eckert, K., Turnbull, D., & MacLennan, A. (2001). Immersion in water in the first stage of labor: A randomized controlled trial. *Birth, 28*(2), 84–93.

Eichenbaum-Pikser, G., & Zasloff, J. S. (2009). Delayed clamping of the umbilical cord: A review with implications for practice. *Journal of Midwifery & Women's Health, 54*(4), 321–326. doi: 10.1016/j.jmwh.2008.12.012

Ethicon. (2004). Wound closure manual. Retrieved from http://www.jnjgateway.com/public/NLDUT/Wound_Closure_Manual1.pdf

Fahy, K. (2009). Third stage of labour care for women at low risk of postpartum haemorrhage. *Journal of Midwifery & Women's Health, 54*, 308–386.

Franchi, M., Cromi, A., Scarperi, S., Gaudino, F., Siesto, G., & Ghezzi, F. (2009). Comparison between lidocaine-prilocaine cream (EMLA) and mepivacaine infiltration for pain relief during perineal repair after childbirth: A randomized trial. *American Journal of Obstetrics & Gynecology, 201*, 186.e1–186.e5. doi: 10.1016/j.ajog.2009.04.023

Fraser, W., Hofmeyr, J., Lede, R., & Faron, G. (2005). Amnioinfusion for the prevention of meconium aspiration syndrome [Electronic version]. *New England Journal of Medicine, 353*, 909–918.

Gabbe, S. G., Niebyl, J. R., & Simpson, J. L. (Eds.). (2007). *Obstetrics: Normal and problem pregnancies* (5th ed.). New York, NY: Churchill Livingstone.

Gregory, K., Main, E., & Lyndon, A. (2009). OB hemorrhage: Definitions and triggers. CMQCC Hemorrhage Task Force. Retrieved from http://www.cmqcc.org/resources/ob_hemorrhage/ob_hemorrhage_best_practice_articles_v1_4_alphabetical_order

Greulich, B., & Tarrant, B. (2007). The latent phase of labor: Diagnosis and management. *Journal of Midwifery & Women's Health, 52*, 190–198.

Habek, D., Habek, J., & Jagust, M. (2003). Acupuncture conversion of fetal breech presentation. *Fetal Diagnosis and Therapy, 18*, 418–421.

Hargitaib, B., Marton, T., & Cox, P. M. (2004). Best practice no. 178: Examination of the human placenta. *Journal of Clinical Pathology, 57*, 785–792.

Hart, J., & Walker, A. (2007). Management of occiput posterior. *Journal of Midwifery & Women's Health, 52*, 508–513.

Hermus, M. A. A., Verhoeven, C. J. M., Mol, B. W., Wolf, G. S., & Fiedeldeij, C. A. (2009). Comparison of induction of labour and expectant management in postterm pregnancy: A matched cohort study. *Journal of Midwifery & Women's Health, 54*, 351–356.

Hofmeyr, G. J. (2010a) Amnioinfusion for meconium-stained liquor in labour. *Cochrane Library, 8.*

Hofmeyr, G. J. (2010b). Amnioinfusion for potential or suspected umbilical cord compression in labour. *Cochrane Database of Systematic Reviews, 8.* doi: 10.1002/14651858.CD000013

Hofmeyr, G. J. (2010c). Amnioinfusion for preterm rupture of membranes. *Cochrane Library, 8.*

Hofmeyr, G. J., & Hannah, M. E. (2007). Planned caesarean section for term breech delivery. *Cochrane Database of Systematic Reviews, 4,* CD000166. doi: 10.1002/14651858.CD000166

ICD9Data.com. (2012). Free 2012 ICD-9 medical coding data. Retrieved from http://www.icd9data.com/

Institute for Clinical Systems Improvement. (2004). *Prevention, diagnosis and treatment of failure to progress in obstetrical labor.* Bloomington, MN: Author.

International Confederation of Midwives. (2006). Management of the third stage of labour to prevent post-partum haemorrhage. Retrieved from http://www.pphprevention.org/files/FIGO-ICM_Statement_November2006_Final.pdf

Jevitt, C. M. (2005). Shoulder dystocia: Etiology, common risk factors, and management. *Journal of Midwifery & Women's Health, 50,* 485–497.

King, T. (2004). Vaginal birth after previous cesarean section [Electronic version]. *Journal of Midwifery & Women's Health, 49,* 68–75.

King, T., & Brucker, M. (Eds.). (2011). *Pharmacology in women's health.* Boston, MA: Jones & Bartlett Learning.

Livingston, J. C., Livingston, L. W., Ramsey, R., Mabie, B. C., & Sibai, B. M. (2003). Magnesium sulfate in women with mild pre-eclampsia: A randomized controlled trial. *Obstetrics & Gynecology, 101,* 217–226.

Lowe, N. K. (2007). A review of factors associated with dystocia and cesarean section in nulliparous women. *Journal of Midwifery & Women's Health, 52,* 216–228.

Macones, G. A., Hankins, G., Spong, C. Y., Hauth, J., & Moore, T. (2008). The 2008 National Institute of Child Health and Human Development workshop report on electric fetal monitoring: Update on definitions, interpretation and research guidelines. *Obstetrics & Gynecology, 112*(3), 661–666. doi: 10.1097/AOG.0b013e3181841395

Marowitz, A., & Jordan, R. (2007). Midwifery management of prelabor rupture of membranes at term. *Journal of Midwifery & Women's Health, 52,* 199–206.

McDonald, S. (2007). Management of the third stage of labor. *Journal of Midwifery & Women's Health, 52,* 254–261.

McDonald, S. J., & Middleton, P. (2009). Effect of timing of umbilical cord clamping of term infants on maternal and neonatal outcomes (review). *Cochrane Library, 3.* doi: 10.1002/14651858.CD004074.pub2

Moses, S. (2004). Indomethacin. Retrieved November 18, 2007, from http://www.fpnotebook.com/PHA37.htm

National Institutes of Health (NIH) Consensus Panel. (2010). Vaginal birth after cesarean section: New insights. Retrieved from http://consensus.nih.gov/2010/vbacstatement.htm

Pistolese, R. (2002). The Webster technique: A chiropractic technique with obstetric implications. *Journal of Manipulative and Physiological Therapeutics, 25,* E1–E9.

Ramirez, N., & Frye, J. (2004). Shoulder dystocia: An evidence-based clinical practice guideline. In C. L. Farley (Ed.), *Final projects database.* Philadelphia, PA: Philadelphia University.

Reedy, N. J. (2007). Born too soon: The continuing challenge of preterm labor and birth in the United States. *Journal of Midwifery & Women's Health, 52,* 281–290.

Riley, C. A., Boozer, K., & King, T. L. (2011). Antenatal corticosteroids at the beginning of the 21st century. *Journal of Midwifery & Women's Health, 56,* 591–597.

Roberts, J. (2002). The push for evidence: Management of the second stage. *Journal of Midwifery & Women's Health, 47,* 2–15.

Romm, A. (2010). *Botanical medicine for women's health.* St. Louis, MO: Churchill Livingstone.

Ross, S. (2007). Chlorhexidine as an alternative treatment for prevention of group B streptococcal disease. *Midwifery Today, 82,* 42–43.

Rouse, D. J., Weiner, S. J., Bloom, S. L., Varner, M. W., Spong, C. Y., Ramin, S. M., & Anderson, G. D. (2009). Second-stage labor duration in nulliparous women: Relationship to maternal and perinatal outcomes. *American Journal of Obstetricians & Gynecologists, 201,* 357.e1–357.e7. doi: 10.1016/j.ajog.2009.08.003

Rx Med. (n.d.) Cytotec. Retrieved from http://www.xmed.com/b.main/b2.pharmaceutical/b2.prescribe.html

Sakala, C., & Corry, M. P. (2007). Listening to Mothers II reveals maternity care quality chasm. *Journal of Midwifery & Women's Health, 52,* 183–185.

Sanchez-Ramos, L., Olivier, F., Delke, I., & Kaunitz, A. M. (2003). Labor induction versus expectant management for postterm pregnancies: A systematic review with meta-analysis. *Obstetrics & Gynecology, 101*(6), 1312–1318.

Sibai, B. M. (2007). Hypertension. In S. G. Gabbe, J. R. Niebyl, & J. L. Simpson (Eds.), *Obstetrics: Normal and problem pregnancies* (5th ed.) (pp. 864–904). New York, NY: Churchill Livingstone.

Simkin, P., & Ancheta, R. (2011). *The labor progress handbook: Early interventions to prevent and treat dystocia.* West Sussex, UK: Wiley.

Simpson, K. R. (2007). Intrauterine resuscitation during labor: Review of current methods and supportive evidence. *Journal of Midwifery & Women's Health, 52,* 229–237.

Simpson, K. R. (2011). Clinician's guide to the use of oxytocin for labor: Induction and augmentation. *Journal of Midwifery & Women's Health, 56,* 214–221.

Soltani, H., Poulose, T. A., & Hutchon, D. R. (2011). Placental cord drainage after vaginal delivery as part of the management of the third stage of labor. *Cochrane Library, 9.* doi: 10.1002/14651858.CD004665.pub3

Soule, D., & Szwed, S. (2000). *The roots of healing: A woman's book of herbs.* Secaucus, NJ: Citadel Press.

Stark, M. A., Rudell, B., & Haus, G. (2008). Observing position and movements in hydrotherapy: A pilot study. *Journal of Obstetric, Gynecologic, & Neonatal Nursing, 37*(1), 116–122.

Tharpe, N. (2004). Holistic evaluation of healing after cesarean birth. *Midwifery Today, 72,* 46–47.

Tharpe, N. (2007). First assisting in obstetrics: A primer for women's healthcare professionals. *Journal of Perinatal & Neonatal Nursing, 21,* 30–38.

Tora, P., & Dunn, J. (2000). Self-collection of antepartum anogenital group B *Streptococcus* cultures. *Journal of the American Board of Family Practice, 13,* 107–110.

Varney, H., Kriebs, J. M., & Gegor, C. L. (2004). *Varney's midwifery* (4th ed.). Sudbury, MA: Jones and Bartlett.

Walls, D. (2007). *Natural families—healthy homes.* LaVergne, TN: Ingram.

5

Care of the Infant and Mother After Birth

The transitions from intrauterine life as a fetus to extrauterine life as an infant, and from pregnant woman to postpartum mother, require rapid adaptations to maintain homeostasis. These changes are enhanced both physiologically and emotionally when mother and baby are kept together as a connected and synergistic dyad.

The baby's birth signals a phase of immense changes when both mother and infant are particularly vulnerable. The newly born infant must make the transition from the intrauterine environment, where nutritional and respiratory needs are met through the umbilicus, to the outside environment, where the newborn must initiate breathing and suckling to survive. Temperature regulation requires the infant to adapt to environmental changes. Maternal–infant interaction is an essential part of this adaptation process. Skin-to-skin contact provides the newborn with warmth, the comfort of the familiar sounds of the maternal heartbeat and gastrointestinal tract, and the tactile stimulation of touch. Fostering mother–baby bonding is an integral part of midwifery practice. Supportive care allows the mother and the baby to focus on each other as they adapt under the watchful eye of the skilled midwife.

Optimal maternity care after birth includes ample in-home help and support, in addition to frequent midwife visits in the early postpartum period. Standard post-partum care as provided to women who give birth in hospitals in the United States is suboptimal as compared to that available in many European and other countries, where in-home help and frequent home visits in the early postpartum days are standard, and paid extended maternity leave is the norm. Extended maternity leave (4 to 12 months) provided in an atmosphere of social support is designed to enable working mothers to form strong bonds with their newborns and have ample time to heal and make a healthy transition after childbirth.

The postpartum period can highlight cultural practices and beliefs about birth and the newborn. For the midwife practicing in a multicultural environment, it provides a wonderful opportunity to explore nurturing in its many forms. Infant feeding and bonding influence each woman's self-image and her view of herself as competent to meet the challenges and tasks of parenting. Changes in intimate relationships are common, because infant care takes time and both physical and emotional energy. Concerns about fertility resurface, providing another opportunity for the midwife to explore women's health within the context of the individual woman's life. Evaluation for postpartum depression, consideration of the effectiveness of infant feeding methods, and thoughtful scrutiny for variations from the norm allow for early intervention to reduce sequelae of potential complications that can result in harm to mother or baby. The guidelines in this section are presented in the order in which they are used if needed for the healthy mother-baby dyad, with acute conditions following in by topic.

CARE OF THE INFANT: ASSESSMENT OF THE NEWLY BORN INFANT

Key Clinical Information

The initial examination of the newborn serves to assess how well the fetus has made the transition from the total support provided within the womb to healthy extrauterine adaptation as a newborn. This evaluation process allows the midwife to identify newborn characteristics and variations that can affect the infant's ability to make this transition successfully or to identify and triage infants that require further evaluation and care by a healthcare professional skilled in neonatal care.

The initial exam is ideally conducted while the baby is nestled in the mother's or other family member's arms, with the practitioner explaining the exam process and findings at each step.

Client History and Chart Review: Components of the History to Consider

(Tappero & Honeyfield, 2009)

- Maternal and family history
  - Genetic disorders
  - Medical conditions, such as
    - Sickle cell
    - Hepatitis
    - Human immunodeficiency virus (HIV)/acquired immunodeficiency syndrome (AIDS)
    - Sexually transmitted infections
    - Thyroid disorders
    - Diabetes
- Contributing pregnancy history
  - Onset of prenatal care
  - Use of drugs, tobacco, and/or alcohol
  - Pregnancy complications
  - Duration of pregnancy
  - Fetal assessment and variation in pregnancy
  - Maternal group B *Streptococcus* (GBS) status
- Labor and birth information
  - Onset and duration of labor
  - Drug or medication exposure
  - Presentation and mode of delivery
  - Complications of labor or birth
    - Cesarean
    - Assisted vaginal birth
    - Fetal distress or evidence of hypoxia
    - Meconium-stained fluid
    - Preterm infant
  - Infant's condition at birth
  - Resuscitative measures, if any
  - Gross evaluation of placenta, cord, and membranes
- Neonatal course
  - Gestational age per Ballard or other validated tool
  - Apgar scores
  - Weight for gestational age
  - Newborn well-being
    - Activity
    - Feeding
    - Bladder and bowel function
  - Significant events or findings since birth

Physical Examination: Components of the Physical Exam to Consider

(Tappero & Honeyfield, 2009)

- Assessment of gestational age using physical parameters
  - Length, weight, and head circumference
  - Breast buds

- ■ Heel creases
- ■ Additional measurements when indicated
- • General appearance
  - ■ Tone, posture, positioning
  - ■ Alertness, vigor (activity), and color (perfusion)
  - ■ Respiratory effort
  - ■ Body proportion and symmetry
- • Skin
  - ■ Vernix, lanugo
  - ■ Pigmentation patterns
  - ■ Lesions, bruising or peeling
  - ■ Rashes, birthmarks
  - ■ Nails
- • Head
  - ■ Shape, symmetry
  - ■ Fontanelles, sutures
  - ■ Molding, caput, cephalohematoma
  - ■ Hair patterning and location of hair whorls
  - ■ Face: Shape and symmetry
  - ■ Eyes
    - ◆ Palpebral fissure inclination and length
    - ◆ Pupils equal, round, reactive to light and accommodation (PERRLA)
    - ◆ Red reflex
    - ◆ Placement, size, and shape of orbits
    - ◆ Color of iris and sclera
    - ◆ Subconjunctival hemorrhage
    - ◆ Conjunctivitis
  - ■ Ears
    - ◆ Location, rotation, configuration, and size
    - ◆ Patency
    - ◆ Placement and shape
    - ◆ Presence of periauricular sinus or skin tags
    - ◆ Universal newborn hearing screening
  - ■ Nose
    - ◆ Shape and position
    - ◆ Patency of nares
    - ◆ Presence of flaring
  - ■ Mouth
    - ◆ Configuration of upper lip, palate, and tongue
    - ◆ Shape and symmetry of lower jaw
    - ◆ Assessment of root, suck, and swallow
    - ◆ Lips, gums, mucous membrane, and uvula
- ■ Neck: Location of posterior hairline
- ■ Presence of sinus tract, masses, torticollis, or webbing
- • Chest and trunk
  - ■ Shape and symmetry
  - ■ Clavicles
  - ■ Nipples and breast buds
    - ◆ Location
    - ◆ Accessory nipples
  - ■ Cardiopulmonary system
    - ◆ Respiratory effort, rate, and breath sounds
    - ◆ Heart rate and rhythm
    - ◆ Murmurs, pulses
  - ■ Abdomen
    - ◆ Number of cord vessels
    - ◆ Muscle tone
    - ◆ Presence of bowel sounds in all four quadrants (1 hour after birth)
    - ◆ Palpation for hernia—umbilical or inguinal
    - ◆ Palpation for enlarged organs or masses
  - ■ Back
    - ◆ Symmetry
    - ◆ Palpate spines
    - ◆ Presence of dimple or hair tuft in intergluteal cleft
- • Genitalia
  - ■ Size, appearance, and presence of ambiguity
  - ■ Female
    - ◆ Configuration
    - ◆ Edema
    - ◆ Discharge
  - ■ Male
    - ◆ Position of urinary meatus
    - ◆ Descent of testes in scrotum
  - ■ Anus: Location and patency
- • Extremities—upper and lower
  - ■ Proportion, appearance, range of motion, and palpation
  - ■ Number of digits, presence of nails
  - ■ Pulses: Femoral, brachial
  - ■ Creases: Palmar, phalangeal, and flexion
  - ■ Hips (Ortolani and Barlow), gluteal folds

- Neurologic
  - Tone, response, alertness
  - Reflexes
    - Rooting
    - Suck
    - Palmar grasp
    - Tonic neck
    - Moro
    - Stepping
    - Plantar grasp
    - Babinski

Clinical Impression: Differential Diagnoses to Consider

(ICD9data.com, 2012)

- Hospital-based history and physical examination (H&P) for the normal newborn
- Out-of-hospital H&P for the normal newborn
- Same-day H&P and discharge for the normal newborn
- Newborn morbidity or mortality related to the following:
  - Maternal conditions unrelated to the present pregnancy
  - Maternal complications of pregnancy
  - Complications of placenta cord and membranes
  - Other complications of labor and delivery
  - Other perinatal conditions
    - Preterm infant
    - Post-term and high-birth-weight infant
    - Birth trauma
    - Respiratory distress syndrome in newborn
- Newborn hearing deficit

Diagnostic Testing: Diagnostic Tests and Procedures to Consider

(Tappero & Honeyfield, 2009)

- Cord blood gases
- Cord blood studies (Rh, ABO)
- Glucose, heel stick (normal value > 45 mg/dL)
- Hematocrit (normal value = 45–65%)

- Total bilirubin (normal value < 13 mg/dL)
- WWW Screening recommendations (March of Dimes, 2011; University of Texas, 2011)
  - Metabolic disorders
  - Fatty acid oxidation disorders
  - Sickle cell diseases
  - Cystic fibrosis
  - Hearing impairment
  - Other disorders
  - Congenital hypothyroidism
  - Biotinidase deficiency
  - Congenital adrenal hyperplasia
  - Classical galactosemia
- Sexually transmitted infection testing
  - RPR, VDRL
  - HIV
  - Herpes simplex (HSV)
  - Hepatitis B
- Drug toxicology (urine or meconium)
- Conjunctivitis
  - Gram stain of eye exudate
  - Culture of eye exudate for gonorrhea/chlamydia (GC/CT) and/or herpes simplex virus
  - Follow-up of prenatal variations, such as fetal hydronephrosis
  - State-mandated testing

Providing Treatment: Therapeutic Measures to Consider

- Infant bath: Verify the parent's cultural preferences for bathing of the infant
- Vitamin K_1 (American Academy of Pediatrics [AAP], 2003/2009)
  - Injection: AquaMEPHYTON (phytonadione)
  - 0.5–1 mg IM within 1 hour of birth
- Prophylactic ophthalmic treatment (Centers for Disease Control and Prevention [CDC], 2010a): Erythromycin ophthalmic ointment 0.5%, for one dose
- Hepatitis B (CDC, 2005)
  - Vaccine prophylaxis (HBsAg-negative mother)
  - Begin soon after birth

- Three-dose series: 0–1, 1–2, and 6–18 months
- May delay first dose up to 1 month
- HBIG (see "Care of the Woman with Hepatitis")
- Phototherapy for hyperbilirubinemia

Providing Treatment: Complementary and Alternative Measures to Consider

- Defer the infant bath or have the parent give the infant bath
- Defer vitamin K
  - Incidence of hemorrhagic disease without vitamin K ranges from 0.25% to 1.7% (AAP, 2003/2009)
  - Greatest incidence is in breastfed infants who do not receive vitamin K
  - Vitamin K is concentrated in colostrum and hindmilk
  - Bifidus factors begin synthesis of vitamin K in the gut after 1 week in breastfed infants
  - Formula-fed infants get significant vitamin K from cow's milk formula
- ⚠ Oral vitamin K
  - There is currently no consistent dosing for oral administration (Lippi & Franchini, 2011)
  - Oral vitamin K is significantly more expensive than injectable vitamin K
  - Konakion MM, mixed micellar preparation: 2 mg PO within 1 hour of birth, followed by additional doses at 7 and 30 days of age
  - For breastfeeding infants: 1 mg Konakion MM Pediatric or Orakay, combined with daily doses of 50 mcg Neokay for 3 months (Strehle, Howey, & Jones, 2010)
  - AquaMEPHYTON (Canadian Pediatric Society & College of Family Physicians of Canada, 1997/2004): 2 mg PO at first feeding, followed by additional doses at 2–4 and 6–8 weeks
- Defer erythromycin ophthalmic ointment
  - Negative maternal GC/CT results
  - Culture and treat if conjunctivitis occurs

- Use plain-water wash as needed
- 🌐 Colostrum drops to each eye (Singh, Sugathan, & Bhujwala, 1982)

Providing Support: Education and Support Measures to Consider

- Discuss physical findings
  - Range of normal
  - Potential or actual concerns
  - Signs and symptoms to watch for
  - Purpose of testing and/or medications
- Encourage questions
- Engage parents in decision making
- Discuss options for care
  - Well-baby care providers
  - Recommended treatments
  - Anticipated results and benefits
  - Risks and side effects
  - Alternatives
- Anticipatory guidance for parenting of newborn
  - Expected feeding and activity levels
  - Evaluation of adequate hydration
  - Common patterns of elimination
  - Planned follow-up for well-baby care
  - When and how to contact pediatric care provider
  - Warning signs (McHugh, 2004b)
    - Poor feeding
    - Lethargy
    - Irritability
    - Jaundice
    - Dehydration
    - Fever
    - Poor color
    - Vomiting

Follow-up Care: Follow-up Measures to Consider

- Daily evaluation first 2–3 days of life
  - Assess adaptation
  - Vital signs
  - Activity
  - Responsiveness

- Observation of feeding
- Determine suck/swallow
- Note latch if breastfeeding
- Maternal–infant interaction
- Document
  - Findings
  - Discussions
  - Recommendations and referrals
  - Plan for continued newborn care
- Weight check at 1 to 2 weeks
- Recheck or follow-up of variations from normal
  - Hearing deficits
  - Feeding issues
  - Bonding concerns
  - Neonatal drug withdrawal (up to 14 days depending on drug)
  - Fetal hydronephrosis

Multidisciplinary Practice: Consider Consultation, Collaboration, or Referral

- Pediatric service: If newborn evaluation is not included in the midwife's practice
- Variations (McHugh, 2004b)
  - Presence of anomalies
  - Evidence of infection
  - Hyperbilirubinemia
  - Hearing impairment
  - Other conditions outside the range of normal or expected findings
- Lactation consultant: Breastfeeding support or difficulties
- Social services: Need for infant supplies or car seat
- For diagnosis or treatment outside the midwife's scope of practice

CARE OF THE INFANT: BREASTFEEDING

Key Clinical Information

Human milk is the ideal food for newborns. Breastmilk is a dynamic and biologically active food that provides the nutritional and immunologic factors necessary for optimal infant health, growth, and brain and organ development. Exclusive breastmilk feedings in the first 6 months of life foster antibody formation to environmental pathogens and support immune system development (Lawrence & Lawrence, 2011). Breastfed infants demonstrate earlier and healthier colonization of the gut, which can contribute to decreased incidence of allergies—in particular, allergies to large proteins such as are found in cow's milk (Riordan & Wambach, 2010).

The process of infant feeding can foster maternal–infant interaction and bonding. The close contact between mother and baby during breastfeeding results in enhanced feelings of security and benefits future social development. However, many social and cultural factors influence a woman's decisions regarding infant feeding. The need to return to full-time work can limit a woman's opportunity to exclusively breastfeed. Many women pump breastmilk or supplement with commercial or homemade formulas when they are not available to breastfeed. Women who are uncomfortable with the sensations of suckling may opt to pump so as to supply their infant with breastmilk.

Evidence shows that breastfeeding a baby has a long-lasting positive impact on the baby's future health, but these effects vary according to the duration of breastfeeding (Riordan & Wambach, 2010). Prenatally, all women should be given information on the benefits of breastfeeding to both mother and infant. Referral to a breastfeeding class is helpful for information on initiating and maintaining lactation.

Client History and Chart Review: Components of the History to Consider

(Riordan & Wambach, 2010)

- Maternal
  - Age, GP TPAL
  - Prenatal history
  - Prenatal risk factors
  - Medications
  - Attendance at childbirth classes
  - Infant feeding plan

- Medical history, surgeries (especially breast surgeries)
- Labor and birth history
  - Medications and interventions
  - Analgesics and anesthetics
  - Oxytocin
  - Intravenous fluids
  - Magnesium sulfate
  - Instrument delivery
  - Postpartum hemorrhage
  - Maternal/newborn separation
- Obstetric/gynecologic history
  - Pregnancy and breastfeeding history
  - Length of breastfeeding
  - Contraceptive preference
- Psychosocial assessment
  - Expressed feelings about breastfeeding
  - Partner & family support of breastfeeding
  - Nutrition patterns
    - Adequacy
    - Eating disorders
  - Perinatal depression
  - Physical activity level
  - Sleep history
  - Alcohol, tobacco, or drug use
  - History of sexual abuse
  - Review of systems
- Family history: Food allergies
- Newborn
  - Birth weight and gestational age
  - Breastfeeding efforts
    - Early breastfeeding
    - Suck/swallow
    - Intensity and duration of breastfeeding
    - Weight loss/gain
    - Frequency of feeds
    - Need for assistance with feeding
  - Sleep–wake patterns
  - Infant temperament
  - Elimination
    - Passage of meconium
    - Number of voids per day
    - Number of stools per day

- Supplementation
  - Indications for supplementation
  - Physical separation of mother and baby
  - Maternal medications incompatible with nursing
  - Insufficient milk supply with baby who nurses well
  - Maternal conditions
    - Psychosis
    - Eclampsia
    - Varicella-zoster infection
    - Breast cancer
  - Infant conditions
    - Inability to effectively suck and swallow
    - Hypoglycemia
    - Weight loss greater than 7–10%
    - Illness or anomalies that prevent effective nursing
- Conditions that can affect breastfeeding
  - Low birth weight
  - Food allergy
  - Gastroesophageal reflux
  - Increased calorie demands
  - Neurologic conditions
  - Congenital anomalies
    - Cleft palate
    - Pierre-Robin syndrome
    - Choanal atresia
  - Disorders
    - Respiratory distress
    - Down syndrome
    - Cerebral palsy
    - Congenital heart defects
    - Phenylketonuria
    - Galactosemia
- ⚠ Contraindications to breastfeeding (CDC, 2007)
  - Infants with galactosemia (a metabolic disorder)
  - Maternal
    - Illicit drug use
    - HIV infection
    - Human T-cell lymphotropic virus infection

- Untreated active tuberculosis
- Antiretroviral medication
- Cancer chemotherapy
- Therapy with radioactive compounds (temporary)

Physical Examination: Components of the Physical Exam to Consider

(Walker, 2006)

- Infant
  - Weight, vital signs
  - Structural evaluation
    - Tongue
    - Jaw
    - Lips and cheeks
    - Palate
    - Airway
  - Reflexes
    - Rooting
    - Suck
    - Swallow
    - Gag
- Maternal
  - Nipples and areola
    - Erect, inverted, or flat
    - Size
  - Presence of the following conditions:
    - Cracks or fissures
    - Blisters
    - Pain
  - Breasts
    - Colostrum or milk present
    - Engorgement
    - Masses
    - Axilla
    - Pain
- Breastfeeding assessment
  - Maternal readiness
    - Attentiveness to infant cues
    - Ability to hold and examine breast
    - Ability to position infant for effective feeding
    - Maternal let-down

- Infant feeding
  - Rooting
  - Effective latch
  - Tongue curved around areola
  - Complete seal with lips
  - No smacking sounds
- Effective feeding
  - Sustained bursts of sucking
  - Audible and/or visible swallowing
  - Coordination of suck, swallow, and breathing
  - Colostrum/milk clearly present
- Post-feeding observations
  - Infant appears satisfied
  - Maternal breasts softer
  - Pre- and post-feeding weights

Clinical Impression: Differential Diagnoses to Consider

(ICD9data.com, 2012)

- Maternal
  - Cracked nipples
  - Engorgement of breasts
  - Nonpurulent mastitis
  - Other disorders of lactation
    - Retracted nipples
    - Suppressed lactation
    - Unspecified disorder of lactation
- Newborn
  - Abnormal loss of weight
  - Abnormal tongue position
  - Cleft palate/lip
  - Dysphagia
  - Failure to thrive
  - Infant feeding difficulty
  - Feeding problems in newborn
  - Neonatal candida infection
  - Suck reflex abnormal

Diagnostic Testing: Diagnostic Tests and Procedures to Consider

- Total serum bilirubin
- Blood glucose
- Metabolic screen

Providing Treatment: Therapeutic Measures to Consider

(Riordan & Wambach, 2010)

- Keep mother and baby together
- Encourage adequate rest and family support
- Relieve breast fullness
  - Breast pump
  - Hand expression
- Allow nipple rest and ensure adequate infant intake
  - Alternate infant feeding positions (see "Education and Support")
  - Alternate infant feeding methods, in conjunction with a lactation consultant or breastfeeding specialist
    - Cup feed
    - Finger feed
    - Nipple shield
    - Tube feeding device such as Lact-Aid
- Provide engorgement pain relief (National Library of Medicine, 2011)
  - Ibuprofen
  - Acetaminophen
  - Avoid use of naproxen or aspirin
- Relieve plugged ducts
  - Gently massage affected breast before and during feeding
  - Breastfeed frequently for short periods
  - Change position to ensure drainage from all sinuses
  - Avoid constricting clothing
  - Oral lecithin 15 mL daily

Providing Treatment: Complementary and Alternative Measures to Consider

- Herbal remedies that support breastmilk production (Laurence, 1998–2011)
  - Fenugreek
  - Blessed thistle
  - Fennel (seed or root only)
- Herbs to avoid while nursing (Straus, 2003)
  - Black cohosh
  - Buckthorn
  - Cascada sagrada
  - Kava kava
  - Sage
  - Senna
  - Wintergreen
- Sore or cracked nipples (Abou-Dakn, Fluhr, Gensch, & Wockel, 2011; Spencer, 2008)
  - Review positioning and latch
  - Reassure the mother that this condition is usually temporary
  - If nipples are slightly red and chapped:
    - Lanolin
    - Expressed milk allow to dry
    - Cool tea bag compresses
  - If nipples are painful throughout feeding, may need antifungal cream
  - If nipples are cracked, may need topical or oral antibiotic
- Engorgement (Mangesi & Dowswell, 2010)
  - Cool cabbage leaves
  - Acupuncture
  - Cool packs or compresses
  - Gentle massage

Providing Support: Education and Support Measures to Consider

- Provide age-appropriate information
- Encourage good nutrition and health habits
  - Ample fluids
  - Well-balanced food choices
  - Avoid alcohol, drugs, and tobacco
- Rest and emotionally supportive care
  - Mother and baby remain together
  - Family support
  - Postpartum doula
- Breastfeeding basics
  - First breastfeeding within 60 minutes of birth
  - Keep the newborn in skin-to-skin contact with the mother until the first feeding is completed
  - Limit stressors that interfere with the let-down reflex

- Feed 8–12 times per day
- Nursing positions
  - Cradle hold
  - Cross cradle
  - Football
  - Side-lying
- Assess for swallowing
- Hand expression or pumping
- In the first postpartum days
  - Mother and baby should remain together
  - Encourage feeding in response to infant cues
  - Assure the mother of the adequacy of colostrum for all newborn nutritional needs
  - Assess for correct latch
    - Wide gape of the mouth
    - Latch far back on the areola
    - Mother feels a tugging sensation
    - Audible swallowing of colostrum
  - Observe for adequate output
- Problem solving
  - Newborn irritability
    - Skin-to-skin contact or swaddle infant
    - Dim lights
    - Create a quiet, peaceful environment
  - Difficulty with latch
    - Feed at first infant cues
    - Place the infant in a position facing the mother
    - Infant is brought to breast
      - ➤ Colostrum at nipple
      - ➤ Gentle traction on chin
      - ➤ Nipple rolling or pumping to make nipple easier to grasp
  - Sleepy infant
    - Keep baby with mother
    - Feed at first infant cues
    - Unwrap and gently stimulate infant
    - Avoid distractions for infant
    - Offer breast frequently
  - Engorgement
    - Nurse frequently
    - Pump or express before feeds to soften breast and allow latch

- Low milk supply
  - Assess infant suck and swallow
  - Nurse frequently
  - Rest with the baby in skin-to-skin contact with the mother
  - Maintain maternal hydration and nutrition
- Plugged ducts
  - Warm compresses
  - Gentle massage during feedings
- Breast infection (see "Care of the Mother: Mastitis")
- Maternal benefits of breastfeeding (AAP, n.d.)
  - Decreased blood loss after delivery
  - Enhanced maternal–infant bonding
  - Stimulation of uterine involution
  - Reduced fertility during exclusive breastfeeding
  - Can foster maternal weight loss postpartum
  - Decreased risk of maternal breast and ovarian cancer
- Infant benefits of breastfeeding (U.S. Department of Health and Human Services, 2011)
  - Enhanced immune responsiveness
  - Decreased incidence of infections and illnesses such as diarrhea, ear infections, and pneumonia
  - Infants less likely to develop asthma
  - Less prone to obesity when breastfed longer than six months
  - Reduced risk of sudden infant death syndrome (SIDS)
- Menstrual cycle and function
  - Breastfeeding and amenorrhea
  - Return to fertility
  - Contraceptive options

Follow-up Care: Follow-up Measures to Consider

- Document
  - Breastfeeding assessment
  - Observation of feeding

- Three to five days of age
  - Assess ability of the infant to remain hydrated
    - Six to eight wet diapers in 24 hours
    - Three to four stools in 24 hours
  - Maintain growth consistent with age
  - Show appropriate physical activity for age
  - Stimulate adequate milk production
  - 🕭 Observe for signs of feeding difficulty
    - Weight loss/gain
    - Dehydration
    - Jaundice
- 🔻 Continued follow-up for infants with:
  - Jaundice
  - Persistent dark stool or urine
  - Ineffective milk transfer (suck and swallow)
  - Infrequent feeding
  - Weight loss of more than 7% of total body weight
  - Requiring formula supplementation
- As indicated for routine well-infant care

Multidisciplinary Practice: Consider Consultation, Collaboration, or Referral

- Pediatric care provider: Infant with significant problems affecting ability to feed
  - Congenital anomalies
  - Infection
  - Metabolic disorders
  - Tight frenulum for frenectomy
- Lactation consultant (Riordan & Wambach, 2010)
  - Early or persistent feeding difficulties
  - Maternal request
  - Flat or inverted nipples
  - Prior breast surgery
  - Nursing infants from a multiple gestation
  - Preterm infant(s)
  - Infant with congenital anomalies or health issues
  - Maternal or infant health issues that temporarily prevent breastfeeding
- OB/GYN provider or gynecologic endocrinologist
  - Dysfunctional lactogenesis
  - Mastitis or breast abscess

- Mental health service
  - Depression
  - Eating disorder
- Nutritionist
- For diagnosis or treatment outside the midwife's scope of practice

CARE OF THE MALE INFANT: INTACT OR CIRCUMCISED PENIS

Key Clinical Information

Medical societies around the world previously recommended against elective circumcision, which is the surgical removal of all or part of the foreskin of the penis without evidence of disease or disorder (Tobian, Gray, & Quinn, 2010). However, recent evidence supports circumcision as being instrumental in limiting transmission of sexually transmitted bacteria and viruses such as HIV, and reducing the initial infection rate in men or the rate of recurrent genital tract infections such as herpes simplex, human papillomavirus, bacterial vaginosis, and *Trichomonas vaginalis* infection in these males' female partners. Nevertheless, evidence demonstrates no clear medical value of nontherapeutic or elective circumcision of the newborn (American Academy of Family Physicians, 2001/2007; AAP, 1999/2005; Circumcision Information and Resource Pages, 2007; College of Physicians and Surgeons of British Columbia, 2007). Elective circumcision of the newborn is typically performed exclusively for religious, cultural, or ethnic reasons.

The American College of Obstetricians and Gynecologists (2001) recommends that parents be provided with "accurate and impartial information" as part of the informed choice process for circumcision. Prenatal discussion allows parents time to thoughtfully weigh the risks of the procedure against the putative future potential benefits. There is insufficient evidence to demonstrate that routine neonatal circumcision offers long-term medical benefits that are greater than the risks of pain, infection, injury, and bleeding that are the most common complications of this procedure. Noninvasive measures and sexual health behaviors exist that are more effective in reducing and preventing the diseases or disorders that circumcision aims to prevent (American Academy of Family Physicians, 2001/2007; AAP, 1999/2005; College of Physicians and Surgeons of British Columbia, 2007).

The midwife who chooses to include circumcision in her or his practice for religious, cultural, or ethnic reasons is obligated to learn and perform the procedure under expert guidance until skilled at the procedure and must perform an adequate number of procedures annually to maintain competence. Use of analgesia and/or local anesthesia is recommended for circumcision to minimize the stress to the infant during this procedure (American College of Obstetricians and Gynecologists, 2001).

Client History and Chart Review: Components of the History to Consider

(Lowenstein, 2004)

- Review the infant's medical record
  - Neonatal course since birth
  - Temperature stability
  - Feeding and voiding
  - Physical examination results
  - Vitamin K administration: ⚠ Oral vitamin K requires up to three doses before it achieves full effectiveness
  - Demonstrated voiding since birth
- ▽ Contraindications to circumcision
  - Hypospadias
  - Abnormality of the penis
  - Medically unstable infant
  - Parents decline procedure

Physical Examination: Components of the Physical Exam to Consider

- Vital signs, including temperature
- Examination of the penis
  - 🕐 Evaluate for epispadias or hypospadias before procedure
  - Evaluate redundancy of the foreskin
  - Identify landmarks for a penile block, if used

Clinical Impression: Differential Diagnoses to Consider

(ICD9data.com, 2012)

Elective or ritual circumcision

Diagnostic Testing: Diagnostic Tests and Procedures to Consider

As indicated to ensure the infant's stability before the procedure

Providing Treatment: Therapeutic Measures to Consider

- Circumcision technique
  - ▽ Obtain informed consent
  - Prepare equipment
    - Gomco clamp
    - Plastibell device
    - Mogen clamp
- Provide for pain relief (AAP, 1999/2005)
  - EMLA cream
  - Dorsal penile block
  - Subcutaneous ring block
  - Parental presence
  - Sucrose on pacifier
  - Swaddling
  - Analgesics
- Perform procedure (Lowenstein, 2004)
  - 🌐 Honor religious or ethnic circumcision rituals
  - Strict aseptic technique
  - Use preferred method (Varney, Kriebs, & Gegor, 2004)
  - Observe for, and treat, active bleeding
- Apply petroleum jelly gauze or other nonadherent dressing
- Comfort the baby and return him to the mother and family

Providing Treatment: Complementary and Alternative Measures to Consider

- Nontherapeutic or ritual circumcision
  - Remove only the very tip of the foreskin
  - Remove the entire foreskin

- Maintain an intact foreskin
- Circumcise later in life if and when indicated

Providing Support: Education and Support Measures to Consider

- Provide information for informed consent (American Academy of Family Physicians, 2001/2007; AAP, 1999/2005)
  - 🌐 Decision is personal and subjective
  - Procedure is not essential to the child's well-being
  - Parents have no obligation to consent to circumcision
  - Parents determine the best option for their infant
  - Religious, cultural, and ethnic considerations
  - Future sexual and psychological considerations
  - Child's right to body integrity
  - Risks associated with circumcision
    - Pain
    - Bleeding
    - Infection
    - Injury
    - Complication rate: 0.2–0.6%
  - Potential benefits of circumcision (Tobian et al., 2010)
    - Decreased incidence or transmission of the following:
      - ➤ Urinary tract infections
      - ➤ Penile cancer (Circumcision Information and Resource Pages, 2008)
      - ➤ Sexually transmitted infections and HIV
    - Number needed to treat based on diagnosis (Singh-Grewal, Macdessi, & Craig, 2005): 111 circumcisions to prevent 1 urinary tract infection
    - Good hygiene and safe sex practices also reduce these risks
- Provide education to parents
  - Care of the infant with an intact foreskin (Sinclair, 2004)

- Keep diaper area clean
- Do not retract foreskin
- If redness or irritation occurs:
  - ➤ Flush area with clear water
  - ➤ Allow to air-dry if possible
  - ➤ Apply diaper ointment to glans
- Care of the infant post-circumcision (Lowenstein, 2004)
  - Crying is common with first voids
  - Head of penis may be quite red
  - Swelling just under the glans is normal
  - A blood clot can form at incision site
  - Pink or yellow serous drainage may occur
  - Instruct in care of circumcised penis
- ⚠ Call for signs or symptoms of complications
  - Active bleeding
  - Infection at incision site
  - Fever
  - Lack of urination within 12–24 hours after circumcision

Follow-up Care: Follow-up Measures to Consider

- Document, as indicated
  - Discussions
  - Informed consent process
  - Parents' decision
  - Procedure (see the "Procedure Note" section earlier in this book)
  - Postprocedure findings
- ⚠ Observe for potential complications
  - 12–24 hours postprocedure
  - At follow-up visit(s)
    - Bleeding
    - Infection or inflammation
    - Urinary retention
    - Tissue trauma or necrosis
    - Cosmetic results
- Criteria for release from care
  - Infant stable and feeding
  - Bleeding minimal
  - Voiding has occurred

Multidisciplinary Practice: Consider Consultation, Collaboration, or Referral

- Mohel/mohelet for Jewish families
  - For information and opinion about circumcision
  - To perform circumcision
- Pediatric service
  - For an infant with congenital defects of the genitals
  - To perform circumcision if this service is not provided by the midwife
- OB/GYN service: To perform circumcision if this service is not provided by the midwife
- For diagnosis or treatment outside the midwife's scope of practice

CARE OF THE INFANT: NEWBORN VARIATIONS FROM NORMAL

Key Clinical Information

Midwives strive to improve the health and well-being of each mother and baby through the provision of excellent midwifery care. As part of this care, the midwife must remain alert to noteworthy maternal or perinatal history and observant for subtle signs or symptoms in the newborn that can indicate a need for gentle assistance or medical intervention. Although most babies born to healthy mothers are themselves healthy, the midwife must consider whether newborn variations represent the wide range of normal or indicate the presence of a condition requiring further evaluation by a clinician skilled in evaluation and care of the newly born infant.

Client History and Chart Review: Components of the History to Consider

(McHugh, 2004a; Tappero & Honeyfield, 2009)

- Maternal medical history
  - Age
  - Illnesses
  - Medications
- Social factors

- Prenatal history
  - Maternal reproductive history
  - Gravida, para, and pregnancy outcomes
  - Preconception folate intake
  - Fetal activity during pregnancy
  - Genetic testing or screening
  - Prenatal test results
  - Complications of pregnancy
  - Drug, alcohol, or tobacco use
  - Teratogenic or environmental exposures
  - Maternal disease or illness
    - Group B streptococcal infection (GBS)
    - Herpes
    - Diabetes
    - Epilepsy
    - HIV
    - Viral and parasitic infections
- Family history (three generations, as applicable)
  - Ethnic background
  - Consanguinity
  - Genetic testing
  - Conditions such as the following:
    - Reproductive losses or infertility
    - Cerebral palsy or mental retardation
    - Congenital anomalies
    - Genetic disorders
- Perinatal history
  - Exposure to medications or environmental toxins
  - Estimated gestational age
  - Labor and birth events
    - Duration
    - Drug or medications in labor
    - Presentation and mode of delivery
  - Abnormal fetal heart rate patterns
  - Complications at birth
    - Presence of meconium
    - Endotracheal intubation or suctioning
    - Instrument or surgically assisted birth
    - Shoulder dystocia
  - Infant's condition at birth
    - Apgar scores
    - Resuscitation
    - Evidence of birth trauma

- Description and disposition of placenta
- Neonatal course
  - Post-resuscitation status
  - Birth weight for gestational age
  - Feeding difficulties
  - Complications or unusual findings
  - Laboratory test results
  - Review symptoms since birth
    - Type of symptom(s)
    - Onset
    - Duration
    - Severity
  - Treatments and infant response

Physical Examination: Components of the Physical Exam to Consider

(McHugh, 2004a)

- ⚠ 📞 Signs and symptoms suggesting the need for further evaluation
  - Respiratory system
    - Presence of apnea
    - Grunting or gasping
    - Retractions
    - Abnormal breath sounds
    - Respiratory rate less than 30 breaths/min or more than 60 breaths/min
  - Heart rate and rhythm
    - Bradycardia < 100 beats/min
    - Tachycardia > 170 beats/min
    - Cardiac instability
  - Temperature instability
  - Color
    - Pallor
    - Cyanosis
    - Rubor
    - Jaundice
      - ➤ Before 24 hours—most likely pathologic
      - ➤ After 24 hours—most likely physiologic
  - Abnormal muscle tone and activity level
    - Poor muscle tone, flaccidity
    - Poor feeding, ineffective suckle
    - Lethargy, poor response to stimulation
    - Irritability

- Hyperactivity
- Seizures
- Failure to move an extremity
- Gastrointestinal adaptation
  - Vomiting
  - Diarrhea
  - Abdominal distention
- Presence of congenital anomalies
- Presence of birth-related conditions
  - Cephalohematoma
  - Brachial plexus injury
  - Pneumothorax
  - Fractured rib or clavicle
  - Subgaleal hemorrhage after vacuum extraction
- 📞 Unusual behavior or findings: Arrange for specialty newborn assessment

Clinical Impression: Differential Diagnoses to Consider

(ICD9data.com, 2012)

- Consider perinatal disorders relating to the following factors and conditions:
  - Family history
  - Congenital anomalies, including genetic disorders
  - Maternal conditions
  - Intrauterine growth retardation
  - Gestational age and birth weight
  - Birth trauma
  - Intrauterine hypoxia and birth asphyxia
  - Respiratory distress syndrome
  - Other respiratory conditions
  - Infection
  - Hemorrhage
  - Hemolytic disease
  - Jaundice
  - Endocrine and metabolic disturbances
  - Hematologic disorders
  - Digestive system disorders
  - Integument and temperature regulation disorders
  - Other perinatal conditions

Diagnostic Testing: Diagnostic Tests and Procedures to Consider

- As indicated by infant presentation *and*
- ⚠ As appropriate for the midwife's scope of practice

Providing Treatment: Therapeutic Measures to Consider

- Provide a neutral thermal environment
  - Skin-to-skin contact with the mother
  - Pre-warmed resuscitation unit
  - Cloth-wrapped hot water bottle for transport
- Provide free-flow oxygen (O_2) as needed for cyanosis (AAP & AHA, 2011)
  - Blow-by or mask
  - Provide positive-pressure ventilation (PPV) for infants with the following signs and symptoms: (AAP & AHA, 2011)
    - Heart rate < 100 beats/min
    - Ineffective or absent respirations
    - Persistent cyanosis with free-flow O_2
  - Failure to attain adequate O_2 saturation per pulse oximetry
- 📞 Access care as indicated by the diagnosis
  - Phototherapy
  - Antibiotic therapy

Providing Treatment: Complementary and Alternative Measures to Consider

🌐 These methods supplement the newborn care processes described previously and are not meant as a substitute for medical care when indicated by the newborn's condition. However, parents retain the right to decline standardized medical care, particularly for their newborns with life-threatening anomalies or conditions associated with a poor quality of life (AAP & AHA, 2011).

- Home phototherapy: bili-lights or sunlight
- Homeopathic rescue remedy to pulse points
- Prayer and acceptance of the infant as a perfect being
- Other remedies as indicated by the infant's condition or presentation

Providing Support: Education and Support Measures to Consider

(American College of Medical Genetics, 2000; CDC, 2010b; Kenner & Lott, 2007)

- 🌐 Offer an interpreter as needed to accommodate ethnocultural and language differences
- Maintain a caring, nonjudgmental environment
  - Provide support to the parents during the following processes:
    - Newborn workup
    - Diagnosis
    - Treatment
  - Assist, as desired by family, to ensure the following:
    - Privacy
    - Autonomy
    - Inclusion of additional family members or clergy
  - Provide acknowledgment of and support during the following:
    - Times of uncertainty
    - Grieving process
- ▽ For an infant with a mild condition, provide information:
  - Warning signs and symptoms of the condition
  - Who to contact if symptoms develop
  - How to contact the infant's healthcare professional
- ▽ For an infant with significant illness or abnormality, provide factual information, as appropriate
  - Working diagnosis
  - Planned diagnostic workup
  - Anticipated prognosis
  - Treatment plan and priorities
  - Recurrence risks
  - Resources

Follow-up Care: Follow-up Measures to Consider

- Reevaluate the infant
  - To establish a baseline or note a change
  - If uncertain regarding the normalcy of the infant's condition

- Documentation
  - Annotated history and physical examination
  - Diagnostic test results
  - Plan for continued care
  - Consultations and referrals
  - Summary of discussions

Multidisciplinary Practice: Consider Consultation, Collaboration, or Referral

- Pediatric or neonatology service
  - Neonate with signs or symptoms of the following:
    - Illness
    - Injury
    - Anomaly
    - Unusual behavior or findings
  - Newborn transport or transfer care of infant as indicated by problem
- Resources
  - Social services assistance during the acute phase
  - Family adjustment
  - Housing and support services
  - Health interpretation and advocacy
  - Long-term needs
  - Early intervention
  - Support groups
  - Psychosocial services
- For diagnosis or treatment outside the midwife's scope of practice

CARE OF THE INFANT: NEWBORN RESUSCITATION

Key Clinical Information

Most infants born into a midwife's hands begin to breathe with nothing more required than gentle supportive care. Occasionally, however, some newly born infants need assistance to successfully make the transition to life outside the womb and breathing on their own. The ideal is for every birth to be attended by one or more individuals who are educated and skilled in resuscitation of the newborn, in addition to one practitioner whose primary responsibility is caring for the mother.

Initiation of ventilation is the single most important aspect of resuscitation of the neonate. The primary goal of positive-pressure ventilation is to provide adequate oxygenated blood to the coronary arteries to allow the heart muscle to effectively pump blood throughout the rest of the baby's body.

When using the stethoscope, both breath sounds and heart rate can be assessed simultaneously, although positive-pressure ventilation may need to be interrupted briefly during such an assessment. Maintenance of an intact umbilical cord during the resuscitation process can provide the baby with a secondary source of oxygen, as well as the volume expansion necessary to fill the infant's pulmonary capillary bed without reducing the baby's blood pressure (Mercer, Erickson-Owens, Graves, & Haley, 2007; Mercer & Skovaard, 2002).

The most effective method of evaluating the newborn's pulse is by auscultation of the infant's chest with a newborn stethoscope. Low neonatal blood pressure or spasm of the cord secondary to cord palpation or tension can inhibit cord blood flow and limit oxygen transport via cord pulsation. As neonatal blood pressure improves with resuscitative measures, umbilical cord pulsation and blood flow frequently resume, thereby enhancing resuscitative efforts through autologous volume expansion.

⚠️ Regular practice is necessary to maintain the skills required for newborn resuscitation. Ideally, resuscitation drills should be performed and documented on a periodic basis.

Client History and Chart Review: Components of the History to Consider

- Presence of risk factors for fetal asphyxia (AAP & AHA, 2011)
  - Cord factors
    - Cord prolapse
    - Cord compression
  - Placental factors
    - Placental abruption
    - Placental insufficiency
    - Placenta previa

- Maternal factors
  - Vascular disease
  - Hypoxia
  - Hypertension
  - Hypotension
  - Uterine hyperstimulation
  - Maternal narcotic use in labor
- Fetal factors
  - Prematurity
  - Meconium aspiration
  - Forceps or vacuum-assisted delivery
  - Nonvertex presentation
  - Shoulder dystocia
- Causes of respiratory distress
  - Hyaline membrane disease
  - Persistent pulmonary hypertension
  - Sepsis
  - Fetal isoimmunization
  - Choanal atresia
  - Diaphragmatic hernia

Physical Examination: Components of the Physical Exam to Consider

- Evaluate for (AAP & AHA, 2011)
  - Gestational age
  - Presence of meconium
  - Respirations
  - Muscle tone
- Evaluate respirations
  - Normal rate: 40–60/min
  - May be irregular
  - No abdominal retractions
  - No grunting, gasping, or wheezing
- Evaluate heart rate
  - Normal rate: 120–160 beats/min
  - Regular rate and rhythm
- Evaluate color
  - Should pink easily with respirations
  - Cyanosis of hands and feet is common
  - Pallor indicates poor perfusion due to either of the following:
    - Volume depletion
    - Inadequate blood pressure

- Central cyanosis indicates the following:
  - Adequate perfusion
  - Hypoxia
- Meconium present
  - Assess vigor
  - Muscle tone (flexion or motion)
  - Respirations (effective)
  - Heart rate (more than 100 beats/min)

Clinical Impression: Differential Diagnoses to Consider

(ICD9data.com, 2012)

- Acute ineffective ventilation or cardiac output
  - Fetus or newborn affected by complications of placenta, cord and membranes
  - Fetus or newborn affected by other complications of labor and delivery
  - Birth trauma
  - Intrauterine hypoxia and birth asphyxia
  - Respiratory distress syndrome in newborn
  - Other respiratory conditions of fetus and newborn
- Newborn resuscitation procedure codes may include the following:
  - Assisted ventilation
    - < 30 minutes
    - > 30 minutes
  - Chest compressions
- Insertion of the following devices:
  - Endotracheal tube
  - Laryngeal mask airway
  - Orogastric tube
  - Oral airway

Diagnostic Testing: Diagnostic Tests and Procedures to Consider

(AAP & AHA, 2011)

- Endotracheal intubation
  - Nonvigorous infant, with meconium
  - Evaluate for meconium below the vocal cords
  - Suctioning of trachea
  - For ventilation and medication administration

- Laboratory testing
  - Cord blood gases
  - Hematocrit
  - Blood glucose
  - Chest x-ray

Providing Treatment: Therapeutic Measures to Consider

(AAP & AHA, 2011)

- Nonvigorous infant with meconium
  - Handle infant gently
  - Suction before giving any stimulation
  - Use a suction method appropriate for the midwife's scope of practice
  - Endotracheal intubation
  - Proceed with ventilation as needed
- Basic steps, with clear amniotic fluid
  - Prevent heat loss
  - Place on a warm surface
    - Maternal abdomen
    - Radiant warmer
  - Dry the infant
  - Remove wet linen
  - Open the infant's airway
    - Position
    - Suction as needed
      - ➤ Gently use a bulb or other suction device
      - ➤ Avoid causing a vagal response
    - Insert oral airway as needed
  - Provide tactile stimulation if the infant is apneic
    - Flick or tap the infant's soles
    - Rub the infant's back
- Free-flow O_2 as indicated by the following signs:
  - Respiratory effort
  - Color
- Positive-pressure ventilation (PPV) with room air or titrated oxygen, for the following newborns:
  - Absent or weak respiratory efforts
  - Heart rate < 100 beats/min
  - Persistent central cyanosis with free-flow O_2
  - Pulse oximetry if O_2 used

- Chest compressions
  - After 30 seconds of effective PPV, if heart rate < 60 beats/min
  - Two-thumb technique
  - Two-finger technique
- Epinephrine 1:10,000
  - Newborns with heart rate < 60 beats/min:
    - After 30 seconds of PPV *and*
    - 30 seconds of PPV and chest compressions
  - Stimulates cardiac contraction and rate
  - Causes peripheral vasoconstriction
  - Dose: 0.1–0.3 mL/kg
  - Route: Umbilical vein (preferred route) or endotracheal tube
  - Give rapidly
  - Heart rate should improve within 30 seconds
- Maintain intact umbilical cord (Coggins & Mercer, 2009)
  - If the cord is pulsing, the infant is getting oxygen
  - The cord pulses with the infant's heart rate
  - Avoid traction or pressure on the cord
  - Supports increase in pulmonary blood flow
  - Provides autologous volume expansion

Providing Treatment: Complementary and Alternative Measures to Consider

These methods supplement the newborn resuscitation process as described previously and are not meant as a substitute for positive-pressure ventilation and chest compressions when indicated by the newborn's condition.

- Head-down position facilitates drainage of fluids
- Encourage the infant to be present through the following measures:
  - Prayer and visualization
  - Talking to the infant
  - Physical touch
- Application of homeopathic remedies (e.g., rescue remedy) to pulse points is considered safe
- Oral administration of any medication, homeopathic, or herbal remedy can cause aspiration and further compromise infant

Providing Support: Education and Support Measures to Consider

- Discuss care of the infant with the parents in the moment as you act and then further when time allows
- Provide information
  - Indication for resuscitation
  - Plan for ongoing infant care
  - Tests or treatments
  - Follow-up evaluation
  - Specialty care
- Listen to the parents' concerns and fears
- Provide information about support groups or services as indicated

Follow-up Care: Follow-up Measures to Consider

- Document resuscitation
  - Indication for resuscitation
  - Respiratory effort, heart rate, color, and tone
  - Sequence of events
  - Resuscitation techniques used
  - Procedures or medication
  - Infant response
  - Consultations
  - Plan for post-resuscitation evaluation and care
- Notify the appropriate personnel that the infant required resuscitation and ensure that the infant is evaluated promptly based on the following considerations:
  - Resuscitation measures required
  - Condition after resuscitation
  - Parent or midwife preferences
- Post-resuscitation care
  - Based on length and extent of resuscitation
  - Evaluate newborn frequently for 24 hours
  - Vital signs: Temperature, pulse, respirations, and blood pressure
  - Color
  - Activity
  - Oxygen saturation
  - Blood glucose

- Renal function
- Presence of encephalopathy
- Transport of newborn, as indicated
  - From a community hospital
  - From a birth center
  - From a home birth

Multidisciplinary Practice: Consider Consultation, Collaboration, or Referral

- OB/GYN service: As indicated during labor and birth
- Pediatric care provider
  - For anticipated need of neonatal resuscitation
  - For an infant who
    - Has a poor response to PPV
    - Requires chest compressions
    - Exhibits signs or symptoms that indicate need for specialty care (AAP & AHA, 2011)
      - Vital signs outside of accepted range
      - Respiratory distress
      - Difficulty with temperature regulation
      - Persistent cyanosis or pallor
      - Seizures or apnea
      - Abnormal tone or activity
      - Diminished urinary output
      - Feeding difficulties
- For diagnosis or treatment outside the midwife's scope of practice

CARE OF THE INFANT: WELL-BABY CARE

Key Clinical Information

Midwives provide well-baby care after the immediate newborn period based on their interest, education, credentials, and scope of practice as defined by their professional association and state regulatory agency. Midwives who continue to provide care to infants after the newborn period (28 days) do so through an integrated practice model by forming collaborative relationships with other infant care professionals, such as pediatricians, pediatric nurse practitioners, and family physicians, who provide medical care or evaluation during times of illness, injury, or deviations from the norm. Routine well-baby care includes periodic screening to assess the infant's health status, growth and development, behavior, and family functioning. Group visits are effective for anticipatory guidance and support during the challenges of parenting and for update of immunizations. The midwife facilitates best care for the infant through information, education, and support for parents, while evaluating the well-being and safety of the child.

Client History and Chart Review: Components of the History to Consider

(McHugh, 2004a; Tappero & Honeyfield, 2009)

- Indication for present evaluation
  - Routine care
  - Problem-oriented care
- Significant perinatal or interim history
  - Pregnancy history
  - Maternal illness
  - Sexually transmitted infection exposure
  - Maternal substance abuse
  - Isoimmunization
  - Gestational age at birth
- Current patterns of behavior
  - Activity and interaction
  - Sleep/wake patterns
  - Feeding method and efforts
  - Elimination patterns
  - Developmental milestones
  - Cognitive/linguistic development
  - Social/emotional development
- Assessment areas
  - Family strengths
  - Parental observations and concerns
  - Parent–child interaction
  - Eye contact
  - Comfort seeking
  - Tone of voice
- ▽ Variations from expected well-baby course
  - Significant findings or events since the last visit
  - Social or developmental delay
  - Infection or injury

- Immunization status
- Review of systems

Physical Examination: Components of the Physical Exam to Consider

(Tappero & Honeyfield, 2009)

- Vital signs
- Growth parameters
  - Head circumference
  - Chest circumference
  - Height/weight
  - Growth pattern
- General appearance
  - Alertness
  - Muscle tone, strength, and activity
  - Nutrition
  - Response to environment and stimuli
- Skin
  - Color and turgor
  - Rashes or lesions
  - Bruises or signs of abuse
- Head, eyes, ears, nose and throat
  - Head shape
  - Torticollis
  - Fontanelles: Size and shape, suture lines
  - Tracking movements of eyes
  - Suck and swallow
  - Tympanic membranes
  - Lymph nodes
- Chest and back
  - Shape and symmetry
  - Heart rate and rhythm
  - Breath sounds
- Abdomen
  - Size and shape
  - Palpation of organs
  - Bowel sounds
  - Muscle tone and integrity
  - Hernias
- Extremities
  - Strength
  - Flexibility and mobility
  - Femoral pulses

- Genitalia and anus
- Neurologic evaluation
  - Reflexes
  - Motor function
- Assessment for signs of illness or injury (McHugh, 2004b)
  - Fever
  - Skin tone variations
    - Pallor
    - Cyanosis
    - Ruddiness
    - Jaundice
    - Rash
  - Cardiopulmonary
    - Heart rate or rhythm abnormalities
    - Respiratory difficulty or wheezing
  - Neurologic
    - Jitteriness or irritability
    - Bulging or sunken fontanelles
    - Unusual sounding cry
  - Musculoskeletal
    - Poor muscle tone
    - Hip clicks or laxity
  - Gastrointestinal
    - Feeding difficulties
    - Abdominal distention
  - Urinary tract
    - Insufficient or unusual elimination pattern
    - Dark color or unusual odor to urine
  - Indications of abuse or neglect
    - Injuries, burns, or bruises
    - Malnutrition
    - Poor hygiene
    - Behavioral disorders

Clinical Impression: Differential Diagnoses to Consider

(ICD9data.com, 2012)

- Well-baby care
- Acute conjunctivitis
- Otitis media

- Developmental delay
- Hearing screening
- Child abuse

Diagnostic Testing: Diagnostic Tests and Procedures to Consider

- Hematocrit
- Lead testing
- Developmental screening
- Hearing screening
- Vision testing
- Oral evaluation
- Other laboratory values or tests as indicated

Providing Treatment: Therapeutic Measures to Consider

- www Childhood immunizations (CDC, 2011a)
  - Hepatitis B immunization: Three (HepB) doses
  - Rotavirus: Three (Rota) doses
  - Diphtheria, tetanus, and acellular pertussis: Five (DTaP) doses
  - *Haemophilus influenzae* type b: Four (Hib) doses
  - Pneumococcal: Four doses
  - Oral polio/inactivated polio vaccine: Four (OPV/IPV) doses
  - Influenza: One dose annually
  - Measles, mumps, and rubella: Two (MMR) doses
  - Varicella: Two doses
  - Hepatitis A: Two doses
- Treatment for underlying disease or illness
  - Antibiotics
  - Congenital hypothyroid treatment
- Other treatments as indicated

Providing Treatment: Complementary and Alternative Measures to Consider

- Nutritional supplementation
  - Goat's milk—fresh, raw
  - Homemade infant formula
  - Commercial infant formula

- www Immunizations
  - Delay in onset of immunizations
  - Lower initial dose of immunizations
  - No immunizations
- Follow-up of oral vitamin K, based on dosing protocol

Providing Support: Education and Support Measures to Consider

- Provide information on anticipated changes
  - Growth and development
  - Behaviors
  - Developmental milestones
- Diet and nutrition recommendations
  - Breastfeeding
  - Formulas
  - Primary feeding method
  - Supplementation
  - Solid foods
- Signs and symptoms of concern
  - Warning signs
  - When to call with concerns
  - How to call in off-hours
- Routine for well-infant care
  - Schedule of visits
  - Immunization recommendations
  - Encourage parental participation in decision making
  - Provide rationale for recommendations
  - Discuss alternatives
  - Provide access to additional resources as needed

Follow-up Care: Follow-up Measures to Consider

- Document
  - Findings, especially any variations from normal
  - Plot growth on appropriate charts
  - Discussions with parents
  - Plan for continued care
  - www Signs and symptoms of vaccine adverse side effects (CDC, 2011b)
  - Consultations or referrals

- Well-child examination schedule (Green & Palfrey, 2002)
  - 1 week of age
  - 1 month of age
  - Every 2 months from 2–6 months of age
  - Every 3 months from 6–18 months of age
  - Every 6 months from 18–24 months of age
  - Annually from 2–5 years of age
- ⚠ www Report adverse vaccine reactions (CDC, 2011b)
  - Vaccine Adverse Event Reporting System form
  - Online: http://www.vaers.hhs.gov
  - Telephone: 1-800-822-7967

Multidisciplinary Practice: Consider Consultation, Collaboration, or Referral

- Pediatric care provider
  - Ongoing well-child care
  - For infants or children with the following:
    - Variations from normal
    - Illness
    - Injury
- For diagnosis or treatment outside the midwife's scope of practice

CARE OF THE MOTHER: ASSESSMENT POSTPARTUM, WEEK 1

Key Clinical Information

During the first days postpartum, daily evaluation of the mother is performed to assess healing. The postpartum woman undergoes a multitude of changes as her body returns to the nonpregnant state and she adapts emotionally to the changes in her family. Although the physiologic process is much the same in each individual, every woman responds differently to the birth of a child and has specific and distinct individual needs that must be met.

In the first week after the birth, most families begin independent care of their newly born infant. Parents must have clear information regarding the expectations and indications for follow-up care, signs of complications, and when and how to access needed services. Fostering family independence requires ongoing access to support, education, and healthcare services.

Client History and Chart Review: Components of the History to Consider

- Age, GP TPAL
- Pregnancy, labor, and birth history
  - Prenatal course
  - Labor and birth information
    - Length of labor
    - Complicating factors for labor and/or birth
    - Manner of birth
    - Lacerations or episiotomy
  - Infant well-being since birth
    - Feeding
    - Sleeping
    - Activity
- Maternal well-being and adaptation
  - Pain
    - Location
    - Severity
    - Relief measures used and results
  - Adaptation to postpartum status
    - Sleep/rest
    - Appetite
    - Amount of lochia
    - Breasts
    - Bowel and bladder function
    - Activity
    - Other symptoms
  - Maternal emotional response
    - To labor and birth
    - To changes postpartum
    - To changes in family dynamics
  - Observe interaction with infant
    - Feeding
    - Bonding
    - Caretaking
  - Cultural traditions/considerations
  - Review of systems

Physical Examination: Components of the Physical Exam to Consider

(Katz, 2007; Varney et al., 2004)

- Vital signs: Blood pressure, temperature, pulse, and respirations
- Weight loss
- Chest and thorax
  - Heart and lungs
  - Breasts and nipples
    - Cracks or fissures
    - Engorgement
    - Colostrum or milk
  - Costovertebral angle (CVA) tenderness
- Abdomen
  - Fundus: Location, consistency, and tenderness
  - Muscle tone: Diastasis, hernia
  - Incision: Dressing, redness, erythema, exudate
  - Bladder: Distention, tenderness
  - Bowel sounds
- Lochia: Type, amount, odor
- Perineum and rectum
  - Redness or inflammation
  - Approximation of tissues
  - Bruising and/or hematoma
  - Edema
  - Discharge
  - Hemorrhoids
- Extremities
  - Edema
  - Reflexes
  - Homans' sign
  - Redness, heat, or pain
  - Varicosities

Clinical Impression: Differential Diagnoses to Consider

(ICD9data.com, 2012)

- Postpartum care and examination
- Postpartum complications
  - Delayed postpartum hemorrhage
  - Postpartum infection
  - Postpartum venous conditions

- Postpartum fever
- Postpartum pulmonary embolism
- Unspecified complications of the puerperium
- Postpartum follow-up of complications
  - Gestational diabetes
  - Postoperative wound infection
  - Preeclampsia
  - Postpartum depression or mood disorders
- Postpartum sterilization
  - Tubal ligation
  - Tubal occlusion with device

Diagnostic Testing: Diagnostic Tests and Procedures to Consider

- Hematocrit and hemoglobin or complete blood count (CBC) first or second postpartum day (Varney et al., 2004)
  - White blood cell count can remain elevated (>15,000 or more) for 48 hours
  - Hematocrit can take 2–5 days to stabilize
- Type and Rh studies of baby's blood
- As indicated for complications
  - Complications of pregnancy
  - Postpartum complications
  - Complications of existing medical condition

Providing Treatment: Therapeutic Measures to Consider

- Laxatives or stool softeners
  - Colace
  - Senokot
  - Milk of magnesia
- Urinary system
  - Encourage frequent voiding
  - Catheterize as needed for urinary retention
  - Insert Foley catheter if unable to void twice
- Heavy lochia and/or uterine atony: Methergine 0.2 mg PO every 4 hours for 6 doses (Botehlo, Emeis, & Brucker, 2011)
- Pain management (see the "Immediate Postpartum Assessment" section)
- Sleep (King, Johnson, & Gamblian, 2011; Mayo Clinic, 2009)

- Use sleep medications with caution in nursing mothers
- Nonbenzodiazepines
  - Zolpidem (Ambien): 5–10 mg at bedtime
  - Eszopiclone (Lunesta): 2–3 mg at bedtime
  - Zaleplon (Sonata): 10 mg at bedtime
- Benzodiazepines
  - Dalmane: 15–30 mg at bedtime
  - Halcion: 0.125–0.25 mg at bedtime
- Immune status (Rhode, 2011)
  - Rh immune globulin: 300 mcg IM
  - Rubella vaccine: Single SQ dose
    - Delay pregnancy for 28 days
  - When giving Rh immune globulin and rubella concurrently, give in separate sites and retest rubella titers at 3 months postpartum
- Antidepressants for at-risk women (see "Care of the Mother: Perinatal Mood Disorders")

Providing Treatment: Complementary and Alternative Measures to Consider

- Home visit(s)
- Bowel care
  - Encourage fiber and fluids
  - Whole grains
  - Flax seed meal, 1–2 Tbs daily
  - Prune juice
  - Dried fruits
- Perineal care (Rhode, 2011)
  - Compresses
  - Epsom salts
  - Witch hazel compresses
  - Comfrey compresses
  - Homeopathic arnica montana PO
  - Sitz baths—plain or herbal
- Urinary care
  - Encourage frequent voiding
  - Urinary retention
  - Oil of peppermint drops in toilet
- Sleep
  - Encourage frequent rest periods
  - Lemon balm tea (University of Maryland, 2011)
  - Chamomile tea

Providing Support: Education and Support Measures to Consider

- Active listening and queries regarding the following topics:
  - Birth experience
  - Maternal and family response to the infant
  - Infant feeding and care
  - Maternal feelings and adaptation
- Provide information
  - Continued care of the infant
  - Return to fertility
  - Contraception options, as needed
  - Medication instructions
  - Vitamin and mineral supplements
  - Other medications as indicated
  - When and how to schedule follow-up care
  - Planned postpartum visit(s)
  - Signs and symptoms of postpartum complications
  - When and how to access the midwife

Follow-up Care: Follow-up Measures to Consider

Ideal maternity care after birth includes ample in-home help and support, in addition to frequent midwife visits in the early postpartum period.

- One- to two-week recheck
  - New mothers
  - Complicated prenatal or postpartum course
  - Incision check post-cesarean section or post-tubal ligation
  - Involution
  - Initiate hormonal contraceptives
- Four- to six-week postpartum examination
  - Involution
  - Lactation
  - Perineum
  - Bowel and bladder function
  - Sleep patterns
  - Family adaptation
  - Postpartum depression screening (see "Care of the Mother: Perinatal Mood Disorders")
  - Concerns and questions

- Eight weeks, as indicated for the following:
  - Intrauterine device (IUD) insertion
  - Diaphragm or cervical cap fitting
- Document all care provided

Multidisciplinary Practice: Consider Consultation, Collaboration, or Referral

- OB/GYN service: As needed for signs of maternal complications
  - Hematoma
  - Endometritis or wound infection
  - Persistent subinvolution of the uterus
  - Thrombophlebitis
  - Pulmonary embolism
- Social services
  - Women, Infant, and Children (WIC) program
  - Aid to Families with Dependent Children (AFDC) program
  - Support groups
- For diagnosis or treatment outside the midwife's scope of practice

CARE OF THE MOTHER: ASSESSMENT POSTPARTUM, WEEKS 2–6

Key Clinical Information

Most women settle into the changes in routines brought about by the birth of their baby without much difficulty. Late postpartum maternal evaluation is directed toward determining the presence of any emerging complications or concerns, addressing needs for birth control information or supplies, and following up on any health issues that were identified or modified during the pregnancy. The midwife tailors information about child spacing, pregnancy prevention methods, infant care, and resources to the woman's cultural background, level of understanding, economic resources, and stated needs.

Some women feel isolated or insecure in the initial weeks after the birth of their baby. The empathetic midwife is able to enhance maternal adaptation by providing care that is culturally acceptable and that fosters social support in the mother's home community. Guidance and support during this time of transition can positively influence maternal self-care and the care the mother provides to her infant by providing a nurturing environment where development of a healthy maternal self-image and feelings of competence and confidence as a woman and mother can result.

Women who have difficulty with postpartum adjustment can benefit from referrals to local resources, such as postpartum or mother's support groups, parenting groups or classes, breastfeeding groups, play groups, counseling, and other support services. Feelings of isolation are not uncommon, and many women need to be given support or actively directed to participate in activities other than newborn care.

Client History and Chart Review: Components of the History to Consider

- Review
  - Labor and birth events and outcomes
  - Initial postpartum course
  - Gynecologic history
  - Medical/surgical history
  - Social history
- Physical return to nonpregnant status (Katz, 2007; Varney et al., 2004)
  - Amount, color, and consistency of lochia
  - Breasts, status of lactation
  - Perineal or abdominal discomfort
  - Bladder and bowel function
  - Physical activity and sleep patterns
  - Resumption of sexual activity
  - Preference for contraception, as indicated
  - Signs or symptoms of delayed involution or medical problems
- Emotional adaptation
  - Cultural practices used during the postpartum period
  - Adjustment to parenting
    - Satisfaction with parenting and sexuality
    - Interactions and support of family and significant others
    - Signs or symptoms of depression or maladaptation

- Infant care
  - Interactions with infant
  - Infant growth and feeding
  - Access to pediatric care
- Review of systems

Physical Examination: Components of the Physical Exam to Consider

- Examination components vary based on the following factors:
  - Timing of visit
  - Indication for visit
  - Client history
- Vital signs, including temperature and weight change since birth
- Thyroid
- Thorax
  - Breast examination
    - Lactation
    - Nipple integrity
    - Masses
    - Axilla
  - Heart
  - Lungs
  - Costovertebral angle tenderness
- Abdominal examination
  - Diastasis recti
  - Muscle tone
  - Cesarean section or tubal ligation incision
- Pelvic examination
  - External genitalia
    - Perineal status
    - Vulvar varicosities
  - Speculum examination
    - Appearance of cervix
    - Specimen collection
  - Bimanual examination
    - Uterine involution
    - Vaginal muscle tone
    - Presence of cystocele or rectocele
  - Rectal examination
- Extremities
  - Edema

- Varicosities
- Phlebitis
- Reflexes

Clinical Impression: Differential Diagnoses to Consider

(ICD9data.com, 2012)

- Normal postpartum course
- Postpartum complications
  - Endometritis
  - Venous complications (i.e., phlebitis)
  - Postpartum fever
  - Mastitis
  - Breastfeeding difficulties
  - Postpartum depression
  - Postpartum adaptation problems
  - Unspecified complications of the puerperium

Diagnostic Testing: Diagnostic Tests and Procedures to Consider

- Sexually transmitted infection testing as indicated by history
- Follow-up testing
  - Pap smear as needed
  - Anemia: Hematocrit and hemoglobin, CBC
  - Gestational diabetes: Fasting blood sugar
  - Postpartum mood disorder: Thyroid testing—thyroid-stimulating hormone (TSH)
- Other laboratory testing as indicated by history

Providing Treatment: Therapeutic Measures to Consider

- Initiation of birth control, as desired (see "Care of the Well Woman Across the Life Span")
  - Natural family planning
  - Nonprescription methods
  - Prescription methods
- Postpartum depression screening
- Vitamin and mineral supplementation (Rhode, 2011)
  - Iron ($FeSO_4$) replacement
  - Calcium
  - Multivitamin

Providing Treatment: Complementary and Alternative Measures to Consider

Provide nutritional support to promote healing and foster well-being:

- Increased fluid and fiber to stimulate regular bowel function
- Well-balanced diet: Adequate protein, vitamins, and minerals

Providing Support: Education and Support Measures to Consider

- Encourage social support
  - Assistance and caring from family and friends
  - Resources in the area for specific needs
    - Play or support groups for new mothers
    - Mothers of twins
    - La Leche League
    - Parenting classes
    - Teen parent groups
- Home or office visit for support and education
  - Infant care and feeding
  - Initiation of physical activity
  - Warning signs or symptoms
  - Recommended diet
  - Anticipated weight changes postpartum
  - Potential decrease in libido and natural lubrication
    - Postpartum
    - With breastfeeding
  - Birth control options

Follow-up Care: Follow-up Measures to Consider

- Validate maternal understanding of recommendations
- Document all care provided, including phone triage
- Make a return visit in 12 months or as indicated by visit
  - Annual gynecologic examination and/or birth control
  - Problem evaluation or follow-up
  - Prenatal care
- Call with questions or concerns

Multidisciplinary Practice: Consider Consultation, Collaboration, or Referral

- Mental health provider
  - Significant postpartum depression
  - Poor maternal adaptation
- OB/GYN service: For poor wound healing or persistent infection
- Medical service: For follow-up of medical problems
  - Diagnosis of diabetes or glucose intolerance
  - Essential hypertension
  - Thyroid disorder
- Social services
  - WIC/AFDC
  - Housing
  - Drug rehabilitation
  - Child welfare
- For diagnosis or treatment outside the midwife's scope of practice

CARE OF THE MOTHER: MASTITIS

Key Clinical Information

Lactation mastitis primarily occurs during the early weeks postpartum but can also occur during long-term breastfeeding (after six months); this condition affects nearly 27% of breastfeeding women. Early identification and prompt treatment at the first signs can preclude the need for antibiotic therapy. Untreated mastitis can result in inadequate milk production, abscess formation, recurrent mastitis, or systemic infection (Riordan & Wambach, 2010). Educating breastfeeding women about presenting signs and symptoms of mastitis, preventive measures, when and how to contact their midwife for evaluation, and treatment options, is an essential part of midwifery practice.

Client History and Chart Review: Components of the History to Consider

- Presence of conditions that can affect immune status
  - Chronic illness
  - Stress and fatigue

- HIV risk assessment
- Breastfeeding history
  - Duration of breastfeeding
  - Infant feeding style
  - Recent changes to nursing patterns
  - Usual breast care
- Previous history of breast problems
  - Mastitis
  - Abscess
  - Breast biopsies
  - Breast reduction or implants
- Presence of risk factors for mastitis (Riordan & Wambach, 2010)
  - Breast trauma
  - Plugged or blocked duct
  - Milk stasis
  - Ineffective breast emptying
  - Engorgement
  - Nipple cracks or fissures
  - Nipple pain
  - Fatigue
  - Stress
  - Previous mastitis
  - Inadequate nutrition
  - Immune factors
  - Pressure on breasts from bra or positioning
  - Manual pump
  - Vigorous upper-body exercise
- Onset, duration, and severity of symptoms (Riordan & Wambach, 2010)
  - Breast symptoms
    - Localized tender/painful breast(s), which worsens when nursing
    - Hot, reddened, tender area of breast
    - Swelling or induration of breast
    - Nipple pain
  - Generalized symptoms
    - Fever and/or chills
    - Malaise or flulike symptoms (muscular aches)
    - Headache
    - Nausea
    - Fatigue

- Self-help measures used and effectiveness
- Review of systems

Physical Examination: Components of the Physical Exam to Consider

- Vital signs, especially temperature, pulse, and pain rating
- General appearance and well-being
- Breast examination
  - Engorgement
  - Tenderness, redness, swelling
  - Induration
  - Warmth—generalized or local
  - Cracks or fissures in nipples
  - Masses
    - Firm or soft
    - Fixed or mobile
    - Tender or nontender
- Axillary examination
  - Engorgement
  - Lymph nodes
- Additional components as indicated by history and physical examination

Clinical Impression: Differential Diagnoses to Consider

(ICD9data.com, 2012)

- Mastitis, acute, postpartum nonpurulent
- Mastitis, acute, postpartum purulent
- Breast abscess
- Breast malignancy

Diagnostic Testing: Diagnostic Tests and Procedures to Consider

- CBC
- Breast ultrasound for mass
  - Abscess suspected
  - Differentiate solid versus cystic mass
- Culture of breastmilk for pathogen
  - Unresponsive to therapy
  - Systemic involvement
- Mammograms are rarely performed during lactation

Providing Treatment: Therapeutic Measures to Consider

- Rest, increased fluids, moist heat, and bed rest
- Fever and pain reducers
  - Ibuprofen
  - Acetaminophen
- Antibiotic therapy for infection, usually for 10–14 days (Rhode, 2011)
  - Dicloxacillin: 125–250 mg IM or PO q6h
  - Cloxacillin: 250–500 mg PO q6h
  - Keflex: 250–500 mg PO q6h
  - Augmentin: 875 mg BID
  - Erythromycin for 10 days
    - ERYC: 250 mg PO q6h
    - Ery-Tab: 333 mg q8h or 500 mg q12h
    - Erythromycin ethylsuccinate: 1.6 g/day in two, three, or four evenly divided doses

Providing Treatment: Complementary and Alternative Measures to Consider

(Romm, 2010)

- Adequate rest, hydration, and nutrition
- Rest with the infant at the breast
- For rest:
  - Chamomile tea
  - Hops infusion
  - Lemon balm infusion
- For fever, infusion of the following herbs:
  - Echinacea
  - Yarrow
  - Peppermint
- To diminish infection:
  - Black walnut
  - Sage
  - Oregano
  - Garlic, fresh uncooked
- Comfrey compresses to affected area

Providing Support: Education and Support Measures to Consider

- Teach careful hand washing and breast care
  - Warm compresses to affected area

- Gentle massage toward nipple
- Frequent nursing and/or pumping
- Vary the infant's suckling positions
  - Cradle
  - Side-lying
  - Football
  - Belly to belly
- Increase fluid intake
- Rest, rest, rest
- Obtain assistance with the following tasks:
  - Housekeeping
  - Child care
  - Promoting rest
- Provide medication instructions
  - Take as directed until medication is gone
  - The infant may develop diarrhea or gastrointestinal upset
  - Continue to nurse unless contraindicated
    - Based on the medication used
    - Because of significant side effects in the infant
    - Because of serious illness of the mother
  - Pumping is an option, but is not as effective as nursing
- Instructions to call or return for care
  - Fever > 100.4°F
  - Chills
  - Worsening symptoms

Follow-up Care: Follow-up Measures to Consider

- Document findings and recommendations
- Reassess within 24 hours
  - To confirm the effectiveness of therapy
  - For evaluation if there is no improvement
  - ⚠ If no improvement occurs, treat the mother empirically for methicillin-resistant *Staphylococcus aureus* (MRSA) infection pending culture results
- Consider hospitalization
  - Persistent fever
  - Systemic symptoms
  - IV antibiotic therapy indicated

Multidisciplinary Practice: Consider Consultation, Collaboration, or Referral

- OB/GYN service
  - For mastitis unresponsive to therapy
  - For breast abscess
- Lactation consultant
  - Mastitis prevention instruction
  - Breast care and feeding during illness
  - Infant positioning
  - Massage techniques
  - Recommendations and support
  - Assistance with supplements if needed
- Social services
  - Home help
  - Visiting nurse
  - Other support services
- Pediatric service: As indicated by infant response to medication
- For diagnosis or treatment outside the midwife's scope of practice

CARE OF THE MOTHER: PERINATAL MOOD AND ANXIETY DISORDERS

Key Clinical Information

Comprehensive midwifery care includes screening each woman for pregnancy-related mood and anxiety disorders. Untreated maternal mood and anxiety disorders have been demonstrated as risk factors for preterm birth and low-birth-weight infants. Perinatal mood and anxiety disorders have also been associated with adverse effects on the infant's cognitive development, as well as behavioral and mental health concerns during childhood (Hackley, 2010; Karsnitz & Ward, 2011). The risks and benefits of medical treatment during pregnancy and breastfeeding must be weighed against the long-term effects on both mother and baby. The midwife is responsible for the screening and identification—with appropriate consultation or referral for diagnosis and treatment—of women with perinatal mood and anxiety disorders during and after pregnancy.

Screening every woman for pregnancy-related mood and anxiety disorders facilitates early identification and treatment of women who require more than simple support to cope with the emotional changes that can occur during pregnancy and after the birth of the infant. Perinatal mood disorders can range from a mild case of "the blues" to significant depression, or postpartum psychosis. Postpartum depression can occur as long as 12 months after giving birth. Perinatal anxiety disorders include generalized anxiety disorder, panic disorder, obsessive–compulsive disorder, and post-traumatic stress disorder (PTSD). Some women feel traumatized by the birth experience and acquire acute stress disorder. Without treatment, over time this condition can develop into PTSD.

Many women may be reluctant to divulge negative feelings about themselves or their baby. Creating a supportive, nonjudgmental environment fosters the trust that many women need to talk about their feelings. Postpartum depression affects 10% to 15% of women who give birth, with as many as 50% to 80% of women experiencing the "postpartum blues" (Hackley, 2010; National Institutes of Health, 2005). Some symptoms of postpartum depression occur in nearly 50% of adolescent women who give birth and are more common in women with history of mood or anxiety disorders (Karsnitz & Ward, 2011; Logsdon & Myers, 2010).

Client History and Chart Review: Components of the History to Consider

(Fernandez, 2005; Hackley, Sharma, Kedzior, & Sreenivasan, 2010; Karsnitz & Ward, 2011)

- Age, GP, TPAL
- Pregnancy, birth, and postpartum history
  - Planned or unintended pregnancy
  - Personal and family response to pregnancy
  - Complications of pregnancy
  - Labor and birth events
  - Perception of birth experience
  - Perception of postpartum period
  - Infant's age
  - Method of infant feeding
  - Sleep patterns and amounts
  - Hormone use

- Social history
  - Absence of support systems
  - Sexual abuse
  - Family discord
  - Socioeconomic stressors
- Risk factors for postpartum mood disorder
  - History of mental health disorder
  - Depression or anxiety during pregnancy
  - Complications of pregnancy
    - Late-onset or erratic prenatal visits
    - History of infertility
    - Miscarriage
    - Perinatal loss
    - Multiple gestation
    - Hyperemesis
  - Social factors
    - Adolescents and single women
    - Social stigma, conflict, or lack of support
    - Poor socioeconomic status
    - Major life events unrelated to pregnancy
- Onset and type of symptoms
  - Postpartum blues
    - Moodiness
    - Tearfulness
    - Elation
    - Heightened reactivity
    - Onset within 3–5 days after birth
    - Occurs across all cultures
    - Transient and self-limiting
    - Resolves in 7–14 days
    - 20% of women with blues progress to depression
  - Adjustment disorder (symptoms present > 2 wks)
    - Greater difficulty with adjustment than normal
    - Decreased coping ability
  - Depression (symptoms present > 2 wks) (Hackley et al., 2010)
    - Agitation
    - Anxiety
    - Sadness
    - Fatigue

- ◆ Sleep disturbances
- ◆ Diminished interest or pleasure
- ◆ Feelings of worthlessness and guilt
- ◆ Feelings of detachment from infant
- ◆ Thoughts of harming infant
- ◆ Suicidal ideation
- ◆ Perinatal up to 12 months postpartum
- ◆ Appetite changes
- ◆ Irritability/mood changes
- ◆ Somatic symptoms or concerns
- ▪ Anxiety (present > 6 months) (Karsnitz & Ward, 2011)
  - ◆ Fatigue
  - ◆ Insomnia
  - ◆ Irritability
  - ◆ Restlessness
  - ◆ Inability to concentrate
  - ◆ Muscular tension
  - ◆ Sleep disturbances
- ▪ Post-traumatic stress disorder (symptoms present > 1 mo.) (Karsnitz & Ward, 2011)
  - ◆ Hyperarousal
  - ◆ Sleep disturbances
  - ◆ Disturbing intrusive thoughts
  - ◆ Vivid and stressful dreams
  - ◆ Feelings of reliving the event
  - ◆ Mania
  - ◆ Euphoria
  - ◆ Decreased need for sleep
  - ◆ Racing thoughts
  - ◆ Distractibility
  - ◆ Can convert into depression or psychosis
- ▪ Psychosis
  - ◆ Medical emergency
  - ◆ Disorganized thinking, behavior, or speech
  - ◆ Perceptual disturbances (auditory or visual)
  - ◆ Delusions
- Assessment
  - ▪ Stressors
  - ▪ Social and economic resources
  - ▪ Sleep–wake patterns
  - ▪ Potential for harming self, infant, or others
- Review of systems (ROS)

Physical Examination: Components of the Physical Exam to Consider

- Vital signs, including temperature and weight
- Signs or symptoms of the following conditions:
  - ▪ Postpartum thyroidosis
  - ▪ Anemia
  - ▪ Infection
- Evaluate for evidence of the following:
  - ▪ Significant weight change
  - ▪ Sleep deprivation
  - ▪ Changes in personal appearance
  - ▪ Peripartum mood disorder
  - ▪ Altered affect
  - ▪ Physical or emotional abuse
  - ▪ Self-neglect

Clinical Impression: Differential Diagnoses to Consider

(ICD9data.com, 2012)

- Perinatal mood disorder
  - ▪ Postpartum blues
  - ▪ Adjustment disorder
  - ▪ Depression
  - ▪ Mania in the postpartum period
  - ▪ Psychosis in the postpartum period
  - ▪ Postpartum codes are applicable within 4 weeks of delivery
- Preexisting mood disorder exacerbated by birth
- Severe sleep deprivation
- Medical illness, such as thyroid disorders

Diagnostic Testing: Diagnostic Tests and Procedures to Consider

(Fernandez, 2005)

- Thyroid profile
- Urinalysis
- CBC with differential
- Comprehensive metabolic panel
- Edinburgh Postnatal Depression Scale
- Postpartum Depression Screening Scale (Beck & Gable, 2000)

Providing Treatment Therapeutic Measures to Consider

(Hackley, 2010; Hackley et al., 2010; Karsnitz & Ward, 2011)

- Referral for diagnosis and treatment may be the best option
- Interpersonal psychotherapy
  - May avoid need for medication
  - Addresses relationships
  - Provides techniques to decrease symptoms
- Antidepressant therapy for mood and anxiety disorders (Hackley, 2010; Karsnitz & Ward, 2011; King et al., 2011) (See "Care of the Woman with Affective Disorders")
  - Medication choice based on the following considerations:
    - Symptom type and severity
    - Method of infant feeding
  - Selective serotonin reuptake inhibitors (SSRIs)
  - Serotonin norepinephrine reuptake inhibitors (SNRIs)
  - Tricyclic antidepressants (TCAs)
  - Late-pregnancy administration for high-risk women
  - Reach therapeutic levels before delivery
  - May result in neonatal behavioral syndrome (Fernandez, 2005)
- Estrogen therapy (National Institutes of Mental Health, 2010)
  - Use for mild to moderate symptoms with early onset
  - Transdermal estradiol 0.1–0.2 mg daily
  - Use 3–6 months if improvement is noted
- Combination hormonal contraceptives may either improve or exacerbate depression

Providing Treatment: Complementary and Alternative Measures to Consider

Alternative therapies should not be a substitute for supervised psychiatric care for the woman who threatens, or appears at risk, to harm herself or her family.

- Omega-3 polyunsaturated fatty acids (King et al., 2011)
- Herbal remedies for depression (Hendrick, 2003; King et al., 2011)
  - St. John's wort: 300 mg TID (but may decrease effectiveness of hormonal contraceptives)
  - Lemon balm tea: 2–3 cups daily
  - Valerian root: 1–3 capsules daily
- Complementary remedies for anxiety (Karsnitz & Ward, 2011)
  - Omega-3 polyunsaturated fatty acids (see "A Nutritional Primer")
  - 5HTP (tryptophan): 8–12 g/day in divided doses
  - Inositol (vitamin B_8): 12–18 g/day
- Light therapy (Hendrick, 2003)
- Home visits by midwife, doula, or nurse (Gjerdingen, 2003)
- Culturally appropriate treatments
- Adequate nutrition
  - Wholesome foods
  - Adequate fluids and fiber
  - Avoid caffeine, alcohol, and cigarettes
- Time scheduled for the following:
  - Sleep
  - Personal care
  - Daily walking or activity
  - Personal time away from the infant
  - Favorite activities
  - Intimate time with the partner
  - Nurturing relationships

Providing Support: Education and Support Measures to Consider

(Fernandez, 2005)

- Shared decision making related to therapies
- Prenatal education
  - Normalcy of feelings associated with postpartum blues

- Signs and symptoms of postpartum mood and anxiety disorders
- Screening process at postpartum visit
- Local resources
  - Self-help or maternal support groups
  - Breastfeeding education and support
  - Parenting organizations
  - Crisis hotline number
  - Mental health professionals
- Postpartum education
  - Review resources
  - Mobilize family support
  - Rest with infant
  - Avoid isolation
  - Maintain nutrition
  - Recognize signs and symptoms of postpartum depression
  - How to access help and support
  - Skills training
  - Family interventions

Follow-up Care: Follow-up Measures to Consider

- Document
  - Screening results
  - Mental health referral
  - Midwife follow-up plan and actions
  - Update plan as condition changes
- Follow-up visits
  - Telephone contact within 24–48 hours
  - Weekly visits (home or office) while acute
  - As needed for adjustment of medication
  - Ensure 24-hour access to care
- During ongoing care, assess the following (Fernandez, 2005):
  - Maternal–child interaction and relationship
  - ⚠ Risk of harm to self or others
  - Infant development
  - Partner relationship
  - With delayed recovery, explore the mother's history for sexual or other forms of abuse, neglect, or trauma

Multidisciplinary Practice: Consider Consultation, Collaboration, or Referral

- Mental health or psychiatric services
  - Psychotherapy or counseling
  - Pharmacologic treatment as indicated by client need and the scope of the midwife's practice
  - Clients who do not respond to midwife-initiated therapy as appropriate for medication
  - 📞 Psychiatric emergency
  - Presence of psychotic symptoms
  - Clients who are suicidal or threaten harm to others
  - Clients or infants who are perceived to be at risk for harm
  - Mother's rejection of or physical aggression (threatened or actual) against the infant
- Support services
  - Lactation consultant
  - Postpartum doula
- Social services
  - Housing
  - Food
  - Finances
  - Child care
- Medical services: For a suspected or confirmed medical condition
- For diagnosis or treatment outside the midwife's scope of practice

CARE OF THE MOTHER: POSTPARTUM ENDOMETRITIS

Key Clinical Information

Postpartum endometritis is a polymicrobial disorder in which bacteria, such as *Streptococcus, Staphylococcus, Ureaplasma,* and *Escherichia coli,* ascend from the lower genital tract and infect the uterus. Postpartum endometritis can occur after either cesarean delivery (3–10% incidence) or vaginal birth (1–3% incidence) (Simmons & Bammel, 2005). The incidence of post-cesarean endometritis is related to the number and types of risk factors present and the use of intraoperative antibiotic prophylaxis (Tharpe, 2008).

Postpartum endometritis can present as early as 48 hours postpartum or up to 6 weeks after the birth (Rhode, 2011). Diagnosis is based primarily on clinical findings, as the physiologic elevation of the white blood cell count that occurs during labor typically persists into the postpartum period. Endometritis should be suspected in the presence of postpartum fever, defined as two temperature elevations to 38°C (100.4°F) or greater on any two days more than 24 hours after and within 10 days after delivery (Tharpe, 2008; Varney et al., 2004).

Client History and Chart Review: Components of the History to Consider

- Duration of postpartum status
- Presence, onset, duration, and severity of symptoms
  - Fever and chills
  - Malaise
  - Uterine pain
  - Foul odor to lochia
  - Change in amount of lochia flow
- General well-being
  - Appetite
  - Urinary function
  - Respiratory function
  - Other associated symptoms
- ▽ Risk factors for postpartum endometritis (Simmons & Bammel, 2005; Tharpe, 2008)
  - Cesarean delivery
  - Manual removal of the placenta
  - Prolonged rupture of membranes
  - Long labor
  - Multiple vaginal examinations
  - Extremes of patient age
  - Prolonged internal fetal monitoring
  - Anemia
  - Poor nutrition
- Medical/surgical history
  - Appendicitis
  - Diverticular disease
  - Immunocompromised condition
- Review of systems

Physical Examination: Components of the Physical Exam to Consider

(Tharpe, 2008)

- Vital signs: Blood pressure, temperature, pulse, respirations, and pain rating
- Cardiopulmonary system
  - Tachycardia
  - Pallor
  - Breath sounds
  - Rales
  - Respiratory effort
- Breast examination
  - Redness
  - Mass
  - Pain
- Abdominopelvic and thoracic examination
  - Uterine size
  - Tenderness with uterine palpation
  - Guarding
  - Rebound tenderness
  - Masses
  - Costovertebral angle tenderness
- Incision or laceration examination
  - Exudate
  - Redness
  - Swelling
  - Masses
- Evaluation of lochia
  - Odor
  - Volume
- Extremities
  - Edema
  - Homans' sign
  - Femoral and pedal pulses

Clinical Impression: Differential Diagnoses to Consider

(ICD9data.com, 2012)

- Genital tract
  - Postpartum endometritis
  - Wound infection
  - Surgical incision

- Episiotomy
- Laceration
- Pelvic or vaginal hematoma
- Retained placental parts
- Breast infection
- Urinary tract
  - Infection
  - Renal calculi
- Cardiopulmonary system
  - Respiratory infection
  - Deep vein thrombosis
  - Pulmonary embolus
- Appendicitis

Diagnostic Testing: Diagnostic Tests and Procedures to Consider

(Tharpe, 2008)

- CBC with differential
- Urinalysis
- O$_2$ saturation
- Cultures as indicated
  - Urine
  - Blood
  - Wound
- Radiology studies as indicated
  - Chest x-ray
  - Ultrasound or computed tomography (CT)
  - Pelvic
  - Hematoma
  - Retained placental fragments
  - Abdominal
  - Appendix
  - Kidney, ureter, and bladder (KUB)
  - Extremities

Providing Treatment: Therapeutic Measures to Consider

- Antimicrobial therapy (Rhode, 2011; Simmons & Bammel, 2005; Tharpe, 2008)
  - IV antibiotic therapy is indicated for serious infection
  - Cefotetan: 1–2 g IV every 12 hours

- Gentamycin: 1.5 mg/kg load, then 1 mg/kg every 8 hours, plus clindamycin 900 mg IV every 8 hours
  - Ampicillin/sulbactam: 3 g IV every 4–6 hours
  - Mezlocillin: 4 g IV every 4–6 hours
  - Ticarcillin/clavulanate: 3.1 g IV every 6 hours
- Hydration
  - Oral fluids
  - IV therapy
- Prevention of deep vein thrombosis
  - Antiembolitic stockings
  - Isometric exercises

Providing Treatment: Complementary and Alternative Measures to Consider

- ⚠ Alternative remedies are not a substitute for prompt medical care
  - Inadequately treated local infection can become systemic
  - Systemic infection can rapidly lead to death
- Rescue remedy to pulse points
- Hot pack to abdomen
- Herbal support
  - Black walnut tincture
  - Sage tea
  - Oregano tea
  - Echinacea tea or tincture
- Homeopathic arnica montana

Providing Support: Education and Support Measures to Consider

- Supportive measures
  - Rest
  - Adequate nutrition
  - Provision for infant care
  - Provide emotional support
  - Listening
  - Updated information as the situation demands
- Discussion with the client and family
  - Working diagnosis
  - Urgency of condition
  - Need for diagnostic testing

- Potential need for
- Medical evaluation
- Hospitalization
- IV antibiotic treatment
- Compatibility of medications with breastfeeding, as needed

Follow-up Care: Follow-up Measures to Consider

- Anticipate response to medication within 48 hours
- ☏ If minimal or no response occurs, evaluate for potential complications
  - Pelvic abscess
  - Pelvic hematoma
  - Wound infection
  - Septic pelvic thrombophlebitis
- Document
  - Clinical evaluation and working diagnosis
  - Consultation(s) and plan of care
  - Update notes frequently, including the following information:
    - ◆ Changes in client status
    - ◆ Rationale for orders
    - ◆ Consultation or transfer of care requests

Multidisciplinary Practice: Consider Consultation, Collaboration, or Referral

- OB/GYN services
  - Evaluation or treatment of postpartum fever or infection
  - Transfer of care from home or birth center for hospitalization
  - Infection that does not respond to treatment within 24–48 hours
- For diagnosis or treatment outside the midwife's scope of practice

CARE OF THE MOTHER: POSTPARTUM HEMORRHOIDS

Key Clinical Information

Hemorrhoids form as a result of dilatation and engorgement of the arteriovenous plexuses of the anal canal.

This condition is often exacerbated during pregnancy, labor, and birth, secondary to direct pressure on the rectal veins. Prompt treatment of hemorrhoids postpartum can prevent thrombosis of external hemorrhoids that have become trapped by the anal sphincter. Thrombosed hemorrhoids are exquisitely painful and can require incision and drainage.

Client History and Chart Review: Components of the History to Consider

- Prior history of hemorrhoids
- Usual diet and bowel function
- Length and positions used during second-stage labor
- Presence of symptoms
  - Itching
  - Aching
  - Severe pain (associated with thrombosis)
- Relief measures used and their effects
- Presence of rectal bleeding

Physical Examination: Components of the Physical Exam to Consider

- Perineal assessment
  - Approximation of repair, if applicable
  - Edema
- Presence of hemorrhoids
  - May be single or circumferential rosette
  - Note the following characteristics:
    - ◆ Size
    - ◆ Location
    - ◆ Edema
    - ◆ Redness
  - Palpate to evaluate for thrombosis
    - ◆ Firm clot felt within vein
    - ◆ Exquisitely painful to touch
- Rectal examination
  - Rectal prolapse
  - Anal fissure, lesions, or mass
  - Undiagnosed third- or fourth-degree laceration

Clinical Impression: Differential Diagnoses to Consider

(ICD9data.com, 2012)

- Hemorrhoids
  - Hemorrhoids, not otherwise specified
  - Hemorrhoids, thrombosed
- Rectovaginal hematoma
- Undiagnosed third- or fourth-degree laceration
- Anal abscess or mass
- Anal fissure

Diagnostic Testing: Diagnostic Tests and Procedures to Consider

- Anoscopy

Providing Treatment: Therapeutic Measures to Consider

- Topical analgesics for discomfort, with or without hydrocortisone (Botehlo et al., 2011; National Library of Medicine, 2006)
  - Pramoxine (Proctofoam/Proctofoam HC/Anusol ointment)
  - Dibucaine (Nupercainal ointment)
  - Benzocaine (Americaine spray or ointment)
- Steroid hemorrhoid preparations for itching
  - Anusol-HC (25 mg hydrocortisone) suppositories
  - Cortifoam (10% hydrocortisone)
  - Proctocort suppositories (30 mg hydrocortisone)
  - May decrease resistance to local infection
- Maintain soft formed stool
  - Stool softeners
    - Colace: 50–200 mg daily
    - Surfak: 240 mg PO daily until normal
  - Laxatives
    - Peri-Colace (softener + stimulant): 1–2 capsules at bedtime
    - Perdiem (fiber + stimulant): 1–2 tsp in 8 oz water at bedtime or in the morning
    - Senokot (senna stimulant): 2 tablets at bedtime

- Fiber supplements
  - Citrucel: 1 Tbs in 8 oz water one to three times daily
  - Metamucil: 1 packet or 1 tsp in 8 oz water one to three times daily
- Glycerin suppositories
- Enemas to avoid straining
  - Fleet enema
  - Soapsuds enema
- Severe hemorrhoids, no thrombosis
  - Manually reduce hemorrhoids as necessary
  - May require rectal packing
    - Provides counterpressure
    - Lubricate with hemorrhoid cream
    - Remove after 12–24 hours
- Thrombosis: May require incision and drainage

Providing Treatment: Complementary and Alternative Measures to Consider

- Topical measures to aid soft tissue healing (Romm, 2010)
  - Sitz baths
  - Warm water
  - Herbal infusions
    - Comfrey
    - Plantain
    - Calendula
  - Ice packs
  - Witch hazel compresses
  - Aloe vera gel
  - Comfrey compresses TID
- Positioning to drain hemorrhoids
  - Hands and knees with head on pillow and hips elevated
  - Back-lying with hips elevated above heart

Providing Support: Education and Support Measures to Consider

- Diet adequate in fluids and fiber
  - Dried fruit
  - Psyllium or flax seed
  - Prune juice

- ▪ Rhubarb
- ▪ Blueberries
- ▪ Whole grains
- ▪ Fresh fruit and vegetables
- • Discussion of treatment options and instructions
  - ▪ Avoidance of the following:
    - ◆ Straining
    - ◆ Prolonged sitting on toilet
    - ◆ Withholding stool
  - ▪ When to call
    - ◆ Bleeding
    - ◆ Increasing pain

Follow-up Care: Follow-up Measures to Consider

- • Reevaluate
  - ▪ 24–48 hours after treatment
  - ▪ Persistent rectal bleeding
  - ▪ Severe pain

- • Document
  - ▪ Examination findings
  - ▪ Recommended treatment plan
  - ▪ Response to treatment

Multidisciplinary Practice: Consider Consultation, Collaboration, or Referral

- • OB/GYN services
  - ▪ Thrombosed hemorrhoids for incision and drainage (I & D)
  - ▪ Suspected third- or fourth-degree laceration
  - ▪ Rectal abscess
  - ▪ Anal fissure
  - ▪ Hematoma
  - ▪ Bleeding
- • For diagnosis or treatment outside the midwife's scope of practice

WEB RESOURCES FOR CLINICIANS

RESOURCE	URL
Ballard gestational scoring	http://www.ballardscore.com/
Searchable drug and lactation database (LactMed)	http://toxnet.nlm.nih.gov/cgi-bin/sis/htmlgen?LACT
Newborn testing	www.babysfirsttest.org, http://www.marchofdimes.com/Baby/bringinghome_screening.html, http://genes-r-us.uthscsa.edu/
Vaccine side effects	http://www.cdc.gov/vaccines/vac-gen/side-effects.htm
Adverse vaccine reaction reporting	http://www.vaers.hhs.gov

REFERENCES

Abou-Dakn, M., Fluhr, J. W., Gensch, M., & Wockel, A. (2011). Positive effect of HPA lanolin versus expressed breastmilk on painful and damaged nipples during lactation. *Skin Pharmacology and Physiology, 24,* 27–35. doi: 10.1159/000318228

American Academy of Family Physicians. (2001/2007). Circumcision: Position paper on neonatal circumcision. Retrieved from http://www.aafp.org/online/en/home/clinical/clinicalrecs/guidelines/Circumcision.html

American Academy of Pediatrics (AAP). (n.d., b) Breastfeeding initiatives. Retrieved from http://www.aap.org/breastfeeding/policyOnBreastfeedingAndUseOfHumanMilk.html

American Academy of Pediatrics (AAP). (1999/2005). Circumcision policy statement. *Pediatrics, 103,* 686–693.

American Academy of Pediatrics (AAP). (2003/2009). Policy statement: Controversies concerning vitamin K and the newborn. *Pediatrics, 112,* 191–192.

American Academy of Pediatrics (AAP) & American Heart Association (AHA). (2011). *Textbook of neonatal resuscitation* (6th ed.). Elk Grove Village, IL: Author.

American College of Medical Genetics. (2000). *Evaluation of the newborn with single or multiple congenital anomalies: A clinical guideline.* Bethesda, MD: Author. Retrieved from http://www.health.state.ny.us/nysdoh/dpprd/exec.htm

American College of Obstetricians and Gynecologists. (2001). Committee opinion no. 260: Circumcision. In 2006 *Compendium of selected publications.* Washington, DC: Author.

Beck, C. T., & Gable, R. K. (2000). Postpartum depression screening scale: Development and psychometric testing. *Nursing Research, 49*(5), 272–282.

Botehlo, N., Emeis, C. L., & Brucker, M. C. (2011). In T. L. King & M. C. Brucker (Eds.), *Pharmacology for women's health* (pp. 629–636). Sudbury, MA: Jones & Bartlett Learning.

Canadian Pediatric Society & College of Family Physicians of Canada. (1997/2004). Joint position statement: Routine administration of vitamin K to newborns. *Paediatrics & Child Health, 2,* 429–431. Retrieved from http://www.cps.ca/ENGLISH/statements/FN/fn97-01.htm

Centers for Disease Control and Prevention (CDC). (2005). A comprehensive immunization strategy to eliminate transmission of hepatitis B virus infection in the United States. *Morbidity and Mortality Weekly Report, 54*(RR16), 1–23. Retrieved from http://www.cdc.gov/MMWR/preview/mmwrhtml/rr5416a1.htm

Centers for Disease Control and Prevention (CDC). (2007). When should a mother avoid breastfeeding? Retrieved from http://www.cdc.gov/breastfeeding/disease/contraindicators.htm

Centers for Disease Control and Prevention (CDC). (2010a). 2010 STD treatment guidelines. Retrieved from http://www.cdc.gov/std/treatment/2010/

Centers for Disease Control and Prevention (CDC). (2010b). Genomics and health. Retrieved from http://www.cdc.gov/genomics/public/index.htm

Centers for Disease Control and Prevention (CDC). (2011a). 2011 child & adolescent immunization schedule. Retrieved from http://www.cdc.gov/vaccines/recs/schedules/child-schedule.htm#printable

Centers for Disease Control and Prevention (CDC). (2011b). Possible side effects from vaccines. Retrieved from http://www.cdc.gov/vaccines/vac-gen/side-effects.htm

Circumcision Information and Resource Pages. (2007). Circumcision: Medical organization official policy statements in Circumcision Reference Library. Retrieved from http://www.cirp.org/library/statements/

Circumcision Information and Resource Pages. (2008). Penile cancer, cervical cancer, and circumcision. Retrieved from http://www.cirp.org/library/disease/cancer/

Coggins, M., & Mercer, J. (2009). Delayed cord clamping offers advantages to infants. *Nursing for Women's Health, 13*(2), 132–139.

College of Physicians and Surgeons of British Columbia. (2007). Circumcision (infant male). In *The physician resource manual.* Retrieved from http://www.cpsbc.ca/cps/physician_resources/publications/resource_manual/malecircum_pf

Fernandez, R. (2005). *Perinatal mood disorders: Psychiatric illnesses during pregnancy and postpartum* [Online video]. Prepared by the Governor's (NJ) Work Group on Postpartum Depression. Retrieved from http://www.vodium.com/MediapodLibrary/index.asp?library=pn100177_fleishman_postpartum&SessionArgs=0U1U0000000100000110

Gjerdingen, D. (2003). The effectiveness of various postpartum depression treatments and the impact of antidepressant drugs on nursing infants. *Journal of the American Board of Family Practice, 16,* 372–382.

Green, M., & Palfrey, J. S. (Eds.). (2002). *Bright futures: Guidelines for health supervision of infants, children, and adolescents* (2nd ed.). Arlington, VA: National Center for Education in Maternal and Child Health.

Hackley, B. (2010). Antidepressant medication use in pregnancy. *Journal of Midwifery & Women's Health, 55*(2), 90–100.

Hackley, B., Sharma, C., Kedzior, A., & Sreenivasan, S. (2010). Managing mental health conditions in primary care settings. *Journal of Midwifery & Women's Health, 55*(1), 9–19.

Hendrick, V. (2003). Alternative treatments for postpartum depression. *Psychiatric Times, 10,* 8. Retrieved from http://www.psychiatrictimes.com/p030850.html

ICD9Data.com. (2012). The Web's free 2012 ICD-9 medical coding data. Retrieved from http://www.icd9data.com/

Karsnitz, D. B., & Ward, S. (2011). Spectrum of anxiety disorders: Diagnosis and pharmacologic treatment. *Journal of Midwifery & Women's Health, 56*(3), 266–281.

Katz, V. L. (2007). Postpartum care. In S. G. Gabbe, J. R. Niebyl, & J. L. Simpson (Eds.), *Obstetrics: Normal and problem pregnancies* (pp. 566–586). Philadelphia, PA: Churchill Livingstone, Elsevier.

Kenner, C., & Lott, J. W. (2007). *Comprehensive neonatal care: An interdisciplinary approach* (4th ed.). Philadelphia, PA: Saunders, Elsevier.

King, T. L., Johnson, R., & Gamblian, V. (2011). Mental health. In T. L. King & M. C. Brucker (Eds.), *Pharmacology for women's health* (pp. 750–791). Sudbury, MA: Jones & Bartlett Learning.

Laurence, R. (1998–2011). Herbs and breastfeeding. Retrieved from http://www.breastfeeding.com/reading_room/herbs.html

Lawrence, R. M., & Lawrence, R. A. (2011). Breastfeeding: More than just good nutrition. *Pediatrics in Review, 32,* 267–280. doi: 10.1542/pir.32-7-267. Retrieved from http://www.ccmcresidents.com/wp-content/uploads/2011/07/Breastfeeding.pdf

Lippi, G., & Franchini, M. (2011). Vitamin K in neonates: Facts and myths. *Blood Transfusion, 9*(1), 4–9.

Logsdon, M. C., & Myers, J. A. (2010). Comparative performance of two depression screening instruments in adolescent mothers. *Journal of Women's Health, 19*(6), 1123–1128.

Lowenstein, V. (2004). Circumcision. In H. Varney, J. M. Kriebs, & C. L. Gegor (Eds.), *Varney's midwifery* (4th ed., pp. 1313–1326). Sudbury, MA: Jones and Bartlett.

Mangesi, L., & Dowswell, T. (2010). Treatments for breast engorgement during lactation. *Cochrane Database of Systematic Reviews, 9,* CD006946. doi: 10.1002/14651858.CD006946.pub2

March of Dimes. (2011). Newborn screening tests. Retrieved from http://www.marchofdimes.com/professionals/bringinghome_screening.html

Mayo Clinic. (2009). Insomnia. Retrieved from http://www.mayoclinic.com/health/sleeping-pills/SL00010

McHugh, M. K. (2004a). Examination of the newborn. In H. Varney, J. M. Kriebs, & C. L. Gegor (Eds.), *Varney's midwifery* (4th ed., pp. 999–1010). Sudbury, MA: Jones and Bartlett.

McHugh, M. K. (2004b). Recognition and immediate care of sick newborns. In H. Varney, J. M. Kriebs, & C. L. Gegor (Eds.), *Varney's midwifery* (4th ed., pp. 1029–1040). Sudbury, MA: Jones and Bartlett.

Mercer, J. S., Erickson-Owens, D. A., Graves, B., & Haley, M. M. (2007). Evidence-based practices for the fetal to newborn transition. *Journal of Midwifery & Women's Health, 52*(3), 262–272.

Mercer, J., & Skovaard, R. (2002). Neonatal transition physiology: A new paradigm. *Journal of Neonatal and Perinatal Nursing, 15,* 56–75.

National Institutes of Health. (2005). Understanding postpartum depression. *News in Health.* Retrieved from http://newsinhealth.nih.gov/2005/December2005/docs/01features_02.htm

National Institutes of Mental Health. (2010). Clinical trial of estrogen for postpartum depression. Retrieved from http://clinicaltrials.gov/ct2/show/NCT00059228

National Library of Medicine (U.S.). (2006). Anesthetics (rectal). *Medline Plus Drug Information.* Thomson Healthcare. Retrieved from http://www.nlm.nih.gov/medlineplus/druginfo/medmaster/a682429.html

National Library of Medicine (U.S.). (2011). LactMed. TOXNET toxicology data network. Retrieved from http://toxnet.nlm.nih.gov/cgi-bin/sis/htmlgen?LACT

Rhode, M. A. (2011). Postpartum. In T. L. King & M. C. Brucker (Eds.), *Pharmacology for Women's Health* (pp. 1117–1145). Sudbury, MA: Jones & Bartlett Learning.

Riordan, J., & Wambach, K. (2010). Breast-related problems. In J. Riordan & K. Wambach (Eds.), *Breastfeeding and human lactation* (4th ed., pp. 291–324). Sudbury, MA: Jones and Bartlett.

Romm, A. (2010). *Botanical medicine for women's health.* St. Louis, MO: Churchill Livingstone.

Simmons, G. T., & Bammel, B. M. (2005). Endometritis. *E-medicine.* Retrieved from http://www.emedicine.com/MED/topic676.htm

Sinclair, C. (2004). *A midwife's handbook.* St. Louis, MO: Saunders.

Singh, M., Sugathan, P. S., & Bhujwala, R. A. (1982). Human colostrum for prophylaxis against sticky eyes and conjunctivitis in the newborn. *Journal of Tropical Pediatrics, 28,* 35–37.

Singh-Grewal, D., Macdessi, J., & Craig, J. (2005). Circumcision for the prevention of urinary tract infection in boys: A systematic review of randomized trials and observational studies. *Archives of Disease in Childhood, 90,* 853–858. doi: 10.1136/adc.2004.049353

Spencer, J. P. (2008). Management of mastitis in breastfeeding women. *American Family Physician, 78*(6), 727–732.

Straus, C. (2003). Herbal and dietary supplements: Be aware of dangers. Retrieved from http://www2.bluecrossca.com/pdf/Health_Articles/herbal%20and%20dietary%20supplements.pdf

Strehle, E. M., Howey, C., & Jones, R. (2010). Evaluation of the acceptability of a new oral vitamin K prophylaxis for breast fed infants. *Acta Paediatrica, 99*(3), 379–383.

Tappero, E., & Honeyfield, M. (2009). *Physical assessment of the newborn: A comprehensive approach to the art of physical assessment* (4th ed.). Santa Rosa: NICU Ink Book Publishers.

Tharpe, N. (2008). Postpregnancy genital tract and wound infections. *Journal of Midwifery & Women's Health, 53*(3), 236–246.

Tobian, A. A. R., Gray, R. H., & Quinn, T. C. (2010). Male circumcision for the prevention of acquisition and transmission of sexually transmitted infections: The case for neonatal circumcision. *Archives of Pediatrics & Adolescent Medicine, 164*(1), 78–84. doi: 10.1001/archpediatrics.2009.232

U.S. Department of Health and Human Services. (2011). The Surgeon General's call to action to support breast-feeding. Retrieved from http://www.surgeongeneral.gov/topics/breastfeeding/factsheet.html

University of Maryland. (2011). Complementary medicine: Lemon balm. Retrieved from http://www.umm.edu/altmed/articles/lemon-balm-000261.htm

University of Texas Health Science Center at San Antonio. (2011). National newborn screening status report. Retrieved from http://genes-r-us.uthscsa.edu/nbsdisorders.pdf

Varney, H., Kriebs, J. M., & Gegor, C. L. (2004). *Varney's midwifery* (4th ed.). Sudbury, MA: Jones and Bartlett.

Walker, M. (2006). *Breastfeeding management for the clinician: Using the evidence*. Sudbury, MA: Jones and Bartlett.

Care of the Well Woman Across the Life Span

Well-woman midwifery care aims to enhance women's health and wellness across the life span, and in the presence of the myriad social and health challenges that many women face.

PREVENTIVE HEALTH CARE FOR WELL WOMEN

Midwives are specialists in primary health care for women. They can cultivate each woman's ability to care for herself by providing women's health care in an environment of support and understanding. Women may look to the midwife for care that includes reproductive health screening and assessment; sports-, college-, or employment-related evaluations; diagnostic testing; family planning services; fertility awareness or infertility issues; care of chronic conditions; and general health maintenance. For many women, the annual reproductive health examination is their only preventive health visit. This possibility necessitates that the midwife be diligent in assessing all body systems, rather than focusing exclusively on reproductive health care.

Some midwives provide well-woman care from menarche through a woman's mature adulthood. Caring for women as they age requires knowledge and understanding of the many changes that occur during the aging process and the effects those changes may have on each woman's life. The changes as women age cannot be quantified simply based on where an individual is on the chart of reproductive life stages but must also take into account how she sees herself and how the challenges of aging affect her.

Adolescence begins with puberty and continues for 8 to 10 years. Chronologically, this phase of development is generally considered to span from ages 11 to 18. Young women may struggle with issues of identity and relationships during this time, as well as a changing body. Adolescence is a time when young women begin to develop judgment and maturity, and strive for independence. The adolescent years are frequently marked by experimentation, including alcohol or drug use, challenging social norms, decorating the body with piercings or tattoos, and a range of health behaviors that can have positive or negative outcomes. Allowing time to build trust with an adolescent woman can be instrumental in facilitating a positive early experience with the healthcare system.

Early and midlife adulthood mark the childbearing and childrearing phases of life for most women. Voluntary childlessness and infertility are important issues that affect life focus and goals of a subset of women. Women in this phase of life may deal with occupational and economic concerns, navigate intimacy versus isolation in relationships, and develop a sense of purpose and contribution to the wider world.

During the perimenopausal period, women may simultaneously have families that include young children, adolescent or adult children, grandchildren, and aging parents. The dream of retirement or financial security may recede with the demands of providing care for aged parents or a diminished ability to work. Health problems may become more prevalent and use up a significant proportion of energy that was previously directed to home, family, or livelihood.

The hormonal changes that occur around the time of menopause influence each woman's response to her life situation. These changes may affect her ability to rest, her emotional well-being, her strength and stamina, and her self-image. Health problems specific to women, such as the vasomotor symptoms of menopause, osteopenia or osteoporosis, and breast cancer, become areas of concern.

Although some women age with grace and dignity, for many others the aging process is beset with challenges. Aging frequently results in or exacerbates physical conditions such as heart disease and hypertension, diabetes, arthritis, and cognitive decline; it may also bring financial difficulty through widowhood, divorce, or limited job opportunities. In addition, isolation may occur as a woman's physical condition and mental abilities decline.

Alternative or complementary therapies may relieve symptoms of menopause, maintain bone integrity, and enhance mental acuity and a woman's overall sense of well-being. Activities such as yoga may provide multiple benefits such as maintenance of balance and bone strength, improved blood pressure,

decreased stress, emotional balance, social interaction, and spiritual solace. Compassionate midwifery care provides women with an opportunity to explore new ways to view themselves as they age while offering health screening and a gateway to needed healthcare services.

In communities across the country, some women have only limited access to healthcare services due to social, cultural, or financial constraints. Midwives frequently reach out to women in the communities where they live to bridge this chasm. Community-based well-woman midwifery practices range from home-based care to neighborhood clinics to complex women's health services delivered within the tertiary care setting. In every environment of care, the individual midwife has the potential to make a difference in the lives of the women who come for care.

In virtually every culture, women have a history of meeting others' needs before attending to their own. Although this trend may be due to social expectations and customs surrounding women's roles, other contributing factors can include limited information or awareness of basic women's reproductive healthcare recommendations, significant communication or language barriers, transportation issues, and/or a lack of resources with which to pay for services. The process of actively listening to women includes validating each woman's experiences, acknowledging her stated needs, offering nonjudgmental support, and considering how any information disclosed may affect this woman within her family and her community.

Opportunities for promoting midwifery care for well women include grassroots encouragement of women's support networks, such as occurs within neighborhoods, cultural enclaves, or ethnic gatherings. Women's health education can be provided as a community service or within the local school system. In areas with limited opportunities for midwives to offer pregnancy and birth care, the provision of well-woman, menopausal, and primary care services for women can be effective in establishing a foothold in the healthcare community by demonstrating the value of midwifery care while providing a much needed service. A commitment to women's health and an inquiring mind are all that is necessary to begin the adventure of improving the health and well-being of women across the life span using the midwifery model of care.

CARE OF THE WELL WOMAN: HEALTH ASSESSMENT AND SCREENING

Key Clinical Information

The well-woman examination provides an opportunity for women of all ages to learn about their bodies while caring for themselves. Each visit offers a chance to develop a partnership within which to address the client's unique concerns. During the initial visit, the client history and physical examination are quite comprehensive. By comparison, on subsequent visits, particularly when the midwife provides ongoing care, a brief update of the history and a limited physical examination may be all that are required.

Midwives caring for adolescent women may be asked to perform a sports or college entry assessment during the annual well-woman visit. Comprehensive health evaluation may also be requested for numerous indications, such as age-related periodic health screening, pre-employment screening, or a preoperative history and physical. Education in the additional components of these examinations is easily obtained through continuing professional education programs.

Client History and Chart Review: Components of the History to Consider

(Bickley & Szilagyi, 2009; Nusbaum & Hamilton, 2002; Schuiling & Likis, 2013)

- Reason for visit
- Reproductive history
  - Last menstrual period (LMP)
  - Pregnancy history
    - GP TPAL
    - Infertility or losses
    - Problems and concerns
    - Plans for future pregnancies

- Gynecologic history
  - Age of menarche
  - Menstrual patterns
  - Vaginal or pelvic infections
  - Gynecologic health practices
    - Reproductive health examinations
    - Genital hygiene practices
    - Female circumcision
- Sexual history (see Box 6-1)
  - Explore what is meaningful to the individual
  - Sexual preference, orientation, and practice
    - Sex with men, women, or both
    - Sexual self-identity
    - Feelings or issues regarding the following:
      - Sexual identity
      - Sexual expression
      - Social support or stigma
    - Emotional response to sexuality and sexual activity
  - Sexual behavior
    - Number of partners
      - In the last 6 months, in the last 5 years, and over her lifetime
      - Recent change in partner(s)
      - Safe sex practices
        - Known partner(s)
        - Sexually transmitted infection (STI) testing
        - Condom use—consistent or erratic
    - Intimate physical contact
      - Frequency and interval of sexual relations
      - Forms of sexual expression
        - Cuddling, fondling, hugging, kissing
        - Intercourse
        - "Outercourse" and oral sex
        - Other physical expressions of intimacy
    - Types of sexual behavior
      - Oral/genital
      - Vaginal penetration
      - Anal penetration

➤ Use of sex toys, dildoes, lubricants, or other sexual aids

➤ Fantasy sexual practices

➤ Participation in potentially harmful practices

- Sexual function
    - Satisfaction with current sexual activity
        - ➤ Frequency of sexual activity
        - ➤ Libido/desire
        - ➤ Foreplay and arousal
        - ➤ Orgasm
        - ➤ Masturbation
        - ➤ Pain with intercourse
        - ➤ Sexuality as marker for relationship/ emotional dynamic
    - Concerns about STIs or HIV

Box 6-1   Asking Intimate Questions

- Invite permission to discuss sexuality and related topics.
- Ask with the woman dressed and in a private setting.
- Explain the purpose of the discussion.
- Emphasize the confidentiality of the discussion.
- Ask permission to record this information.
- Acknowledge the client's or your own discomfort.
- Use specific appropriate language to refer to body parts.
- Be matter-of-fact and nonjudgmental.
- Use open-ended questions and active listening.
- Reflect back what you hear.
- Provide factual information in a supportive manner.
- Offer recommendations for specific concerns.
- Offer referral for complex issues.

- Presence or absence of trusting relationship
    - Consensual sexual intimacy
    - Coercive sexual contact
    - Sex trade or exploitation

- Emotional, sexual, or verbal abuse
    - ➤ Current
    - ➤ Past
    - ➤ Childhood
- Medical/surgical history
    - Allergies
    - Medications and remedies
        - Over-the-counter (OTC) products
        - Prescription products
        - Herbal/homeopathic remedies
    - Current immunization status
    - Diseases, conditions, or problems
    - Hospitalizations and/or surgeries
- Current health care
    - Health philosophy
    - Health screening
        - Dental care
        - Eye care
        - Hearing testing
        - Mental health
        - Skin cancer
    - Primary care provider
    - Specialty care providers
    - Illnesses or diseases
    - Treatments
- Age-appropriate social history
    - Social influences on health and sexual behaviors
    - Cultural influences on health care
    - Use of alcohol, tobacco, and drugs
    - Family and community support systems
    - Intimate-partner violence screen
    - Emotional well-being screen
    - Health and personal safety habits
    - Diet and physical activity
    - Occupational stressors or requirements
- Family history
    - Medical conditions
    - Hereditable conditions
- Review of systems (ROS)
    - Client impression of her own health and well-being
        - Physical
        - Emotional

- General symptoms
  - ◆ Changes in weight or appetite
  - ◆ Weakness, fatigue, or malaise
  - ◆ Fever or chills
  - ◆ Change in bowel or bladder function
  - ◆ Shortness of breath/palpitations
- Other symptoms by body system
  - ◆ Head, eyes, ears, nose, and throat (HEENT)
  - ◆ Cardiopulmonary
  - ◆ Gastrointestinal
  - ◆ Neurologic
  - ◆ Reproductive
  - ◆ Musculoskeletal
  - ◆ Endocrine
  - ◆ Integumentary

Physical Examination: Components of the Physical Exam to Consider

(Schuiling & Likis, 2013; Varney, Kriebs, & Gegor, 2004)

- Vital signs
  - Height, weight, and body mass index (BMI)
  - Blood pressure, pulse, and respirations
- General appearance
  - Hygiene and dress
  - Speech and communication patterns
  - Body language and posture
  - Affect or emotional state
- Developmental assessment
  - Physical (Tanner stages) (Marshall & Tanner, 1969); see Figure 6-1
  - Emotional
  - Sociocultural
- Skin
  - Texture
  - Lesions
  - Scars
  - Bruises
  - Cyanosis or pallor
  - Tattoos
  - Body piercings/body jewelry

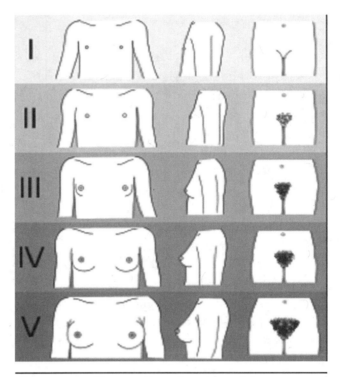

Figure 6-1 Tanner Developmental Stages

- Head, eyes, ears, nose, and throat
  - Eyes
    - ◆ Visual acuity
    - ◆ Ophthalmic examination
    - ◆ Nystagmus
  - Ears
    - ◆ Hearing
    - ◆ Canals
    - ◆ Tympanic membranes
  - Nose
    - ◆ Patency of nares
    - ◆ Lesions
  - Mouth
    - ◆ Lesions
    - ◆ Condition of teeth and gums
    - ◆ Tonsils
- Neck
  - Range of motion
  - Lymph nodes
  - Thyroid
    - ◆ Symmetry
    - ◆ Size
    - ◆ Masses or nodules

- Back and chest
  - Lesions
  - Configuration and symmetry
  - Costovertebral angle tenderness
  - Scoliosis or kyphosis
- Lungs
  - Rate, rhythm, and depth of respirations
  - Breath sounds
  - Changes with percussion
- Heart
  - Rate and rhythm
  - Murmurs or bruits
  - Extra or unusual sounds
- Breasts
  - Shape and symmetry
  - Presence of masses, dimples, or scars
  - Nipple discharge
  - Axillary nodes
- Abdomen
  - Configuration
  - Masses or pain
  - Diastasis recti
  - Hernia
  - Bowel sounds
  - Palpation of organs
- Extremities
  - Configuration
  - Range of motion
  - Peripheral pulses
  - Reflexes
  - Symmetry
  - Strength
  - Joint stability or mobility
  - Edema
  - Varicosities
- Pelvic examination
  - External genitalia and rectum
    - Configuration
    - Lesions, discharge
    - Bartholin's glands, urethra, and Skene's gland (BUS)
    - Hemorrhoids
  - Speculum examination
    - Vagina
      - Lesions
      - Discharge
      - Odor
    - Cervix
      - Discharge
      - Lesions
      - Configuration
      - Specimen collection
  - Bimanual examination
    - Uterine position
    - Size and shape
    - Pain on cervical motion
    - Adnexal
      - Masses
      - Pain
      - Mobility
  - Rectal examination
    - Hemorrhoids
    - Masses
    - Bleeding
    - Specimen collection

Clinical Impression: Differential Diagnoses to Consider

(ICD9data.com, 2012)

- Well-woman preventive health examination
- Preventive immunizations
- Well-woman examination with an additional diagnosis
  - Gynecologic examination
  - Health issues related to personal or family history
  - Health screening for STIs
  - Contraceptive care
  - Diagnosis based on symptoms

Diagnostic Testing: Diagnostic Tests and Procedures to Consider

- Testing performed or collected during visit
  - Dip urinalysis
  - Pregnancy testing
  - Fingerstick hematocrit or hemoglobin

- Pap smear
- Chlamydia culture or nucleic acid amplification
- Gonorrhea culture or nucleic acid amplification
- Oral in-office HIV testing
- Wet prep
  - Bacterial vaginosis (BV)
  - Trichomoniasis
  - Candidiasis
- Stool for occult blood
- Mantoux test or purified protein derivative (PPD) for tuberculosis (TB)
- Laboratory-based testing
  - Complete blood count (CBC) or hematocrit and hemoglobin (H&H)
  - Hepatitis profile
  - Human immunodeficiency virus (HIV) testing
  - Syphilis testing: VDRL or rapid plasma reagin (RPR)
  - Quantitative or qualitative β-human chorionic gonadotropin (HCG)
  - Sickle cell prep
  - Fasting blood glucose or 2-hour postprandial glucose
- Urinalysis or urine culture
- Thyroid screening
- Cholesterol/lipid panel screening
- Radiology
  - Ultrasound
  - Mammogram
  - Bone density testing
  - Chest x-ray, with history of the following:
    - Positive purified protein derivative (PPD)
    - BCG vaccine

Providing Treatment: Therapeutic Measures to Consider

- Administer immunizations as indicated (Table 6-1) and desired by client (Centers for Disease Control and Prevention [CDC], 2012)
- Treatments are based on diagnosis and lifestyle choices
- Provide support for healthy choices
  - Provide information and rationale to change unhealthy choices
  - Encourage attaining or maintaining a healthy weight

Table 6-1   Immunization Schedule for Adult Women

VACCINE	AGE RANGES AND INDICATIONS		
	19–49 YEARS	50–64 YEARS	≥ 65 YEARS
Tetanus, diphtheria, pertussis	1 dose every 10 years; may substitute Tdap for Td		
Measles, mumps, rubella	1–2 doses Contraindicated in pregnancy	1 dose if a risk factor is present	
Human papillomavirus	3 doses for females aged ≤ 26		
Varicella	2 doses given 4–8 weeks apart	2 doses given 4–8 weeks apart	
Influenza	1 dose annually	1 dose annually	
Hepatitis A	2 doses given 6–18 months apart, if risk factors are present		
Hepatitis B	3 doses given 1–3 months apart, if risk factors are present		
Pneumococcal	1–2 doses if risk factors are present		1 dose
Meningococcal	1+ doses if risk factors are present		
Zoster			1 dose at ≥ 60 years

Source: CDC, 2012.

- Encourage attaining or maintaining nonsmoking status
- Reinforce good diet and exercise habits

Providing Treatment: Complementary and Alternative Measures to Consider

Treatment is based on the specific diagnosis but may include the following measures:

- Vitamin and mineral supplements
- Omega-3 supplements

Providing Support: Education and Support Measures to Consider

- Address client concerns
- Provide preventive health recommendations
  - Diet and nutrition
  - Physical activity
  - Weight management
  - Safety counseling
  - Smoking cessation
  - Emotional wellness
  - Depression screening
  - Screening for drug or alcohol abuse
  - Screening for intimate-partner violence
- Notification process for results
- Recommendations for ongoing care

Follow-up Care: Follow-up Measures to Consider

- Return for care
  - Reading of Mantoux or PPD test results
  - Periodic health maintenance
  - Follow-up of illness, disease, or disorder
- Document the encounter
- Notify the client of her test results
- **www** Report adverse reactions to vaccines

Multidisciplinary Practice: Consider Consultation, Collaboration, or Referral

- OB/GYN services
  - Abnormal Pap smear
  - Abnormal breast examination
  - Other gynecologic problems

- Specialty services
  - Screening colonoscopy
  - Thyroid disorder
  - Diabetes
  - Hypertension
  - Heart disease
  - Other medical or surgical problems
- Social services
  - Transportation services
  - Mental health services
  - Addiction detoxification services
  - Homeless shelters
  - Protective services for women in abusive relationships
  - Community food bank
  - Fuel assistance
  - Health program enrollment
- For diagnosis or treatment outside the midwife's scope of practice

CARE OF THE WELL WOMAN: HEALTH ASSESSMENT AND SCREENING DURING MENOPAUSE

Key Clinical Information

The woman who stands on the threshold of menopause is entering a new phase of her life. In addition to being a time of marked physiologic changes, the physiologic perimenopausal period is frequently a time of introspection, reappraisal, and personal growth. Each woman responds differently to the precursors of menopause—one may sigh with relief that her time of menstruation is nearly done, whereas another may be dismayed by the passing of her fertility. The onset of menopause can be portrayed using negative terms or, alternatively, celebrated as a healthy life stage that honors the accomplishments and strengths of women and ushers in a new generative phase of life.

Although physiologic menopause is typically defined as the day when it has been 12 months since the last menstrual period, the time of transition can last several years, during which a woman can experience multiple signs and symptoms, such as hot flashes, night sweats, and menstrual changes (Schuiling & Likis, 2013). Early signs of pregnancy can be erroneously dismissed as perimenopausal menstrual irregularity. For this reason, the midwife seeks to ensure that women have access to safe and reliable contraception as they approach menopause. Health-related visits during the perimenopausal and early postmenopausal period represent a time when the midwife can assess individual women's health beliefs and practices while screening for health problems that become more common as women age. Providing information and education related to the "change of life" can ease the transition for many women, particularly in the early postmenopausal period when women experience the greatest incidence of troublesome symptoms (Schuiling & Likis, 2013).

Client History and Chart Review: Components of the History to Consider

(Schuiling & Likis, 2013)

- Age, race, and cultural heritage
- Reproductive and sexual history
  - GP TPAL
  - Pap history
  - STIs
  - Breast changes or pain
  - Menstrual status
  - Frequency, duration, and flow
  - Changes in menses
    - Pattern of bleeding
    - Intermenstrual bleeding
    - Prolonged
    - Excessive or scanty flow
  - Vasomotor symptoms
    - Hot flashes or flushes
    - Night sweats
    - Flushing
  - Urogenital symptoms
    - Vaginal dryness or thinning of tissues
    - Urinary symptoms such as incontinence or urgency
  - Other symptoms
    - Insomnia or sleep pattern changes
    - Emotional changes
      - Emotional lability
      - Depression or anxiety
      - Diminished coping ability
    - Dry eyes or visual changes
    - Forgetfulness
  - Sexual activity and practices
    - Sexual activity
    - Sexual orientation
    - Sex-related changes
      - Libido
      - Vaginal lubrication
      - Sexual functioning
    - Dyspareunia
- Medical/surgical history
  - Allergies
  - Medications and herbal supplements
  - Complementary and alternative therapies
  - Presence or absence of cervix, uterus, and ovaries
  - Recent diagnostic testing with other healthcare practitioner(s)
    - Dental examination
    - Hearing testing
    - Vision examination
    - Medical screening tests
  - Chronic illness or disease
  - Surgeries
- Risk factor assessment
  - Coronary artery disease
  - Osteoporosis
  - Thyroid disorder
  - Diabetes mellitus
  - Malignancy
  - Intimate-partner violence
  - Smoking is associated with earlier age at menopause
- Family history
  - Age of menopause in close female relatives
  - Osteoporosis
  - Female reproductive cancers

- Colon or gastrointestinal malignancy
- Heart disease
- Diabetes
- Social history
  - Attitudes toward menopause
  - Family support systems
  - Social activities
  - Tobacco, alcohol, or drug use
- Ability to care for self
  - Food, shelter, and social support
  - Activities of daily living
  - Ability to seek assistance as needed
  - Physical activity
  - Nutritional assessment
- Review of systems
  - Integumentary
    - Skin changes
    - Lesions
  - HEENT
    - Hearing loss
    - Visual changes
  - Cardiopulmonary
    - Shortness of breath (SOB)
    - Palpitations
    - Edema
  - Gastrointestinal
    - Bowel changes
    - Rectal bleeding
    - Rectocele
  - Genitourinary
    - Urinary frequency
    - Incontinence
    - Dyspareunia
  - Endocrine
    - Fatigue
    - Intolerance to cold or heat
  - Neurologic
    - Confusion
    - Headaches
  - Musculoskeletal
    - Pain
    - Range of motion
    - Joint enlargement

Physical Examination: Components of the Physical Exam to Consider

- Vital signs, including blood pressure
  - Height, weight, and BMI
  - Changes in height or weight
- General
  - Evidence of self-care
  - Affect and responsiveness
  - Skin turgor and thickness
  - Presence of bruises, cuts, or signs of trauma
  - Posture
  - Physical strength
  - Balance
- HEENT
  - Hearing
  - Vision
  - Thyroid
  - Cervical nodes
  - Nasal patency
  - Teeth and gums
- Back
  - Costovertebral angle tenderness
  - Evaluate for kyphosis, lordosis, and low back pain
  - Respiratory examination: Auscultate lung fields bilaterally
- Cardiac examination
  - Rate and rhythm
  - Murmurs
  - Pulses
  - Peripheral edema
- Breast examination
  - Masses
  - Discharge
  - Axillary nodes
- Abdomen
  - Bowel sounds
  - Liver margins
  - Central obesity
- Extremities
  - Edema
  - Varicosities

- Range of motion
- Joint swelling, redness, or pain
- Genital examination
  - Genital atrophy and skin changes
  - Vaginal dryness
  - Lesions or abrasions
  - Speculum examination
  - Bimanual examination
    - Uterus
      - Size
      - Consistency
      - Contour
      - Mobility
    - Adnexa
      - Size
      - Consistency
      - Mobility
    - Presence of cystocele or rectocele
- Rectal examination
  - Hemorrhoids
  - Palpate for lesions and masses

Clinical Impression: Differential Diagnoses to Consider

(ICD9data.com, 2012)

- Well-woman examination
- Amenorrhea
- Mastalgia
- Premenopausal menorrhagia
- Postmenopausal bleeding (PMB)
- Sleep disturbances
- Urinary incontinence
- Vasomotor symptoms

Diagnostic Testing: Diagnostic Tests and Procedures to Consider

(American College of Obstetricians and Gynecologists [ACOG], 1995, 2006a; U.S. Preventive Services Task Force, 2011)

- Women's health screening
  - Endometrial biopsy
  - Mammogram

- Bone density testing
- Pap smear
- STI testing
  - Hepatitis testing
  - HIV testing
- General medical testing
  - Depression screening
  - Fasting blood sugar
  - Hemoglobin
  - Liver function tests
  - Lipid profile or cholesterol
  - Thyroid testing (TSH)
  - Urinalysis
  - Colorectal cancer screening
  - Electrocardiogram
  - Tuberculosis testing

Providing Treatment: Therapeutic Measures to Consider

(ACOG, 2006a; U.S. Preventive Services Task Force, 2011)

- Immunization update (CDC, 2012)
  - Tetanus, diphtheria, and pertussis
  - Influenza
  - Pneumococcal
  - Meningococcal
  - Varicella
  - Zoster
- Contraception as indicated for carefully selected women: Low-dose triphasic oral contraceptive pills (OCPs)
  - Reliable contraception
  - Relief from vasomotor symptoms
- Vitamin and mineral supplements
  - Calcium: 1200–1500 mg daily
  - Magnesium: 400 mg daily
  - Vitamin E: 400 IU BID with meals
  - Omega fats in fatty fish, flaxseed, and supplements
- Hormone therapy for carefully selected women (see "Care of the Woman Interested in Hormone Replacement Therapy")

- Local treatment for symptomatic relief of vaginal atrophy
- Systemic for severe vasomotor symptoms
  - Estrogen replacement therapy (post hysterectomy)
  - Combination HRT (intact uterus)
  - Estrogen/androgen therapy (decreased libido post hysterectomy)
- Treatment for medical conditions (see "Primary Care in Women's Health")
  - Hypertension
  - Diabetes
  - Hypothyroidism
  - Breast cancer prevention
  - Stroke prevention (low-dose aspirin)
  - Obesity

Providing Treatment: Complementary and Alternative Measures to Consider

- Dietary changes
  - Decrease consumption of fat, caffeine, sugar, and alcohol
  - Increase consumption of soy, whole grains, and dietary fiber
  - Vitamin E, vitamin D, calcium, and magnesium
- Maintain regular weight-bearing exercise
  - Walking or jogging
  - Weight training
  - Aerobics
- Non–weight-bearing exercise for joint mobility
  - Swimming
  - Biking
- Sleep aids
  - Valerian root
  - Chamomile
  - Melatonin
  - Develop a sleep routine
    - Create a comforting pre-sleep routine
    - Go to bed at the same time each night
    - Arise at the same time each day
    - Keep electronics out of the bedroom

- Utilize creative outlets
  - Journal writing
  - Dance, drawing, or singing
  - Prayer or meditation
- Community involvement and groups
  - Schools or child care
  - Religious affiliation
  - Library or school
  - Nature preserves
  - Homeless shelters
  - Soup kitchens
  - Nonprofit organizations
  - Municipal organizations
- Sexual comfort
  - Vaginal lubricants
  - Alternative sexual practices

Providing Support: Education and Support Measures to Consider

- Review signs and symptoms of the following conditions:
  - Perimenopause and postmenopause
  - Thyroid dysfunction
  - Diabetes
- Screening recommendations
  - Benefits and drawbacks to testing
  - Preparation for testing, when indicated
  - Interpretation of test results
- Discuss medical therapies for symptoms
  - Anticipated benefits
  - Potential harms
  - Complementary and alternative therapies
- Discuss complementary and alternative therapies for symptoms
  - Risks
  - Benefits
- Maintain mental acuity
  - Puzzles and word games
  - Adult education classes
  - Change daily routines
  - Seek mental challenges and new experiences
  - Avoid isolation

- Physical activity (20 minutes or more daily)
  - Releases endorphins
  - Maintains strength and flexibility
    - Yoga, Tai Chi
    - Dance
    - Aerobic activities
- Dietary recommendations
  - Flaxseed meal
  - Whole grains
  - Dark, leafy green vegetables
  - Citrus fruits (except grapefruit)
  - Sea vegetables
  - Protein from legumes, nuts, and seeds
  - Limited organic animal proteins and fats
- ⚠ Teach warning signs of female reproductive cancers
  - Bleeding
  - Pain
  - Masses
  - Lesions

Follow-up Care: Follow-up Measures to Consider

- Document findings
- Return for continued care
  - Annually
  - As indicated by test results
  - With the onset of problem or symptoms

Multidisciplinary Practice: Consider Consultation, Collaboration, or Referral

- OB/GYN services: For abnormal reproductive findings or test results
- Medical services: For diagnostic workup or ongoing care of medical problems
- Support services
  - Smoking cessation
  - Drug or alcohol rehabilitation
  - Stress management
  - Housing assistance
- Support groups
  - Diabetes
  - Intimate-partner violence
  - Substance abuse

- For diagnosis or treatment outside the midwife's scope of practice

CARE OF THE WOMAN INTERESTED IN BARRIER METHODS OF BIRTH CONTROL

Key Clinical Information

Barrier contraceptives include both mechanical devices and chemical agents that act as barriers to prevent motile sperm from reaching the cervical os. Barrier methods are an effective and low-cost form of birth control that is particularly well suited for women who do not engage in intercourse on a frequent basis. Some barrier methods provide contraception while simultaneously reducing the risk of contracting STIs. The primary drawback of barrier methods is that they require using the method correctly and consistently for each and every act of intercourse. The effectiveness of each barrier method is related to the method type, use of spermicide, parity of the woman, and actual method use patterns. Efficacy ranges from 60% to 93%. Multiparous women tend to have higher failure rates than nulliparous women. Barrier methods may be used as an adjunct to other methods, used with other barrier methods, or used alone (Hatcher et al., 2011).

Client History and Chart Review: Components of the History to Consider

(Hatcher et al., 2011; Johnson, 2004)

- Allergies, including latex allergy
- Medications
- Gynecologic history
  - Contraindications to hormonal contraceptives or IUDs
  - Preference for nonhormonal or relations-based barrier contraceptive
  - LMP and typical menstrual pattern
    - Recent abnormal Pap smear or cervical procedure
    - Last examination, Pap smear, and STI testing, as applicable
    - History of STIs—diagnosis and treatment

- Pregnancy history
  - GP TPAL
  - Recent childbirth or abortion
- Past and current medical and surgical history
- Social history
  - Drug and/or alcohol use
  - Living situation and resources
  - Sexual-partner support for method of birth control
  - Client ability to negotiate for barrier use
- Method-related considerations
  - Frequency of sexual relations
  - Ability to learn and use the method reliably
  - Impact of an unplanned pregnancy
  - Previous reaction to spermicides

Physical Examination: Components of the Physical Exam to Consider

The well-woman examination focuses, as indicated, on the following:

- Vaginal and cervical anatomy and position
- Fit of the diaphragm or cap
- The woman's ability to insert and remove the device

Clinical Impression: Differential Diagnoses to Consider

(ICD9data.com, 2012)

- Contraceptive management includes the following considerations:
  - General counseling and advice
  - Diaphragm or cap fitting
  - Counseling on initiation of OTC methods
  - Unspecified contraceptive management

Diagnostic Testing: Diagnostic Tests and Procedures to Consider

- Pap smear
- Urinalysis
- Serum or urine pregnancy test
- STI screening
- Other screening tests according to age and health history

Providing Treatment: Therapeutic Measures to Consider

(Hatcher et al., 2011; Johnson, 2004)

- Diaphragms and cervical caps
  - Both have the potential to increase the woman's risk of urinary tract infections
  - Female superior position during intercourse can dislodge these devices
  - Spermicide use is recommended
  - A prescription is needed for these devices in the United States
- Cervical caps
  - Prentif cavity rim cervical cap: No longer available in the United States
  - FemCap, nonlatex: Three sizes are available, based on parity
    - Small, for women who have never been pregnant
    - Medium, for women who have had an abortion or a cesarean delivery
    - Large, for women who have given birth vaginally
  - Lea's shield, nonlatex: One size, no fitting required
  - Oves cap, nonlatex
    - Single-use cap
    - Available in Canada and online
    - Requires fitting
    - Three sizes
- Diaphragms
  - Sizes ranging from 50 to 95 mm
  - Flat spring, for women with firm vaginal tone
  - Arcing spring, for women with lax muscle tone
  - Wide seal provides a greater surface area for the seal
- Reality female condom, nonlatex
  - Allows female control for STI protection and contraception
  - Offers greater protection than the male condom
- Male condom
  - Provides some measure of protection against STIs

- ■ Can contribute to latex allergy
- ■ Requires male cooperation to use effectively
- • Contraceptive sponges: 83–91% effective
  - ■ Today sponge: Nonoxyl-9
  - ■ Protectaid
    - ◆ Available in Canada and online
    - ◆ F5 gel (sodium cholate, nonoxy-9, and benzalkonium chloride)
  - ■ Pharmatex sponge
    - ◆ Available in Canada
    - ◆ Benzalkonium chloride

Providing Treatment: Complementary and Alternative Measures to Consider

- • Fertility awareness
- • Abstinence
- • Nonpenetrating sexual relations ("outercourse")
- • Withdrawal

Natural Spermicide

The following natural spermicide (Trapani, 1984) may be used with a cervical cap or diaphragm (instead of nonoxyl-9):

- • 1 cup water
- • 1 tsp fresh lemon juice
- • 5 tsp table salt
- • 10 tsp cornstarch
- • 10 tsp glycerin

Mix the solids, and then add the liquids slowly while stirring to form a smooth paste. Cook, over low heat, stirring constantly, until thick. Store refrigerated in a sealed container. Discard unused portions after 30 days.

Providing Support: Education and Support Measures to Consider

(Hatcher et al., 2011; Johnson, 2004)

- • Review use and effectiveness of the chosen method(s)

- • Review other birth control methods and their effectiveness
- • Help clients learn to negotiate for safe sex
- • Condoms are recommended to protect against STIs
  - ■ Use for every act of penile contact
  - ■ Apply before any penile genital, oral, or anal contact
  - ■ Hold the rim during withdrawal
  - ■ Use only water-soluble lubricants
- • Diaphragm or cervical cap
  - ■ Have the client demonstrate device insertion and removal
  - ■ Instruct the client in proper use, cleaning, and care of reusable devices
    - ◆ Wash hands before insertion or removal
    - ◆ Insertion or removal is easier with one leg bent on chair or toilet or in the squatting position
    - ◆ Wear the cap or diaphragm during every act of intercourse
    - ◆ Use with a spermicidal gel or cream
    - ◆ Wear until at least 6 hours after intercourse
    - ◆ Check for correct placement before removing the device; if it becomes dislodged, seek emergency contraception as soon as possible
    - ◆ Use in conjunction with a condom
      - ➤ Until confident that the device is placed and fits correctly
      - ➤ With concern about the risk of STIs
- • ⚠ Educate regarding signs and symptoms of toxic shock syndrome (Deresiewicz, n.d.)
  - ■ Caused by *Staphylococcus aureus*
  - ■ May occur with use of vaginal barriers
    - ◆ Avoid use during menses
    - ◆ Remove within recommended time frame
  - ■ Sudden onset of symptoms
    - ◆ Fever
    - ◆ Sunburn-like rash
    - ◆ Hypotension
  - ■ Seek care immediately

Follow-up Care: Follow-up Measures to Consider

- Document
  - Discussions
  - Method choice(s)
  - Client teaching
  - Fitting and client demonstration of prescription devices
  - Planned follow-up
- Call or return for care
  - Two-week evaluation of diaphragm or cervical cap use
  - In 3 to 4 months, repeat the Pap smear for cap users
  - Annual well-woman visit
  - Method-related problems
  - Amenorrhea
  - Positive pregnancy test

Multidisciplinary Practice: Consider Consultation, Collaboration, or Referral

- Signs or symptoms of the following conditions:
  - Toxic shock syndrome
  - Latex allergy reaction
- For diagnosis or treatment outside the midwife's scope of practice

CARE OF THE WOMAN INTERESTED IN EMERGENCY CONTRACEPTION

Key Clinical Information

Emergency contraception (EC) offers women an opportunity to effectively prevent pregnancy from occurring in the event of unprotected intercourse or contraceptive failure, such as when a condom breaks during intercourse. EC is most effective when initiated as soon as possible after unprotected sex. Available options include emergency contraceptive pills (ECPs) and the copper-T intrauterine device (IUD) (Hatcher et al., 2011).

ECPs are available in two forms: progestin-only pills (POP), such as Plan B One-Step, Next Choice (levonorgestrel), Ella (ulipristol acetate), or combined oral contraceptive pills (OCPs) formulated with both estrogen and progestin (Fine et al., 2010; Schuiling & Likis, 2013). ECPs are available without a prescription for women and men ages 17 and older, although they may be kept behind the pharmacy counter (Duramed Pharmaceuticals, 2006a). The requirement to show identification and proof of age to obtain EC is a barrier for many women and their partners, and at the time of this book's revision was hotly under dispute.

Although research has demonstrated that ECPs are approximately 74% effective when taken as long as 120 hours after unprotected sexual exposure, the manufacturer of Plan B One-Step recommends administration within 24 hours and up to 72 hours after exposure (Duramed Pharmaceuticals, 2006a; Ellertson et al., 2003). Side effects of ECPs include nausea and vomiting, and an antiemetic can be helpful (ACOG, 2001a). Clients can access an emergency contraceptive website at www.not-2-late.com; midwives can be listed as ECP providers by clicking on the "For Providers" tab on this site and completing the provider form.

A copper-T IUD, such as ParaGard, can be placed as long as 5 days after unprotected intercourse as an EC measure and will provide continued contraception for up to 10 years. Although postcoital IUD insertion reduces the risk of pregnancy by more than 99%, IUD insertion is not readily available in this time frame and may not be suitable for many women.

Client History and Chart Review: Components of the History to Consider

- Pregnancy and gynecologic history
  - LMP and typical menstrual pattern
  - GP TPAL
  - Sexual history
    - Number of hours since unprotected intercourse
    - Reasons for unprotected sexual exposure
      - Contraceptive failure
      - Lack of contraceptive planning
      - Missed or forgotten pills
      - Lost patch or ring

- ➤ Date rape or sexual assault/abuse
- ➤ Judgment altered by substance abuse
  - Current or recent use of contraception
    - ◆ Ability to use ECP as directed
    - ◆ Plans for long-term birth control
  - Contraindications to ECP use
    - ◆ Pregnancy
    - ◆ Undiagnosed genital bleeding
  - Contraindications to IUD insertion (see "Care of the Woman Interested in an Intrauterine Device or Intrauterine System")
  - Most recent examination, Pap smear, and STI testing, if applicable
    - ◆ History of STIs
    - ◆ History of abnormal Pap smears
- Medical history
  - Allergies
  - Medications
  - Medical conditions
- Social history

Physical Examination: Components of the Physical Exam to Consider

- Not required for ECP, but can be useful in the following circumstances:
  - The woman's history is unclear
  - STI testing is indicated
  - Other symptoms are present
  - The woman has not had any examinations within past 12 months
- Limited reproductive examination
- Complete well-woman examination
- Requiring an office visit for ECP creates a barrier to access of ECP for many women; ECP is available without a prescription behind the counter in many areas

Clinical Impression: Differential Diagnoses to Consider

(ICD9data.com, 2012)

- Encounter for emergency contraceptive counseling and prescription

- Counseling related to contraceptive pills
- Copper-T IUD insertion

Diagnostic Testing: Diagnostic Tests and Procedures to Consider

- Pregnancy testing: If menstrual history is uncertain or unclear
- STI screening
- Other screening tests, according to age and health history

Providing Treatment: Therapeutic Measures to Consider

- Provide an antiemetic 1 hour before the first ECP dose (ACOG, 2001a; Trussell & Raymond, 2006)
  - Meclizine (OTC): two 25-mg tablets
  - Compazine: 5- to 10-mg tablet or 15 mg spansule
  - Phenergan: 25-mg tablet or suppository
  - Benadryl: 25–50 mg PO
- Emergency contraceptive pills
  - Nonprescription (levonorgestrel)
    - ◆ Plan B One Step
    - ◆ Next Choice
  - Prescription only (ulipristal acetate) (Fine, Mathe, Ginde, Cullins, Morfesis, & Gainer, 2010)
    - ◆ Ella: 30 mg
    - ◆ Greater efficacy than levonorgestrel in women 48–120 hours post exposure
  - Use of prescription oral contraceptives (Table 6-2)
- Copper-T IUD insertion (see "Care of the Woman Interested in an Intrauterine Device or Intrauterine System")

Providing Treatment: Complementary and Alternative Measures to Consider

- Nausea
  - Seabands
  - Ginger tea

Table 6-2   Oral Contraceptives Used for Emergency Contraception in the United States

BRAND	COMPANY	FIRST DOSE	SECOND DOSE (12 HOURS LATER)	ETHINYL ESTRADIOL PER DOSE (MCG)	LEVONORGESTREL PER DOSE (MG)
Progestin-Only Pills					
Plan B, option 1	Barr/Duramed	2 white pills	None	0	1.5
Plan B, option 2	Barr/Duramed	1 white pill	1 white pill	0	1.5
Combined Progestin and Estrogen Pills					
Alesse	Wyeth-Ayerst	5 pink pills	5 pink pills	100	0.50
Aviane	Barr/Duramed	5 orange pills	5 orange pills	100	0.50
Cryselle	Barr/Duramed	4 white pills	4 white pills	120	0.60
Enpresse	Barr/Duramed	4 orange pills	4 orange pills	120	0.50
Jolessa	Barr/Duramed	4 pink pills	4 pink pills	120	0.60
Lessina	Barr/Duramed	5 pink pills	5 pink pills	100	0.50
Levlen	Berlex	4 light-orange pills	4 light-orange pills	120	0.60
Levlite	Berlex	5 pink pills	5 pink pills	100	0.50
Levora	Watson	4 white pills	4 white pills	120	0.60
Lo/Ovral	Wyeth-Ayerst	4 white pills	4 white pills	120	0.60
Low-Ogestrel	Watson	4 white pills	4 white pills	120	0.60
Lutera	Watson	5 white pills	5 white pills	100	0.50
Nordette	Wyeth-Ayerst	4 light-orange pills	4 light-orange pills	120	0.60
Ogestrel	Watson	2 white pills	2 white pills	100	0.50
Ovral	Wyeth-Ayerst	2 white pills	2 white pills	100	0.50
Portia	Barr/Duramed	4 pink pills	4 pink pills	120	0.60
Quasense	Watson	4 white pills	4 white pills	120	0.60
Seasonale	Barr/Duramed	4 pink pills	4 pink pills	120	0.60
Seasonique	Barr/Duramed	4 light-blue-green pills	4 light-blue-green pills	120	0.60
Tri-Levlen	Berlex	4 yellow pills	4 yellow pills	120	0.50
Triphasil	Wyeth-Ayerst	4 yellow pills	4 yellow pills	120	0.50
Trivora	Watson	4 pink pills	4 pink pills	120	0.50

Source: Office of Population Research & Association of Reproductive Health Professionals, 2006.

- Herbs that foster the onset of menstruation (Romm, 2010)
  - Black cohosh
  - Dong quai
  - Ginger
  - Motherwort
  - Pennyroyal
  - Rue
  - Vitex or chasteberry
  - Evening primrose oil
- Vitamin C

⚠️ Herbal abortifacients are not recommended due to their potential for toxicity and the safety of medical termination of pregnancy.

Providing Support: Education and Support Measures to Consider

- Verify that the client does not want to become pregnant
- Emergency contraceptive pills (Office of Population Research & Association of Reproductive Health Professionals, 2006)
  - Emphasize that ECPs are not recommended for regular use as contraception
  - Common side effects of ECPs
    - Nausea and vomiting
    - Breast tenderness
    - Menses may be earlier or later than usual
    - Antiemetics may cause drowsiness
  - Take ECP dose(s) as instructed
    - Dose within 48 hours improves efficacy
    - Dose within 72 hours is recommended
    - Dose within 120 hours is the outer range of effectiveness
    - Preventive antiemetic recommended
    - Take exact number of ECPs per protocol
    - Repeat the dose if vomiting occurs within 1 hour
  - Breastfeeding women should discard milk for 6 hours after each dose
  - Return for care if menses do not occur within 21 days
    - Provide options counseling
    - ECPs are nonteratogenic

- 🔺 Call immediately for onset of warning signs or symptoms
    - Abdominal or pelvic pain
    - Chest pain
    - Headache
    - Eye problems or visual disturbances
    - Severe pain in legs, or numbness or tingling of extremities
- IUD (see "Care of the Woman Interested in an Intrauterine Device or Intrauterine System")
- Discussion
  - Mechanism of action
  - Safe sexual practices
  - Pregnancy and STI prevention
  - Long-term contraceptive options

Follow-up Care: Follow-up Measures to Consider

- Document instructions and prescriptions, if provided
- Improve access to emergency contraception (Trussell & Raymond, 2006)
  - Educate the office staff in OTC and prescription EC options
  - Add discussion of emergency contraception to routine visits
    - Provide ECPs and instruction in advance
    - Provide women younger than 17 years old with prescriptions and instructions for EC
    - Provide prescriptions by phone for known clients
    - Offer prescriptions without clinical examination
- Follow-up visit for information, counseling, or care
  - Initiation of regular contraception
  - Gynecologic examination and STI screening
  - Amenorrhea 21 days or more after ECP
  - Symptoms suggesting complications or adverse effect

Multidisciplinary Practice: Consider Consultation, Collaboration, or Referral

- For diagnosis or treatment outside the midwife's scope of practice

CARE OF THE WOMAN INTERESTED IN FERTILITY AWARENESS

Key Clinical Information

Every woman can benefit from increased awareness and understanding of her body. Fertility awareness offers women a means of becoming attuned to the functioning of their reproductive system and its impact on their overall health and well-being throughout the life span.

Awareness of changes throughout the menstrual cycle gives many women a greater sense of control over their lives and can be useful in recognizing ovulation, identifying menstrual dysfunction, and understanding changes during breastfeeding and perimenopause. Cycle tracking can be done through charting of symptoms or use of a tool such as cycle beads, which can be easily incorporated into daily routines.

Teaching fertility awareness to adolescents provides a wonderful outreach opportunity for midwives, while building the midwife's prospective client base. The knowledge provided can be incredibly empowering to adolescent women; clearly presented factual information on reproductive function can be instrumental in adolescent women delaying the onset of sexual activity and can motivate them to make appropriate use of safe sex practices.

Heterosexual couples interested in the nuances of the female cycle can enhance their relationship while seeking pregnancy prevention or conception through discussions centered on the menstrual cycle and sexual activity. Fertility awareness requires interactive dialogue between partners, acceptance of physiologic phases, and willingness to create mutual goals. This process fosters development of a respectful and an emotionally intimate relationship and places sex at the periphery rather than at the center of the union (Singer, 2004).

Fertility awareness can also be helpful for the woman who desires pregnancy in determining the best times for intercourse to result in conception. For women who have difficulty achieving pregnancy and for lesbian or single women using artificial insemination, awareness of fertility can help identify when assisted reproductive technologies are recommended to achieve pregnancy.

Client History and Chart Review: Components of the History to Consider

- Social history
  - Goals of learning fertility awareness
  - Partner interest, if applicable
- Menstrual history
  - LMP
  - Frequency of menses
  - Duration of menses
  - Mid-cycle pain or discharge
- Sexual history
  - Age at onset of sexual activity
  - Frequency of sexual activity
  - Type of sexual activity
  - Safe sex practices
    - Abstinence
    - STI testing
    - Condom use
    - Monogamy
  - Sexual relationships
    - Long-term monogamy
    - Serial monogamy
    - Multiple partners
    - Same-sex and/or opposite-sex partner(s)
  - Current method of birth control, if any
- Pregnancy history: GP TPAL
  - Difficulty achieving pregnancy
  - Difficulty maintaining pregnancy
- Medical/surgical history
- Assessment of fertility awareness techniques and practices
- Review of systems (ROS)

Physical Examination: Components of the Physical Exam to Consider

- Not required for fertility awareness education
- Weight, height, and BMI
- Physical examination components as indicated by the following considerations:
  - Age and health status
  - History and client interview

- Screening recommendations (see "Care of the Well Woman: Health Assessment and Screening")

Clinical Impression: Differential Diagnoses to Consider

(ICD9data.com, 2012)

- Family planning advice and counseling
- Health education
- General medical examination

Diagnostic Testing: Diagnostic Tests and Procedures to Consider

- Pap smear
- STI testing
- Thyroid testing
- Over-the-counter (OTC) testing options
  - Ovulation predictor tests
  - Luteinizing hormone tests
  - Electronic fertility monitors

Providing Treatment: Therapeutic Measures to Consider

- Fertility awareness (Pallone & Bergus, 2009): Appropriate for women
  - From menarche through menopause
  - During breastfeeding
  - With menstrual irregularities
- Fertility awareness methods
  - Cervical mucus
  - Basal body temperature
  - Menstrual cycle charting
  - Ovulation sensations
  - Electronic hormonal fertility monitoring

Providing Treatment: Complementary and Alternative Measures to Consider

- Nonpharmacologic methods of birth control (Hatcher et al., 2011)
  - Abstinence
    - Periodic abstinence (rhythm method)
    - Avoid intercourse during fertile times

- Withdrawal
  - May work for some couples
  - May expose women to sperm in pre-ejaculatory fluid
  - May interrupt sexual satisfaction
- Natural spermicides (see "Care of the Woman Interested in Barrier Methods of Birth Control")
- "Outercourse"
  - Hugging and kissing
  - Holding and fondling
  - Oral sex
  - Sexual activity that excludes the following acts:
    - Penetration
    - Genital-to-genital contact

Providing Support: Education and Support Measures to Consider

- Provide fertility awareness education (Singer, 2004)
  - Physiologic and hormonal changes
    - During the menstrual cycle
    - During breastfeeding
    - During perimenopause
  - Primary fertility signals
    - Basal body temperature
    - Cervical fluid
    - Cervical changes
  - Secondary fertility signals
    - Mid-cycle pain
    - Ferning of salivary fluid
    - Spotting
    - Breast tenderness
    - Libido changes
  - Benefits, drawbacks, and use of resources
    - Basal body thermometer
    - Cycle beads
    - Cycle charts
    - Ovulation predictors
  - Implementing the method
    - Resources
    - Charts and notations
    - Interpretation of data
    - Application to the client's personal situation

- When using fertility awareness for birth control
  - Engage the partner in the discussions
  - Discuss the best method for the couple
  - Consider use of optional barrier methods or spermicide at mid-cycle
  - Consider the lack of STI protection
  - Use of emergency contraception

Follow-up Care: Follow-up Measures to Consider

- Document
  - Education process and components
  - Recommended resources
  - Discussions
  - Plan to verify client understanding and correct use of method
- Return for care
  - For fertility chart review
  - As recommended by age and sexual activity
  - For Pap smear and STI testing as indicated
  - With pregnancy

Multidisciplinary Practice: Consider Consultation, Collaboration, or Referral

- Assistive reproductive technologies
  - When pregnancy is not achieved after 1 year of trying
  - After 6 months in women older than age 35
- For diagnosis or treatment outside the midwife's scope of practice

CARE OF THE WOMAN INTERESTED IN HORMONAL CONTRACEPTION

Key Clinical Information

Hormonal contraceptives offer women protection against unplanned pregnancy through suppression of ovulation, mechanisms to inhibit sperm motility and penetration of the cervical canal and ovum, and/or thinning of the endometrium (Hatcher et al., 2011; Organon, 2011b). Reliable hormonal contraceptives for women are available in a wide array of delivery methods.

Oral contraceptive pills offer a well-established, woman-controlled method of hormonal birth control. Contraceptive rings and patches provide an easily reversible, steady state of contraceptive hormones on a cyclical basis, avoiding the peaks and valleys associated with OCPs. Contraceptive injections, implants, and hormonal IUDs offer long-acting contraception for women who are not candidates for estrogen-containing contraceptives or who prefer continuous protection for extended intervals.

Hormonal contraceptives reduce ovarian and endometrial cancer risk, improve dysmenorrhea, decrease menstrual blood loss, and result in a lighter menstrual flow (Dhont, 2011; Hatcher et al., 2011). Some women report premenstrual syndrome symptoms when using progestin-only contraceptives. Moreover, contraceptive hormones pass into breastmilk, which is a concern for breastfeeding women. Although estrogen has been demonstrated to decrease milk production, long-term effects of estrogen and progesterone on the infant remain poorly documented (Hatcher et al., 2011).

Client History and Chart Review: Components of the History to Consider

(Hatcher et al., 2011)

- Age
- GYN history
  - LMP and typical menstrual pattern
  - Results of last examination, Pap smear, and STI testing if applicable
  - Incidence of the following conditions:
    - Dysmenorrhea
    - Menorrhagia
    - Dysfunctional uterine bleeding
  - Frequency of intercourse
  - Risk factors for STIs: Diagnosis and treatment
  - Abnormal Pap smears: Diagnosis and treatment
  - Breast, mammogram abnormalities: Diagnosis and treatment

- Pregnancy history
  - Plans for pregnancy
  - GP TPAL; date of most recent birth if postpartum
- Past and current health history
  - Allergies
  - Medications and supplements: Potential for interaction with hormonal contraceptives (Hatcher et al., 2011)
    - Anticonvulsants: Can decrease hormonal contraceptive efficacy and medication therapeutic levels
    - Anti-HIV protease inhibitors: Can alter hormonal contraceptive efficacy
    - Diazepam and chlordiazepoxide: Can increase medication effects
    - Griseofulvin (antifungal): Can decrease hormonal contraceptive efficacy
    - Rifamycin and rifabutin: Can decrease hormonal contraceptive efficacy
    - St. John's wort: Can decrease hormonal contraceptive efficacy
    - Theophylline: Can increase medication effects
  - Personal or family history
    - Contraindications to hormonal contraceptive use (ACOG, 2006b; Organon, 2011a)
      - Pregnancy
      - Liver disease
      - Undiagnosed abnormal genital bleeding
      - Thrombophlebitis or thromboembolitic disease
      - Coronary heart disease or cerebrovascular disease
      - Cancer of the reproductive organs or breast
      - Migraine with aura
    - Relative contraindications (see full prescribing information)
      - Breastfeeding and less than 6 weeks postpartum
      - Women older than age 35 years old who smoke

- Hypertension
- Hyperlipidemia
- Depression or mood disorder
- Gallbladder disease
- Abnormal glucose metabolism or diabetes
- Asthma
- Kidney disease
- Seizure disorder
- Lupus
- Sickle cell disease
- Obesity

- Assessment of the woman's ability and motivation to use client-regulated hormonal contraception (Raine et al., 2011)
  - Motivation to prevent pregnancy
  - Ability and motivation to comply with the recommendations for care
    - Daily routine for pill taking
    - Weekly routine for patch
    - Three-week cycle for ring
    - Thirteen-week cycle for injections
  - Ability to cope with side effects while adjusting to hormones
- Social history
  - Cigarette smoking
  - Drug and/or alcohol use
  - Living situation and resources
  - Payment method for contraception
  - Sexual-partner support for method of contraception
- Risk factors for osteoporosis
  - Low-calcium diet
  - Sedentary
  - Small frame
  - History of anorexia-related amenorrhea
  - Family history
  - Duration of injectable contraceptive use

Physical Examination: Components of the Physical Exam to Consider

- Blood pressure
- Height, weight, and BMI

- Comprehensive well-woman examination
  - Focus on reproductive system
    - Thyroid
    - Breasts
    - Pelvic examination
      - Speculum examination
      - Bimanual examination
      - Collection of texting specimens as indicated by history
  - Method-specific focus
    - Inner aspect of upper arm (implant)
    - Depth of uterine cavity (IUD)

Clinical Impression: Differential Diagnoses to Consider

(ICD9data.com, 2012)

- Gynecologic examination
- OCPs
  - Counseling and prescription of OCPs
  - Repeat prescription of OCPs
  - Follow-up care for OCPs
- Intrauterine system (IUS)
  - Insertion of hormonal IUS
  - Follow-up care for IUS
- Implants
  - Insertion of subdermal contraceptive implant
  - Follow-up care for subdermal contraceptive implant
- Other hormonal contraceptive methods
  - Initiation of other contraceptive measures
  - Follow-up care for other contraceptive measures

Diagnostic Testing: Diagnostic Tests and Procedures to Consider

(Hatcher et al., 2011; Organon, 2011a)

- Pregnancy testing
- Pap smear
- Urinalysis
- STI testing
- Screening tests according to age and health history

- Lipid profile
  - Family history of coronary artery disease
  - Smoker on hormonal contraceptives
- Fasting blood sugar
- TSH
- Mammogram
- Bone density testing

Providing Treatment: Therapeutic Measures to Consider

(Hatcher et al., 2011; Pfizer, 2011)

- Progestin-only contraceptives
  - Injectable contraceptives
    - Amenorrhea is common
    - May delay return to fertility
    - May contribute to osteoporosis
    - May diminish risk of sickle cell crisis and symptoms of endometriosis
    - Initial injection given
      - Within first 5 days of normal menses
      - Within first 5 days postpartum if not breastfeeding
      - At 4–6 weeks postpartum if breastfeeding
    - Depo-Provera given deep IM
    - Depo SubQ given in anterior thigh or abdomen
  - Hormonal IUD (see "Care of the Woman Interested in an Intrauterine Device or Intrauterine System")
    - Insert per manufacturer's recommendations
    - May reduce incidence of menorrhagia and dysmenorrhea
  - Progestin-only pills (POP)
    - Have lower effectiveness than combination OCPs
    - Breakthrough bleeding (BTB) is common
    - If pregnancy occurs, there is greater risk of ectopic implantation
    - Good choice for a breastfeeding woman who wants an OCP

- Implanon (Organon, 2011a)
  - Insert subdermally according to the manufacturer's instructions
  - Timing is based on the woman's current method of contraception
  - Palpate immediately after insertion
  - Rod is palpable when inserted correctly
- Combination contraceptives (estrogen and progestin)
  - Can decrease breastmilk production in some women
    - Avoid during breastfeeding *or*
    - Delay use until breastfeeding is well established or the infant is taking additional foods
  - OCPs
    - Use the lowest effective dose
    - Higher doses are used for specific indications
    - Very-low-dose birth control pills
      - BTB may occur
      - May have improved side-effect profile over low-dose OCPs
    - Low-dose birth control pills
      - Slightly higher dose
      - Less BTB
      - Increased side-effect profile
    - Ninety-day pills (Seasonale)
      - Take for 84 days continuously
      - Initial high rate of BTB
      - Menses four times per year
    - 365 days/year pill (Lybrel) (Wyeth, 2008)
      - Low combined daily dose of the hormones levonorgestrel (LNG, 90 mcg) and ethinyl estradiol (EE, 20 mcg)
      - Effectiveness is approximately 98–99%
      - Amenorrhea occurs in 60% of women at the end of a year of use
      - Initial high rate of BTB
  - Transdermal patch: Ortho Evra
    - Patch lasts 7 days; three patches per prescription-cycle carton

- Effectiveness is approximately 99%
- Decreased effectiveness in women weighing more than 198 lb / 90 kg
- NuvaRing contraceptive vaginal ring
  - Lower effective dose of hormones
  - Effectiveness is approximately 98–99%

Providing Treatment: Complementary and Alternative Measures to Consider

- Fertility awareness/natural family planning
- Outercourse
- Abstinence
- Withdrawal
- Natural spermicides
- Barrier methods

Providing Support: Education and Support Measures to Consider

(Hatcher et al., 2011)

- Information and instruction
  - Use of hormonal contraceptives
  - Effectiveness
  - Side effects
  - Warning signs
  - Return schedule
- ⚠ Ascertain whether the health plan covers the chosen method or whether the client can self-pay: Some companies offer assistance for economically disadvantaged women
- Smoking cessation information and support (see "Care of the Woman in Need of Smoking Cessation")
- OCPs
  - Start methods
    - Quick start: Take first pill at office visit
    - First-day start: Take first pill on the first day of menses
    - Sunday start: Take first pill on the Sunday after the onset of menses
  - Use of a barrier or alternate method is recommended for the first cycle
  - Condoms are recommended to protect against STIs

- Breakthrough bleeding is common in the first cycles
- Take the pill daily at the same time; link with another daily activity such as brushing the teeth
- Take pills as soon as possible if forgotten
- Use a backup method or ECP if more than two pills are missed
- NuvaRing (Organon, 2011b)
  - Insert by following the manufacturer's instructions
    - Ring is inserted into the vagina
    - Remains in place for 3 weeks
    - The woman then goes ring-free for 1 week
    - Side effects are same as for OCPs
    - May use tampons with the ring
    - Start instructions
      - If no hormonal contraceptive
        - Start on cycle day 1 *or*
        - Start on cycle days 2–5
      - Requires nonhormonal contraception for first 7 days of use
    - Combination OCP or patch: Start within 7 days of the last pill or patch
- Progestin-only method (pills, injection, or IUD)
  - Requires nonhormonal contraception for first 7 days of use
  - Pills: Start any day
  - Injection: Start when next injection is due
  - Implant: Start on day of removal
  - After first-trimester spontaneous or induced abortion
    - Start on days 1–5 *or*
    - Start with first menses
    - Requires nonhormonal contraception first 7 days
- Ortho Evra (Janssen Pharmaceuticals, 2011)
  - Patches release 60% more estrogen than the 35-mg OCPs
  - Side effects similar to OCPs
    - Greater risk of deep vein thrombosis
    - Patch users are urged not to smoke

- First day or Sunday start
- Replace patch each week for three patches
- The woman then goes patch-free for 1 week (maximum 7 days)
- Apply the patch to clean dry skin in one of the following areas:
  - Buttocks
  - Upper outer arm
  - Lower abdomen
  - Upper torso
- Use additional method or abstinence
  - During the first week of use
  - If patch falls off or is forgotten
- Replace the patch if full or partial detachment occurs
- Injections (Pfizer, 2011)
  - Significant bone mineral loss may occur
    - Limit use to less than 2 years unless other methods prove inadequate
    - Ensure adequate calcium and vitamin D intake
  - Side effects
    - Weight gain and fluid retention
    - Delayed return to fertility (range: 4–31 months)
    - Bleeding irregularities
- Implanon (Organon, 2011a)
  - Side effects
    - Bleeding irregularities
    - Mood changes, including depression
    - Headache
    - Weight gain
- ⚠️ All methods: Call or return for care in the following circumstances:
  - Unexpected amenorrhea or menorrhagia
  - Persistent intermenstrual bleeding
  - Depression
  - Suspected pregnancy
  - Persistent side effects
    - Nausea
    - Irregular menses
    - Mood changes

- Seek emergency care immediately for the following side effects:
    - Abdominal or pelvic pain
    - Chest pain
    - Headache
    - Eye problems or visual disturbances
    - Severe pain in legs, or numbness or tingling of extremities
- Potential health benefits of oral contraceptives (Dhont, 2011)
    - Regulation of menses
    - Decreased cramping and flow
    - Protection against uterine and ovarian cancer
    - Decreased incidence of the following conditions:
        - Colon cancer
        - Benign breast disease
        - Ectopic pregnancy
        - Functional ovarian cysts
    - Decreased risk of bone loss (except Depo-Provera)
- Potential risks of oral contraceptives
    - User or method failure may result in pregnancy
    - Exacerbation of gallbladder disease
    - Stroke or blood clots
    - Estrogen-dependent cancers
    - Osteoporosis (Depo-Provera)
    - Uterine perforation (IUD)
    - Pelvic inflammatory disease (IUD)
    - Local infection (injection and implants)

Follow-up Care: Follow-up Measures to Consider

- Document
    - Pertinent history and physical examination
    - Verification of nonpregnant state
    - Method-related education and counseling
    - Plan for continued care
- Follow-up visit
    - Timing
        - Implant: 2–4 weeks to assess healing
        - Injectable contraceptive: 11–13 weeks for next injection

- Combined contraceptives: 3 months to assess continued use
    - IUD: After first menses to verify placement
- Blood pressure and weight
- Laboratory tests
    - Hemoglobin and hematocrit
    - Triglycerides
    - Glucose
- The client's satisfaction with the method
- Questions or concerns
- Review warning signs: ACHES
    - **A**bdominal or pelvic pain
    - **C**hest pain
    - **H**eadache
    - **E**ye problems
    - **S**evere leg pain
- Problem solving (Hatcher et al., 2011)
    - Amenorrhea
        - Choose increased estrogenic OCP
        - Basal body temperature charting
    - Acne or hirsutism
        - Ortho Tri-Cyclen
        - Estrostep
        - Yasmin
        - Mircette
    - Breakthrough bleeding
        - Rule out nonhormonal contraceptive causes
            - Pregnancy
            - Cervical abnormalities
            - Infection
        - Progestin-only contraceptives
            - Offer one or more cycles of combined OCP use if estrogen is not contraindicated
            - Counsel that BTB typically diminishes over time
        - Combined hormone contraceptives: Change OCP formulation
            - BTB on active pills
                - Increase progestin throughout the cycle *or*

➧ Increase progestin at the end of the active pills (triphasic)

➤ BTB after withdrawal bleed

➧ Increase estrogen *or*

➧ Decrease progestin in early pills

■ Breast tenderness
- ◆ Low-dose OCPs
- ◆ Extended-cycle OCPs
- ◆ Continuous-dose method (ring or patch)

■ Headaches
- ◆ Monitor blood pressure
- ◆ Determine type of headache
  - ➤ Timing, duration, location, and severity
  - ➤ Evaluate potential causes and refer as needed
- ◆ Lower dose of estrogen or progestin
- ◆ Discontinue OCPs

■ Mood swings or depression
- ◆ Recommend B vitamin supplement
- ◆ Discontinue injection or implant
- ◆ Continuous-dose method (ring or patch)
- ◆ Low-dose or extended-cycle OCPs
- ◆ Avoid levonorgestrel-containing OCPs

■ Nausea
- ◆ Take OCP at bedtime
- ◆ Decrease estrogen dose
- ◆ Take missed pills at 12-hour intervals
- ◆ Continuous-dose method (ring or patch)
- ◆ Increase fresh fruit, vegetable, and fluid intake

Multidisciplinary Practice: Consider Consultation, Collaboration, or Referral

- OB/GYN services: Clients with relative contraindications to hormonal contraceptives who wish to try this method
- Specialty care: Development of significant complication(s) related to hormonal contraceptive use
  - ■ Severe headache, stroke, or neurologic symptoms
  - ■ Depression or mood disorder

- ■ Acute abdomen
- ■ Cardiac or vascular symptoms
- For diagnosis or treatment outside the midwife's scope of practice

CARE OF THE WOMAN ON HORMONE REPLACEMENT THERAPY

Key Clinical Information

Hormone replacement therapy includes both estrogen replacement therapy (ERT) and combination hormone replacement therapy (HRT). For women with severe vasomotor symptoms associated with surgical or natural menopause, short-term low-dose HRT use (for less than 5 years) in the immediate postmenopausal period and in the absence of significant risk factors for breast cancer or heart disease can moderate symptoms while minimizing adverse effects.

HRT offers significant benefits to a carefully selected group of women, yet for other women poses considerable risk. Women who use long-term HRT have an increased risk of heart disease and breast cancer over women who decline HRT. Monotherapy with estrogen (ERT) is not recommended for women with an intact uterus due to the substantially elevated risk of endometrial cancer when compared with women who use combination HRT or women who decline HRT. In women with an intact uterus who use estrogen or estrogen-like substances, it is recommended that the estrogenic effects be balanced with progestin (combination therapy). Women who use combination HRT are also at greater risk for breast cancer, although this risk is small for women on short-term therapy and diminishes once therapy has been concluded (Institute for Clinical Systems Improvement [ICSI], 2008). Whereas an increase in cardiovascular events such coronary artery disease and stroke is associated with oral HRT, the use of low-dose transdermal estrogen moderates this risk (ICSI, 2008; Renoux, Dell'Aniello, Garbe, & Suissa, 2010).

Discussion of the risks, benefits, and alternatives to HRT, as well as each woman's personal indications and preferences, is an integral part of providing hormone therapy. Providing women with the most current information allows each woman the opportunity to make the best personal decision while being an active participant in this process. Other treatment modalities exist for the treatment of vasomotor symptoms, osteoporosis, and the physiologic changes associated with postmenopausal status.

Client History and Chart Review: Components of the History to Consider

(ICSI, 2008)

- Age
- Reproductive history
  - GP TPAL
  - Menstrual history
    - Current menstrual status
    - Age at menopause
    - Hysterectomy
  - Presence of vasomotor symptoms
    - Hot flashes
    - Night sweats
  - Symptoms related to estrogen decline
    - Sleep changes
    - Mood changes
    - Urinary changes
    - Skin changes
      - Development of fine lines
      - Increase in facial hair
      - Vaginal atrophy and dryness
    - Sexual changes
      - Diminished libido
      - Decreased lubrication
      - Dyspareunia
  - Reproductive cancers and disorders (e.g., leiomyomata)
- Review most recent results
  - Physical examination
  - Pap smear
  - Mammogram
  - Bone mineral density (BMD) testing
- Medical/surgical history
  - Allergies
  - Medications
  - Heart disease

- Coronary artery disease
- Hypertension
- Prior thromboembolus or thrombosis
  - Risk factors for osteoporosis (see "Care of the Woman at Risk for Osteoporosis")
  - Mood disorder
  - Gallbladder disease
  - Liver disease
- Family history
  - Osteoporosis
  - Heart disease
  - Alzheimer's disease
  - Colon cancer
  - Breast cancer
- Social history
  - Tobacco and alcohol use
  - Physical activity patterns
  - Nutritional status
  - Intimate partner violence
- Contraindications to HRT
  - History of estrogen-sensitive tumors
  - Breast cancer
  - Endometrial hyperplasia
  - Endometrial cancer
  - Hypertriglyceremia
  - Undiagnosed postmenopausal bleeding
  - Chronic liver disease
  - History of thromboembolus or thrombosis
  - Heart disease
- Review of systems (ROS)

Physical Examination: Components of the Physical Exam to Consider

- Vital signs, including blood pressure
- Height and weight
  - BMI
  - Height: Compare with previous measurements
- Thyroid
- Breast examination
  - Presence of masses
  - Documentation of contour
- Cardiopulmonary evaluation

- Pelvic examination
    - Genital atrophy or pallor
    - Uterine size and contour
    - Presence of masses
- Bony integrity
    - Range of motion
    - Arthritis
    - Kyphosis
- Rectal examination

Clinical Impression: Differential Diagnoses to Consider

(ICD9data.com, 2012)

- HRT
- Flushing
- Menopausal and postmenopausal disorders
- Sleep disturbance

Diagnostic Testing: Diagnostic Tests and Procedures to Consider

- Serum or salivary hormone levels
- Pap smear
- Blood lipid evaluation
- Electrocardiogram
- BMD testing
- Mammogram
- Pelvic ultrasound
- Postmenopausal women: Before initiation of HRT, consider the following steps:
    - Endometrial biopsy
    - Progestin challenge
        - Provera: 5–10 mg daily for 10 days
        - Anticipate withdrawal bleed within 10 days of completion of medication
        - If little or no bleeding, consider continuous HRT
        - If vigorous bleeding, consider cyclic HRT

Providing Treatment: Therapeutic Measures to Consider

- Indications for HRT
    - Severe vasomotor symptoms

- Osteoporosis: Consider nonhormonal therapies first
    - ASC-US Pap smear: Local therapy is preferred
    - Mood disturbance related to hormone changes: Consider other medications first
- Initiation of treatment regimens
    - Offer short-term therapy
    - Review benefits and harms
    - Link therapy with breast and coronary artery disease (CAD) screening
    - Use the lowest effective dose
    - Use progestin only in women with intact uteri
- Perimenopausal woman with moderate to severe vasomotor symptoms in whom contraception is needed
    - Combination hormonal contraceptives
        - Low-dose triphasic oral contraceptives
        - NuvaRing
        - Do not use in women who smoke and are 35 years or older
    - Progestogen: Depo-medroxyprogesterone acetate (DMPA)
        - 150 mg IM monthly
        - Oral 20 mg/day
    - Transdermal estrogen
- Abnormal Pap smear (ASC): Estrogen vaginal cream
- Transdermal estrogen
    - Estraderm 0.5 to 1.0 mg
    - Progestin not required with regular monthly menses
    - Add progestin when menses is irregular
        - Provera: 5–10 mg for 5–10 days
        - Prometrium: 200 mg at bedtime for 12 days
- Postmenopausal woman with an intact uterus
    - Continuous combination HRT
    - Use for as brief a period as possible
- CombiPatch (estradiol/norethindrone acetate transdermal system): Apply the patch at a twice-weekly interval

- Prempro (oral conjugated estrogens/progestin): Use the lowest effective dose
  - 0.3 mg/1.5 mg once PO daily
  - 0.45 mg/1.5 mg once PO daily
  - 0.625 mg/2.5 mg once PO daily
  - 0.625/5 once PO daily
- Estrogen: Daily
  - Conjugated estrogen: 0.3–0.625 mg
  - Estropipate: 0.625 mg
  - Esterified estrogen: 0.3–0.625 mg
  - Micronized estradiol: 0.5–1 mg
  - Transdermal estrogen: 0.05 mg
- Progestin: Daily—Provera 2.5 mg
- Cyclic HRT
  - Estrogen: days 1–25 of month
  - Dose range: 0.3–1.25 mg daily; varies with brand and indication
  - 0.625 mg is the lowest dose recommended to treat osteoporosis
- Plant-based estrogens
  - Estrace
  - Cenestin
  - Gynodiol
  - Estratab
  - Ogen
- Progestin use with cyclic estrogen
  - Provera: 5–10 mg for 5–10 days
  - Prometrium: 200 mg at bedtime for 12 days
  - Use progestin on days 11–25 to 16–25 of the cycle month
- Estrogen–androgen therapy
  - For decreased libido
  - Given cyclically (e.g., 3–4 weeks on, 1 week off)
  - Short-term therapy
  - Virilization may occur
  - Must use progestin in a client with an intact uterus
  - Products available
    - Esterified estrogen 0.625 mg/ methyltestosterone 1.25 mg
    - Esterified estrogen 1.25 mg/ methyltestosterone 2.5 mg

- Conjugated estrogen 0.625 mg/ methyltestosterone 5 mg
- Conjugated estrogen 1.25 mg/ methyltestosterone 10 mg

Providing Treatment: Complementary and Alternative Measures to Consider

- Use of bioidentical hormones
- Vitamin and mineral supplements
  - Calcium and magnesium supplementation
  - Vitamin E supplements: 400 IU BID with meals

Providing Support: Education and Support Measures to Consider

- Provide information for informed choice (ICSI, 2008), including the risks, benefits, and alternatives to HRT
- HRT recommendations
  - In perimenopause to early postmenopause
  - Short-term use
  - Indications for HRT
    - Osteoporosis
    - Significant vasomotor symptoms
- Limitations and risks of HRT, including the following increased risks:
  - Stroke
  - Breast cancer
  - Coronary artery disease
  - Thromboemboli
- Methods of HRT, dose, timing, and side effects
- Osteoporosis prevention and evaluation
- Provide medications instructions
  - Dose
  - Timing and method of use
  - Anticipated results
  - Warning signs and symptoms
- Reinforce need to return for evaluation in the following circumstances:
  - Unscheduled vaginal bleeding
  - Symptoms of complications related to HRT
- Dietary recommendations

- Limit intake of caffeine, fats, refined sugar, flour, and alcohol
- Increase intake of whole grains, dark leafy green vegetables, and sea vegetables
- Obtain protein from legumes, nuts, and seeds
- Recommended lifestyle changes
  - Smoking cessation
  - Regular exercise, rest, and relaxation
  - Support acceptance of life stage

Follow-up Care: Follow-up Measures to Consider

- Document
  - Indication for HRT
  - Discussions with the client
  - Treatment plan
- Return for evaluation
  - Three months after initiating HRT and/or estrogen replacement therapy
    - Weight and blood pressure
    - Reduction in symptoms
    - Bleeding patterns
    - Satisfaction with treatment
    - Concerns or unexpected side effects
  - Annual well-woman examination
  - Unanticipated or unscheduled vaginal bleeding
  - Breast changes

Multidisciplinary Practice: Consider Consultation, Collaboration, or Referral

- OB/GYN services
  - Symptoms that do not respond to standard HRT regimens
  - Unexplained or persistent vaginal bleeding
  - Gynecologic complications of HRT
- Medical services
  - Diagnosis of osteoporosis (see "Care of the Woman at Risk for Osteoporosis")
  - Signs or symptoms of heart disease, heart attack, or stroke
  - Medical complications of HRT

- Breast specialist: Breast mass or abnormal mammogram
- For diagnosis or treatment outside the midwife's scope of practice

CARE OF THE WOMAN INTERESTED IN AN INTRAUTERINE DEVICE OR INTRAUTERINE SYSTEM

Key Clinical Information

The intrauterine device and/or system (IUD/IUS) offers women a highly effective, reversible method of birth control that can be either hormonal or non-hormonal in nature. The ParaGard (Copper-T 380A) IUD is impregnated with copper and is effective for 10 years. The Mirena (LNG-IUS) releases the progestin levonorgestrel into the intrauterine cavity and is effective for 5 years. As with any method of birth control, careful evaluation to determine who is an appropriate candidate for this method is required. Benefits of IUD/IUS use include its effectiveness (more than 99%) and ease of use (Hatcher et al., 2011).

In a new mother, the IUD/IUS can be inserted immediately following birth of the placenta or as early as four weeks postpartum. While there is a higher expulsion rate with post-placental insertion, women can be lost to care when interval insertion is planned, or unintended pregnancy may occur in the interim. The ParaGard IUD, when inserted before resumption of sexual intercourse, offers breastfeeding women a reliable nonhormonal method of contraception.

The common IUD side effect of heavy bleeding can be minimized by insertion of the Mirena IUS; its continual release of a low dose of progestin thins the lining of the uterus and can be used to treat menorrhagia or dysmenorrhea (Fraser, 2010; Schuiling & Likis, 2013). Risks associated with IUD/IUS use include uterine perforation during or following insertion, increased risk of pelvic infection, greater incidence of ectopic pregnancy, and contraceptive failure secondary to IUD or IUS expulsion (Hatcher et al., 2011).

Client History and Chart Review: Components of the History to Consider

- Age
- GP TPAL
- Allergies
- Medications
- Medical/surgical history: An IUD/IUS is appropriate for women with the following conditions (ACOG, 2011a):
  - Diabetes
  - Thromboembolism (copper IUD)
  - Bleeding disorders or anticoagulant therapy (hormonal IUS)
  - Menorrhagia/dysmenorrhea (hormonal IUS)
  - Breastfeeding (prior to 6 weeks postpartum: copper IUD only)
  - Breast cancer (copper IUD)
  - Liver disease (copper IUD)
- Reproductive history
  - LMP or date of delivery
  - Contraceptive history and current use
  - Pap smear and/or human papillomavirus (HPV) history
  - STI diagnosis and treatment history
  - History of fibroids or unusual configuration of uterus
  - Menstrual history
- The ideal candidate for IUD/IUS use (ACOG, 2011a)
  - Low risk for STIs
  - Preference for long-term contraception
  - One or more full-term pregnancies
  - Comfortable with the thought of an IUD/IUS in her uterus
  - Able to check for the IUD/IUS string
- ⚠ Contraindications to IUD/IUS insertion (ACOG, 2011a; Hatcher et al., 2011)
  - Pregnancy
  - Unexplained vaginal bleeding
  - Genital tract infection
    - STIs
    - Pelvic inflammatory disease
    - Postpartum endometritis
    - Recent septic abortion
  - Untreated malignancy
    - Cervix
    - Endometrium
    - Molar pregnancy
    - Breast cancer
  - Distortion of the uterine cavity (i.e., fibroids)
- Before removal, determine the following:
  - Indication for removal
  - Birth control method desired, if any

Physical Examination: Components of the Physical Exam to Consider

- Physical examination as indicated by client history
  - Breast exam
  - Pelvic exam
- Before insertion
  - Obtain Pap smear and STI testing as needed
  - Perform a bimanual examination to determine the following:
    - Uterine size and contour
    - Uterine position
    - Involution if postpartum
  - Assess for presence of the following:
    - Cervical motion or adnexal tenderness
    - Cervical discharge
    - Genital tract lesions
    - Cervical friability
    - Uterine masses (fibroids)
  - Consider cervical priming for nulligravid women
    - Insertion of osmotic dilator 1 day before insertion *or*
    - Misoprostol 400 mg PO 4–12 hours before insertion
  - Speculum examination
  - Sound uterus: 6–9 cm depth is recommended
- Before removal
  - Speculum examination for visualization of strings
  - Based on indication for removal

Clinical Impression: Differential Diagnoses to Consider

(ICD9data.com, 2012)

- Contraceptive counseling, including use of an IUD
- Emergency contraceptive counseling
- IUD insertion
- IUD follow-up post procedure
- Surveillance of the IUD in situ
- IUD removal and/or reinsertion
- Complications of IUD insertion and use
  - Failed IUD insertion: Cervical stenosis
  - Discontinued procedure
    - Vasovagal syncope
    - Perforation of the uterus
  - Displaced IUD
  - Infection secondary to IUD
  - Menorrhagia, secondary to IUD in situ

Diagnostic Testing: Diagnostic Tests and Procedures to Consider

- Pregnancy testing
- Pap smear and/or HPV testing
- Chlamydia and gonorrhea testing
- Hepatitis profile
- HIV testing
- Other laboratory tests as indicated by health status
  - Blood glucose
  - Liver function tests

Providing Treatment: Therapeutic Measures to Consider

(Hatcher et al., 2011; Yen, Saah, & Hillard, 2010)

- Preprocedure prophylaxis
  - Misoprostol 400 mg PO or bucally 2–4 hours before the procedure
  - Ibuprofen 600 mg or naproxen sodium 550 mg PO 1–2 hours before the procedure
  - Paracervical or intracervical block using local anesthetic
    - Prevents pain with insertion
    - Reduces incidence of vagal response
- ⚠ Have atropine sulfate available for treatment of vagal response
  - Give IM when the IV route is not available
  - Give 0.4–0.6 mg IM for bradycardia (Varney et al., 2004)
- Antibiotic prophylaxis is not indicated
- Obtain informed consent
- Timing of insertion (Hatcher et al., 2011)
  - Immediately after abortion or delivery
  - Four to eight weeks postpartum
  - During menses
  - As emergency contraception (copper IUD only)
  - Anytime, as long as pregnancy is ruled out
- To sound uterus before insertion
  - Position tenaculum gently
    - Close slowly to decrease cramping
    - Position on the anterior lip for an anteverted uterus
    - Position on the posterior lip for a retroverted uterus
    - Avoid vessels at the 3 and 9 o'clock positions
  - Apply traction to tenaculum
    - Straighten uterine curvature
    - Gently insert a sterile sound until slight resistance is felt
      - ➤ Do not use force
      - ➤ Dilate the cervix if needed
    - Note the depth of the sound: 6–9 cm is recommended (Bayer HealthCare Pharmaceuticals, 2009; Duramed Pharmaceuticals, 2006b)
  - Use the sound to prepare the IUD/IUS insertion device per the manufacturer's instructions
- IUD insertion under sterile technique
  - Swab the cervix with an antiseptic solution (e.g., Betadine)
  - Load the IUD/IUS into the insertion device
  - Apply gentle traction to the tenaculum

- ◆ Straighten the uterine curvature
- ◆ Carefully place the IUD/IUS according to the manufacturer's instructions to avoid uterine perforation
- ◆ Remove the insertion device
  - ▪ Remove the tenaculum
  - ▪ Obtain hemostasis
    - ◆ Apply pressure to bleeding sites
    - ◆ Apply silver nitrate to bleeding sites (may cause cramping)
  - ▪ Trim strings to approximately 3–4 cm (1.5–2 in.) in length
  - ▪ A vagal response may occur during or after procedure and requires treatment (Varney et al., 2004)
    - ◆ Stop the procedure
    - ◆ Place the client in the Trendelenburg position
    - ◆ Administer smelling salts
    - ◆ Administer atropine sulfate 0.4–0.6 mg IM
- IUD/IUS removal
  - ▪ Swab the cervix with an antiseptic solution (e.g., Betadine)
  - ▪ Grasp the strings with ring forceps and pull gently but firmly
  - ▪ If the strings are not visible at the os
    - ◆ Probe cervical canal with sterile forceps, grasp the string or IUD/IUS if felt, and pull gently
    - ◆ If unable to identify IUD/IUS
      - ➤ Evaluate for presence of IUD/IUS with ultrasound
      - ➤ Removal under anesthesia may be required
  - ▪ Initiate another form of birth control as needed

Providing Treatment: Complementary and Alternative Measures to Consider

- Fertility awareness/natural family planning
- Outercourse
- Abstinence
- Withdrawal

- Natural spermicides
- Barrier methods

Providing Support: Education and Support Measures to Consider

- Review all birth control options appropriate for this woman
- Review her history with the client and her partner as needed
- Ascertain whether the client's health plan will cover the chosen method or whether the client can self-pay: Some companies offer assistance for economically disadvantaged women
- Discuss the risks, benefits, and effectiveness of IUD/IUS (Bayer HealthCare Pharmaceuticals, 2009; Duramed Pharmaceuticals, 2006b; Hatcher et al., 2011)
  - ▪ Risks
    - ◆ Uterine perforation or expulsion
    - ◆ Embedment in the uterus
    - ◆ Pelvic inflammatory disease
    - ◆ Ectopic pregnancy
    - ◆ Increased incidence of ovarian cysts (hormonal IUS)
  - ▪ Benefits
    - ◆ Effectiveness
      - ➤ Mirena: 99.9%
      - ➤ ParaGard: 99.2%
    - ◆ Use unrelated to sexual activity
    - ◆ May decrease menses and dysmenorrhea (hormonal IUS)
- Provide information
  - ▪ Preprocedure preparation
  - ▪ IUD/IUS cost
  - ▪ Details of insertion procedure
  - ▪ Potential side effects and complications
    - ◆ Signs and symptoms
    - ◆ When to call
    - ◆ How to call during off-hours
- Teach the client to feel the strings
  - ▪ After insertion
  - ▪ Before intercourse for the first cycle
  - ▪ After menses or monthly

Follow-up Care: Follow-up Measures to Consider

- Document insertion and/or removal (see the "Procedure Note" section)
- Return for care (Bayer HealthCare Pharmaceuticals, 2009; Duramed Pharmaceuticals, 2006b)
  - Two to six weeks post insertion or after next menses
  - With onset of the following conditions:
    - Fever, abdominal pain, or heavy bleeding
    - Malodorous vaginal discharge
    - Signs or symptoms of pregnancy
    - Inability to locate the IUD/IUS strings
    - Other significant side effects
  - Scheduled well-woman care
  - Exposure to STIs
  - Desired return to fertility
  - Scheduled IUD/IUS replacement
    - Five years for Mirena
    - Ten years for ParaGard
- IUD/IUS troubleshooting (Hatcher et al., 2011)
  - Cramping: Nonsteroidal anti-inflammatory drugs (NSAIDs)
  - Expulsion
    - Verify nonpregnant status
    - Insert a new IUD/IUS
  - Suspected uterine perforation
    - Ultrasound or CT to verify the IUD/IUS location
    - Refer for laparoscopy for intra-abdominal IUD/IUS
  - Positive pregnancy test
    - Confirm location of pregnancy
    - Remove IUD/IUS promptly: Decreases risk of spontaneous abortion due to IUD/IUS
    - Influenza-like illness may signal septic abortion
  - Suspected salpingitis
    - Treat empirically per current CDC recommendations
    - May leave IUD/IUS in situ
    - Male partner examination and treatment indicated

Multidisciplinary Practice: Consider Consultation, Collaboration, or Referral

- OB/GYN services
  - Relative contraindications for IUD/IUS insertion
    - Uterine anomalies
    - History of postpartum endometritis or pelvic inflammatory disease (PID) in past 3 months
  - For complications of IUD/IUS insertion
    - Difficulty sounding uterus
    - Perforation of uterus
  - Complications of IUD/IUS use
    - IUD/IUS strings not visible or palpated and removal of IUD/IUS is desired
    - Septic abortion with IUD/IUS in situ
    - PID with IUD/IUS in situ
- For diagnosis or treatment outside the midwife's scope of practice

CARE OF THE WOMAN INTERESTED IN PRECONCEPTION CARE

Key Clinical Information

Every well-woman visit with a woman of childbearing age provides an opportunity for preconception care. The planned preconception visit offers the midwife a chance to address the client's health needs that can affect pregnancy before pregnancy occurs. This type of client-initiated visit indicates a hunger for information related to preconceptual health, pregnancy and parenting resources, and labor and birth options. However, midwives should also seek information regarding pregnancy goals at routine gynecologic examinations so that preconception education can begin far in advance of pregnancy. This consideration is especially important given that half of all pregnancies are unintended, making a formal preconception visit unlikely for many women. Midwife-initiated screenings and discussions related to preconception care can spark awareness and interest in women not previously motivated to modify health behaviors before considering pregnancy. The woman may, in fact, choose to delay attempts at pregnancy until particular healthcare concerns are addressed and remediated. This option is especially important for women with chronic health conditions such as diabetes, seizure disorders, or hypertension; women with exposure to teratogens or toxic substances; and those women with genetic concerns.

Client History and Chart Review: Components of the History to Consider

(ACOG, 2008; Kent, Johnson, Curtis, Hood, & Atrash, 2006; March of Dimes, n.d.)

- Age
- Pregnancy history
  - GP TPAL
  - Outcome of previous pregnancies
    - Term births
    - Preterm births
    - Pregnancy losses
    - Infertility
- Gynecologic history
  - LMP
  - Length of cycle and menses
  - STIs or pelvic infections
  - HIV status
  - Abnormal Pap smears and cervical treatment
  - Most recent method of birth control
  - Female genital cutting (FGC) status
- Medical/surgical history
  - Immunization history
  - Oral health and dentition
  - Tattoos or body piercings
  - Usual weight and dietary patterns
  - Medical conditions, such as
    - Asthma
    - Diabetes
    - Heart disease
    - Hepatitis
    - HIV/AIDS
    - Hypothyroidism
    - Maternal phenylketonuria
    - Obesity
    - Rubella immune status
    - Seizure disorders
  - Previous surgery

- Medications and supplements
  - Antiepileptic drugs
  - Isotretinoins
  - Oral anticoagulants
  - Folic acid supplementation
  - Over-the-counter medications and supplements
  - Herbs
- Mental well-being
- Social history
  - Partner/family support
  - Substance abuse
  - Intimate-partner violence
  - Occupational hazards
    - Chemicals or toxins
    - Work hours or conditions
- Family history: Client and partner
  - Birth defects
  - Genetic disorders
  - Multiple births
  - Pregnancy losses
  - Familial health disorders
- Personal concerns
  - Readiness (self and partner)
  - Financial concerns
  - Partner and/or family concerns
  - Cultural considerations for childbearing
  - Health habits
    - Physical activity patterns
    - Assess for nutritional deficits
      - Eating disorders
      - Bariatric surgery
      - BMI extremes
      - Pica
      - Vegan diet
      - Lactose or gluten intolerance
      - Calcium or iron deficiency
- Review of systems (ROS)

Physical Examination: Components of the Physical Exam to Consider

- Complete physical examination as indicated by
  - History
  - Interval since last physical

- Primary focus
  - Appropriate weight for height
  - Thyroid
  - Breast examination
  - Gynecologic examination
  - Cardiopulmonary evaluation

Clinical Impression: Differential Diagnoses to Consider

(ICD9data.com, 2012)

- Preconception counseling
- Genetic counseling
- Genetic screening
- Other related screening
- General medical examination
- Additional diagnoses as indicated

Diagnostic Testing: Diagnostic Tests and Procedures to Consider

(ACOG, 2008, 2011b; Heath & Acevedo, 2000–2007)

- Tuberculosis testing
  - Purified protein derivative or Mantoux testing
  - Chest x-ray
- Cervicovaginal screening
  - Pap smear
  - Wet prep
  - Group B *Streptococcus* (GBS)
  - Chlamydia
  - Gonorrhea
- Blood tests
  - Complete blood count
  - Rubella titer
  - Hepatitis B and C titers
  - Blood type and Rh
  - Hematocrit and hemoglobin
  - Complete blood count
  - Thyroid-stimulating hormone (TSH) or thyroid panel
  - Toxoplasmosis screen
  - Varicella
  - HIV testing
  - VDRL or RPR

- Genetic studies
  - Genetic counseling
  - Cystic fibrosis screening for all women
- Additional screening of one or both partners
  - African heritage: Sickle cell anemia
  - Mediterranean heritage: β-Thalassemia
  - Southeast Asian or Chinese: α-Thalassemia
  - Jewish descent: Tay-Sachs disease and Canavan disease
- Other as indicated by history

Providing Treatment: Therapeutic Measures to Consider

(ACOG, 2008)

- Medical conditions
  - Adjust medications according to benefit/risk profile and potential effects on pregnancy
  - Consult for those medications and medical conditions outside the midwife's scope of practice
- Vitamin and mineral supplements (U.S. Preventive Services Task Force, 2009)
  - Folic acid 0.4–0.8 mg (400–800 mcg) PO daily
    - Begin 1 to 12 months before planned conception
    - Continue through at least 13 weeks' gestation
  - Consider multivitamin with or without iron
  - Women with previous child with neural tube defect
    - Consider the presence of a folic acid deficit
    - Folic acid 4 mg (4000 mcg) to 5 mg (5000 mcg) daily (Health Canada, 2010)
    - Include vitamin B_{12} supplement
    - Begin 1 to 3 months before conception
    - Continue through 3 months' gestation
- Update immunization status
  - Hepatitis B
  - HPV (women up to age 26)
  - Influenza

- Tetanus and diphtheria
- Avoid pregnancy for 1 month after administration of live virus vaccines
  - Varicella
  - Rubella

Providing Treatment: Complementary and Alternative Measures to Consider

- Healthy well-balanced diet
- Minerals and folic acid from the following sources:
  - Dietary sources
  - Organic prenatal vitamins
  - Supplements such as Floradix
- Fertility awareness methods for determining ovulation

Providing Support: Education and Support Measures to Consider

(ACOG, 2008; Heath & Acevedo, 2000–2007)

- Preconception counseling related to risk factors
  - Medications
  - Diabetes
  - Hypertension
  - Genetic disorders
  - Neural tube defects
  - Maternal age
  - HIV infection
  - Drug or alcohol use
- Pregnancy health risk awareness
  - Age-related risks
  - Hyperthermia from hot tubs
  - Toxoplasmosis
  - *Listeria*
  - Mercury from selected fish
  - Domestic violence
- Fertility awareness
  - Menstrual cycle and ovulation
  - Signs of fertility
  - Fertility charting
  - Postcontraception fertility rates
  - Signs of conception

- Health promotion
  - Weight goals and physical activity patterns
  - Nutrition: Protein, vitamins, minerals, and folate
  - Counseling regarding pertinent issues as determined by the client's history
  - Encourage dental work before conception
  - Avoidance of cigarettes, alcohol, and recreational drugs
  - Moderation in caffeine use (200 mg or less daily)
- Environmental concerns
  - Occupational hazards
  - Toxic chemicals
  - Radiation contamination
- Health concerns
  - Effects of maternal health on the developing fetus
  - Recommendations for optimal care
  - Pregnancy information and resources
  - Labor and birth options, locations, and services

Follow-up Care: Follow-up Measures to Consider

- Document care provided
- Return for the following reasons:
  - Reading of Mantoux test
  - Review of fertility charts
  - Onset of amenorrhea for HCG testing
  - Follow-up per recommendations
  - If pregnancy does not occur within 6–12 months
  - Questions or concerns

Multidisciplinary Practice: Consider Consultation, Collaboration, or Referral

- OB/GYN services
  - Infertility evaluation or treatment
  - Based on risk assessment
- Genetic counseling
- Social services
  - Substance abuse centers
  - Physical abuse
  - Psychosocial issues

- Nutritional risk assessment by a dietician
- Medical or perinatology services: Management of disease or illness
  - Diabetes
  - Hypertension
- For diagnosis or treatment outside the midwife's scope of practice

CARE OF THE WOMAN AT RISK FOR OSTEOPOROSIS

Key Clinical Information

Women, especially postmenopausal women and women who use Depo-Provera for an extended period of time (2 or more years), have an increased chance of developing osteoporosis as they age. Osteoporosis affects an estimated one in three women older than age 50. It is defined as a disorder of bone metabolism that is characterized by a decrease in the level of bone mass itself, resulting in bones that are more porous. This process leads to deterioration of the structural integrity of the bone and results in fragile bones that are prone to fracture with even minimal trauma.

Diagnosis of osteoporosis or osteopenia (the onset of bone loss at a lesser degree than occurs in osteoporosis) is made using bone mineral density (BMD) evaluation. All women with a history of a fracture after age 40 should consider BMD testing (National Osteoporosis Foundation, 2010). Osteoporosis is diagnosed when the BMD is more than 2.5 standard deviations (SD) below the mean. Measures to maintain bone mass and sustain muscle strength to support the bone include adequate calcium and vitamin D intake, regular weight-bearing physical activity, fall prevention, smoking cessation, and minimal or no alcohol use. Medical treatment of osteoporosis is aimed at both slowing the loss of bone demineralization and rebuilding bone mass (Schuiling & Likis, 2013).

Client History and Chart Review: Components of the History to Consider

(National Osteoporosis Foundation, 2010)

- Age

- Reproductive history
  - LMP, GP TPAL
  - Age at menarche
  - Age at menopause
  - Length of time post menopause or on Depo-Provera
  - Use of hormonal medications
    - Contraceptives
    - Replacement therapy
    - Herbs or plant extracts
  - Breastfeeding history
- History of screening
  - Previous BMD or Osteomark screening
  - Oral examinations and x-rays: Tooth loss may indicate osteoporosis
- Medical/surgical history
  - Allergies
  - Medications
  - Herbs, homeopathics, and nutritional supplements
  - Health conditions
    - Breast disorders
    - Gallbladder disease
    - Heart disease
- Risk factors for osteoporosis (National Osteoporosis Foundation, 2010)
  - History of fragility fracture
  - Sedentary lifestyle or immobility
  - Poor lifetime calcium intake
  - Postmenopausal status
  - White or Asian race
  - Small or thin frame or body size
  - Personal or family history of osteoporosis
  - Frequent falls
  - Cigarette smoker
  - Alcohol use (more than 7 oz/week)
  - History of estrogen deficiency
    - Medical or surgical oophorectomy
    - Premature menopause
    - Endocrine disorders leading to amenorrhea
    - Amenorrhea
      - Long-term breastfeeding
      - Anorexia
      - Extended Depo-Provera use

- Breast cancer treatment
  - ➤ Chemotherapy
  - ➤ Radiation
- Contributing factors for osteoporosis
  - ◆ High cola intake, especially during bone formation
  - ◆ Medications
    - ➤ Corticosteroids
    - ➤ Thyroxine
    - ➤ Heparin
    - ➤ Anticonvulsants
    - ➤ Methotrexate
    - ➤ Chemotherapy
  - ◆ Medical conditions
    - ➤ Cushing's disease
    - ➤ Hyperthyroidism
    - ➤ Hyperparathyroidism
    - ➤ Diabetes
    - ➤ Malignancy
    - ➤ Cerebral palsy
    - ➤ Multiple sclerosis
    - ➤ Major depression
- Assess for symptoms of osteoporosis in the following circumstances:
  - Complaints of back pain
  - Changes in posture or height
  - Fractures after perimenopausal period
  - Inability to perform activities of daily living
- Current prevention measures
  - Mineral supplementation
    - ◆ Vitamin D intake/sun exposure
    - ◆ Calcium intake
  - Weight-bearing exercise
  - Safety measures to prevent falls
- Health habits
  - Daily physical activity
  - Nutrition
  - Alcohol and tobacco use

Physical Examination: Components of the Physical Exam to Consider

- Vital signs
- Height, weight, and BMI: Compare to previous findings

- Musculoskeletal system
  - Presence of kyphosis ("dowager's hump")
  - Palpation of vertebrae for pain
  - Muscle strength
  - Posture and gait
- Evidence of increased risk for falls
  - Weakness or physical limitations
  - Diminished balance and coordination
  - Visual or auditory limitations
  - Cognitive limitations
- Other examination components as indicated by history

Clinical Impression: Differential Diagnoses to Consider

(ICD9data.com, 2012)

- Estrogen deficiency
- Kyphosis
- Osteopenia
- Osteoporosis, drug induced
- Osteoporosis, idiopathic
- Osteoporosis, postmenopausal

Diagnostic Testing: Diagnostic Tests and Procedures to Consider

- Serum vitamin D levels
- [www] Risk assessment with FRAX fracture risk assessment tool
- Biochemical markers of bone remodeling (Inverness Medical, n.d.)
  - Osteomark enzyme-linked immunosorbent assay (ELISA) testing
  - Urine or serum
  - Screens for bone collagen breakdown
  - Can be used to assess the effectiveness of treatment
- BMD testing: Dual x-ray absorptiometry (DXA) (National Osteoporosis Foundation, 2010)
  - Low radiation dose
  - T-score: Bone mass score in relation to young adult reference population
    - ◆ Normal: T-score of −1; less than 1 SD decrease in bone mass

- ◆ Osteopenia: T-score of –1 to –2.5; between 1 and 2.5 SD decrease in bone mass is associated with a twofold higher risk in fracture
- ◆ Osteoporosis: T-score less than –2.5; more than 2.5 SD decrease in bone mass is associated with a fourfold higher risk of fracture

Providing Treatment: Therapeutic Measures to Consider

(National Osteoporosis Foundation, 2010)

- Address pain issues that limit mobility
- Calcium and vitamin D therapy for women older than age 50
  - Calcium: 1200 mg daily
  - Vitamin D: 800–1000 international units (IU)
    - ◆ Titrate vitamin D supplementation based on serum levels
    - ◆ Maximum recommended vitamin D dose: 2000 IU
- Initiate fall prevention measures
  - Regular lifelong physical activity or exercise
  - Avoidance of tobacco use
  - Moderation of alcohol use
  - Fall risk assessment and education
  - 🕮 Physical or occupational therapy
    - ◆ Weight-bearing aerobic activities for the skeleton
    - ◆ Postural training
    - ◆ Progressive resistance training for muscle and bone strengthening
    - ◆ Stretching for tight soft tissues and joints
    - ◆ Balance training
- Osteoporosis treatment is initiated for postmenopausal women who meet the following criteria:
  - A hip or vertebral (clinical or morphometric) fracture
  - T-score ≤ –2.5 at the femoral neck or spine after evaluation for secondary causes

- T-score between –1.0 and –2.5 at the femoral neck or spine (low bone mass) *and*
  - ◆ A 10-year probability of a hip fracture ≥ 3% *or*
  - ◆ A 10-year probability of a major osteoporosis-related fracture ≥ 20% (www based on WHO algorithm [FRAX])
- Clinician's judgment and/or patient preferences may indicate treatment for people with 10-year fracture probabilities above or below these levels
- For women with no contraindications to hormone therapy
  - Single or combination hormone therapy (see "Care of the Woman on Hormone Replacement Therapy")
  - Short-term therapy (less than 5 years)
  - Weigh benefits versus risks
  - Consider nonhormonal treatments
- Nonhormonal treatment
  - Bisphosphonates
    - ◆ Alendronate (Fosamax)
      - ➤ Osteopenia: 5 mg PO every day, or 35 mg/week
      - ➤ Osteoporosis: 10 mg PO every day, or 70 mg/week
      - ➤ Fosamax plus D contains 2800 or 5600 IU vitamin D
    - ◆ Ibandronate sodium (Boniva)
      - ➤ 2.5 mg PO daily, or 150 mg PO monthly
      - ➤ Requires 60-minute upright posture and fast after administration
      - ➤ Also available as 3 mg dose given IV every 3 months
    - ◆ Risedronate (Actonel)
      - ➤ 5 mg PO daily, or 35 mg/week
      - ➤ Actonel with Ca[1] for weekly dosing includes Actonel 35 mg (1 tablet) plus calcium carbonate 1250 mg (6 tablets)
      - ➤ Monthly dosing
        - ▸ 75 mg PO 2 consecutive days per month *or*
        - ▸ 150 mg PO once per month

- May cause irritation of upper gastrointestinal mucosa
- Contraindications
  - Esophageal abnormalities that delay esophageal emptying (e.g., stricture or achalasia)
  - Inability to stand or sit upright for 30–60 minutes
  - Hypocalcemia or hypercalcemia
  - Creatinine clearance rate of 30–35 mL/min
- Instructions
  - Take upon arising after 6- to 8-hour fast
  - Swallow whole with 6–8 oz plain water
  - Remain upright and fasting for 30–60 minutes
  - Medications or dietary supplements may be taken after 60 minutes
  - Avoid simultaneous use with aspirin or NSAIDs
  - Take adequate calcium and vitamin D
  - Report the following symptoms:
    - Gastrointestinal symptoms
    - Bone, joint, or muscle pain
- Zoledronic acid (Reclast)
  - 5 mg IV once per year (treatment)
  - 5 mg IV once every 2 years (prevention)
  - Administer over 15 minutes or more
  - Approved for treatment of individuals on steroid therapy
  - Increased incidence of atrial fibrillation compared to other bisphosphonates
- Selective estrogen receptor modulator: Raloxifene (Evista) 60 mg PO daily
  - Contraindications
    - History of deep vein thrombosis
    - Liver disease
    - Cholestyramine use
  - Side effects
    - May cause hot flashes and blood clots
    - Lowers risk of breast cancer in at-risk women

- Carries a lower risk of endometrial cancer than estrogen
  - Instructions: Discontinue use at least 72 hours before surgery
- Calcitonin-salmon (Miacalcin, Calcimar, Fortical)
  - For women who are more than 5 years post menopause
  - 200 units intranasally daily *or*
  - 50–100 IU IM or SC every other day
- Parathyroid hormone (teriparatide)
  - 20 mcg SC daily
  - Supplied in 28-dose delivery system
  - ⚠ Contraindications
    - Inability to perform self-injection
    - Primary or secondary malignancy of bone
    - Prior radiation therapy of bone
    - Hypercalcemia
    - Paget's disease of bone, as this medication may increase the risk of osteosarcoma
  - Side effects
    - Orthostatic hypotension
    - Muscle spasms
    - Nausea and vomiting
  - Instructions
    - Administer per the manufacturer's instructions
    - Refrigerate the medication
    - The client should sit or recline if orthostatic hypotension develops
    - Treatment period should last less than 2 years

Providing Treatment: Complementary and Alternative Measures to Consider

(National Osteoporosis Foundation, 2010)

- Nutritional support
  - High-calcium foods (see "A Nutritional Primer")
  - Vitamin and mineral supplements

- Isoflavones
  - ◆ Soy
  - ◆ Red clover
  - ◆ Prunes (Hooshmand, Chai, Saadat, Payton, Brummel-Smith, & Arimandi, 2011)
  - ◆ Omega-6 fatty acids
- Sunlight exposure for vitamin D synthesis
  - Use sunscreen on the hands and face
  - Minimum 10 minutes daily
- Improve or maintain balance and strength
- Acupuncture
- Stress reduction
  - Biofeedback
  - Yoga or meditation

Providing Support: Education and Support Measures to Consider

- Provide information
  - Calcium sources and intake (see "A Nutritional Primer")
  - Physical activity options
- Regular lifelong physical activity or exercise
  - Maintains strength, balance, and agility
  - Benefits overall health
  - Weight-bearing physical activities
    - ◆ Walking
    - ◆ Dancing
    - ◆ Tai-Chi
    - ◆ Stairs
    - ◆ Tennis
    - ◆ Yoga
    - ◆ Rocker board
  - Muscle-strengthening physical activities
    - ◆ Weight-training
    - ◆ Swimming
    - ◆ Vacuuming
    - ◆ Gardening
- Fall prevention measures
  - Address visual or auditory deficits
  - Evaluate neurologic status
  - Review medications for side effects affecting balance

- Provide a checklist for fall safety measures that can be implemented at home or at work
- Recognition of limitations
  - Ask for and accept help
  - Use mechanical devices as needed
    - ◆ Cane or walker for balance
    - ◆ Reaching tools
    - ◆ Shower chair
- Identify modifiable risks
  - Lifestyle factors
  - Fall risks
    - ◆ Throw rugs
    - ◆ Uneven or slippery surfaces
    - ◆ Lack of grab bars
    - ◆ Balance issues
- Formulate a prevention plan
  - Risk reduction actions
  - Access to help in case of a fall
  - Screening or treatment
  - Follow-up plan
- Community preventive health programs
  - Smoking cessation
  - Alcoholics Anonymous
  - Exercise programs and opportunities
- Avoid or limit use of the following substances:
  - Tobacco
  - Alcohol
  - Caffeine
  - Phosphorus-containing soft drinks (i.e., colas)

Follow-up Care: Follow-up Measures to Consider

- Document
  - Care provided
  - Screening results
  - Recommendations
- Reevaluate for modifiable osteoporosis risk factors
  - Medication use
  - Smoking
  - Alcohol use
  - Physical activity patterns
  - Changes in physical strength and balance
- Review risk status during well-woman examination

- BMD testing at 1- to 2-year intervals
- Women undergoing treatment: Monitor effectiveness of the treatment
  - Central DXA
  - Quantitative computed tomography (QCT densitometry)
  - Biochemical markers of bone turnover (urinary or serum assays)

Multidisciplinary Practice: Consider Consultation, Collaboration, or Referral

- OB/GYN, medical, orthopedic, or endocrine services: Treatment for osteoporosis
- Physical or occupational therapy
  - Assess for risk of falls
    - Strengthening program
    - Balance improvement program
  - Ability to maintain activities of daily living
- Social services
  - Smoking cessation
  - Alcohol treatment program
- Nutritionist: Evaluation of dietary status
- For diagnosis or treatment outside the midwife's scope of practice

CARE OF THE WOMAN WITH PERIMENOPAUSAL OR POSTMENOPAUSAL BLEEDING

Key Clinical Information

Perimenopausal bleeding and postmenopausal bleeding (collectively known as PMB) require a thorough directed history and evaluation of the genital tract for cervical, vaginal, and endometrial causes of bleeding. Causes of PMB may include hormone use, polyps, fibroids, trauma, and malignant or premalignant genital tract lesions (Burbos et al., 2010; Menzies et al., 2011). Midwives who have expanded their skill set after obtaining their basic education can perform the two recommended initial diagnostic tests for abnormal uterine bleeding—that is, office-based endometrial biopsy and transvaginal ultrasound. In women with abnormal uterine bleeding, an endometrial thickness of less than 5 mm excludes endometrial cancer, while a thickness of greater than 5 mm requires further diagnostic testing (Menzies et al., 2011).

The perimenopausal period is a time of transition that typically lasts 2 to 4 years. During this time, fluctuations in hormone levels can result in heavy or irregular menses so frequently that they are considered normal. Menstrual irregularity can have a significant effect on women's productivity, physical and social well-being, and sexual function. Hormone imbalance is the most common cause of perimenopausal bleeding; if necessary, it can be treated with cyclical hormone therapy or herbal support. Persistent perimenopausal bleeding requires further evaluation for nonhormonal causes such as fibroids, uterine polyps, or endometrial cancer.

Use of natural estrogen precursors or estrogen-containing products for the treatment of menopausal symptoms can result in PMB. Women should be encouraged to report any unexpected or unusual bleeding. Recurrent PMB bleeding is also frequently associated with endometrial cancer. Cyclic use of a progestin can diminish the growth of the endometrium in women with intact uteri using estrogen or an estrogen-like product (Burbos et al., 2010). When prescribed for clinical indications, the use of combination HRT decreases risk of endometrial cancer as compared with both nonhormone users and those women with a uterus who take only estrogen. Endometrial cancer is diagnosed in approximately 10% of women with PMB and often remains undetected until abnormal bleeding occurs (Burbos et al., 2010; Menzies et al., 2011). When found early, cancer of the endometrium is highly treatable.

Client History and Chart Review: Components of the History to Consider

- Age
- Reproductive history
  - GP TPAL
  - LMP or age at menopause
  - Presenting symptoms
    - Onset, duration, and severity of bleeding

- Bleeding intervals
  - Random
  - Cyclic
  - Postcoital
  - Isolated or recurrent
- Amount, consistency, and color of bleeding
- Other accompanying symptoms
  - Pain and cramping
  - Diarrhea
  - Backache
  - Respiratory symptoms
- Medical history
  - Diabetes
  - Clotting dysfunction
    - Coagulopathy
    - Liver disorder
  - Endocrine disorders
    - Thyroid
    - Polycystic ovary syndrome (PCOS)
  - Heart disease
- Medication and supplement use
  - Tamoxifen therapy
  - Estrogen replacement therapy
  - Hormone replacement therapy
  - Aspirin or anticoagulant use
  - Estrogen precursors
- Factors contributing to PMB (American Cancer Society, 2007; Burbos et al., 2010)
  - Early menarche
  - Late menopause
  - Nulliparous status
  - Infertility
  - Polycystic ovary syndrome
  - Estrogen-producing tumors
  - Dietary estrogen precursors
  - Diabetes
  - Hereditary non-polyposis colorectal cancer
  - Hypertension
  - Increasing age
  - Obesity
  - Tamoxifen use

- Thyroid disorders
- Previous or current breast cancer
- Family history
  - Northern European
  - North American
- Review of systems (ROS)
  - Jaundice
  - Easy bruising
  - Abdominal enlargement
  - Persistent cough

Physical Examination: Components of the Physical Exam to Consider

- Vital signs, including blood pressure, weight, height, and BMI
- Speculum examination
  - Blood in vaginal vault
  - Appearance of the cervix
  - Presence of lesions or masses
- Bimanual examination
  - Uterine size and contour
  - Cervical contour
  - Adnexal masses
  - Presence of pain
  - Firmness and mobility of reproductive organs
- Inguinal lymph nodes
- Rectovaginal examination
  - Confirm pelvic examination
  - Evaluate the posterior pelvis
  - Check for masses
  - Assess the mobility of tissues

Clinical Impression: Differential Diagnoses to Consider

(ICD9data.com, 2012)

- Perimenopausal vaginal bleeding
- Postmenopausal vaginal bleeding
- Endometrial hyperplasia
- Endometrial hyperplasia, with atypia
- Uterine fibroid, location unspecified
- Uterine polyp

Diagnostic Testing: Diagnostic Tests and Procedures to Consider

(Burbos et al., 2010)

- Pelvic ultrasound
  - Routes
    - Transvaginal
    - Transuterine (sonohysterography)
    - Abdominal
  - Evaluation of endometrial stripe: A visible stripe less than 5 mm is considered within normal limits
- Histology
  - Endometrial biopsy
  - Endometrial curettage (D&C)
  - Sonohysterography with biopsy
  - Hysteroscopy with biopsy
- Pap smear
- Complete blood count (CBC)
- Clotting studies

Providing Treatment: Therapeutic Measures to Consider

- Perimenopausal bleeding (see "Care of the Woman with Dysfunctional Uterine Bleeding")
  - Nonhormonal therapies
    - NSAIDs
    - Tranexanic acid
  - Combination hormone therapy (see "Care of the Woman Interested in Hormonal Contraceptives")
  - Progesterone hormone therapy
    - Mirena IUS
    - Cyclic progestin therapy
  - Surgical therapies
    - Endometrial ablation
    - Hysterectomy
- Consult or refer for treatment of malignancy
- Treatment of endometrial cancer (American Cancer Society, 2007)
  - Hysterectomy

- Oophorectomy
- Pelvic lymph nodes for staging
- Additional surgery may be required
- Radiation therapy
- Chemotherapy

Providing Treatment: Complementary and Alternative Measures to Consider

- ⚠️ The use of alternative therapies should not delay evaluation and treatment of the client with PMB.
- Support during irregular perimenopausal bleeding: Red raspberry leaf tea
- Nutritional support for healing
  - Healthy balanced low-fat diet
    - Maintain healthy BMI
    - Increase dietary intake of
      - Whole grains
      - Legumes, including soy
      - Vitamins C and E
      - Antioxidant foods, such as blueberries and green tea
      - Omega-3 fatty acids
      - Live-culture yogurt
    - Avoid hormone-containing foods:
      - Meats and poultry
      - Dairy products
  - Herbal support (Sallamander Concepts, 1998–2011)
    - Alfalfa
    - Astragalus root
    - Chamomile
    - Garlic
- Avoid herbs that may decrease clotting ability for 7–14 days before surgery (Sallamander Concepts, 1998–2011)
  - Astragalus
  - Feverfew
  - Garlic
  - Ginseng
  - Ginkgo

- Acupuncture
- Emotional immune support
  - Laughter
  - Visualization
  - Meditation
  - Prayer

Providing Support: Education and Support Measures to Consider

- Discussion of the following topics:
  - Potential significance of symptoms
  - Need for diagnostic workup
  - Results
    - ◆ Physical examination
    - ◆ Diagnostic testing
  - Referrals and ongoing care
  - Options for support services
- Active listening
  - Client fears and concerns
  - Questions
  - Preferences for care

Follow-up Care: Follow-up Measures to Consider

- Document
  - Clinical findings
  - Discussions and teaching
  - Client preferences
  - Plan for ongoing care
  - Referrals
- Offer continued support, as appropriate
- Assess for the following conditions:
  - Depression
  - Altered self-image
  - Barriers to healing
- Offer encouragement
  - Positive attitude
  - Use of healing modalities
- Return visits based on the following criteria:
  - Diagnosis and treatment needs
  - Client need for support
  - Scope of practice

Multidisciplinary Practice: Consider Consultation, Collaboration, or Referral

- OB/GYN services
  - Evaluation of persistent perimenopausal or postmenopausal bleeding
  - Diagnosis of the following conditions:
    - ◆ Endometrial atypia
    - ◆ Endometrial hyperplasia
    - ◆ Endometrial cancer
- Support services
  - Social services
  - Nutritionist
  - Support groups
- For diagnosis or treatment outside the midwife's scope of practice

CARE OF THE WOMAN IN NEED OF SMOKING CESSATION

Key Clinical Information

Approximately 19.6% of working adult Americans older than age 18 are cigarette smokers (CDC, 2012). Smoking significantly increases preventable risks associated with cancer, heart and lung disease, stroke, and early death (CDC, 2008; National Cancer Institute, 2011). Cigarette smoking is addictive both physically and psychologically. Women who succeed at smoking cessation demonstrate a determination to quit. Success can be enhanced by offering effective methods of treating the physical symptoms of nicotine withdrawal, by providing emotional support, and by cultivating positive coping skills and habits. The midwife's caring, concern, and counseling can be critical components in a woman's decision to quit smoking and persistence in remaining tobacco free. Asking about smoking is the first step in identifying individuals who smoke and initiating a brief intervention.

Client History and Chart Review: Components of the History to Consider

(Fiore et al., 2008)

- Reproductive status: Pregnant women are encouraged to quit without medications

- Smoking history and assessment
  - When and why started
  - Packs per day
  - Current desire to quit
  - Prior attempts to quit
- Personal and/or family medical history
  - Diabetes
  - Heart disease
    - Coronary artery disease
    - Elevated cholesterol
    - Hypertension
  - Respiratory disorders
    - Asthma
    - Chronic cough
    - Bronchitis
    - Chronic obstructive pulmonary disease
    - Emphysema
  - Seizure disorders
- Mental health disorders
  - Eating disorders
  - Depression
  - Bipolar disorder
  - Psychosis
- Medication use
  - Antihypertensive medications
  - Seizure medications
  - Estrogen products
    - Oral contraceptives
    - Hormone replacement therapy
  - Antidepressants
    - Wellbutrin (same as Zyban)
    - Monoamine oxidase (MAO) inhibitors
- Social history
  - Partner/family support
  - Coping skills
  - Stress levels
  - Work environment
  - Other smokers in the family
- Personal factors
  - Assessment of nicotine dependence
  - Coping skills
  - Weight gain
- Review of systems (ROS)

Physical Examination: Components of the Physical Exam to Consider

- Vital signs
- Height, weight, and BMI
- Note the presence or absence of a tobacco odor
- Perform an exam as indicated by
  - History and review of systems
  - Interval since last examination
- Cardiopulmonary system
  - Blood pressure and carotid pulses
  - Heart rate and rhythm
  - Evaluation of heart sounds
  - Lung fields
  - Respiratory rate
- Integumentary system: Note tobacco staining on the fingers

Clinical Impression: Differential Diagnoses to Consider

(ICD9data.com, 2012)

- Tobacco dependence
- Preventive medicine counseling and risk factor reduction intervention services
- Medical diagnosis codes as appropriate
- Healthcare Common Procedure Coding System (HCPCS [Medicare]) codes (American College of Physicians, 2005): Smoking cessation counseling
  - 3–10 minutes
  - > 10 minutes

Diagnostic Testing: Diagnostic Tests and Procedures to Consider

- Lipid profile
- Electrocardiogram (ECG)
- Chest x-ray

Providing Treatment: Therapeutic Measures to Consider

(Fiore et al., 2008)

- www. Brief interventions
  - 1–3 minutes

- Ask about or otherwise assess the client's readiness to quit
- Advise the client using a clear, strong personal message
- Agree on a goal with the client to
  - Set a quit date
  - Tell her social group and engage their support
  - Anticipate challenges
  - Seek out smoke-free environments
- Assist with quitting and offer medication
- Arrange follow-up
  - Problem-solving/skills training
    - Identify smoking triggers
    - Develop coping skills
  - Inquire about quitting process
  - Provide encouragement
- Motivational interview techniques
  - Express empathy
  - Highlight the discrepancy between the client's behavior and priorities
  - Use reflection if the client expresses resistance
  - Support self-efficacy
  - Find the personal relevance in quitting
  - Personalize the smoking-related risk
  - Engage the client in identifying the rewards of quitting
- Varenicline (Chantix)
  - First-line prescription medication
  - Pregnancy Category C: Not recommended
  - Reduces symptoms associated with smoking cessation
  - Decreases the urge to smoke
  - Decreases nicotine cravings
  - Can cause vivid, disturbing dreams and depression
  - Begin 1 week before the "stop smoking" date
  - Dosage
    - Days 1–3: 0.5 mg PO daily
    - Days 4–7: 0.5 mg PO BID
    - Day 8 to end of treatment: 1 mg PO BID

- Bupropion HCl (Zyban)
  - First-line prescription medication
  - Pregnancy Category C: Not recommended
  - 150 mg PO for 3 days, then 150 BID with 8 hours between doses
  - Stop smoking within 1–2 weeks of initiation
  - May use with nicotine medications
  - Contraindicated for women who meet the following criteria:
    - Eating disorders
    - Seizures
    - Prescribed use of Wellbutrin or MAO inhibitors
- Nortriptyline
  - Second-line medication
  - Pregnancy Category D: Not recommended
  - Starting dose: 25 mg/day
  - Usual dose: 75 mg/day
  - Titrate to serum level 50–150 ng/mL
- Clonidine
  - Second-line medication
  - Off-label use
  - Pregnancy Category C: Not recommended
  - Usual dose: 0.10–0.20 mg PO or transdermal
  - Begin up to 3 days before quit date
- Nicotine-containing medications
  - Pregnancy Category D: Not recommended
  - Provide informed consent
  - Nicoderm or Habitrol
    - 7 mg/24 hours, 14 mg/24 hours, or 21 mg/24 hours
    - Begin with 21- or 14-mg patch
    - Use 2–6 weeks, then decrease dose
    - Repeat with decreased dose
  - Nicotrol step-down patch (transdermal)
    - 5–15 mg/16-hour patch *or*
    - Use during waking hours
  - Nicorette gum
    - 2 mg or 4 mg strength
    - Use 2 mg if less than one pack per day smoker
    - Maximum: 24 pieces/day

- Nicotrol NS, inhaler
  - 0.5 mg/spray or 10 mg/cartridge inhaler
  - One to two doses per hour

Providing Treatment: Complementary and Alternative Measures to Consider

- Herbal support: Lobelia
- 🌐 Engage in learning positive coping skills
  - Avoid situations that increase the desire to smoke
  - Keep gum or healthy "finger foods" available for oral satisfaction
  - Increase physical activity
- Behavior modification techniques

Providing Support: Education and Support Measures to Consider

- Review smoking cessation benefits
- Provide clear medication instructions
- Bupropion HCl
  - May treat concomitant depression
  - May decrease appetite
  - Absence of negative sexual side effects
  - ⚠ May cause medication interactions
- Nicotine-containing medications
  - Stop smoking before or with onset of use
  - Use lower dose in the following individuals:
    - Coronary artery disease history
    - Body weight less than 100 lb
  - Patches
    - Apply new patch daily
    - Place the patch on the upper torso or arm
    - Do not reuse skin sites for at least 1 week
    - Apply a new patch each 24 hours
- Nortriptyline
  - May treat concomitant depression
  - Potential side effects
    - Dry mouth
    - Sedation
    - Cardiac arrhythmias
    - Decreased libido

- Counsel as determined by history and readiness to change
  - Encourage regular physical exercise
  - Provide nutrition information
  - Provide support for quitting
- Provide information
  - Local resources for developing healthy coping mechanisms
  - Smoking support groups

Follow-up Care: Follow-up Measures to Consider

- Document
  - Discussions and education
  - Client plan for smoking cessation
- Revisit 2 weeks after the smoking cessation start date
  - Client support and counseling
  - Evaluation
    - Current smoking patterns
    - Blood pressure and weight changes
    - Symptoms or side effects of medication
    - Assess for signs of depression or suicidal ideation
    - Confirm continued desire to be smoke free
    - Explore challenges and successes

Multidisciplinary Practice: Consider Consultation, Collaboration, or Referral

- Medical services
  - Cardiopulmonary history
  - Adverse medication reaction
  - Onset of cardiac symptoms with use of nicotine-containing medications
- Mental health service: Exacerbation or onset of depression symptoms
- Social services
  - Smoking cessation support services in the local community
    - American Cancer Society
    - American Lung Association
    - Public Health Department
  - Other services as necessary to address social issues

- For diagnosis or treatment outside the midwife's scope of practice

CARE OF THE WOMAN WITH AN UNINTENDED PREGNANCY

Key Clinical Information

Women experience unintended or unwanted pregnancies because of many factors, such as birth control failure, issues of access to reproductive services or education, impaired judgment or cognitive ability, poor self-image resulting in limited contraceptive or sexual negotiating skills, and sexual coercion or assault. The role of the midwife is to provide sound, unbiased information regarding reproductive choices and supportive, nonjudgmental care that allows each woman the opportunity to make an informed personal decision when confronted with this difficult situation (American College of Nurse–Midwives [ACNM], 2011).

Many women will come to terms with their unintended pregnancy and become mothers, adapting their lives to all the changes that this pregnancy brings. A few women will continue their unplanned pregnancies and make plans to relinquish the infant for adoption. Other women opt for early termination of unplanned pregnancies. Each woman's decision to continue or terminate a pregnancy has both short- and long-term emotional, financial, and social consequences.

Adoption options range from traditional "closed record" adoptions, in which the infant is removed from the mother immediately after birth, to "open adoption," in which the birth mother has more control over the process. During open adoptions, the birth mother may meet the prospective parent(s) to determine whether she deems them suitable for her child. The adoptive parents may be present for the birth and may receive the infant directly from the birth mother shortly after the birth. Open adoption allows the mother the potential to have future contact with her child and provides adoptive parents with information such as the birth parents' medical and family histories. In all forms of adoption, a post-adoption waiting period is typical to allow the birth mother an opportunity to review her choice before it becomes legally binding.

Early termination of pregnancy offers women another choice for unplanned pregnancy. Medical abortion using mifepristone is approved by the U.S. Food and Drug Administration (FDA) for women less than 49 days from the LMP (FDA, 2011). It offers women the opportunity to end pregnancy without undergoing a surgical procedure and is successful in 95–98% of cases (FDA, 2005). Surgical abortion represents an option for women who desire termination of pregnancy beyond 8 weeks' gestation or prefer the timeliness and efficacy (99–100% effectiveness) of surgical abortion.

Participation in pregnancy termination procedures by the midwife is a highly individual choice often based on the midwife's moral and ethical values and her beliefs regarding women's right to reproductive choice (ACNM, 2011). The process for expanding midwifery practice to include abortion services follows the ACNM Standards for the Practice of Midwifery (ACNM, 2011). In many states, abortion services are limited by statute to physician-provided services.

Client History and Chart Review: Components of the History to Consider

(Hatcher et al., 2011)

- Age
- Pregnancy history
  - GP TPAL
  - Verify pregnancy
    - LMP and cycle history
    - Date of conception, if known
    - Most recent method of birth control
    - Date of pregnancy test
    - Signs and symptoms of pregnancy
  - Blood type and Rh factor, if known
- Gynecologic history
  - STI screening and results
  - Last Pap smear and examination
  - Gynecologic procedures

- Medical/surgical history
  - Allergies
  - Medications—prescription and OTC
  - Medical conditions, such as
    - Asthma
    - Inflammatory bowel disease
    - Seizure disorders
    - Cardiac valvular disease
    - Bleeding disorders
  - Family history of genetic disorders
  - Prior surgery
- Social issues
  - Feelings about pregnancy
  - Personal support systems
  - Financial concerns regarding pregnancy options
  - Cultural considerations affecting response to pregnancy
  - Drug, alcohol, and tobacco use
  - Sexual coercion or rape
  - Mental health concerns
  - Tentative plans regarding pregnancy
- Contraindications to medical abortion
  - Allergy to medication
  - Confirmed or potential ectopic pregnancy
  - IUD in situ
  - Potential for noncompliance with required follow-up
  - Presence of significant medical problems
    - Chronic adrenal failure
    - Bleeding disorders or anticoagulant therapy
    - Long-term corticosteroid therapy
    - Inherited porphyria
  - Refusal to follow up with definitive surgical treatment if medical treatment fails

Physical Examination: Components of the Physical Exam to Consider

- Vital signs
- Speculum and bimanual examination
  - Cervical discharge
  - Uterine size, position, contour, and consistency
  - Presence of adnexal mass
  - Presence of cervical motion tenderness
  - Estimate of gestational age
- Other evaluations as indicated by history

Clinical Impression: Differential Diagnoses to Consider

(ICD9data.com, 2012)

- Pregnancy examination with immediate confirmation
- Pregnancy examination or test, pregnancy unconfirmed
- Legally induced abortion without complication
- Legally induced abortion with complication

Diagnostic Testing: Diagnostic Tests and Procedures to Consider

(Hatcher et al., 2011)

- Serum or urine human chorionic gonadotropin (HCG)
- Complete blood count, or hematocrit and hemoglobin
- Screening for genital tract infections
  - Bacterial vaginosis
  - Candidiasis
  - Trichomoniasis
  - Chlamydia
  - Gonorrhea
- Blood type and Rh screen
- Pelvic ultrasound
  - Vaginal or abdominal
  - Rule out ectopic pregnancy
  - Estimate gestational age
- Genetic testing

Providing Treatment: Therapeutic Measures to Consider

For the woman choosing to maintain her pregnancy and parent her child, see "Care of the Woman During Pregnancy."

For the woman choosing to maintain her pregnancy and relinquish her child, see "Care of the Woman During Pregnancy" and refer her to an adoption agency.

For the woman who is undecided, counsel her regarding her options and schedule a return visit within a week.

For the woman who requests a medical or surgical termination of pregnancy:

- Obtain informed consent
- Initiate treatment as needed for genital tract infection
- Remove IUD/IUS, if one is present
- FDA-approved regimen for medical abortion through 49 days post-LMP (FDA, 2011; Hatcher et al., 2011; Mackenzie & Yeo, 1997)
  - ■ 🕐 Verify surgical coverage
    - ◆ Client preferences
    - ◆ Retained products of conception (POC)
  - ■ ⚠ Obtain informed consent
  - ■ Prophylactic antibiotics are not indicated
  - ■ Day 1: Mifepristone administration
    - ◆ Dose: 600 mg PO in the presence of the provider
    - ◆ Observation for 30 minutes
    - ◆ Provide for pain relief
      - ➤ Acetaminophen
      - ➤ Acetaminophen with codeine
      - ➤ Nonsteroidal anti-inflammatory drugs
        - ▶ Compatible with mifepristone
        - ▶ Provide significant pain relief
  - ■ Day 3: Misoprostol administration
    - ◆ Dose: 400 mg PO in the presence of the provider
    - ◆ Observe for 4 hours (expulsion of POC occurs during this time in 60% of clients)
    - ◆ Send tissue to pathology for verification of POC
    - ◆ Provide RhIG if indicated: One dose (full or mini) post abortion
  - ■ Day 14: Post treatment
    - ◆ Client returns to confirm complete expulsion of POC
    - ◆ Suction aspiration offered for retained POC
- The safety and effectiveness of other mifepristone dosing regimens, including use of oral misoprostol tablets intravaginally, has not been established by the FDA (2011)
- Evidence-based regimen for medical abortion through 63 days after LMP (Hatcher et al., 2011)
  - ■ Include off-label use in informed consent
  - ■ Day 1: Mifepristone administration
    - ◆ Dose: 200 mg PO in the presence of the provider
    - ◆ Misoprostol 800 mg provided and self-administered
      - ➤ Buccally: 24–36 hours post mifepristone
      - ➤ Vaginally: 6–72 hours post mifepristone
  - ■ Post-treatment follow-up: 2–14 days post mifepristone
  - ■ Advantages
    - ◆ Comparable efficacy to the FDA-approved regimen
    - ◆ Extended window for treatment
    - ◆ Shorter time to completion
    - ◆ Decreased medication costs
    - ◆ Fewer office visits
    - ◆ Decreased side effects
  - ■ Disadvantages: Theoretical increase in risk of anaerobic infection with vaginal misoprostol
- Vacuum aspiration abortion (Hatcher et al., 2011)
  - ■ Obtain informed consent
  - ■ Ensure the presence of emergency medications and equipment
  - ■ Local anesthesia and/or sedation may be used
  - ■ The cervix is dilated with osmotic or mechanical dilators
  - ■ The evacuation cannula is inserted through the cervix: Size is equivalent to the number of weeks' gestation (e.g., 5-mm cannula for 5 weeks' gestation)
  - ■ Uterus is evacuated using a vacuum pump or syringe
  - ■ Provide for tissue examination of POC
- Second trimester: Dilatation and evacuation
- Second trimester: Induction abortion

Providing Treatment: Complementary and Alternative Measures to Consider

- Herbal remedies to foster initiation of menses (see "Care of the Woman Interested in Emergency Contraception")
- Remedies to support the reproductive system during medical or surgical abortion
  - Herbal products (Soule, 1996; Zeus, 2007)
    - Echinacea
    - Red raspberry leaf
    - Dong quai
    - Vitex
    - Lemon balm
    - Alfalfa leaf
    - Nettle leaf
    - Yellow dock
  - Homeopathic support (Smith, 1984)
    - Arnica
    - Sabina
    - Pulsatilla
    - Other remedies as indicated by client symptom presentation
  - Bach flower remedies
    - Rescue remedy
    - Other remedies as indicated by the client's emotional presentation
- Herbal abortifacients are not recommended due to their potential for toxicity and the safety of medical termination of pregnancy

Providing Support: Education and Support Measures to Consider

- Provide or ensure access to the following services:
  - Factual unbiased information during options counseling
  - Support and guidance to allow an informed choice
  - Culturally appropriate information and care
- Available options may differ based on the following issues:
  - Age of the client
  - Availability of services

- Cultural factors
- Duration of gestation
- Maternal medical factors
- Financial considerations
- Clear information should be provided regarding the following topics:
  - Prenatal care and birth options
    - Adoption outside the family
    - Adoption within the family
    - Keeping and caring for the infant
  - Voluntary termination of pregnancy
    - Medical
    - Surgical
- Termination procedure(s)
  - Access to services
  - Medical abortion process: Provide written information and instructions
    - Medication dose and administration schedule
    - Anticipated sequence of events
    - Plan for follow-up visits
    - Medication side effects
      - Nausea and vomiting
      - Diarrhea
      - Malaise
    - Warning signs
    - How to contact the practitioner
  - Surgical abortion process: Provide written information and instructions
    - Procedure
    - Sedation or anesthesia available
    - Anticipated sequence of events
    - Warning signs
    - How to contact the practitioner
  - Identify surgical coverage for suction aspiration if needed

Follow-up Care: Follow-up Measures to Consider

- Following options counseling
  - Schedule prenatal care *or*
  - Schedule termination after verification of gestation
  - Offer support services as needed

- Post-termination examination: 4–14 days after the procedure (Hatcher et al., 2011)
  - Examination to verify complete abortion
  - Post-abortion counseling
  - Referral for retained POC
- Emotional after-care as needed: Assess the client's emotional response to the procedure
  - Short-term responses (Lemkau, 1988)
    - Ambivalence
    - Relief
    - Depression or anxiety
    - Regret or doubt
  - Long-term responses/sequelae (Goodwin & Ogden, 2007)
    - Linear recovery
    - Persistent upset
    - Negative reappraisal
    - Never upset
- ⚠️ 📞 Presence of warning signs after medical abortion (Emma Goldman Clinic, 2007; FDA, 2011)
  - Consider sepsis
  - Obtain complete blood count
  - Initiate immediate antibiotic treatment for anaerobic bacteria such as *Clostridium sordellii*
- Contraceptive management

Multidisciplinary Practice: Consider Consultation, Collaboration, or Referral

- OB/GYN or women's health services
  - If the midwife cannot provide objective options counseling
  - If the midwife does not offer termination services
  - For surgical coverage for clients undergoing medical abortion
- Social services
  - Parenting resources
  - Adoption resources
  - Mental health services
  - Support groups
- For diagnosis or treatment outside the midwife's scope of practice

CARE OF THE WOMAN WITH VASOMOTOR SYMPTOMS OF MENOPAUSE

Key Clinical Information

During menopause, hot flashes, night sweats, and mood swings occur in some women as a result of the physiologic decline in ovarian function or secondary to medical or surgical ablation of the ovaries. At the time of physiologic menopause, many women still have one-third of their life ahead of them. Vasomotor symptoms peak approximately 12 months after menopause or oophorectomy and can persist for several years, frequently affecting the quality of a woman's life. These symptoms may be particularly troubling for women who undergo oophorectomy prior to physiologic menopause and for women treated with tamoxifen for a personal or family history of breast cancer. The severity of vasomotor symptoms is affected by women's age, cultural perceptions of menopause, lifestyle factors, stress levels, and the presence of preexisting anxiety or depression (Melby, Anderson, Sievert, & Obermeyer, 2011).

Women seek relief from troublesome symptoms to enhance their quality of life and overall well-being. Practitioners are encouraged to invite women to actively participate in selection of their preferred treatment approach after consideration of the associated benefits, risks, and costs. Treatment choices include lifestyle changes, hormone-based therapies, and alternative therapies (Garcia, Gonzaga, Tan, Ng, Oei, & Chan, 2010; North American Menopause Society, 2010; Schuiling & Likis, 2013).

Client History and Chart Review: Components of the History to Consider

- Age
- Reproductive history
  - GP TPAL
  - LMP or age at menopause
  - Current menstrual status
- Menopausal symptoms and perceived severity
  - Identify the following items:
    - Frequency
    - Severity

- ◆ Effect of symptoms on the woman's lifestyle
  - ➤ Self-image
  - ➤ Emotional well-being
  - ➤ Relationships
  - ➤ Stamina and physical well-being
  - ◆ Previous treatment(s) and results
- ■ Vasomotor symptoms (North American Menopause Society, 2010)
  - ◆ Hot flashes or flushes
  - ◆ Night sweats
  - ◆ Seven to eight hot flashes a day or more than 60 per week: Classified as severe symptoms
  - ◆ Contributing factors
    - ➤ Elevated ambient temperature
    - ➤ Cigarette smoking
    - ➤ Elevated BMI
    - ➤ Sedentary lifestyle
    - ➤ Low socioeconomic status
    - ➤ Alcohol or caffeine
    - ➤ Stress
    - ➤ Anxiety or depression
- ■ Sleep disorders
  - ◆ Sleep habits
  - ◆ Insomnia
  - ◆ Wakefulness
  - ◆ Night sweats
  - ◆ Daytime sleepiness: Relationship to vasomotor symptoms
- ■ Urogenital and sexual symptoms
  - ◆ Decreased libido
  - ◆ Vaginal atrophy and dryness
  - ◆ Urinary frequency or urgency
  - ◆ Dyspareunia
- ■ Skin changes
  - ◆ Fine wrinkles
  - ◆ Increase in facial hair
  - ◆ Thinning of vulvar tissues
  - ◆ Thinning of pubic hair
- ■ Mood disturbance or mental status changes
  - ◆ Mood swings
  - ◆ Depression
  - ◆ Irritability
  - ◆ Confusion
  - ◆ Cognitive changes
- • Medical/surgical history
  - ■ Allergies
  - ■ Medications
  - ■ Herbs or nutritional supplements
  - ■ Change in weight
  - ■ Prior surgeries
    - ◆ Oophorectomy
    - ◆ Hysterectomy—complete or partial
  - ■ Health conditions or symptoms of disorders, such as
    - ◆ Breast disorders or pain
    - ◆ Diabetes
    - ◆ Fractures
    - ◆ Gallbladder disease
    - ◆ Heart disease or stroke
    - ◆ Hypertension or hypercholesterolemia
    - ◆ Blood clots
    - ◆ Liver or kidney disease
    - ◆ Other chronic illness
    - ◆ Mood disorder
- • Family history
  - ■ Heart disease
  - ■ Diabetes
  - ■ Cancer
- • Social history
  - ■ Self-efficacy and self-image
  - ■ Coping ability and strategies
  - ■ Support systems
    - ◆ Partner
    - ◆ Friends
    - ◆ Social activities
  - ■ Significant life stressors
  - ■ Alcohol, tobacco, and substance use
  - ■ Intimate-partner violence or abuse
- • Physical activity patterns
- • Nutritional assessment
- • Review of systems (ROS)

Physical Examination: Components of the Physical Exam to Consider

- • Vital signs, including blood pressure
- • Weight, height, and BMI

- Observation for vasomotor symptoms
  - Hot flashes or flushing
  - Mood and affect
  - Changes in cognition
- General physical examination with focus on the following areas:
  - Thyroid
  - Cardiopulmonary status
  - Breast examination
  - Pelvic examination
    - Observe for atrophy of tissues
      - Pale
      - Thin
      - Fragile
    - Size, position, and consistency of uterus, cervix, and adnexa

Clinical Impression: Differential Diagnoses to Consider

(ICD9data.com, 2012)

- Symptoms related to physiologic menopause
- Symptoms related to medical or surgical menopause
- Medical conditions with similar symptoms
  - Thyroid disorders
  - Mood disorders
  - Sleep disorders
  - Tuberculosis

Diagnostic Testing: Diagnostic Tests and Procedures to Consider

- TSH
- Mantoux TB testing
- Follicle-stimulating hormone (FSH) and luteinizing hormone (LH)
- Other diagnostic tests as indicated

Providing Treatment: Therapeutic Measures to Consider

- Lifestyle changes (North American Menopause Society, 2010)
  - Reduce ambient temperature
  - Wear light clothing

  - Mindfulness relaxation techniques
  - Smoking cessation
  - Small, non-spicy meals
  - Limit alcohol intake
  - Daily moderate physical activity
  - Treatment of underlying mood disorders
- Antidepressants (Pachman, Jones, & Loprinzi, 2010; Thacker, 2011): Effective for hot flashes and mood changes
  - Celexa (citalopram): 20 mg/day
  - Effexor (venlafaxine): 75 mg/day
  - Paxil (paroxetine): 12.5–25 mg/day
  - Pristiq (desvenlafaxine): 100–150 mg/day
  - Prozac (fluoxetine): 20 mg/day
- Hormonal treatment (see "Care of the Woman Interested in Hormone Replacement Therapy")
  - Oral, vaginal, or transdermal
  - Contraindicated for women with breast cancer
- Other nonhormonal medical treatments (Pachman et al., 2010; Schuiling & Likis, 2013): Indicated when hormones are contraindicated and other treatments are ineffective
  - Gabapentin: 900 mg/day
  - Lyrica (pregabalin): 75 mg/day
  - Megace: 20 mg/day
- Sleep aids: Short-term therapy (King & Brucker, 2011)
  - Use caution in the following circumstances:
    - Suspected clinical depression
    - Alcohol or substance use
    - Hepatic or renal disease
  - Reevaluate in 2–3 weeks
  - Options
    - OTC medications, such as Tylenol PM or Advil PM
    - Ambien: 5–10 mg at bedtime
    - Dalmane: 15–30 mg at bedtime
    - Lunesta: 1–3 mg at bedtime
    - Sonata: 5–10 mg at bedtime
- Urogenital symptoms
  - Vaginal lubricants
  - Hormone therapy (see "Care of the Woman Interested in Hormone Replacement Therapy")

- Urinary treatments (see "Care of the Woman with Urinary Tract Symptoms")

Providing Treatment: Complementary and Alternative Measures to Consider

- Bioidentical hormones: Hormones that are chemically identical to endogenous hormones
  - Custom compounding of hormone blends
  - Prepared by professional compounding pharmacies
  - Hormone creams, absorbed via the skin
- Phytoestrogens (Pachman et al., 2010)
  - Reduce symptoms in some women
  - May stimulate endometrial hyperplasia
  - Contraindicated in women with breast cancer
  - Isoflavones
    - Soy derivatives
    - Flaxseed meal
  - Food sources (ACOG, 2001b)
    - Peanuts, soy, and other legumes
    - Whole grains such as oats and corn
    - Berries
    - Vegetables
- Vaginal dryness
  - Lubrication
    - Water-based lubricants
    - Massage oil
  - Evening primrose oil
    - 500 mg PO two to four times daily
    - Apply vaginally
      - Capsule
      - Oil-soaked tampon
  - Slippery elm oral capsules
- Herbal treatments have not been found to be effective for hot flash relief in double-blind studies but many women still use them and gain relief (Pachman et al., 2010)
  - Black cohosh herb or extract
    - Hot flashes
    - Affective changes
    - Estroven
    - Remifemin
    - Contraindicated in women with a history of breast cancer

- Don quai
  - Hot flashes
  - Affective changes
  - Contraindicated in some women
    - On warfarin
    - With a history of breast cancer
  - May cause skin sensitivity to sunlight
- Ginkgo biloba: Mental acuity and memory
- St. John's wort: Affective changes
- Vitex or chasteberry (Chopin, 2003)
  - Hot flashes
  - Affective changes
  - Breast tenderness
- Red clover

Providing Support: Education and Support Measures to Consider

- Provide information
  - Menopause and common symptoms
  - Treatment recommendations
  - Lifestyle recommendations
  - Indications to return for evaluation
  - Local resources for women
- ▽ Reinforce suggested practices for symptom relief (North American Menopause Society, 2010)
  - Maintain cool ambient temperatures
    - Fan or air conditioner
    - Cool drinks
    - Dress in layers
  - Maintain optimal BMI
  - Reduce or eliminate cigarette smoking
  - Controlled diaphragmatic breathing at onset of a hot flash
  - Active relaxation techniques
    - Yoga
    - Meditation
    - Massage
  - Allow time for self-care
    - Moderate daily exercise
    - Cool-down period following physical activity
    - Rest and relaxation

- Limit intake of the following substances:
  - Caffeine
  - Saturated fats
  - Refined foods, sugar, and flour
  - Cigarettes and alcohol
  - Phosphorus-containing soft drinks
- Develop a sleep routine

Follow-up Care: Follow-up Measures to Consider

- Document
  - Care provided
  - Discussion of options
  - Recommendations and client choices
  - Plan for continued care
- Return for continued care
  - As needed to provide ongoing support
  - Unexpected vaginal bleeding
  - Breast mass, pain, or changes
  - Osteoporosis prevention and evaluation
  - Ineffective coping or mood disorder
  - Worsening symptoms
    - Mood disorders
    - Mental status changes
    - Vasomotor symptoms
  - Evaluation of treatment and its side effects
  - Annual evaluation

Multidisciplinary Practice: Consider Consultation, Collaboration, or Referral

- OB/GYN services
  - Symptoms that do not respond or worsen with treatment
    - Nonpharmaceutical therapy
    - Standard HRT regimens
    - Complementary and alternative therapy
  - Unexplained or persistent vaginal bleeding
- Medical or surgical services
  - Breast mass
  - Osteoporosis
  - Abnormal liver or renal function test results
  - Symptoms of chronic medical conditions
    - Heart disease
    - Diabetes
- Mental health or social services
  - Depression
  - Ineffective coping
  - Psychosis
  - Support groups
- Sleep specialist
  - Persistent wakefulness
  - Severe insomnia
- For diagnosis or treatment outside the midwife's scope of practice

WEB RESOURCES FOR CLINICIANS

RESOURCE	URL
Abortion information by state	http://www.prochoiceamerica.org/government-and-you/state-governments/
Collaborative management of women in menopause with HRT	http://www.icsi.org/menopause_and_hormone_therapy/menopause_and_hormone_replacement_therapy_ht___collaborative_decision_making_and_management_.html
Fertility awareness	http://www.irh.org/?q=resources
	• Taking Charge of Your Fertility: http://www.tcoyf.com
	• Garden of Fertility: http://www.gardenoffertility.com
	• Billings Ovulation Method: http://www.billingsmethod.com
	• Institute for Reproductive Health: http://irh.org
	• Institute for Natural Family Planning: http://www.marquette.edu/nursing/NFP/

- Couple to Couple League International: http://www.ccli.org
- Downloadable fertility charts: www.fertilityawareness.net
- Additional sites for fertility monitoring supplies
  - http://www.fertile-focus.com
  - http://www.ovulation-predictor.com
  - http://www.birthcontrol.com

Herbal information	http://www.herbmed.org
Hormone replacement medications charts	http://www.menopause.org/htcharts.pdf
	http://www.menopause.org/PSht10.pdf
	http://www.menopause.org/PSvagestrogen07.pdf
	http://www.ncbi.nlm.nih.gov/pmc/articles/PMC2971731/
	http://www.jabfm.com/content/24/2/202.full
Medical abortion protocol	http://www.reproductiveaccess.org/med_ab/mife_protocol.htm
Osteoporosis prevention and treatment	http://www.nof.org/professionals/clinical-guidelines
	FRAX: http://www.shef.ac.uk/FRAX/index.jsp
Smoking cessation	http://www.cdc.gov/tobacco/quit_smoking/cessation/practical_guide/index.htm
Vaccine recommendations	http://www.cdc.gov/vaccines/default.htm
	Vaccine Adverse Event Reporting: http://vaers.hhs.gov/
WHO medical eligibility criteria for contraceptive use	http://www.fhi.org/NR/rdonlyres/e7kii7aodskp2exshxcjsom7we7wkxuolmsdnr7r2wd5fr55twscwzb42ce5mpmcfcmzgoz2vhv2xl/FPQuickReferenceChart1.pdf
	http://www.fhi.org/en/RH/Pubs/servdelivery/quickreferencechart.htm

REFERENCES

American Cancer Society. (2007). Detailed guide: Endometrial cancer. Retrieved from http://www.cancer.org/docroot/CRI/CRI_2_3x.asp?rnav=cridg&dt=11

American College of Nurse–Midwives (ACNM). (2011). *ACNM position statement: Reproductive choices.* Silver Spring, MD: Author. Retrieved from http://www.midwife.org/siteFiles/position/Reproductive_Choices_05.pdf

American College of Obstetricians and Gynecologists (ACOG). (1995). Health maintenance for perimenopausal women. In *2002 compendium of selected publications* (Technical Bulletin no. 210). Washington, DC: Author.

American College of Obstetricians and Gynecologists (ACOG). (2001a). Emergency oral contraception. In *2005 compendium of selected publications* (Practice Bulletin no. 25). Washington, DC: Author.

American College of Obstetricians and Gynecologists (ACOG). (2001b). Use of botanicals for management of menopausal symptoms. In *2005 compendium of selected publications*. Washington, DC: Author.

American College of Obstetricians and Gynecologists (ACOG). (2006a). Primary and preventive care: Periodic assessments (Committee Opinion no. 357). *Obstetrics & Gynecology, 108,* 1615.

American College of Obstetricians and Gynecologists (ACOG). (2006b). *Use of hormonal contraception in women with coexisting medical conditions* (Practice Bulletin no. 73). Washington, DC: Author.

American College of Obstetricians and Gynecologists, District II/NY. (2008). *Preconception care.* Albany, NY: Author. Retrieved from http://mail.ny.acog.org/website/PreconBooklet.pdf

American College of Obstetricians and Gynecologists. (2011a). Practice Bulletin no. 121: Long-acting reversible contraception: implants and intrauterine devices. *Obstetrics & Gynecology, 118,* 184–196.

American College of Obstetricians and Gynecologists. (2011b). Committee Opinion no. 486: Update on carrier screening for cystic fibrosis. *Obstetrics & Gynecology, 117,* 1028–1031.

American College of Physicians. (2005). Medicare ushers in new smoking cessation coverage. *ACP Observer.* Retrieved from http://www.acponline.org/journals /news/may05/smoking.htm

Bayer HealthCare Pharmaceuticals. (2009). *Mirena package insert.* Wayne, NJ: Author. Retrieved from http:// berlex.bayerhealthcare.com/html/products/pi/ Mirena_PI.pdf

Bickley, L. S., & Szilagyi, P. S. (2009). *Bates' guide to physical examination and history taking* (10th ed.). Philadelphia, PA: Wolters Kluwer.

Burbos, N., Musonda, P., Giarenis, I., Shiner, A. M., Giamougiannis, P., Morris, E. P., & Nieto, J. J. (2010). Predicting the risk of endometrial cancer in postmenopausal women presenting with vaginal bleeding: The Norwich DEFAB risk assessment tool. *British Journal of Cancer, 102,* 1201–1206. doi: 10.1038/sj.bjc.6605620. Retrieved from http://www.ncbi.nlm.nih.gov/pmc/ articles/PMC2856001/pdf/6605620a.pdf

Centers for Disease Control and Prevention (CDC). (2008). Smoking prevalence among women of reproductive age—United States, 2006. *Morbidity and Mortality Weekly Report, 57*(31), 849–852. Retrieved from http://www.cdc.gov/mmwr/preview/mmwrhtml/ mm5731a2.htm

Centers for Disease Control and Prevention (CDC). (2012a). Recommended adult immunization schedule— United States, 2012. *Morbidity and Mortality Weekly Report, 61*(04), 1–7. Retrieved from http://www.cdc .gov/vaccines/recs/schedules/downloads/adult/adult- schedule.pdf

Centers for Disease Control and Prevention (CDC). (2011). Current cigarette smoking prevalence among working adults: United States, 2004–2010. *Morbidity and Mortality Weekly Report, 60*(38), 1305–1309. Retrieved from http://www.cdc.gov/mmwr/preview /mmwrhtml/mm6038a2.htm?s_cid=%20mm6038a2 .htm_w

Chopin, L. B. (2003). Vitex agnus castus essential oil and menopausal balance: A research update. *Complementary Therapies in Nursing and Midwifery, 8,* 148–154.

Deresiewicz, R. (n.d.). Toxic shock syndrome: A health professional's guide. Retrieved from http://www .toxicshock.com/

Dhont, M. (2011). Non-contraceptive benefits of oral contraceptives. *Open Access Journal of Contraception, 2,* 119–126. Retrieved from http://www.dovepress.com /non-contraceptive-benefits-of-oral-contraceptives- peer-reviewed-article-OAJC

Duramed Pharmaceuticals. (2006a). *ParaGard® T380A intrauterine copper contraceptive prescribing information.* Pomona, NY: Barr Pharmaceuticals. Retrieved from http://www.paragard.com/hcp/custom_images /ParaGard_HCP_PI.pdf

Duramed Pharmaceuticals. (2006b). Plan B® prescribing information. Retrieved from http://www.go2planb.com /PDF/PlanBPI.pdf

Ellertson, C., Evans, M., Ferden, S., Leadbetter, C., Spears, A., Johnstone, K.,... & Trussell, J. (2003). Extending the time limit for starting Yuzpe regimen of emergency contraception to 120 hours. *Obstetrics & Gynecology, 101,* 1168–1171.

Emma Goldman Clinic. (2007). *Post-abortion care.* Iowa City, IA: Author. Retrieved from http://www .emmagoldman.com/services/abortion/care.htm

Fine, P., Mathe, H., Ginde, S., Cullins, V., Morfesis, J., & Gainer, E. (2010). Ulipristal acetate taken 48–120 hours after intercourse for emergency contraception. *Obstetrics & Gynecology, 115,* 257–263. Retrieved from http://ec.princeton.edu/news/Fine%202010%20-% 20UPA.pdf

Fiore, M. C., Jaen, C. R., Baker, T. B., Bailey, W. C., Benowitz, N. L., Curry, S. J.,... & Wewers, M. E. (2008). *Treating tobacco use and dependence: 2008 update.* Clinical Practice Guideline. Rockville, MD: U.S. Department of Health and Human Services, Public Health Service. Retrieved from http://www.surgeongeneral.gov/tobacco /treating_tobacco_use08.pdf

Food and Drug Administration (FDA). (2011). Mifeprex (mifepristone) information. Retrieved from http://www .fda.gov/drugs/drugsafety/postmarketdrugsafety informationforpatientsandproviders/ucm111323.htm

Fraser, I. S. (2010). Non-contraceptive health benefits of intrauterine hormonal systems. *Contraception, 82,* 396–403. doi: 10.1016/j.contraception.2010.05.005

Garcia, J. T., Gonzaga F., Tan, D., Ng, T. Y., Oei, P. L., & Chan, C. (2010). Use of a multibotanical (Nutrafem) for the relief of menopausal vasomotor symptoms: A double-blind, placebo-controlled study. *Menopause, 17,* 303/308. doi: 10.1097/gme.0b013e3181bf8e92

Goodwin, P., & Ogden, J. (2007). Women's reflections upon their past abortions: An exploration of how and why emotional reactions change over time. *Psychology & Health, 22*(2), 231–248.

Hatcher, R. A., Trussell, J., Stewart, F., Nelson, A. L., Cates, W., Kowal, D., & Policar, M. (2011). *Contraceptive technology* (20th ed.). New York , NY: Ardent Media.

Health Canada. (2010). High dose folic acid supplementation: Questions and answers for health professionals. Retrieved from http://www.hc-sc.gc.ca/fn-an/nutrition /prenatal/fol-qa-qr-eng.php

Heath, C., & Acevedo, R. (2000–2007). Preconception screening and counseling. *The Female Patient.* Retrieved from http://www.femalepatient.com/html/arc /sig/screening/articles/029_10_052.asp

Hooshmand, S., Chai, S. C., Saadat, R. L., Payton, M. E., Brummel-Smith, K., & Arimandi, B. H. (2011). Comparative effects of dried plum and dried apple on bone in postmenopausal women. *British Journal of Nutrition, 106,* 923–930.

ICD9data.com. (2012). ICD-9 codes. Retrieved from http://www.ICD9data.com

Institute for Clinical Systems Improvement (ICSI). (2008). Menopause and hormone therapy (9th ed.). Retrieved from http://www.icsi.org/menopause_and_hormone_ therapy/menopause_and_hormone_replacement_ therapy_ht___collaborative_decision_making_and_ management_.html

Inverness Medical. (n.d.). Bone therapy monitoring. Author. Retrieved from: http://www.osteomark.com/pdf /BoneTherapy.pdf

Janssen Pharmaceuticals. (2011). Ortho Evra. Retrieved from http://www.orthoevra.com/

Johnson, J. (2004). Diaphragms, caps and shields. Planned Parenthood. Retrieved from http://www.planned parenthood.org/birth-control-pregnancy/birth-control /diaphragms-caps-andshields.htm

Kent, H., Johnson, K., Curtis, M., Hood, J. R., & Atrash, H. (2006). *Proceedings of the preconception health and health care clinical, public health, and consumer workgroup meetings.* Atlanta , GA: Centers for Disease Control and Prevention. Retrieved from http://www.cdc.gov /ncbddd/preconception/documents/Workgroup%20 Proceedings%20June06.pdf

Lemkau, J. (1988). Emotional sequelae of abortion. *Psychology of Women Quarterly, 12,* 461–472.

Mackenzie, S. J., & Yeo, S. (1997). Pregnancy interruption using mifepristone (RU-487): A new choice for women in the USA. *Journal of Nurse–Midwifery, 42,* 86–98.

March of Dimes. (n.d.). Preconception screening and counseling checklist. Retrieved from http://www .marchofdimes.com/professionals/19583_4182.asp

Marshall, W. A., & Tanner, J. M. (1969). Variations in pattern of pubertal changes in girls. *Archives of Disease in Childhood, 44*(235), 291–303. doi: 10.1136 /adc.44.235.291

Melby, M. K., Anderson, D., Sievert, L. L., & Obermeyer, C. M. (2011). Methods used in cross-cultural comparisons of vasomotor symptoms and their determinants. *Maturitas, 70,* 110–119.

Menzies, R., Wallace, S., Ennis, M., Bennett, A., Jacobson, M., Yip, G., & Wolfman, W. (2011). Significance of abnormal sonographic findings in postmenopausal women with and without bleeding. *Journal of Obstetrics and Gynaecology Canada, 33,* 944–951. Retrieved from http://jogc.org/abstracts/full/201109_Gynaecology_3 .pdf

National Cancer Institute. (2011). Cigarette harms of smoking and benefits of quitting. Retrieved from http://www.cancer.gov/cancertopics/factsheet/Tobacco /cessation

National Osteoporosis Foundation. (2010). *Clinician's guide to prevention and treatment of osteoporosis.* Washington, DC: Author. Retrieved from http://www.nof.org /sites/default/files/pdfs/NOF_ClinicianGuide2009_ v7.pdf

North American Menopause Society. (2010). Estrogen and progestogen use in postmenopausal women: 2010 position statement of the North American Menopause Society. *Menopause, 17,* 242–255. doi: 10.1097 /gme.0b013e3181d0f6b9

Nusbaum, M. R. H., & Hamilton, C. D. (2002). The proactive sexual health history. *American Family Physician, 66,* 1705–1712.

Office of Population Research & Association of Reproductive Health Professionals. (2006). Types of emergency contraception. Retrieved from http://ec.princeton.edu /questions/dose.html#dose

Organon. (2011a). *Implanon provider insert.* Roseland, NJ: Author. Retrieved from http://www.implanon-usa.com /HCP/prescribingImplanon/index.asp

Organon. (2011b). *NuvaRing provider insert.* Roseland, NJ: Author. Retrieved from http://www.nuvaring.com/hcp /index.asp

Pachman, D. R., Jones, J. M., & Loprinzi, C. L. (2010). Management of menopause-associated vasomotor symptoms: Current treatment options, challenges and future directions. *International Journal of Women's Health, 2,* 123–135. Retrieved from http://www.ncbi .nlm.nih.gov/pmc/articles/PMC2971731/

Pallone, S. R., & Bergus, G. R. (2009). Fertility awareness-based methods: Another option for family planning. *Journal of the American Board of Family Medicine, 22,* 147–157. doi: 10.3122/jabfm.2009.02.080038

Pfizer. (2011). Depo Provera contraceptive injection prescribing information. Retrieved from http://www.pfizer.com/products/rx/rx_product_depo_provera.jsp

Raine, T. R., Foster-Rosales, A., Upashyay, U. D., Boyer, C. B., Brown, B. A., Sokoloff, A., & Harper, C. H. (2011). One-year contraceptive continuation and pregnancy in adolescent girls and women initiating hormonal contraceptives. *Obstetrics & Gynecology, 117*, 363–371. doi: 10.1097/AOG.0b013e31820563d3. Retrieved from http://www.ncbi.nlm.nih.gov/pmc/articles/PMC3154007/pdf/nihms-313509.pdf

Renoux, C., Dell'Aniello, S., Garbe, E., & Suissa, S. (2010). Transdermal and oral hormone replacement therapy and the risk of stroke: A nested case-control study. *British Medical Journal, 340*. doi: 10.1136/bmj.c2519. Retrieved from http://www.bmj.com/content/340/bmj.c2519.long

Romm, A. (2010). *Botanical medicine for women's health.* St. Louis, MO: Churchill Livingstone.

Sallamander Concepts. (1998–2011). Herbal encyclopedia. Retrieved from http://www.ageless.co.za/herbal-encyclopedia.htm

Schuiling, K., & Likis, F. (2013). *Women's gynecologic health* (2nd ed.). Burlington, MA: Jones & Bartlett Learning.

Singer, K. (2004). *The garden of fertility.* New York: Avery.

Smith, T. (1984). *A woman's guide to homeopathic medicine.* New York, NY: Thorsons.

Soule, D. (1996). *The roots of healing.* Secaucus, NJ: Citadel Press.

Thacker, H. L. (2011). Assessing risks and benefits of nonhormonal treatments for vasomotor symptoms in perimenopausal and postmenopausal women. *Journal of Women's Health, 20*, 1007–1016. doi: 10.1089/jwh.2010.2403

Trapani, F. J. (1984). *Contraception naturally.* Coopersburg, PA: C. J. Frompovich.

Trussell, J., & Raymond, E. (2006). *Emergency contraception: A cost-effective approach to preventing unintended pregnancy.* Princeton, NJ: Office of Population Research. Retrieved from http://ec.princeton.edu/questions/ec-review.pdf

U.S. Preventive Services Task Force. (2009). Folic acid for the prevention of neural tube defects: U.S. Preventive Services Task Force recommendation statement. *Annals of Internal Medicine, 150*, 626–631. Retrieved from http://www.uspreventiveservicestaskforce.org/uspstf09/folicacid/folicacidrs.htm

U.S. Preventive Services Task Force. (2011). The guide to clinical preventive services 2011: Recommendations for adults. Retrieved from http://www.uspreventiveservicestaskforce.org/adultrec.htm#obstetric

Varney, H., Kriebs, J. M., & Gegor, C. L. (2004). *Varney's midwifery* (4th ed.). Sudbury, MA: Jones and Bartlett.

Wyeth. (2008). Lybrel: Inhibition of menses. Retrieved from http://www.wyeth.com/hcp/lybrel/efficacy/inhibitionofmenses

Yen, S., Saah, T., & Hillard, P. J. (2010). IUDs and adolescents: An under-utilized opportunity for pregnancy prevention. *Journal of Pediatric and Adolescent Gynecology, 23*, 123–128. Retrieved from http://peds.stanford.edu/Rotations/adolescent_medicine/documents/IUDsandTeens.pdf

Zeus, S. (2007). Taking care after abortion, miscarriage or herbally induced abortion. Retrieved from http://www.sisterzeus.com/post_ca.htm

Care of the Woman with Reproductive Health Problems

When faced with reproductive health problems, women look to midwives for continued care and appropriate referrals.

Many women routinely rely on midwives for reproductive health care unrelated to pregnancy. In addition to routine well-woman care, professional midwifery practice often includes providing care to women with reproductive health problems and variations from normal. The scope of care provided to women with reproductive health issues is based not only on the midwife's education and training, but also on additional factors such as the location and type of practice, clinical site expectations, and the needs of the population of women served.

The expert midwife develops the ability to differentiate those conditions or findings that represent the wide spectrum of "normal" from those that are subtle presentations of abnormal conditions. Skill as a diagnostician is vital to midwifery practice and is an integral component of providing comprehensive care to women. A problem-oriented directed history is essential to accurate diagnosis and validation of the woman's concerns. Physical examination centers on pertinent body systems and the organs that influence them. The resulting clinical impression, or list of potential differential diagnoses, guides the midwife's decisions regarding appropriate diagnostic studies and situations in which consultation or referral is indicated. The optimal midwifery plan of care clearly delineates anticipatory thinking and addresses planned follow-up both with and without resolution of symptoms.

Maintaining competency in women's reproductive health care requires ongoing professional education to keep up with changes in diagnostic techniques and terminology and with current treatment methods. A wide range of resources is available to develop, maintain, and improve competence in the diagnosis and treatment of commonly encountered women's health problems.

The American College of Nurse–Midwives (ACNM, 2011) recently revised its definition and scope of midwifery practice to include "treatment of male partners for sexually transmitted infections [STIs]." Although this chapter is primarily concerned with variations in women's health, it begins with assessment of the male for STIs. Because many treatments for STIs are similar for women and men, therapies are addressed in the specific clinical practice guideline for women. Treatments, tests, or other issues unique to men within those clinical practice guidelines will be highlighted with the following male icon: ♂.

ASSESSMENT AND CARE OF THE MAN CONCERNED ABOUT SEXUALLY TRANSMITTED INFECTION

Key Clinical Information

Although the primary focus of midwifery care is for women, the sexual health of the male partner or partners is of direct and immediate importance to a woman's health. Midwives care for men in STI clinics and sometimes treat the male through patient-delivered partner treatment (PDPT), also known as expedited partner management (FitzMaurice, Keller, Trebbin, & Wilson, 2011; Hatcher et al., 2011). With the recent inclusion of males noted in the ACNM (2011) definition and scope of practice, it is expected that more midwives will include assessment and care of men for STIs in their range of services.

Client History and Chart Review: Components of the History to Consider

- Age
  - Review previous STI history
  - STI testing
  - STI treatments
- Sexual history
  - Sexual practices
    - Number of partners for self or partner(s)
    - Vaginal, oral, anal intercourse
    - Condom use
      - ➤ Male condom
      - ➤ Female condom
- Problem-focused history
  - Onset, duration, and severity of symptoms
  - Last unprotected intercourse
  - Partner diagnosed with STI
  - Symptom profile
    - May be asymptomatic
    - Urinary frequency and dysuria
    - Urethritis
    - Anal discharge
    - Sore throat
    - Urethral discharge
    - Genital pain and discharge
    - Fever
- Medical/surgical history
  - Allergies
  - Medications
  - Chronic health conditions
- Social history
  - Behavioral risk factors
    - Alcohol and drug use
    - Exposure to more than five sexual partners
    - Male partner or bisexual
  - Social support
  - Access to health care
- Review of systems (ROS)

Physical Examination: Components of the Physical Exam to Consider

- Vital signs, including temperature
- Oral examination for lesions and discharge, if indicated
- Male genitalia examination (Bickley & Szilagyi, 2009)
  - Inspection of the skin
    - Note lesions of the penis, testicles, and inguinal areas
    - Prepuce or foreskin—if present, ask the patient to retract it
    - Note the location of the urinary meatus; compress the glans
    - Note penile or anal discharge
  - Palpate for abnormalities, nodules, or swelling
    - Shaft
    - Testes and epididymis
    - Inguinal area for lymph nodes

Clinical Impression: Differential Diagnoses to Consider

(ICD9data.com, 2012)

- Gonorrhea
- Chlamydia
- Urethritis

- Nongonococcal urethritis
- Trichomoniasis
- Herpes simplex virus, type 1 or 2
- Human papillomavirus
- Human immunodeficiency virus
- Syphilis

Diagnostic Testing: Diagnostic Tests and Procedures to Consider

- Gonorrhea testing (Centers for Disease Control and Prevention [CDC], 2010)
  - Gram stain
    - Diagnostic for male urethral specimen only
    - Gram-negative intracellular diplococci, plus polymorphonuclear leukocytes
  - Culture test types
    - DNA probe
    - Enzyme-linked immunosorbent assay (antigen specific)
    - Nucleic acid amplification tests
  - Culture specimen sites
    - Oropharyngeal
    - Rectal
    - Urethral
    - Urine
- Chlamydia testing
- Syphilis testing
- HIV counseling and testing

Providing Treatment: Therapeutic Measures to Consider

(FitzMaurice et al., 2011; Hatcher et al., 2011)

- See the specific relevant clinical practice guideline, noting the male icon for any differences in treatment of male patients
- Consider patient-delivered partner treatment (PDPT)

Providing Treatment: Complementary and Alternative Measures to Consider

- ⚠ Alternative therapies are not a substitute for medical treatment

- Supportive measures to promote healing
  - Adequate rest
  - Nutritional support
    - Live culture yogurt
    - Blue-green algae
    - Vitamins C and E

Providing Support: Education and Support Measures to Consider

- Diagnosis
  - Potential sequelae of infection
  - Treatment recommendations
  - Partner notification and referral for treatment
    - PDPT can be considered
    - Give prescription and written materials
    - [www] Legal regulations vary; check www.cdc.gov/std/ept
  - State reporting requirements
- Treatment instructions: Avoid sexual relations
  - Until treatment is completed
  - Until symptoms have resolved
  - Until partner treatment is completed
- When and how to access care
- STI transmission and prevention: Emphasize use of condoms

Follow-up Care: Follow-up Measures to Consider

- Document
  - Confirmation of diagnosis
  - Medication administration
  - Epidemiologic reporting
- Indications to return for care (CDC, 2010)
  - Persistent symptoms
  - Reinfection
  - Drug-resistant organism
  - Noninfectious process
- Repeat testing only in the following circumstances:
  - Persistent symptoms
  - New partner for self or for partner
- Offer HIV and other STI counseling and testing

Multidisciplinary Practice: Consider Consultation, Collaboration, or Referral

- Urology service or infection specialist
- Public Health Department
- For diagnosis or treatment outside the midwife's scope of practice

CARE OF THE WOMAN WITH AN ABNORMAL MAMMOGRAM

Key Clinical Information

Abnormalities found on mammography include breast lesions that may be either benign or malignant. With an abnormal mammogram, further evaluation of the client is needed to determine whether treatment is indicated. Most women with abnormal results are understandably anxious and may not accurately take in information presented by the clinician. Many practitioners prefer to give abnormal results in person, offering women an opportunity to ask questions and take written information home to discuss with loved ones.

Digital mammography is an emerging technology that performs better as a screening modality in younger women, who typically have denser breast tissue (Fritz & Speroff, 2011). When digital images are compared with prior film mammograms, however, some women may be called back for further testing to differentiate artifact from abnormality as a consequence of differences between the two methods. Digital mammography uses lower doses of radiation but may require more images for screening.

Mammography frequently identifies women with premalignant lesions or early signs of breast cancer before a palpable mass is present. Prompt evaluation and treatment of women with early breast malignancy provides the best chance for long-term survival. Many communities now have breast centers where women with breast abnormalities can obtain specialty care.

Client History and Chart Review: Components of the History to Consider

(Aliotta & Schaeffer, 2013)

- Reproductive history
  - Current menstrual status
  - Pregnancy history
    - GP TPAL
    - Age at first birth
    - Breastfeeding history
      - ➤ Number of children breastfed
      - ➤ Duration of breastfeeding
  - Contraceptive history
  - Breast history
    - Mastitis
    - Prior breast masses
    - Prior breast surgery
    - Prior treatment for breast disease
- Current symptoms
  - Pain (mastalgia)
  - Skin changes
  - Presence of mass
  - Spontaneous nipple discharge
    - Sexual history
    - Breast stimulation
  - Symptom history
    - Location
    - Onset
    - Duration
    - Severity
- Family history
  - Breast cancer
  - Ovarian cancer
  - Benign breast disease
  - Ethnic heritage
- **www** Breast cancer risk assessment (American Cancer Society [ACS], 2010)
  - Most breast cancer occurs randomly
  - Contributing factors
    - Older age
    - Early menarche
    - Alcohol use
    - Postmenopausal hormone therapy
    - Eastern European Jewish heritage
    - Nulliparous women
    - Never having breastfed
    - Significant family history
    - Personal history of breast cancer or certain benign breast conditions
    - Exposure to radiation
    - Overweight or obesity

Physical Examination: Components of the Physical Exam to Consider

(Aliotta & Schaeffer, 2013)

- Complete breast examination
  - Positioning
    - Seated, arms at sides
    - Seated, arms raised
    - Seated, leaning forward
    - Supine
  - Evaluate for the following:
    - Mass
    - Dimpling
    - "Orange peel" sign
    - Nipple retraction
    - Nipple discharge
    - Redness
    - Induration
    - Axillary lymphadenopathy
    - Breast or axillary tenderness
  - Note characteristics of any mass found
    - Size and contour
    - Mobility
    - Definition of borders
    - Firmness
    - Associated signs and symptoms
      - Pain or tenderness
      - Skin changes
      - Distortion of breast contour
  - Note characteristics of nipple discharge
    - Presence in one or both breasts
    - Color and consistency
    - Spontaneous emission

Clinical Impression: Differential Diagnoses to Consider

(ICD9data.com, 2012)

- Abnormal mammogram, unspecified
- Abnormal mammogram, microcalcifications
- Other abnormal findings on radiologic examination of breast
- Benign breast conditions
- Breast malignancy
- Axillary lymphadenopathy

Diagnostic Testing: Diagnostic Tests and Procedures to Consider

- Follow-up mammogram: Based on radiologist recommendations
  - Magnification views
  - Three- to six-month follow-up
- Ultrasound
  - Benign process suspected
  - Differentiates solid from cystic mass
- 🕿 Biopsy
  - Based on the following:
    - Clinical findings
    - Radiologist recommendations
    - Client preference
  - Biopsy methods
    - Fine-needle aspiration
    - Core-needle biopsy
    - Stereotactic biopsy
    - Excisional biopsy
- Genetic testing
  - BRCA1
  - BRCA2
- Magnetic resonance imaging (MRI)

Providing Treatment: Therapeutic Measures to Consider

- Treatment depends on the diagnosis and the client's risk profile
- 🕿 Excisional biopsy
  - Definitive treatment for benign masses
  - Treatment for small malignancies, combined with the following measures:
    - Chemotherapy
    - Radiation treatment
- Cancer treatments
  - Surgery
    - Lumpectomy
    - Mastectomy
      - Partial
      - Simple
      - Modified radical
      - Radical
    - Axillary node evaluation
      - Sentinel node(s)
      - Axillary node dissection

- Medical therapy
  - Chemoprevention
    - Tamoxifen
    - Raloxifene
  - Radiation treatment
  - Chemotherapy
- Prophylactic mastectomy for women at high risk for breast cancer

Providing Treatment: Complementary and Alternative Measures to Consider

(Romm, 2010)

- ⚠ Alternative therapies should not delay diagnostic measures or substitute for medical or surgical treatment
- Healthy whole-foods diet
  - Avoid foods and other substances with the following:
    - Hormones (meat, milk)
    - Hormone-like activity
    - Pesticides or herbicides
    - Preservatives
  - Avoid microwaving food in plastic containers
  - Limit consumption of the following:
    - Animal fats
    - Caffeinated products, coffee, and tea
    - Dairy products
    - Alcohol
    - Refined sugar and flour
    - Processed foods
- ⚠ Herbal remedies may interact with medications
- Vitamin supplementation
  - Vitamin B_6: 50–100 mg daily
  - Vitamin E: 400–800 IU daily
- Emotional support, which in turn provides immune support
  - Love and laughter boost the immune response
    - Rent comedy videos
    - Enjoy time with friends
  - Cultivate a positive attitude
    - Meditation or prayer
    - Enjoy each day as a gift
    - Seek healing and optimal health

- Warm breast compresses
  - With castor oil
  - With poke root
- Aromatherapies, see "An Herbal Primer"
- Bach flower essences, such as rescue remedy
- Herbal remedies
  - Chasteberry
  - Dong quai
  - Blue cohosh
  - Flaxseed
  - Evening primrose oil

Providing Support: Education and Support Measures to Consider

- Advise the client of any abnormal screening test results
- Provide information
  - An abnormal mammogram is *not* indicative of cancer; it indicates need for additional testing
  - Review the recommendations of the radiologist for further testing
  - Written information is helpful
- 🌐 Allow time for the client to express her concerns
  - Acknowledge concerns
  - Address fears and feelings
  - Help her stay grounded in the moment
- Develop a management plan
  - Schedule for the following tests as indicated:
    - Repeat mammogram
    - Ultrasound
    - MRI
  - Referral for biopsy
  - Plan for follow-up
- 📞 With a cancer diagnosis, provide information on community resources
  - Reach to Recovery
  - American Cancer Society (ACS)
  - Cancer support groups

Follow-up Care: Follow-up Measures to Consider

- Document
  - Characteristics of clinical findings

- Discussions with the client
- Referral indication and plan
- Provide the client with referral information
  - Appointment time and date
  - Directions
  - Anticipated sequence of events
- Return for care
  - To review findings
  - To provide client education
  - For support and counseling
  - For well-woman care

Multidisciplinary Practice: Consider Consultation, Collaboration, or Referral

- Surgery or breast care service
  - Suspicious mammogram result
  - Evaluation of lesion
  - Second opinion
- Community resources
  - Social services
  - Transportation
  - Counseling
  - Support groups
- For diagnosis or treatment outside the midwife's scope of practice

CARE OF THE WOMAN WITH AN ABNORMAL PAP SMEAR

Key Clinical Information

Of the 50 to 60 million Pap smears done in the United States each year, approximately 3.5 million will return abnormal results. Recent advances in understanding of the role of the human papillomavirus (HPV) in the development of cervical cancer and the ability of the body's immune system to clear this virus at certain developmental stages, combined with screening techniques that allow for identification of high-risk HPV subtypes, have led to revisions in the recommended management of abnormal Pap smear results (American Society for Colposcopy and Cervical Pathology, 2011). Many providers who perform cervical cancer screenings have been slow

to adopt these new guidelines due to a lack of understanding of the evidence behind these recommendations. Midwives will appreciate that overtreatment of abnormal Pap smears with invasive procedures in young women can lead to problems in subsequent pregnancies without improving cervical cancer outcomes. Widespread use of the HPV vaccine has the potential to change cervical screening practices in the future. As midwives are often primary providers of cervical cancer screening for both their pregnant and well-woman clients, it is important for every midwife to understand and implement evidence-based guidelines in this area of practice.

Client History and Chart Review: Components of the History to Consider

- Age
- Last menstrual period (LMP), GP TPAL
- Special circumstances
  - Pregnant client
  - Adolescent client
  - Postmenopausal client
- Related history
  - Abnormal Pap smears
  - Diagnostic testing
  - Treatment
- Sexual history
  - Age at onset of sexual activity
  - Number of sexual partners
  - Condom use
  - History of STIs
    - ◆ HPV
    - ◆ HIV
- Medical history
- Surgical history: Hysterectomy
  - Complete or partial
  - Indication
- Social history
  - Smoking
  - Drug and alcohol use
- Family history
  - Cervical disease
  - Diethylstilbestrol (DES) exposure in utero

- Risk factors for abnormal Pap smear
  - More than three sexual partners
  - History of STIs, especially HPV and HIV
  - Prior abnormal Pap smears
  - Lack of self-care
  - Cigarette smoking
  - Presence of cervical intraepithelial neoplasia (CIN) grades 2 and 3
- Symptoms consistent with cervical cancer
  - Persistent watery discharge
  - Intermenstrual bleeding

Physical Examination: Components of the Physical Exam to Consider

- Examination of the external genitalia for HPV lesions
  - Visible HPV is considered low risk for CIN
  - External HPV may contribute to the following conditions:
    - Vulvar intraepithelial neoplasia (VIN)
    - Vaginal intraepithelial neoplasia (VaIN)
- Visualization of the cervix and vaginal vault
  - Presence of gross lesions
  - Signs of genital atrophy
  - Cervical cuff in women with hysterectomy
- Colposcopic examination, if indicated
  - Squamocolumnar junction
  - Presence of acetowhite lesions
    - Punctation
    - Mosaicism
    - Abnormal vessels
  - Lesion borders
  - Abnormal Lugol's solution

Clinical Impression: Differential Diagnoses to Consider

(ICD9data.com, 2012)

- Cervicitis
- Vaginitis, nonspecific
- Atypical glandular cells of unknown significance (AGC-US)
- Atypical squamous cells of unknown significance (ASC-US)

- Atypical squamous cells, cannot exclude high grade (ASC-H)
- Low-grade squamous intraepithelial lesion (LSIL)
- High-grade squamous intraepithelial lesion (HSIL)
- Positive test results for high-risk HPV DNA
- Pap smear suspicious for cervical cancer

Diagnostic Testing: Diagnostic Tests and Procedures to Consider

(Bond, 2009; Ribaldone, Capuano, & Di Oto, 2010; Wright, Massad, Dunton, Spitzer, Wilkinson, & Solomon, 2007a)

- Based on Pap smear results
- Negative Pap smear with obscuring—repeat in 6 months in women with the following characteristics:
  - Previous abnormal Pap smear within 2 years
  - Previous Pap smear with AGC
  - High-risk HPV diagnosed within 12 months
  - Inability to sample the endocervix
  - Immunosuppression
  - Similar obscuring on a previous Pap smear
  - Irregular, infrequent screening
- Specimen unsatisfactory
  - Treat any underlying infection
  - Repeat Pap smear in 2–4 months
  - ⚠ Persistent unsatisfactory results
    - Associated with progressive lesions
    - Colposcopy
    - Biopsy
- Atypical squamous cells of undetermined significance (ASC-US)
  - HPV DNA testing *or*
  - Repeat Pap smear every 6 months for 2 years *or*
  - Colposcopic evaluation
  - If follow-up testing/evaluation is within normal limits:
    - Repeat Pap smear in 12 months
    - Liquid cytology preferred
  - Evaluation abnormal: Colposcopy indicated

- Adolescent women (up to age 20): Repeat Pap smear in 12 months
  - Less than HSIL: Repeat Pap smear in 12 months
    - ➤ Negative: Routine screening
    - ➤ ASC or greater: Colposcopy
  - HSIL: Perform colposcopy
- Atypical squamous cells, cannot exclude high-grade (ASC-H): Colposcopy
- Low-grade squamous intraepithelial lesion (LSIL)
  - Colposcopic evaluation
    - Identification of lesions
    - Directed biopsy
    - Endocervical curettage
  - Adolescents
    - See the previous discussion of ASC-US
    - ⚠ High-risk HPV testing is unacceptable
  - Pregnancy
    - Colposcopy *or*
    - Defer colposcopy until postpartum
    - Endocervical curettage is not acceptable
  - Postmenopausal women
    - Triage with high-risk HPV testing *or*
    - Repeat cytology in 6 and 12 months *or*
    - Colposcopy
    - In case of negative testing/evaluation, repeat cytology in 12 months
    - With ASC or greater, or positive HPV, perform colposcopy
- High-grade squamous intraepithelial lesion (HSIL)
  - Colposcopic evaluation
    - Identification of lesion
    - Directed punch biopsy
    - Endocervical curettage
  - ⚠ Loop electrical excision procedure (LEEP) biopsy is unacceptable for the following groups:
    - Pregnant women
    - Adolescent women
- Atypical glandular cells (AGC) or adenocarcinoma in situ
  - Colposcopic evaluation
  - Biopsy of lesions
  - Endocervical sampling

- Endometrial sampling in patients older than age 35
  - With unexplained vaginal bleeding
  - With diagnosed chronic anovulation
- High-risk HPV DNA testing
- Atypical endometrial cells
  - Endocervical sampling
  - Endometrial sampling
  - Normal results: Colposcopy

Providing Treatment: Therapeutic Measures to Consider

- Menopausal clients with ASC or LSIL
  - Vaginal estrogen for 3 months
  - Repeat cytology as indicated
- Ablation therapies
  - Cryotherapy
  - Laser
- 🔧 Excisional therapies
  - LEEP procedure
  - Cold-knife cone

Providing Treatment: Complementary and Alternative Measures to Consider

(Romm, 2010)

- ⚠ Alternative therapies are not a substitute for prompt evaluation and treatment
- Nutritional support
  - Beta-carotene: 50,000 IU BID with meals
  - Vitamin C: 1000–2000 mg TID
  - Vitamin E: 400 IU daily
  - Folic acid: 2 mg daily for 3 months, then 0.4 mg daily
  - Selenium: 200 mg daily
  - Zinc: 30 mg daily
  - Essential fatty acids
- Herbs to support the immune system
  - Echinacea
  - Reishi mushroom
  - St. John's wort
  - Ginseng
  - Licorice
- Stress management techniques

Providing Support: Education and Support Measures to Consider

(Mortensen & Adeler, 2010)

- Provide information about cervical disease
  - Written information is preferred
  - Explain the meaning of abnormal Pap smear result
  - Give information about diagnostic testing options
  - Explain potential treatment measures
  - Acknowledge concerns and provide support
- Importance of, and schedule for, follow-up
- Smoking cessation, as needed
- Recommended vitamin and mineral supplements
- Safe sexual practices

Follow-up Care: Follow-up Measures to Consider

- Document
  - Cytology result
  - Discussion with the client

- Plan for continued care
- Consultations and referrals
- Manage the client as recommended by American Society for Colposcopy and Cervical Pathology (see Figures 7-1 to 7-10)
- Treat and follow up according to results

Multidisciplinary Practice: Consider Consultation, Collaboration, or Referral

- OB/GYN services
  - Unusual cervical configuration or appearance
    - Visually
    - By palpation
    - By colposcopy
  - Colposcopy for HSIL lesions
  - Evaluation and treatment of AGC-US lesions
    - CIN lesions
    - Malignancy
- For diagnosis or treatment outside the midwife's scope of practice

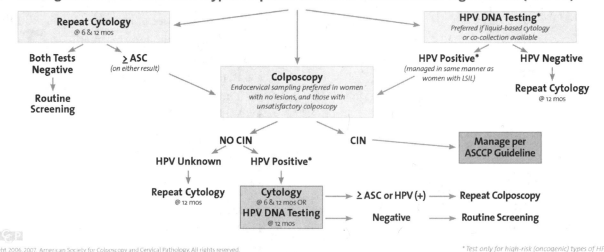

Figure 7-1   Management of Women with Atypical Squamous Cells of Undetermined Significance (ASC-US)

Source: Copyright 2006, 2007. American Society for Colposcopy and Cervical Pathology. All rights reserved.

Management of Adolescent Women with Either Atypical Squamous Cells of Undetermined Significance (ASC-US) or Low-grade Squamous Intraepithelial Lesion (LSIL)

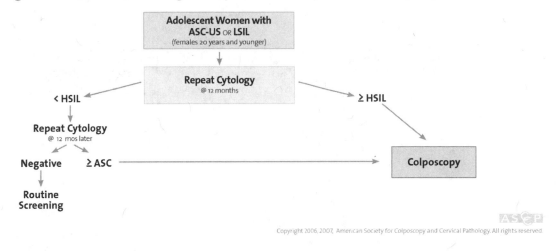

Figure 7-2   Management of Adolescent Women with Either Atypical Squamous Cells of Undetermined Significance (ASC-US) or Low-grade Squamous Intraepithelial Lesion (LSIL)

Source: Copyright 2006, 2007. American Society for Colposcopy and Cervical Pathology. All rights reserved.

Management of Women with Atypical Squamous Cells: Cannot Exclude High-grade SIL (ASC - H)

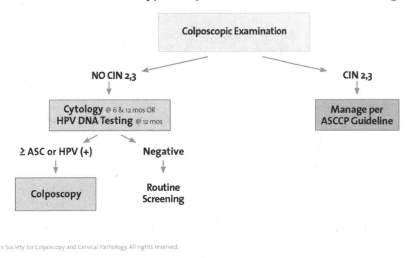

Figure 7-3   Management of Women with Atypical Squamous Cells: Cannot Exclude High-grade SIL (ASC-H)

Source: Copyright 2006, 2007. American Society for Colposcopy and Cervical Pathology. All rights reserved.

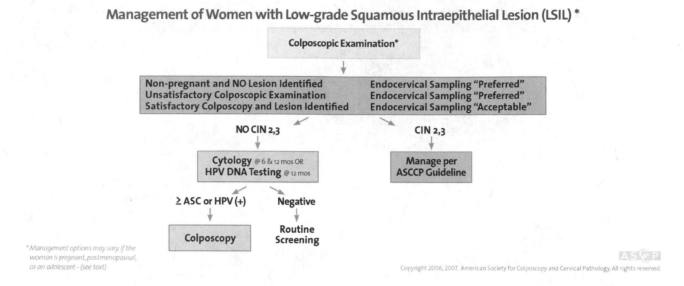

Figure 7-4 Management of Women with Low-grade Squamous Intraepithelial Lesion (LSIL)

Source: Copyright 2006, 2007. American Society for Colposcopy and Cervical Pathology. All rights reserved.

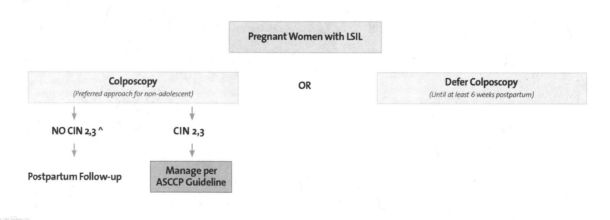

Figure 7-5 Management of Pregnant Women with Low-grade Squamous Intraepithelial Lesion (LSIL)

Source: Copyright 2006, 2007. American Society for Colposcopy and Cervical Pathology. All rights reserved.

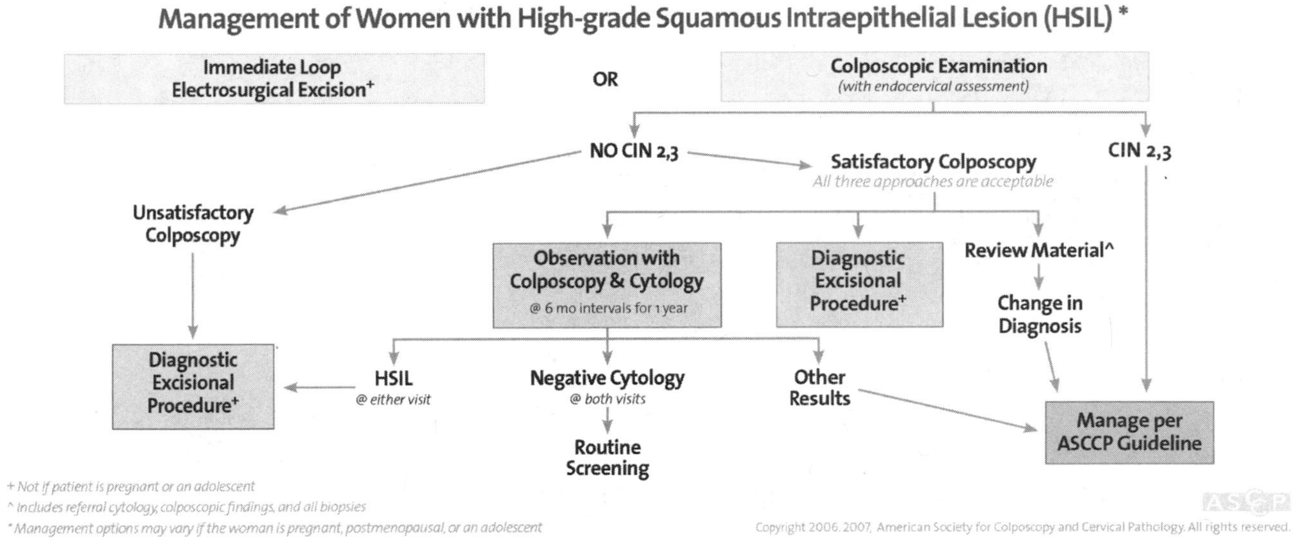

Management of Women with High-grade Squamous Intraepithelial Lesion (HSIL) *

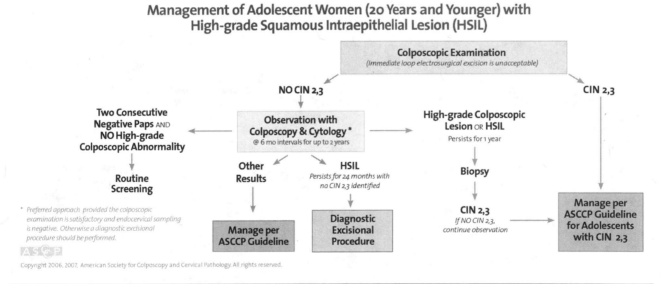

Figure 7-6 Management of Women with High-grade Squamous Intraepithelial Lesion (HSIL)

Source: Copyright 2006, 2007. American Society for Colposcopy and Cervical Pathology. All rights reserved.

Management of Adolescent Women (20 Years and Younger) with High-grade Squamous Intraepithelial Lesion (HSIL)

Figure 7-7 Management of Adolescent Women (20 Years and Younger) with High-grade Squamous Intraepithelial Lesion (HSIL)

Source: Copyright 2006, 2007. American Society for Colposcopy and Cervical Pathology. All rights reserved.

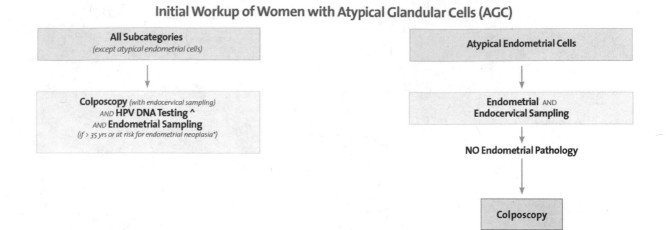

Figure 7-8 Initial Workup of Women with Atypical Glandular Cells (AGC)
Source: Copyright 2006, 2007. American Society for Colposcopy and Cervical Pathology. All rights reserved.

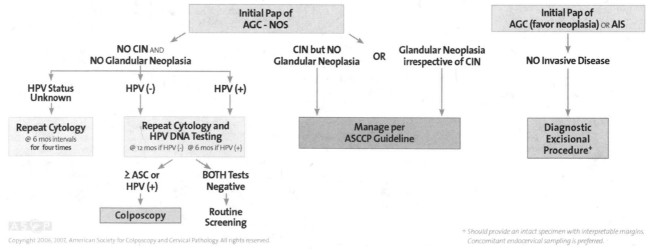

Figure 7-9 Management of Women with Atypical Glandular Cells (AGC)
Source: Copyright 2006, 2007. American Society for Colposcopy and Cervical Pathology. All rights reserved.

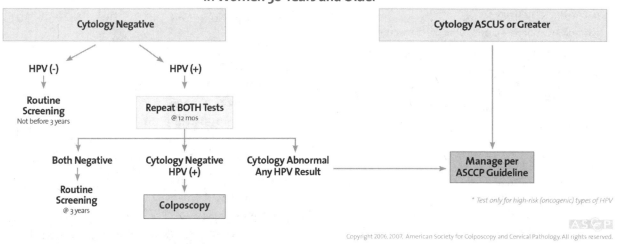

Figure 7-10 Use of HPV DNA Testing* as an Adjunct to Cytology for Cervical Cancer Screening in Women 30 Years and Older

Source: Copyright 2006, 2007. American Society for Colposcopy and Cervical Pathology. All rights reserved.

CARE OF THE WOMAN WITH AMENORRHEA

Key Clinical Information

Primary amenorrhea is an uncommon condition that is defined as an absence of menarche in a young woman who by age 14 has not begun developing secondary sex characteristics, or who by age 16 or older has developed secondary sex characteristics but not started menstruation (Fritz & Speroff, 2011). Primary amenorrhea may result from genetic and congenital disorders or from medical conditions such as malnutrition or hyperthyroidism. As many as 10% of young women with primary amenorrhea have a constitutional delay of menarche, with onset of menarche as late as age 18. Secondary amenorrhea is defined as the absence of menses for 3–6 months in a woman who has previously menstruated and is not pregnant, breastfeeding, or menopausal, frequently secondary to anovulation (Faucher & Schuiling, 2013). As a diagnostic strategy, pregnancy should be considered in any woman of childbearing potential presenting with amenorrhea. If pregnancy is not confirmed, then disorders of the genital outflow tract and uterus, ovary, pituitary, hypothalamus, and the central nervous system should be considered (Fritz & Speroff, 2011).

Client History and Chart Review: Components of the History to Consider

(Faucher & Schuiling, 2013; MedlinePlus, 2006)

- Age
- Menstrual history
  - Age at menarche
  - Previous menstrual pattern
  - Onset and duration of amenorrhea
  - Presence of associated symptoms
    - Galactorrhea
    - Hirsutism
    - Headache
    - Vaginal dryness
    - Visual changes

- ◆ Cyclic pelvic or lower abdominal pain
- ◆ Cyclic urinary complaints
- Gynecologic history
  - Presence of secondary sex characteristics
  - Gynecologic surgery
    - ◆ Cervical cryosurgery
    - ◆ Dilation and curettage (D&C)
    - ◆ Dilation and evacuation (D&E)
    - ◆ Endometrial ablation
  - Sexual history
    - ◆ Sexual activity
    - ◆ Sexual abuse
  - Contraceptive history
    - ◆ Depo-Provera
    - ◆ Mirena
    - ◆ Continuous oral contraceptives
    - ◆ Implanon
  - Pregnancy and breastfeeding history
    - ◆ Pregnancy terminations
    - ◆ Length of breastfeeding
- Medical and surgical history
  - Thyroid disorders
  - Weight changes
    - ◆ Loss or gain
    - ◆ Distribution
  - Systemic illness
- ▽ Medications that may contribute to amenorrhea (MedlinePlus, 2006)
  - Busulfan
  - Chlorambucil
  - Cyclophosphamide
  - Phenothiazines
  - Oral contraceptives
  - Non–oral contraceptives
    - ◆ Depo-Provera
    - ◆ Mirena intrauterine device (IUD)
- Psychosocial assessment
  - Stressors
  - Nutrition patterns
    - ◆ Adequacy of diet
    - ◆ Eating disorders
  - Physical activity level: Competitive sports
  - Effects of amenorrhea on self-image
- Review of systems

Physical Examination: Components of the Physical Exam to Consider

(Faucher & Schuiling, 2013; Fritz & Speroff, 2011)

- Vital signs
- Height and weight
  - Body mass index
  - Weight changes
  - Weight distribution
  - Ratio of muscle to adipose tissue
  - Short stature
- Thyroid examination
  - Enlargement
  - Nodularity
  - Physical findings consistent with thyroid disorders (see "Assessment of the Woman with Endocrine Symptoms")
- www Tanner staging (Vermont Public Health Department, n.d.)
  - Age-appropriate height increases
  - Acne vulgaris
  - Pubic hair development
    - ◆ Texture
      - ➤ Fine villus hair
      - ➤ Minimal coarse, pigmented hair
      - ➤ Dark, curly, coarse hair
    - ◆ Distribution
      - ➤ Labia
      - ➤ Mons
      - ➤ Axilla
      - ➤ Medial thigh
  - Breast development
    - ◆ Breast buds
    - ◆ Areolar enlargement
    - ◆ Development of breast mound
    - ◆ Areola forms secondary mound
    - ◆ Adult contour

Pubertal Growth

Breast development is a reliable indicator of exposure to endogenous or exogenous estrogen (Fritz & Speroff, 2011).

- Pelvic examination
  - Examination for physical cause of amenorrhea
    - Outflow tract disorders
      - ➤ Imperforate hymen
      - ➤ Labial fusion
      - ➤ Cervical stenosis
    - Absence of vagina, cervix, or uterus
    - Ambiguous genitalia
  - Signs of endocrine/central nervous system disorders
    - Vaginal atrophy
    - Clitoral hypertrophy
- (☎) Visual field examination: Pituitary tumor

Clinical Impression: Differential Diagnoses to Consider

(ICD9data.com, 2012)

- Amenorrhea, primary or secondary
- Amenorrhea, due to the following causes:
  - Asherman's syndrome
  - Ovarian dysfunction
  - Pregnancy
  - Hormonal contraception use
  - Premature menopause
  - Hypothalamic dysfunction secondary to the following:
    - Low body fat
    - Stress
  - Endocrine disorders
    - Premature ovarian failure
    - Polycystic ovary syndrome
    - Androgen-producing tumors
    - Hyperprolactinemia
    - Hypothyroidism
    - Pituitary disease
    - Cushing's syndrome
  - Genetic factors
    - Constitutional rate of maturation
    - Congenital anomalies
      - ➤ Congenital anomalies of genital tract
      - ➤ Congenital adrenal hyperplasia
- Galactorrhea

Diagnostic Testing: Diagnostic Tests and Procedures to Consider

(Fritz & Speroff, 2011)

- Primary amenorrhea
  - Normal secondary sex characteristics: Pelvic sonography
  - Uterus present
    - Serum human chorionic gonadotropin (HCG)
    - Serum T_4 and TSH
    - Prolactin level (less than 100 ng/mL = normal)—if elevated:
      - ➤ MRI of head/pituitary *or*
      - ➤ Computed tomography (CT) of sella turcica
  - (☎) Uterus absent
    - Evaluate testosterone level
    - Evaluate karyotype
- Secondary amenorrhea
  - Serum β-human chorionic gonadotropin (β-HCG)
  - Negative β-HCG test
    - Thyroid-stimulating hormone (TSH): Elevated TSH = hypothyroidism
    - Prolactin level (less than 100 ng/mL = normal)
  - Consider progesterone trial
- No secondary sex characteristics: Check follicle-stimulating hormone (FSH)/luteinizing hormone (LH) levels
  - FSH: Normal is 5–30 IU/L
  - LH: Normal is 5–20 IU/L
  - (☎) Abnormalities:
    - Elevated FSH/LH: Evaluate karyotype
    - Normal or low FSH/LH: Refer for trial of gonadotropin-releasing hormone

Providing Treatment: Therapeutic Measures to Consider

- Progesterone trial
  - Medication options
    - Provera 10 mg for 10 days or
    - Prometrium 400 mg at bedtime for 10 days *or*

- ◆ Crinone 4%, progesterone gel 45 mg vaginally QID for six doses
  - ▪ Expect withdrawal bleeding within 10 days after medication is begun
- Refer for treatment based on working diagnosis
  - ▪ Gynecologic
  - ▪ Endocrine
  - ▪ Congenital

Providing Treatment: Complementary and Alternative Measures to Consider

(Romm, 2010)

- Herbal remedies that support menstruation
  - ▪ Red raspberry leaf tea
  - ▪ Vitex tea, tincture, or capsules
  - ▪ Dong quai tea (not to be used while nursing)
  - ▪ Wild yam root tea or tincture
  - ▪ Blue cohosh root tea or tincture
  - ▪ Use for 3 months, even after menstrual cycle resumes
- Acupuncture
- Exercises to increase pelvic blood flow
  - ▪ Yoga
  - ▪ Belly dancing
- Stress management techniques
- Achieve and maintain normal BMI

Providing Support: Education and Support Measures to Consider

- Provide age-appropriate information
  - ▪ Menstrual cycle and function
  - ▪ Potential causes
    - ◆ Breastfeeding
    - ◆ Exercise and low body fat
    - ◆ Endocrine disorders
    - ◆ Chromosomal abnormalities
    - ◆ Congenital anomalies
- Plan for testing and results
- Expectation for treatment
- Potential for associated
  - ▪ Infertility
  - ▪ Endometrial hyperplasia
  - ▪ Osteopenia and osteoporosis

Follow-up Care: Follow-up Measures to Consider

(Faucher & Schuiling, 2013)

- Document
  - ▪ Working diagnosis
  - ▪ Plan for continued care
- Office follow-up
  - ▪ As indicated by results and diagnosis:
    - ◆ Results of progestin challenge
      - ➤ Withdrawal bleed with normal prolactin and TSH = anovulation
      - ➤ Negative withdrawal bleed requires further workup
  - ▪ For support during gynecologic workup
  - ▪ As indicated for routine care

Multidisciplinary Practice: Consider Consultation, Collaboration, or Referral

- OB/GYN or gynecologic endocrinologist
  - ▪ Primary amenorrhea
    - ◆ Presence of anomalies
    - ◆ Abnormal laboratory results
    - ◆ Reproductive
    - ◆ Endocrine
    - ◆ Genetic
  - ▪ Secondary amenorrhea
    - ◆ Primary evaluation
    - ◆ After progestin challenge, if no withdrawal bleed occurs
- Mental health services: Presence of eating disorder
- Social services: Evidence of malnutrition
- For diagnosis or treatment outside the midwife's scope of practice

CARE OF THE WOMAN WITH BACTERIAL VAGINOSIS

Key Clinical Information

Bacterial vaginosis (BV) is one of the most commonly occurring forms of vaginitis, characterized by the classic "fishy" odor and accounting for as many as 50% of vaginitis diagnoses. BV results from an imbalance in the vaginal flora—specifically, a reduction of lactobacillus species and an overgrowth of anaerobic bacteria. This state can represent a transient change in some women as the body's defenses restore balance, or it may persist longer in other women (CDC, 2010).

Although this condition is not considered to be an STI, incidence of BV is higher in women with new or multiple sexual partners. Untreated BV can contribute to endometritis and reproductive postoperative wound infections and can increase susceptibility to STIs, including HIV (CDC, 2010). Although controversy exists as to whether BV contributes to the onset of preterm labor, persistent recurrent BV has been linked to background *Mycoplasma* infection that can contribute to risk for pregnancy complications. However, screening and treating asymptomatic pregnant women for BV has not resulted in improved perinatal outcomes (CDC, 2010).

Lesbian and bisexual women get BV more often than heterosexual women for reasons not fully understood (Cochran, 2011). Treatment of the male partner in a heterosexual couple has not been beneficial in preventing BV recurrence in the woman (CDC, 2010).

Client History and Chart Review: Components of the History to Consider

(CDC, 2010)

- Onset and duration of symptoms
  - BV can be asymptomatic
  - Vulvovaginal irritation or burning
  - Presence of discharge
    - Copious
    - Homogenous
    - Thin
    - Grayish white
  - Odor
    - Described as foul or "fishy"
    - Stronger after menses and intercourse
  - Treatments used and results
- Pregnancy/gynecologic history
  - LMP
  - Birth control method

- Previous BV infection
  - Testing
  - Treatment
- BV associated with the following conditions:
  - Endometritis/pelvic inflammatory disease (PID)
  - STIs
  - Postoperative wound infection
- Sexual practices that can contribute to BV (CDC, 2010)
  - Oral–genital contact
  - Vaginal contact after anal penetration
  - Multiple partners (woman or partner): Inquire about discharge or symptoms in partner(s)
  - Female partner(s)
- Medical history
  - Allergies
  - Medications
    - Antibiotics
    - Hormones
  - Systemic illness
    - Diabetes
    - HIV
- Hygiene practices
  - Douching
  - Toileting habits

Physical Examination: Components of the Physical Exam to Consider

- Pelvic examination
- External examination
  - Redness
  - Erythema
  - Lesions
  - Discharge
  - Odor
- Speculum examination
  - Discharge
  - Lesions
  - Retained tampon or foreign body
- Bimanual examination
  - Cervical motion tenderness
  - Adnexal masses

Clinical Impression: Differential Diagnoses to Consider

(ICD9data.com, 2012)

- Bacterial vaginosis
- Candida vaginitis
- Cervicitis
- Foreign body
- Chlamydia
- Gonorrhea
- *Mycoplasma*
- Trichomoniasis
- Vaginitis complicating pregnancy

Diagnostic Testing: Diagnostic Tests and Procedures to Consider

(CDC, 2010)

- Wet preparation (provider performed microscopy); see Table 7-1
  - Vaginal pH greater than 4.5
  - KOH preparation
    - Positive KOH whiff test
    - Negative mycelia or branching hyphae
  - Saline preparation
    - Positive clue cells
    - Rare lactobacilli
    - Occasional white blood cells
- Gram stain
- DNA probe, such as BD Affirm VPIII
- Point-of-service rapid tests
  - QuickVue Advance
  - Osom BV test

- ⚠ Note: Visual inspection of vaginal discharge is nonspecific and cannot be used alone for diagnosis. Multiple pathogens may be present. Perform additional testing as required for accurate diagnosis.

Providing Treatment: Therapeutic Measures to Consider

(CDC, 2010)

- Metronidazole
  - Pregnancy Category B
  - Pregnancy dosing
    - 500 mg PO BID for 7 days *or*
    - 250 mg orally TID for 7 days
  - Nonpregnancy dosing
    - 500 mg PO BID for 7 days
    - MetroGel-Vaginal 0.75%
      - One applicator (5 g) per vagina
      - At bedtime for 5 days
- Cleocin (clindamycin)
  - Pregnancy Category B
  - Pregnancy dosing: Clindamycin 300 mg PO BID for 7 days
  - Nonpregnancy dosing
    - Vaginal cream 2%: 5 g intravaginally at bedtime for 7 days
    - Clindamycin 300 mg PO BID for 7 days
    - Clindamycin ovules 100 mg intravaginally at bedtime for 3 days
- Tindamax (tinidazole): Nonpregnancy dosing
  - 2 g PO QD for 2 days
  - 1 g PO QD for 5 days

Table 7-1 Amstel's Criteria to Diagnose Bacterial Vaginosis	
Qualities of vaginal discharge	Thin, white, homogenous, smoothly coats vaginal walls
pH of vaginal discharge	Greater than 4.5
Odor	Fishy odor before or after KOH
Microscopic findings	Clue cells present

Note: Must meet three of the four criteria for diagnosis.

Providing Treatment: Complementary and Alternative Measures to Consider

(Romm, 2010)

- Infection of imbalance
  - Provide immune support
  - "Tincture of time" to allow spontaneous resolution
- Black walnut tincture
- Boric acid capsules
  - Boric acid powder
  - Slippery elm powder, one applied per vagina at bedtime for 5 nights
  - Follow with lactobacillus capsules, one applied per vagina at bedtime for 5 nights
- Garlic vaginal suppository
  - One clove garlic, peeled
  - Attach 6-inch length of dental floss
  - Use nightly for 5 nights
- Herbal sitz bath or peri-wash
  - Tincture of
    - Calendula: 2 parts
    - Echinacea root: 2 parts
    - Myrrh: 2 parts
  - Place 50 gtts in 1 cup warm calendula tea
  - Use for 6 nights

Providing Support: Education and Support Measures to Consider

- Review genital hygiene
  - Limit alkaline soaps
  - Wipe front to back
  - Urinate after sexual relations
  - Cotton panties or liners
  - Avoid close-fitting clothing
  - Avoid douching
- Provide information about BV
- Treatment instructions
  - Avoid alcohol consumption when taking metronidazole
  - Avoid sexual relations during treatment
  - Return for care for persistent symptoms
  - Additional testing may be needed
  - Partner may need treatment

- Diagnosis during pregnancy: Risk and benefits of treatment

Follow-up Care: Follow-up Measures to Consider

- No follow-up is needed if the symptoms resolve
- Return if the symptoms recur or persist
  - Consider testing for the following:
    - *Chlamydia*
    - *Mycoplasma*
    - Trichomoniasis
  - Retreat patient
    - Using repeat or other standard therapy *or*
    - MetroGel twice weekly for 4–6 months

Multidisciplinary Practice: Consider Consultation, Collaboration, or Referral

- OB/GYN services: For persistent or unresponsive vaginitis
- For diagnosis or treatment outside the midwife's scope of practice

CARE OF THE WOMAN WITH A BREAST MASS

Key Clinical Information

Approximately 90% of breast masses are benign (Aliotta & Schaefer, 2013). Nevertheless, every breast mass must be considered suspicious for breast malignancy until shown to be otherwise. Breast cancer is second only to lung cancer as a cause of cancer mortality in women. While more white women get breast cancer than black women, mortality rates are higher for African American women with this disease (National Cancer Institute, 2011). Breast cancer rates have been dropping slowly since 2000, this trend attributed to a decrease in the widespread use of hormone replacement therapy in perimenopausal and postmenopausal women. Pregnancy does not exclude breast cancer from the differential diagnosis; 2% of all breast cancers are diagnosed during pregnancy (Ulery, Carter, McFarlin, & Giurgescu, 2009).

Client History and Chart Review: Components of the History to Consider

(Klein, 2005)

> **Breast Cancer Risk Assessment Tool**
>
> Calculate risk of breast cancer for individual women using the interactive tool at http://www.cancer.gov/bcrisktool/.

- Age
- GP TPAL
- Diet history
  - Caffeine intake
  - Fat intake
  - Alcohol consumption
  - Overcooked or charred meat
  - Unwashed fruits and vegetables (pesticides)
- Medications
  - Oral contraceptives
  - Hormone replacement therapy
- LMP and menstrual status
- Location and onset of breast mass
  - When first noted
  - Relation to menstrual cycle
  - Characteristics of mass
    - Location
    - Consistency
    - Mobility
    - Pain
- Associated breast changes
  - Nipple discharge
  - Dimpling
  - "Orange peel" sign
  - Skin changes
- Axillary masses
- Previous mammography
- Presence of risk factors for breast cancer (ACS, 2010)
  - Female gender
  - Age
  - Presence of BRCA1 or BRCA2 gene
  - Positive family history
  - Previous history of breast cancer
  - Atypical hyperplasia on biopsy
  - Exposure to high-dose radiation
  - High postmenopausal bone density
  - Early menarche/late menopause
  - Nulliparous, or first child born after age 30
  - Long-term hormone replacement therapy
  - Obesity, diabetes, or high-fat diet
  - Tall women
  - Jewish heritage
  - Alcohol consumption
- Previous or current breast conditions
  - Lactation
  - Benign disorders
    - Fibrocystic breasts
    - Mastitis
    - Breast abscess
  - Biopsies
- Self-breast examination habits and techniques
- Review of systems

Physical Examination: Components of the Physical Exam to Consider

(ACS, 2010; Klein, 2005)

- Height, weight, and BMI
- Complete breast examination, sitting and supine
- Visual findings
  - Scarring
  - Dimpling and retraction
  - Skin changes
    - "Orange peel" sign
    - Paget's disease
  - Asymmetry
  - Nipple retraction
  - Redness
- Palpation of superficial, intermediate, and deep tissue
- Palpable findings of mass(es)
  - Single or multiple
  - Location(s)
    - The upper outer quadrant is the most common site of cancer
    - Diffuse distribution is more common with cystic breasts

- Contour
  - ◆ Smooth
  - ◆ Stellate
- Size: Describe in centimeters
- Round, oval, or irregular
- Mobility
  - ◆ Mobile
  - ◆ Fixed
- Consistency
  - ◆ Firm
  - ◆ Hard
  - ◆ Soft
- Heat
- Nipples
  - Palpate for masses
  - Spontaneous nipple discharge
  - Expression of discharge
- Palpation for lymph nodes
  - Axilla
  - Supraclavicular
  - Neck

Clinical Impression: Differential Diagnoses to Consider

(ICD9data.com, 2012)

- Breast mass(es)
- Breast abscess, postpartum
- Breast abscess
- Breast cyst, solitary
- Fibrocystic breasts
- Fibroadenosis of breast
- Traumatic hematoma of breast
- Mastitis, postpartum
- Mastitis
- Nipple discharge
- Enlarged lymph node(s)
- Malignancy of breast

Diagnostic Testing: Diagnostic Tests and Procedures to Consider

(Kearney & Murray, 2009; Klein, 2005)

- Screening mammogram: Difficult to interpret in some clients

- Young women
- During lactation
- Dense breast tissue
- Diagnostic mammogram
  - Indications (Madigan Army Medical Center, 2006)
    - ◆ Persistent breast mass
    - ◆ Spontaneous unilateral nipple discharge
    - ◆ Nipple or skin retraction
  - Lesion marked with radiopaque marker
    - ◆ Spot compression
    - ◆ Magnified views
  - Digital mammogram: Allows for image enhancement
- Ultrasound
  - Young women with dense breast tissue
  - Cyst or abscess suspected
  - May support or oppose physical findings
  - Shows fluid-filled soft-tissue changes best
  - Differentiates palpable solid masses
- MRI
  - Women at high or moderately high risk for breast cancer
  - Women with silicone breast implants
  - Women in whom it is difficult to interpret mammogram or ultrasound results
    - ◆ Dense or scarred breast tissue
    - ◆ Breast cancer follow-up
    - ◆ Axillary metastasis with unknown primary site
- Biopsy
  - Definitive diagnosis with tissue specimen
  - Each technique has limitations
    - ◆ Fine- or core-needle aspiration biopsy
    - ◆ Stereotactic biopsy
    - ◆ Excisional biopsy
- Genetic screening
  - BRCA1 and BRCA2 genes
  - Family history
    - ◆ Breast cancer
    - ◆ Ovarian cancer
  - Ashkenazi Jewish heritage
  - A negative screen does not exclude a person from risk of breast cancer

Providing Treatment: Therapeutic Measures to Consider

(Klein, 2005)

- Cystic mass
  - Observation for one cycle
  - Aspiration
  - Excision
- Abscess
  - Treat with oral antibiotics (see "Care of the Mother with Mastitis")
  - May require incision and drainage
- Solid mass
  - With sharp margins by ultrasound
  - With uniform shape
  - With no characteristics of malignancy
    - Reevaluation within 1–3 months
    - Needle or stereotactic biopsy
    - Excision of mass
  - Characteristics of malignant or premalignant lesions
    - Needle or stereotactic biopsy
    - Excisional biopsy
- Breast cancer treatments (ACS, 2010)
  - Surgery
  - Radiation
  - Biologic therapy
  - Chemotherapy
  - Hormone therapy

Providing Treatment: Complementary and Alternative Measures to Consider

- ⚠ Alternative measures are not a substitute for prompt evaluation and treatment
- Improve the diet
  - Decrease or eliminate intake of the following foods:
    - Caffeine
    - Chocolate
    - Alcohol
    - Carbonated beverages
  - Avoid products from hormone-fed animals
    - Meat
    - Poultry
    - Milk
    - Cheese
  - Avoid grains, fruits, and vegetables grown with chemical treatments:
    - Pesticides
    - Herbicides
  - Limit fat intake
  - Increase vitamin intake
    - Vitamin C
    - Beta-carotene
    - Vitamin E
    - Vitamin B complex
- Increase intake of the following foods:
  - Deep green vegetables
  - Grains
  - Legumes
  - Sea vegetables
  - Fruit
- Red clover tea

Providing Support: Education and Support Measures to Consider

- Teach self-breast examination (SBE) techniques
  - Review the benefits and limitations of SBE (ACS, 2010)
  - Become familiar with one's own breast changes through the menstrual cycle
  - Perform SBE in the bath or shower
  - Soap the hands to allow deeper palpation
- ▽ Provide information
  - Working diagnosis
  - Informed choice
  - Evaluation modalities
  - Testing recommendations
  - Treatments
  - Support services and options
- Prevention measures (ACS, 2010)
  - Maintain optimal BMI
  - Regular physical activity
  - Reduction of alcohol consumption to fewer than two drinks per day
  - Hormone replacement therapy

- ◆ Avoid *or*
- ◆ Use as short a time as possible
- ◆ Take the lowest effective dose
- ■ High-risk women (positive for the BRCA gene or assessed as high risk on a screening tool)
  - ◆ Tamoxifen therapy
  - ◆ Prophylactic mastectomy
  - ◆ Prophylactic oophorectomy

Follow-up Care: Follow-up Measures to Consider

- • Document
  - ■ Findings
  - ■ Discussion
  - ■ Plan for continued care
    - ◆ Follow-up
    - ◆ Referral
- • Screening recommendations (ACS, 2010; Kearney & Murray, 2009)
  - ■ Age 40 and older
    - ◆ Mammogram annually for women in good health
    - ◆ Clinical breast examination annually
    - ◆ Regular self-breast examination: Report any changes to healthcare provider
  - ■ Ages 20–39, low risk
    - ◆ Clinical breast examination at least every 3 years
    - ◆ Regular self-breast examination: Report any changes to healthcare provider
  - ■ Women at high risk for breast cancer: Annual mammogram and MRI
    - ◆ Lifetime risk of 20% or greater by risk assessment tool
    - ◆ Known BRCA1 or BRCA2 gene mutation
    - ◆ First-degree relative with BRCA 1 or BRAC 2 gene mutation
    - ◆ Radiation therapy to chest between ages of 10 and 30
  - ■ Women at moderately increased risk for breast cancer: Annual mammogram and consider MRI

- ◆ Lifetime risk of 15–20% by risk assessment tool
- ◆ Personal history of breast cancer or atypical hyperplasia
- ◆ Extremely or unevenly dense breast tissue by mammogram
- • Assess
  - ■ Emotional state
  - ■ Understanding of information
  - ■ Ability to proceed with recommendations
  - ■ Need for counseling/support
- • Return for care
  - ■ Cystic mass
    - ◆ One to three cycles
    - ◆ After menses
    - ◆ Immediately if enlargement occurs
  - ■ Solid masses, not referred for biopsy
    - ◆ Must appear benign by the following methods:
      - ➤ Clinical findings *and*
      - ➤ Mammogram and/or ultrasound
    - ◆ One-month rechecks
      - ➤ After menses (if cycling)
      - ➤ No growth or regression
      - ➤ ⚠ A benign mass can mask a malignancy
  - ■ Women post-biopsy for benign lesion: Unilateral mammogram in 6 months to establish a new baseline

Multidisciplinary Practice: Consider Consultation, Collaboration, or Referral

- • Breast center or surgery service
  - ■ Breast mass that is suspicious for cancer
  - ■ Diagnostic evaluation
    - ◆ Abnormal mammogram
    - ◆ Abnormal ultrasound
    - ◆ Persistent mass
  - ■ For excision if a cyst recurs after its aspiration
  - ■ Client preference for definitive therapy (e.g., excisional biopsy)
- • For diagnosis or treatment outside the midwife's scope of practice

CARE OF THE WOMAN WITH CHLAMYDIA

Key Clinical Information

Chlamydia remains the most common STI in the United States. Women with chlamydial infection can present with symptoms that range from mucoid discharge to fulminant PID. Chlamydial infection contributes to decreased tubal patency, which can in turn result in infertility and ectopic pregnancy. Chlamydial infection is also associated with persistent pelvic pain, preterm labor and rupture of membranes, and neonatal conjunctivitis and trachoma. Chlamydia frequently coexists with gonorrhea or other STIs, such as *Mycoplasma* infection, and can be asymptomatic. Routine annual chlamydia screening is recommended for women younger than 25 and for women older than 25 with a new sexual partner or multiple partners. Screening is a cost-effective means of reducing the incidence of chlamydia (CDC, 2010). For healthcare providers, it is important to reach out to high-risk adolescents, as they account for approximately half of all chlamydia diagnoses (Foulkes, Pettigrew, Livingston, & Niccolai, 2009).

Client History and Chart Review: Components of the History to Consider

(Ross, Judlin, & Nilas, 2007)

- Age
- GP TPAL
- LMP
  - Onset and duration
  - Abnormal bleeding
    - Intermenstrual
    - Postcoital
  - Potential for pregnancy
    - Current method of birth control
    - Ectopic pregnancy may mimic chlamydia
    - Gestational age, if pregnant
- Onset, duration, and type of symptoms
  - Pain
    - Location
      - Urethral
      - Adnexal
      - Suprapubic
    - Severity
    - Precipitating factors
  - Discharge
    - Amount
    - Color
    - Consistency
- Sexual history
  - New sexual partner for self or for partner
  - Multiple sexual partners
  - Previous diagnosis of STIs
  - Presence of IUD
  - Condom use
- Medical/surgical history
  - Allergies
  - Medications
  - Chronic health problems
- Social history
  - Alcohol or drug use
  - Non-white ethnicity
- Review of systems

Physical Examination: Components of the Physical Exam to Consider

(Ross et al., 2007)

- Vital signs, including temperature
- Abdominal palpation
  - Rebound tenderness
  - Guarding
- Pelvic examination
  - External genitalia
  - Speculum examination
    - Vaginal discharge
    - Appearance of cervix
      - Presence of mucopurulent cervical discharge
      - Edema or erythema of cervix
  - Bimanual examination
    - Cervical motion tenderness
    - Uterine enlargement or tenderness
    - Adnexal mass
    - Adnexal pain

Clinical Impression: Differential Diagnoses to Consider

(ICD9data.com, 2012)

- Chlamydia
- Gonorrhea
- PID
- Endometriosis
- Ectopic pregnancy
- Ovarian cyst
- Cervicitis
- Pelvic malignancy
- Irritable bowel
- Appendicitis

Diagnostic Testing: Diagnostic Tests and Procedures to Consider

(CDC, 2010; Meyers et al., 2008)

- Chlamydia testing
  - Urine
  - Cervical swab
  - Patient collected vaginal swab (CDC, 2010)
  - Rectal swab
  - Oropharyngeal swab
  - ♂ Urethral swab
- Gonorrhea testing
- Vaginal wet preparation
- Serum/urine pregnancy testing
- Serum testing
  - HIV
  - Hepatitis B
  - Syphilis
- Pelvic ultrasound
- ⚠ Note: Visual inspection of the vaginal discharge is nonspecific and cannot be used alone for diagnosis. Multiple pathogens may be present. Perform additional testing as required for accurate diagnosis.

Providing Treatment: Therapeutic Measures to Consider

(CDC, 2010; FitzMaurice et al., 2011; Hatcher et al., 2011; Ross et al., 2007)

- Recommended treatments
  - Single-dose treatment under observation is ideal
  - Azithromycin: 1 g PO single dose
    - First-line therapy
    - Acceptable for use in pregnancy
    - Pregnancy Category B
  - Doxycycline: 100 mg PO BID for 7 days
    - First-line therapy for nonpregnant women
    - ⚠ Do not use in pregnancy
    - Pregnancy Category D
  - Amoxicillin: 500 mg TID for 7 days
    - First-line therapy for pregnant women
    - Pregnancy Category B
- Alternative treatments
  - Erythromycin base: 500 mg PO QID for 7 days (Pregnancy Category B)
  - Erythromycin ethylsuccinate: 800 mg PO QID for 7 days (Pregnancy Category B)
  - Ofloxacin: 300 mg PO BID for 7 days (Pregnancy Category C)
  - Levofloxacin: 500 mg PO QID for 7 days
- Consider patient-delivered partner treatment (PDPT) (Pavlin et al., 2010)
- Intrauterine device or system
  - If desired: Delay insertion until treatment is given and verified as effective
  - If present at time of diagnosis: Remove
  - Provide an alternative method of birth control
- Analgesia for pain relief

Providing Treatment: Complementary and Alternative Measures to Consider

- ⚠ Alternative measures are not a substitute for antibiotic therapy
- Promote well-being
  - Rest
  - Balanced diet
- Herbal remedies to boost immune response: Echinacea
- Acidophilus to offset effects of antibiotics on the gut
  - Capsules
  - Yogurt
  - Probiotics

Providing Support: Education and Support Measures to Consider

- Provide age-appropriate information
  - Infection cause and transmission
  - Effects on reproductive organs and future fertility
  - Reportable infection
  - Treatment plan and follow-up
    - Need to evaluate and/or treat partner(s)
    - Medication instructions
  - Avoidance of intercourse
    - Until the partner has been tested and treated *and*
    - Until 7 days after medication is begun (CDC, 2010)
  - Prevention measures
    - Risk behaviors
    - Safe sexual practices
  - Partner notification and referral for treatment
    - PDPT can be considered
    - Give prescription and written materials
    - www Legal regulations vary; check www.cdc.gov/std/ept
- Education particularly important in high-risk adolescent populations

Follow-up Care: Follow-up Measures to Consider

- Document
  - Results
  - Treatment
  - Reporting
  - Client discussion and education
  - Plan for follow-up
- Further STI testing, including *Mycoplasma* infection
- Return to office or clinic
  - Three to four weeks after treatment for test of cure
    - Pregnancy
    - Lack of concordance with plan of care
    - High-risk behaviors (CDC, 2010)
  - For continued symptoms
  - For persistent pain
  - New partner for self or for partner
  - Client preference for testing
- Rescreen within 3–6 months
- With new diagnosis of pregnancy
  - Test all clients
  - Perform early ultrasound after PID to rule out ectopic pregnancy
- Assess postpartum and newborn clients
  - Endometritis
  - Salpingitis
  - Newborn ophthalmic infection
  - Newborn respiratory infection (CDC, 2010)

Multidisciplinary Practice: Consider Consultation, Collaboration, or Referral

- OB/GYN services: For complicated infection
  - Persistent symptoms
  - Pelvic infection
  - Unresponsive infection
  - Positive HIV or hepatitis B status
  - Persistent pelvic pain
  - Ectopic pregnancy
- Urology services
- Pediatric services: Imminent delivery
  - With chlamydia infection or symptoms
  - Preterm labor
  - Newborn with signs of the following conditions:
    - Chlamydia
    - Ophthalmia neonatorum
    - Pneumonia
- For diagnosis or treatment outside the midwife's scope of practice

CARE OF THE WOMAN UNDERGOING COLPOSCOPY

Key Clinical Information

Colposcopy is a directed examination of the uterine cervix and genitals for areas of abnormality, including the cervix, vagina, and vaginal opening (vulva).

In this procedure, a special binocular microscope (colposcope) is used to illuminate and magnify the area of examination by 10 to 40 times (Frank, 2008). During the procedure, one or more solutions are applied to the tissues, and colored filters may be used to help delineate or highlight abnormal lesions and allow detailed examination. Directed biopsies are then taken from the most abnormal area(s). Neither cytology nor histology reliably predicts the biologic potential of a lesion to progress to invasive cancer (Wright, Massad, Dunton, Spitzer, Wilkinson, & Solomon, 2007b); instead, colposcopy remains the gold standard for the evaluation of abnormal Pap smear results and genital tract lesions. Colposcopy skills are considered an expanded clinical skill appropriate for midwives after additional education and supervised practicum are successfully mastered.

Client History and Chart Review: Components of the History to Consider

- Age
- Indications for colposcopy (Wright et al., 2007b)
  - ASC-US
    - Recurrent ASC-US
    - High-risk HPV-positive status
  - ASC-H
  - LSIL
  - Adolescent women younger than age 20 with the following:
    - Persistent ASC-US
    - HSIL
  - HSIL
  - AGC
  - Vulvar or vaginal lesions
- Presence of symptoms
  - Vaginal discharge
  - Postcoital bleeding
  - Postmenopausal bleeding
  - Pelvic pain
- Reproductive history
  - GP TPAL
  - LMP and pregnancy status

- Method of birth control
- History of STIs
- Prior abnormal Pap smears
  - HPV test results
  - Diagnostic procedures
  - Treatment
- Intermenstrual or postcoital bleeding
- Medical history
  - HIV infection
  - Decreased immune response
- Social history
  - Smoking
  - Diet
  - Support
- Factors that contribute to risk (ACS, 2006b)
  - High-risk HPV infection
  - Multiple sexual partners (self or partner)
  - Unprotected sex
  - Chlamydia
  - Smoking
  - Diet low in fruits and vegetables
  - Low socioeconomic status
  - Grand multipara
  - Immune deficiency
  - Long-term oral contraceptive use
  - Family history
  - Diethylstilbestrol (DES) exposure in utero
- Verify client preparation for procedure
  - Explain the procedure to the woman
  - Obtain informed consent
  - Answer questions and address concerns
  - Offer premedication (discussed later in this section)

Physical Examination: Components of the Physical Exam to Consider

(Moses, 2007; Sellors & Sankaranarayanan, 2003)

- Colposcopy is an expanded midwifery skill; further education and training are needed to perform it
- Vulvar examination
  - Apply 5% acetic acid–soaked pads (white vinegar may be used)

- Examine for evidence of potential vulvar intraepithelial lesion (VIN)
  - Pigmented or acetowhite lesions
  - Visible warts
  - Discharge
- Vaginal examination
  - Apply 5% acetic acid wash
  - Examine for evidence of vaginal intraepithelial lesion (VaIN)
    - Acetowhite lesions
    - Warts or other signs of HPV
    - Punctation or mosaicism
  - Visible lesion present
    - Gentle biopsy *or*
    - 🕐 Refer for biopsy
    - ⚠ The posterior vaginal wall is very thin
- Cervical examination
  - Obtain specimens only if indicated
    - May cause tissue disruption and limit examination
    - Pap smear
    - HPV testing
  - Apply 5% acetic acid wash
    - Examine without magnification
    - Examine colposcopically
      - No filter
      - Green filter
    - Satisfactory examination includes visualization of the following areas:
      - Squamocolumnar junction
      - Transformation zone
    - Evaluate lesion(s)
      - Size
      - Location
      - Clarity of margins
      - Thickness of edge
      - Brightness of acetowhite tissue
      - Presence of punctation and/or mosaicism
        - Intercapillary distance
        - Fine versus coarse changes
        - Abnormal vessels
    - Apply Lugol's solution if needed to clarify the presence of a lesion or its borders
    - Obtain biopsies as indicated

- After biopsies of lesion(s)
- Ensure hemostasis
  - Pressure
  - Monsel's paste
    - Ferric subsulfate solution
    - Leave open so that it thickens to a paste
  - Silver nitrite application
    - Insert one to three sticks into the biopsy wound
    - Apply gentle, steady pressure
    - Release the pressure
    - Do not pull on the sticks
    - Tap gently until the sticks spontaneously release
- Allow the patient to rest supine for several minutes

Clinical Impression: Differential Diagnoses to Consider

(ICD9data.com, 2012)

- Abnormal Pap smear
- HPV
  - High risk, DNA test positive
  - Low risk, DNA test positive
- Condyloma acuminatum
- Postcoital bleeding
- Postmenopausal bleeding
- Leukoplakia of cervix
- Vaginal discharge, noninfectious
- Cervical dysplasia
- Carcinoma in situ of cervix
- Procedures (CPT codes apply)
  - Colposcopy, no biopsy
  - Colposcopy, with biopsy
  - Cervical biopsy
  - Endocervical biopsy

Diagnostic Testing: Diagnostic Tests and Procedures to Consider

(Frank, 2008; Wright et al., 2007b)

- Pap smear—rarely indicated
  - Obtaining a Pap smear may obscure the lesion

- Benefit is seen with HSIL, for correlation of results
- HPV DNA testing
- STI testing per client history
- Biopsies as indicated by colposcopic examination
  - Directed biopsies of lesion(s)
  - Endocervical curettage
    - If unsatisfactory examination *or*
    - All clients

Providing Treatment: Therapeutic Measures to Consider

- Treatment options
  - Expectant management
  - Cryotherapy (ablative therapy)
  - LEEP procedure (excisional therapy)
  - Laser (ablative therapy)
  - Cold-knife cone (excisional therapy)
- Treatment triage (Wright et al., 2007b): Client with consistent results
  - No high-risk HPV, no lesion, ASC-US Pap smear
    - No treatment indicated
    - Observation with close follow-up for 2 years
  - ASC-US, ASC-H, or LSIL Pap smear
    - Pap, lesion, and biopsy consistent with CIN grade 1
    - Conservative management: Close follow-up
    - Ablative treatment acceptable
      - Persistent CIN grade 1 lesion
      - Satisfactory examination
      - Negative endocervical sampling
    - Excisional treatment
      - Persistent CIN grade 1 lesion
      - Unsatisfactory examination
      - Positive endocervical sampling
      - Previous treatment
  - HSIL or AGC—not otherwise specified (NOS) Pap smear
    - Pap smear, lesion, and biopsy consistent with CIN grade 1

- Conservative management: Close follow-up for 1 year
  - Satisfactory examination *and*
  - Negative endocervical sampling
  - Follow-up
    - Pap smear every 6–12 months or
    - HPV test every 12 months
  - Negative follow-up: Return to routine screening
  - HSIL noted on follow-up
    - Colposcopy
    - Excisional biopsy
- Excisional treatment
- Adolescents with CIN grade 1: Repeat cytology in 12 months
  - Less than HSIL: Pap smear in 12 months
    - Normal Pap smear: Routine screening
    - ASC or greater: Colposcopy
  - HSIL: Colposcopy
- Pregnant women with CIN grade 1: Follow without treatment until after delivery
- CIN grades 2 and 3
  - Satisfactory colposcopy
    - Ablative treatment
    - Excisional treatment
  - Unsatisfactory colposcopy: Diagnostic excision
  - Two follow-up options
    - Cytology every 6 months twice
      - Routine screening after two negative results
      - Colposcopy and endocervical curettage for ASC or greater
    - HPV DNA testing every 6 months twice
      - Routine screening after two negative results
      - Colposcopy and endocervical curettage for high-risk HPV
  - Adolescents with CIN grades 2 and 3
    - Observation or treatment acceptable
    - Cytology and colposcopy every 6 months
    - Repeat biopsy for persistent or worsening lesion

➤ Treatment
- ◗ CIN grade 3 *or*
- ◗ CIN grades 2 and 3 that persist greater than or equal to 24 months

Providing Treatment: Complementary and Alternative Measures to Consider

- Supplements or food sources for the following nutrients:
  - Folic acid
  - Vitamins C and E
  - Selenium
- Whole foods diet
  - Dark yellow and orange vegetables
    - ◆ Winter squash
    - ◆ Carrots
    - ◆ Rutabaga
  - Tomatoes
- Support immune system (short-term therapy)
  - Echinacea
  - Goldenseal
  - Yarrow
- Visualization of healing

Providing Support: Education and Support Measures to Consider

- Provide information
  - Indication for colposcopy
  - Colposcopic procedure
  - Performed with the client in stirrups, using a speculum
  - Takes 5–20 minutes
  - May cause cramping
  - Occasional vagal response (syncope)
- Decrease stress during the procedure (Galaal, Deane, Sangal, & Lopes, 2007)
  - Play music during the procedure
  - Use video colposcopy if available
  - Premedicate with a nonsteroidal anti-inflammatory drug (NSAID)
- Postcolposcopy instructions
  - Brownish discharge is common
  - Vaginal rest for 7 days
  - Call with bright bleeding
- Postcolposcopy information
  - Working diagnosis
  - Anticipated treatment and/or follow-up
  - Provide written information
    - ◆ Abnormal Pap smears
    - ◆ HPV
- Decrease risk of progression
  - Smoking cessation
  - Healthy diet
  - Safe sex practices

Follow-up Care: Follow-up Measures to Consider

- Document
  - Indication for colposcopy
  - Findings: Pictorial and descriptive
  - Anticipated biopsy result(s)
  - Actual biopsy result(s)
  - Correlate results to formulate a plan of care
    - ◆ Pap smear
    - ◆ HPV test
    - ◆ Clinical picture
    - ◆ Biopsy results
- Close follow-up per American Society for Colposcopy and Cervical Pathology recommendations (see Figures 7-11 to 7-16)

Multidisciplinary Practice: Consider Consultation, Collaboration, or Referral

- OB/GYN or colposcopy service
  - If colposcopy is not within the midwife's scope of practice
  - For high-grade lesions
  - For confirmed CIN grades 2 and 3 or greater for treatment
  - Clients with demonstrated progression of disease
  - Clients with lack of concordance to treatment plan
  - For development of a management plan for a woman in whom results are not consistent
- For diagnosis or treatment outside the midwife's scope of practice

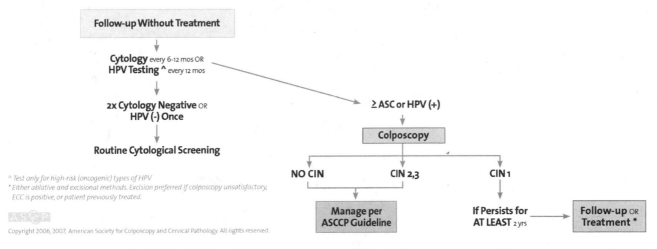

Figure 7-11   Management of Women with a Histological Diagnosis of Cervical Intraepithelial Neoplasia Grade 1 (CIN 1) Preceded by ASC-US, ASC-H, or LSIL Cytology

Source: Copyright 2006, 2007. American Society for Colposcopy and Cervical Pathology. All rights reserved.

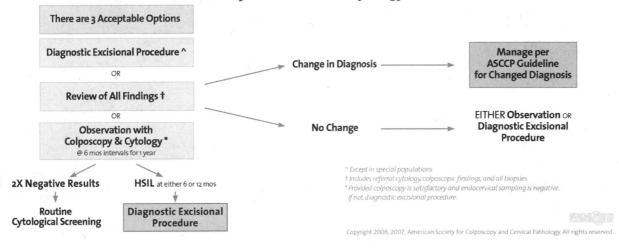

Figure 7-12   Management of Women with a Histological Diagnosis of Cervical Intraepithelial Neoplasia—Grade 1 (CIN 1) Preceded by HSIL or AGC-NOS Cytology

Source: Copyright 2006, 2007. American Society for Colposcopy and Cervical Pathology. All rights reserved.

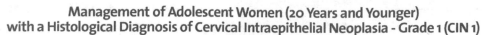

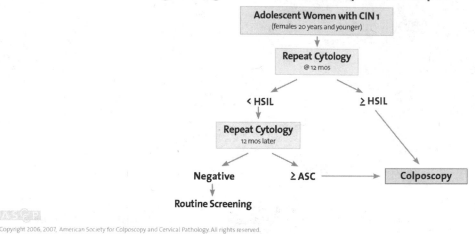

Figure 7-13   Management of Adolescent Women (20 Years and Younger) with a Histological Diagnosis of Cervical Intraepithelial Neoplasia—Grade 1 (CIN 1)

Source: Copyright 2006, 2007. American Society for Colposcopy and Cervical Pathology. All rights reserved.

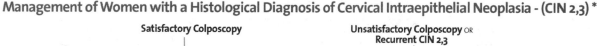

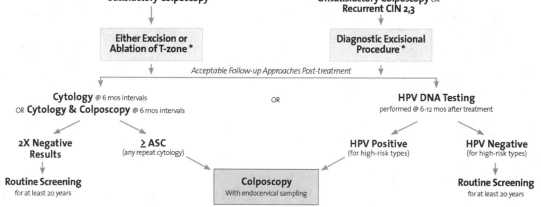

Figure 7-14   Management of Women with a Histological Diagnosis of Cervical Intraepithelial Neoplasia—(CIN 2, 3)

Source: Copyright 2006, 2007. American Society for Colposcopy and Cervical Pathology. All rights reserved.

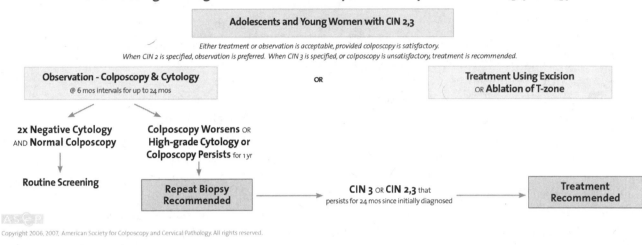

Figure 7-15 Management of Adolescent and Young Women with a Histological Diagnosis of Cervical Intraepithelial Neoplasia—Grade 2, 3 (CIN 2, 3)

Source: Copyright 2006, 2007. American Society for Colposcopy and Cervical Pathology. All rights reserved.

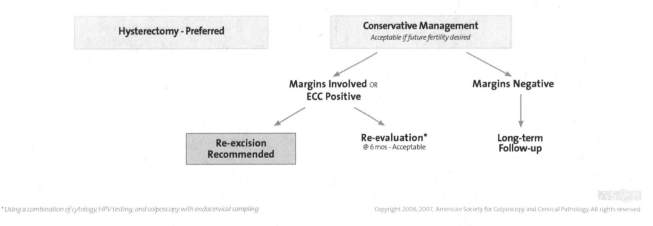

Figure 7-16 Management of Women with Adenocarcinoma in-situ (AIS) Diagnosed from a Diagnostic Excisional Procedure

Source: Copyright 2006, 2007. American Society for Colposcopy and Cervical Pathology. All rights reserved.

CARE OF THE WOMAN WITH DYSFUNCTIONAL UTERINE BLEEDING

Key Clinical Information

Dysfunctional uterine bleeding (DUB), defined as noncyclic bleeding that occurs in anovulatory women, is diagnosed by the exclusion of uterine pathology or underlying medical causes (Fritz & Speroff, 2011). DUB is characterized by irregular menstrual cycles with bleeding that ranges from light to heavy and occurs in approximately 10% of American women at some point in their lives (King, 2011). A sustained high level of estrogen, as tends to occur with adolescence, perimenopause, obesity, and polycystic ovary syndrome, is associated with heavy bleeding (Fritz & Speroff, 2011). Unopposed estrogen from anovulation can lead to endometrial hyperplasia if left untreated. Successful management of DUB requires understanding the mechanisms involved and ruling out other conditions that can lead to similar symptoms.

Client History and Chart Review: Components of the History to Consider

(Fritz & Speroff, 2011; Taylor, Schuiling, & Sharp, 2013)

- Age
- Pregnancy history: GP TPAL
- Current method of contraception
  - IUD
  - Hormonal methods
- Menstrual history
  - LMP
  - Onset of menarche or menopausal symptoms
  - Usual flow patterns
  - Changes in menses/bleeding
    - Onset, frequency, and duration of bleeding
    - Number of pads/tampons per day
    - Incidence of the following:
      - Clots
      - Heavy blood flow
      - Odor
  - Association of bleeding with the following:
    - Menstrual cycle
    - Intercourse
    - Pain
  - Other associated signs and symptoms
    - Tachycardia
    - Pallor
    - Fatigue or breathlessness
    - Weight changes
    - Change in hair texture or distribution
    - Pain with intercourse
    - Urinary frequency
    - Abdominal bloating
    - Premenstrual symptoms (molimina)
    - Menopausal symptoms
- Medical history
  - Allergies
  - Medications
  - Herbal or over-the-counter remedies
  - Medical conditions
  - History of and risk for STIs
  - Results of prior Pap smears: Date of last Pap smear and examination
- Social history: Potential for hypothalamic suppression
  - Stress
  - Anorexia
  - High level of physical activity
- Directed history to potential causes of DUB
  - Pregnancy-related conditions
    - Spontaneous abortion
    - Ectopic pregnancy
    - Placenta previa or abruption
  - Gynecologic conditions
    - Infection
    - Benign lesions, such as fibroids
    - Trauma
    - Malignant or premalignant lesions
    - Polycystic ovary syndrome
    - Polyps
    - Adenomyosis
  - Systemic conditions
    - Thyroid disease

- ◆ Hypothalamic suppression
- ◆ Diabetes
- ◆ Hypertension
- ◆ Adrenal disorders
- ◆ Blood dyscrasias and coagulopathies, such as von Willebrand's disease
- ◆ Liver disease
- ◆ Pituitary adenoma
- ◆ Kidney disease
- ◆ Malignancy
- ◆ Systemic lupus erythematosus
- ■ Prescription medications
  - ◆ Hormones
  - ◆ Tamoxifen
  - ◆ Selective serotonin reuptake inhibitors
  - ◆ Anticoagulants
  - ◆ Antipsychotics
  - ◆ Corticosteroids
- ■ Herbal or over-the-counter remedies
  - ◆ Aspirin
  - ◆ Blue or black cohosh
  - ◆ Ginkgo biloba
  - ◆ Ginseng
  - ◆ Soy
  - ◆ Bromelain
- • Review of systems

Physical Examination: Components of the Physical Exam to Consider

(Schorge, Schaffer, Halvorson, Hoffman, Bradshaw, & Cunningham, 2008; Taylor et al., 2013)

- • Vital signs
  - ■ Hypotension
  - ■ Tachycardia or bradycardia
  - ■ Subnormal temperature
- • Weight: Note changes
- • Body habitus
- • Skin and mucous membranes
  - ■ Pallor
  - ■ Dry, coarse texture
  - ■ Diaphoresis
  - ■ Petechiae

- ■ Hirsutism
- ■ Acne
- ■ Alopecia
- ■ Acanthosis nigricans
- • Thyroid
  - ■ Size
  - ■ Symmetry
  - ■ Nodules
- • Breasts: Presence of galactorrhea
- • Speculum examination
  - ■ Origin of bleeding
  - ■ Cervix and vagina
    - ◆ Erosion
    - ◆ Lesions
    - ◆ Friability
    - ◆ Presence of IUD strings
  - ■ Presence of polyps
  - ■ Evidence of trauma or foreign body
- • Bimanual examination
  - ■ Uterine, cervical, and adnexal
    - ◆ Position
    - ◆ Size
    - ◆ Contour
    - ◆ Consistency
  - ■ Masses
  - ■ Pain
  - ■ Cervical motion tenderness
- • Rectal or rectovaginal examination
  - ■ Hemorrhoids
  - ■ Masses

Clinical Impression: Differential Diagnoses to Consider

(ICD9data.com, 2012)

- • Pregnancy (see "Care of the Pregnant Woman with Vaginal Bleeding, First Trimester")
  - ■ Threatened or missed abortion
  - ■ Ectopic pregnancy
- • Functional DUB (ovarian dysfunction)
- • Cervicitis
- • Cervical polyps
- • Endometrial hyperplasia

- Uterine fibroids
- Menorrhagia, primary
- Menorrhagia, adolescent
- Menorrhagia, perimenopausal
- Menorrhagia, postmenopausal
- Premature ovarian failure
- Polycystic ovary syndrome
- Thyroid dysfunction
- Coagulopathy
- Malignancy
- Infection

Diagnostic Testing: Diagnostic Tests and Procedures to Consider

- Office testing
  - Pregnancy testing
  - Pap smear
  - Chlamydia and/or gonorrhea testing
  - Wet prep
  - Endometrial biopsy
    - Older than age 35
    - Elevated BMI
    - Endometrial stripe greater than 12 mm on ultrasound
- Endocrine testing
  - Thyroid testing: TSH, thyroid antibodies, T3, T4
  - Hormonal evaluation
    - FSH and LH
    - Prolactin
    - Estradiol
    - Testosterone
    - Progesterone
- Hematology
  - Complete blood count (CBC) with differential
  - Hematocrit and hemoglobin
  - Serum ferritin
  - Bleeding time, prothrombin time (PT), and partial thromboplastin time (PPT)
- Pelvic imaging
  - Abdominal or vaginal ultrasound
    - Threatened or missed abortion
    - Uterine fibroids

- Thickness of endometrial stripe
- Intrauterine polyps
- Ovarian or adnexal masses
  - CT of abdomen and pelvis
- Surgical biopsy methods
  - Saline-infusion sonohysterography
  - Hysteroscopy
  - Dilation and curettage

Providing Treatment: Therapeutic Measures to Consider

(Fritz & Speroff, 2011; King & Brucker, 2011; Taylor et al., 2013)

- For acute, heavy DUB
  - High-dose estrogen
    - 1.25 mg conjugated estrogen *or*
    - 2.0 mg micronized estradiol
      - Take q 4–6 hr × 24 hr
      - Taper after bleeding is controlled to 1 PO qd × 7–10 days
      - Followed by combined oral contraceptives or progesterone
  - Combined oral contraceptives: Low-dose monophasic pill
    - One pill PO BID until bleeding slows
    - Daily to complete pack
    - May cause nausea
    - May use extended regimen after taper
  - High-dose progestin
    - Provera: 10–20 mg BID PO, or
    - Norethindrone: 5 mg BID PO, or
    - Megestrol acetate: 20–40 mg BID PO
    - Take for 7–10 days, then qd for 2 weeks
- For chronic DUB
  - NSAIDs
    - Begin up to 3 days before or with onset of menses
    - Continue through menses
      - Naproxen: 550 mg PO loading dose, then 275 mg q 6 hr for 3–5 days
      - Ponstel: 500 mg PO TID for 3–5 days
      - Ibuprofen: 400 mg PO TID for 3–5 days

- Combination hormonal contraceptives
  - Pills, patch, or vaginal ring
  - Best choice for women who occasionally ovulate and desire contraception
- Cyclical progestins
  - Begin on the first day of the month or 14–15 days before the next anticipated menses
  - Provera: 5–10 mg/day for 12–14 days each month
  - Aygestin: 2.5–10 mg/day for 12–14 days each month
  - Prometrium: 200–400 mg for 12–14 days each month
    - Take in the evening
    - May cause drowsiness
- Mirena IUD
- DepoProvera
- Tranexamic acid
  - 1–1.5 mg PO 3–4 times QD
  - With menses onset, continue 4–7 days
- Iron replacement therapy
- ⚠️ 📞 For severe, acute DUB
  - Refer to emergency services
  - IV estrogen to control bleeding
  - Surgical treatment measures
    - Dilation and curettage
    - Endometrial ablation
    - Hysterectomy
    - Uterine artery embolization
- 📞 Additional treatment as indicated by the differential diagnosis

Providing Treatment: Complementary and Alternative Measures to Consider

- Balanced nutrition
  - Iron foods to treat anemia (see "Food Sources of Iron")
  - Vitamins A, C, E, and K
  - Bioflavonoids
  - Phytoestrogens
- Moderate physical activity
- Stress management

- Planned time for the following:
  - Regular physical activity
  - Rest and recreation
  - Personal time
- Counseling for emotional issues
- Herbal remedies (Hudson, 2008)
  - Milk thistle
  - Red raspberry
  - Blue cohosh
  - Squaw vine
  - Shepherd's purse
  - Vitex
  - Purslane
  - Ginger
- Acupuncture

Providing Support: Education and Support Measures to Consider

- Client education
  - Normal menstrual functioning
  - Workup related to working diagnosis
- Maintain menstrual calendar
- Results and diagnosis
  - Informed choice regarding treatment options
  - Follow-up plan
  - Treatment instructions
  - When and how to contact healthcare providers for problems
  - Consultation and/or referral criteria

Follow-up Care: Follow-up Measures to Consider

- Document
  - Working diagnoses
  - Evaluation plan
  - Discussions with the client
  - Referral criteria
- Return for continued care
  - Hyperplasia (no atypia): Follow-up endometrial biopsy in 6–12 months
  - For persistent or worsening symptoms
  - For support during evaluation and/or treatment
  - For well-woman care after treatment

Multidisciplinary Practice: Consider Consultation, Collaboration, or Referral

- OB/GYN services
  - Diagnostic testing, such as sonohysteroscopy
  - Women with acute bleeding
    - Hemodynamic stabilization
    - Parenteral estrogen therapy
    - Surgical treatment
  - Presence of the following:
    - Uterine fibroids
    - Reproductive cancer or precancerous condition
    - Ectopic pregnancy
    - Incomplete abortion
  - DUB
    - Persistent and progressive bleeding
    - Unresponsive to herbal or hormone therapy
    - Unknown cause
  - Client preference
- Medical or endocrinology services: Bleeding secondary to the following:
  - Systemic condition
  - Endocrine dysfunction
- For diagnosis or treatment outside the midwife's scope of practice

CARE OF THE WOMAN WITH DYSMENORRHEA

Key Clinical Information

Painful menstrual periods may be related to functional uterine contractions in ovulatory women (primary dysmenorrhea) or can be caused by endometriosis, adenomyosis, pelvic adhesions, infection, hormonal dysfunction, or enlarging uterine fibroids (secondary dysmenorrhea). Primary dysmenorrhea occurs in approximately 60% of adolescent women (Fritz & Speroff, 2011). When dysmenorrhea does not respond to treatment, evaluation for endometriosis should be considered. The pain of endometriosis frequently begins before the onset of menses, unlike physiologic pain, which is caused by uterine contractions

expelling the menstrual flow (Fritz & Speroff, 2011). Pain with menstruation is often accompanied by heavy flow, headache, nausea, vomiting, diarrhea, or other symptoms; it can cause women lost days from school or work, and limit their ability to care for themselves or their families. Careful investigation into this common problem may provide options for relief or a decrease in symptoms.

Client History and Chart Review: Components of the History to Consider

- Age: Dysmenorrhea is common in adolescent women with onset of ovulatory cycles (Fritz & Speroff, 2011)
- Pregnancy history
  - GP TPAL, LMP
  - Dysmenorrhea is common in nulliparous women
- Gynecologic history
  - Menstrual history
    - Age of menarche
    - Usual menstrual patterns
      - Interval
      - Duration
      - Flow
    - Age at onset of dysmenorrhea
    - Characteristics of discomfort
      - Location
      - Duration
      - Severity
      - Timing in cycle at onset
      - Progression over time
      - Association with other body functions
      - Bowel and bladder changes with pain
      - Other associated symptoms, including premenstrual symptoms
      - Occurrence of symptoms at times other than menses
    - Relief measures used and results
    - Impact on lifestyle and daily functioning
  - Current method of birth control
    - Hormonal contraceptive use
    - IUD use and type of device

◆ History of surgical sterilization
- PID/STIs
- Endometriosis
  ◆ Symptoms
  ◆ Diagnosis
- Previous pelvic surgery
- Congenital pelvic anomaly
• Medical/surgical history
  - Medications
  - Allergies
  - Health conditions
• Family history
  - Dysmenorrhea
  - Endometriosis
• Social history
  - 🌐 Cultural attitudes regarding menstruation
  - Marital/relationship status
  - Tobacco use
  - Exercise patterns
  - History of sexual assault
• Review of systems

Physical Examination: Components of the Physical Exam to Consider

• Vital signs
• Body mass index
• Abdominal palpation
  - Lower abdominal tenderness
  - Costovertebral angle tenderness
• Pelvic examination
  - Speculum examination
    ◆ Appearance of cervix
    ◆ Appearance of vagina
    ◆ Specimen collection as needed
  - Bimanual examination
    ◆ Uterine size, position, and contour
    ◆ Uterine or cervical motion tenderness
    ◆ Uterine and adnexal mobility
    ◆ Adnexal tenderness
    ◆ Pelvic masses
    ◆ Cystocele or rectocele
• Rectal examination

Clinical Impression: Differential Diagnoses to Consider

(ICD9data.com, 2012)

• Functional dysmenorrhea
• Endometriosis
• Adenomyosis
• Pelvic adhesions
• Neoplasia
• PID
• Pelvic anomaly
• Uterine fibroids
• Pelvic organ prolapse
• Premenstrual syndrome
• Urinary tract infection
• Bowel disorder or disease

Diagnostic Testing: Diagnostic Tests and Procedures to Consider

• Pap smear
• Chlamydia/gonorrhea testing
• Urinalysis
• Stool for occult blood after rectal examination
• Pelvic ultrasound based on pelvic examination findings

Providing Treatment: Therapeutic Measures to Consider

• Functional dysmenorrhea: First-line therapies (Fritz & Speroff, 2011)
  - Ibuprofen: 400 mg q 6 hr
  - Naproxen: 500 mg, then 250 mg q 6–8 hr
  - Mefenamic acid: 500 mg, then 250 mg q 4 hr
  - Timing
    ◆ Begin with onset of menses *or*
    ◆ Begin 24–48 hours before menses is expected for severe cases
    ◆ Take with food to avoid gastrointestinal symptoms
• Hormonal control (King, 2011)
  - Combination hormonal birth control
    ◆ Extended cycling doses
    ◆ NuvaRing

- Mirena IUD
- Depo-Provera
- Implanon
- Suspected endometriosis: See "Care of the Woman with Endometriosis"
- ⏱ Other diagnoses: Evaluate and treat as appropriate

Providing Treatment: Complementary and Alternative Measures to Consider

(Dennehy, 2006; Romm, 2010)

- Heat to abdomen
- Balanced diet
  - Vegetarian diet
  - Vitamin E
    - ◆ 200 IU BID 2 days prior to menses and 3 days after
    - ◆ Do not exceed 400 IU daily
    - ◆ ⚠ Exercise caution with anticoagulant use
  - Omega-3 fatty acids: ⚠ Exercise caution with anticoagulant use
  - Vitamin B_1: 100 mg daily
  - Vitamin B_6
  - Magnesium
  - Decrease salt intake
  - Natural diuretics
    - ◆ Tea or coffee
    - ◆ Asparagus
  - Plenty of fiber
- Vigorous exercise for endorphin release
- Acupuncture
- Herbal remedies
  - Vitex tea, tincture, or capsules
  - Evening primrose oil: 3–6 capsules/day
  - Dong quai tea: ⚠ Use with caution in the following situations:
    - ◆ Anticoagulant use
    - ◆ Pregnant or nursing mothers
    - ◆ Hormone use
  - Crampbark and black haw tea

Providing Support: Education and Support Measures to Consider

- Provide age-appropriate information
  - Reproductive anatomy and physiology
    - ◆ Symptoms may improve after pregnancy
    - ◆ Teach fertility awareness
      - ➤ Foster awareness of cycle
      - ➤ Consider NSAID use before onset of menses
  - Working diagnosis
    - ◆ Evaluation options
    - ◆ Testing and treatment recommendations
    - ◆ Self-help measures
    - ◆ When to return for care
  - Indications for consultation or referral
- Validate client concerns

Follow-up Care: Follow-up Measures to Consider

- Document
- Return for care
  - After treatment to evaluate effectiveness
  - As indicated by test results
  - For worsening symptoms

Multidisciplinary Practice: Consider Consultation, Collaboration, or Referral

- OB/GYN services
  - For evaluation and treatment of suspected endometriosis
  - For symptoms that do not improve with treatment
  - For abnormal ultrasound, prolapse, or occult bleeding
- For diagnosis or treatment outside the midwife's scope of practice

CARE OF THE WOMAN UNDERGOING ENDOMETRIAL BIOPSY

Key Clinical Information

Endometrial biopsy is the removal of small samples of uterine endometrial tissue via suction aspiration or curettage for laboratory analysis. Evaluation of a woman's uterine endometrium can be easily and safely accomplished in the office setting with endometrial biopsy. This form of tissue sampling is commonly used to evaluate for endometrial hyperplasia, atypia, or malignancy. Endometrial cancer is the most common cancer of the female reproductive tract, with 41,000 women affected annually in the United States (McFarlin, 2006).

The woman who presents with persistent DUB can be evaluated using endometrial biopsy. Evaluation of Pap smear results with endometrial cells or atypical glandular cells (AGC-US) requires endometrial biopsy; however, in this scenario, endometrial biopsy is best performed in conjunction with colposcopy performed by an expert colposcopist because of the possibility that the woman may have highly aggressive disease (Wright et al., 2007a). Gentle technique minimizes discomfort during the procedure and helps prevent complications. Endometrial biopsy skills are considered an expanded practice clinical skill appropriate for midwives after additional education and supervised practicum are successfully mastered.

Client History and Chart Review: Components of the History to Consider

(Grube & McCool, 2004)

- Age
- GP TPAL
- History of cervical trauma
  - May contribute to cervical stenosis
  - Abnormal Pap smear treatment
  - Abortion
  - Dilation and curettage
- Indications for endometrial biopsy
  - DUB
  - Rule out endometrial cancer or premalignant lesions
    - Abnormal uterine bleeding
    - Postmenopausal bleeding
    - Endometrial stripe greater than 5 mm
  - Infertility investigation

- Pap smear results (Wright et al., 2007a)
  - Atypical glandular cells
  - Adenocarcinoma in situ
  - Endometrial cells
- Contraindications for endometrial biopsy
  - Positive HCG or suspected pregnancy
  - Genital tract infection
  - Cervical cancer
- Risk factors for endometrial cancer (ACS, 2006a)
  - Age older than 50 years
  - Polycystic ovary syndrome
  - Elevated BMI
  - Prolonged exposure to estrogen
    - Nullipara
    - Unopposed estrogen therapy
    - Delayed menopause (age 52 or older)
  - Diabetes mellitus
  - Tamoxifen
- LMP or menstrual status
  - Luteal phase for infertility investigation: Confirmation of ovulation on days 22–23
  - Potential for pregnancy
  - Method of birth control if applicable
- Last Pap smear and results
- Medical history
  - Allergies
  - Medications
    - Hormone replacement
    - Hormonal contraception
    - Tamoxifen
    - Aspirin
  - Medical conditions
    - Current undiagnosed fever
    - Bleeding or clotting disorders
    - Heart valve replacement
    - Coronary artery disease
- Verify client preparation
  - Questions or concerns
  - Informed consent obtained
  - Premedication, as needed
  - Nutritional intake
  - Support person available

Physical Examination: Components of the Physical Exam to Consider

- Vital signs, both before and after the procedure
- Bimanual examination
  - Verify the size and position of the uterus
  - Check for cervical motion tenderness
- Speculum examination
  - Vaginal or cervical discharge
  - Cervical scarring
- Reproductive tract infection: If present, treat the condition and reschedule the biopsy

Clinical Impression: Differential Diagnoses to Consider

(ICD9data.com, 2012)

- Endometrial biopsy, procedure (CPT codes apply)
- Indications
  - Postmenopausal bleeding
  - Postmenopausal hormone replacement therapy
  - Endometrial hyperplasia
  - Persistent DUB
  - Luteal-phase defect
  - Atypical glandular cells

Diagnostic Testing: Diagnostic Tests and Procedures to Consider

(Grube & McCool, 2004)

- Urine or serum HCG
- Vaginal wet preparation slide
- STI testing
- Pelvic ultrasound
  - Transvaginal (McFarlin, 2006)
    - Can be used as the initial screening for endometrial abnormalities
    - Hyperplasia is a common finding without abnormal cellular changes
    - Normal endometrium with thickness less than or equal to 4 mm: No need for endometrial biopsy
  - Abdominal
- Sonohysteroscopy

- Hysteroscopy with directed biopsy
- Endometrial biopsy procedure
  - Cleanse cervix with a prep solution
  - Use careful aseptic technique
  - Apply a tenaculum to straighten the uterus
    - Apply 20% benzocaine gel to the application site, if desired
    - Slow application decreases cramping
    - Apply to the upper lip of the cervix for an anteverted/anteflexed uterus
    - Apply to the posterior lip of the cervix for a retroverted/retroflexed uterus
    - Avoid the 3 and 9 o'clock positions
  - Apply gentle, steady traction to the tenaculum
  - Sound the uterus
    - Helps to dilate the cervix
    - Determines depth
      - Of the endometrial cavity
      - Of the biopsy collection device
    - Gently insert the sound or device in the direction of uterine curvature
    - Apply gentle pressure at the os to relax it
    - When resistance releases:
      - Gently advance the sound to the fundus
      - Do not force the sound
      - If perforation occurs, remove the sound and do not proceed
      - Remove the sound
      - Note the centimeter marking on the sound
  - Insert the endometrial biopsy collection device to the fundus
    - Determine the depth by sound measurement
    - Apply suction according to the manufacturer's instructions
    - Rotate the device 360 degrees while gently moving it along the length of the uterus several times
    - Suction is lost when the tip is removed from the uterus

- Deposit the specimen into formalin
  - Label the formalin container
  - Cut off the end of the collection device (into the formalin)
  - Expel the remainder of the specimen into the formalin
- Remove the tenaculum and provide hemostasis of the puncture sites
  - Pressure
  - Silver nitrate
- Assessment
  - Bleeding
  - Vasovagal response
- Allow the client to rest supine
- Obtain postprocedure vital signs

Providing Treatment: Therapeutic Measures to Consider

(Grube & McCool, 2004)

- Preprocedure medication
  - Ibuprofen: 600–800 mg PO
  - Give 1 to 2 hours before the procedure
- Vasovagal syncope
  - Atropine sulfate: Indicated for a heart rate less than 40
    - The preferred route is IV, but may be given IM
    - Dose: 0.4 mg
  - Be prepared for cardiopulmonary resuscitation
  - Call for additional help
- Uterine perforation (Patel, 2005)
  - Rate: 1–2 events per 1000 procedures
  - Expectant management
    - Stable, no hemorrhage
    - Empiric antibiotics
  - Surgical intervention
    - Unstable, hemorrhage
    - Bowel visible

Providing Treatment: Complementary and Alternative Measures to Consider

- Alternative measures are not a substitute for evaluation of abnormal uterine bleeding

- Herbal support
  - Red raspberry leaf
    - Yarrow
    - Dong quai
    - Black cohosh

Providing Support: Education and Support Measures to Consider

- Provide information
  - Potential side effects
  - Cramping
  - Light bleeding
  - Vasovagal syncope
  - Potential complications
    - Cervical stenosis preventing adequate biopsy
    - Uterine perforation
    - Postprocedure infection
- Plan for continued care
  - Obtaining results
  - Warning signs of complications
  - Indications for consultation or referral
  - When to return for care

Follow-up Care: Follow-up Measures to Consider

- Document the procedure; see "Procedure Note"
  - Depth of the uterus
  - Client response
  - Adequacy of the sample
- Return for continued care
  - As indicated by biopsy results
  - Treatment based on diagnosis
  - With bleeding, pain, or fever
  - Recurrent or unresolved symptoms
- Interpretation of results
  - Negative findings
    - Atrophic endometrium
    - Proliferative endometrium
    - Secretory endometrium
  - Positive findings
    - Luteal-phase defect
    - Simple or complex hyperplasia, without atypia

- ◆ Simple or complex hyperplasia with atypia
- ◆ Endometrial adenocarcinoma

Multidisciplinary Practice: Consider Consultation, Collaboration, or Referral

- OB/GYN services
  - ■ Cervical stenosis
  - ■ Uterine perforation
  - ■ Treatment recommendations
  - ■ Diagnostic testing
    - ◆ Sonohysteroscopy
    - ◆ Hysteroscopy with directed biopsy
  - ■ Postprocedure infection
  - ■ Pathology result diagnostic of the following:
    - ◆ Endometrial hyperplasia
    - ◆ Endometrial atypia
    - ◆ Endometrial cancer
- Medical services
  - ■ Clearance for clients
    - ◆ With heart valve replacement: Antibiotic prophylaxis recommendations
    - ◆ With coronary artery disease
  - ■ Follow-up of clients with coronary artery disease or significant vagal response
- For diagnosis or treatment outside the midwife's scope of practice

CARE OF THE WOMAN WITH ENDOMETRIOSIS

Key Clinical Information

Endometriosis is a disorder in which endometrial glands and stroma are implanted in areas outside the uterus (Schorge et al., 2008). Endometriosis implants are most commonly found on the pelvic peritoneum, ovaries, and rectovaginal septum. Because definitive diagnosis of this condition is made through laparoscopic surgery, and because women with endometriosis can present with no symptoms or only mild and vague symptoms, incidence of this disease is difficult to quantify. The prevalence of endometriosis in reproductive-age women ranges from 3% to 10% but is higher in selected subgroups. In women with pelvic pain, the rate of endometriosis is 40% to 50%;

in women with infertility, endometriosis is found in 20% to 50%; and an estimated 50% of adolescent women with chronic pelvic pain or dysmenorrhea have endometriosis (Fritz & Speroff, 2011; Schorge et al., 2008). The treatment options offered for endometriosis will take into account the severity of the woman's pain and her desire for future fertility.

Client History and Chart Review: Components of the History to Consider

- Age
- Pregnancy history
  - ■ GP TPAL
  - ■ Desire for future pregnancy
- Gynecologic history
  - ■ Menstrual history
    - ◆ Age at menarche
    - ◆ LMP
    - ◆ Usual menstrual patterns
  - ■ Sexual activity
    - ◆ Contraception
      - ➤ Hormonal contraceptives
      - ➤ IUD
    - ◆ STIs
- Onset, duration, severity and frequency of symptoms (Schorge et al., 2008; Verga, 2013)
  - ■ Age at onset of symptoms
  - ■ Presence of symptoms related to endometriosis
    - ◆ Significant cyclic premenstrual and perimenstrual pain
      - ➤ Onset in adolescence is common
      - ➤ Limits the woman's ability to perform daily activities
      - ➤ Associated with a sacral-area backache
    - ◆ Dyspareunia: Deep pain
    - ◆ DUB
    - ◆ Infertility
    - ◆ Effect on bowel and bladder function
      - ➤ Diarrhea or gastrointestinal upset with menses
      - ➤ Pain with defecation
      - ➤ Urinary urgency or frequency
  - ■ ▽ Risk factors for endometriosis

- Early menarche (before age 12)
- Shorter, more frequent menstrual cycles, less than 26 days
- Heavy prolonged menstrual bleeding, greater than 7 days
- Family history of endometriosis
- Allergies or autoimmune disorders
- Protective factors for endometriosis
  - Pregnancy
  - Breastfeeding
  - Regular exercise
- Associated factors linked to autoimmune disorders (Fritz & Speroff, 2011)
  - Chronic fatigue syndrome
  - Allergic responses
  - Headaches
  - Arthralgias and myalgias
  - Eczema
  - Hypothyroidism
  - Frequent vulvocandidiasis
- Relief measures used and their effect
- Medical/surgical history
  - Allergies
    - Environmental
    - Food
    - Atopic
  - Medications
  - Cystitis
  - Pelvic surgery
  - Diverticular disease
  - Appendicitis
- Family history
  - Prenatal exposure
    - Diethylstilbestrol exposure
    - Dioxin
  - Dysmenorrhea
  - Infertility
  - Endometriosis
  - Diabetes
  - Bowel disorders
- Social history: Risk factors
  - PID
  - Ectopic pregnancy
- Review of systems

Physical Examination: Components of the Physical Exam to Consider

- Vital signs
- Weight and BMI
- Body habitus
- Thyroid
- Abdominal examination
  - Tenderness
  - Rebound
  - Guarding
  - Masses
- Speculum examination
  - Cervical lesions: Blue or red-powder burn
  - Friable cervix
- Bimanual examination
  - Uterine position, size, and consistency
  - Cervical motion tenderness
  - Adnexal size, location, and tenderness
    - Mobility
    - Masses
- Findings suggestive of endometriosis (Schorge et al., 2008; Verga, 2013)
  - Findings on the physical exam may be normal or vague
  - Fixed, retroverted uterus
  - Adnexal thickening, nodularity, or irregularity in the following structures:
    - Uterosacral ligaments
    - Cul-de-sac
    - Rectovaginal septum
  - Limited mobility of the following structures:
    - Uterus
    - Adnexa

Clinical Impression: Differential Diagnoses to Consider

(ICD9data.com, 2012)

Pelvic pain may occur secondary to any of the following conditions:

- Endometriosis
- Uterine fibroids
- Salpingitis
- Ectopic pregnancy

- Interstitial cystitis
- Appendicitis
- Abdominal adhesions related to the following:
  - PID
  - Pelvic surgery
  - Peritonitis
  - Diverticular disease

Diagnostic Testing: Diagnostic Tests and Procedures to Consider

(Fritz & Speroff, 2011; Schorge et al., 2008)

- 🕐 Laparoscopy for definitive diagnosis
  - Visualization of pelvic lesions
  - Tissue sample for histology
  - Classification of disease
    - Endometrial Fertility Index (Adamson & Pasta, 2010)
    - Clinical description: Minimal, mild, moderate, or severe
- Pelvic ultrasound
  - May be suggestive of endometriosis
  - May demonstrate endometrioma
  - Used to rule out other differential diagnoses
- MRI
- Serum markers
  - CA125
  - CA19-9

Providing Treatment: Therapeutic Measures to Consider

(Fritz & Speroff, 2011; Schorge et al., 2008; Verga, 2013)

- Women with no or minimal pain, or perimenopausal status: Expectant management
- Medical treatments: NSAIDs
  - Ibuprofen
  - Naproxen sodium
  - Ponstel
  - Ketoprofen
- Ovulation suppression (King, 2011)
  - Combined oral contraceptives
  - Progestins
    - Mirena IUD

- Depot medroxyprogesterone
- Oral progestins
- Selective progesterone receptor modulators: Mifepristone
- Androgens: Danazol
- Gonadotropin-releasing hormone (GnRH) agonists
  - Lupron
    - 3.75 mg IM depot monthly for 3–6 months *or*
    - 11.25 mg IM for 1 month (lasts 3 months)
  - Decapeptyl: 3.75 mg IM depot monthly for 3–6 months
  - Zoladex: 3.6 mg SC monthly for 3–6 months
  - Synarel
    - 200 mg BID
    - Given intranasally in alternating nostrils for morning and evening doses
  - Add-back therapy
    - Concerns about extended use of hypoestrogenic agents
      - Vasomotor symptoms
      - Bone mineral density
    - Add combined oral contraceptives to GnRh therapy
- Aromatase inhibitors
- 🕐 Surgical treatments
  - Laparoscopy for diagnosis and preliminary treatment
    - Ablation, excision, or lysis of endometrial implants
    - Can be repeated for symptom recurrence
    - Fertility sparing
  - Endometrioma resection
  - Presacral neurectomy
  - Hysterectomy with oophorectomy

Providing Treatment: Complementary and Alternative Measures to Consider

- Dietary support
  - Shiitake mushroom
  - Low-glycemic diet

- Essential fatty acids
  - Fish oil
  - Primrose oil
  - Borage oil
- Vitamin/mineral supplements
  - Vitamins C and E
  - Vitamin B complex
  - Magnesium
- Live culture yogurt or probiotics
- Digestive enzymes
- Limit dairy and meat
- Avoid food allergens
- Symptomatic treatment (see "Care of the Woman with Dysmenorrhea")
  - Local heat with heating pad or rice pack
  - Castor oil packs
  - Massage
  - Acupuncture
- Herbal support (Romm, 2010)
  - Dong quai
  - Pulsatilla
  - Ginger
  - Black cohosh
- Exercise: Aerobic and weight-bearing
- Stress reduction
  - Support groups
  - Meditation

Providing Support: Education and Support Measures to Consider

- Encourage participation in the evaluation and treatment process
  - Active listening
  - Women may opt to live with their symptoms
- Provide information
  - Endometriosis
  - 🔲 Endometriosis Association
  - Fertility awareness
  - Evaluation process
  - Potential modes of treatment
- 📞 Indications for surgery
  - Diagnosis
    - Severe endometriosis

- Infertility
- Failed medical management
- 📞 Surgical options: Conservative, fertility-sparing surgery
  - Ablation or excision of implants
    - Laser
    - Cautery
    - Scalpel
  - Lysis of adhesions
  - Resection of endometriomas
  - Pregnancy rates after surgery: 5–50%
  - Recurrence rates: 10–44%
- Definitive treatment: Hysterectomy with bilateral salpingo-oophorectomy

Follow-up Care: Follow-up Measures to Consider

- Document
  - Criteria used for diagnosis
  - Discussions with the client
  - Treatment plan
  - 🔻 Referrals
- Return for care
  - As needed during diagnosis and/or treatment
  - For well-woman care
  - With pregnancy

Multidisciplinary Practice: Consider Consultation, Collaboration, or Referral

- OB/GYN services
  - Suspected endometriosis
  - Persistent pelvic pain
  - Pain accompanied by bowel or bladder involvement
  - Pain accompanied by fever or elevated white blood cell levels
- For diagnosis or treatment outside the midwife's scope of practice

CARE OF THE WOMAN WITH FIBROIDS

Key Clinical Information

Fibroids, also known as leiomyomas or myomas, are a common benign tumor of the uterus, with an incidence of 20% to 25% of women and 1% to 2% of pregnant women (Fritz & Speroff, 2011; Schorge et al., 2008). Fibroids are often discovered as an incidental finding during a pelvic exam, radiologic test, or surgery for other indications. Histologic and sonographic studies suggest the incidence of fibroids may be as high as 80%. These estrogen- and progesterone-sensitive tumors are initially found in women of childbearing age and typically regress during menopause. Fibroids are classified by location and direction of their growth; they typically occur in multiple locations in and around the uterine tissue. Expectant management is appropriate in most cases, with more aggressive treatments reserved for women with symptoms of pain, bleeding, or infertility (Verga, 2013).

Client History and Chart Review: Components of the History to Consider

- Age
- Menstrual history
  - LMP
  - Menstrual status
    - Duration, frequency, and length
    - Amount of flow
    - Dysmenorrhea
    - Intermenstrual bleeding
    - Dysfunctional uterine bleeding
    - Perimenopausal or postmenopausal
  - Previous clinical findings
    - Uterine size and contour
    - Previous pelvic ultrasounds
  - Pregnancy history
    - GP TPAL
    - Infertility
  - Hormone use
    - Contraception
    - Hormone replacement therapy
- Current symptoms: Onset, duration, and severity
- Symptoms of uterine fibroids
  - Pelvic pressure or pain
    - Suprapubic pain
    - Lower back pain
    - Dypareunia

- Abdominal enlargement
  - Rapid enlargement suggests malignancy
  - May experience pressure sensations in legs
    - Varicosities
    - Edema
- Changes in bowel or bladder function
  - Urinary frequency
  - Constipation
- Menorrhagia with anemia
- Pregnancy losses
- Risk factors for uterine myoma (Schorge et al., 2008)
  - African American ethnicity
  - Late-reproductive-age and perimenopausal women
  - Early menarche
  - Elevated BMI
  - Family history of uterine fibroids
- Medical history
- Review of systems

Physical Examination: Components of the Physical Exam to Consider

(Verga, 2013)

- Vital signs, including blood pressure and weight
- Abdominal palpation
  - Uterine size and shape if palpable abdominally
  - Abdominal girth
  - Guarding or rebound tenderness
- Pelvic examination
  - Cervical or vaginal discharge
  - Uterus
    - Size and position
    - Contour
    - Consistency
  - Cervical motion tenderness
  - Adnexal issues
    - Masses or fullness
    - Pain
- Rectal or rectovaginal examination
  - Rectal lesions
  - Palpate posterior uterus
  - Stool for occult blood

Clinical Impression: Differential Diagnoses to Consider

(ICD9data.com, 2012)

- Enlarged uterus
- Uterine fibroids
- Pregnancy
- Menorrhagia, premenopausal
- Postmenopausal bleeding
- Gastrointestinal bleeding
- Anemia, iron deficiency

Diagnostic Testing: Diagnostic Tests and Procedures to Consider

(Schorge et al., 2008)

- Pelvic ultrasound
  - Vaginal
  - Abdominal
  - Saline-infusion sonography
- ⏱ Hysteroscopy or hysterosalpinogography
- Color flow Doppler imaging
- Magnetic resonance imaging

Providing Treatment: Therapeutic Measures to Consider

(King, 2011; Schorge et al., 2008)

- Expectant management
  - Annual pelvic examination
  - Annual sonographic evaluation
- Hormonal regulation of menses
  - Combined oral contraceptives
  - Mirena IUS
  - May inhibit development of myoma
  - Indicated for fibroids with the following symptoms:
    - Dysmenorrhea
    - Menorrhagia
- ⏱ Gonadotropin-releasing hormone (GnRH) agonists (Schorge et al., 2008)
  - Short-term treatment of 3–6 months
  - Surgical pretreatment to decrease myoma size *or*
  - Temporizing agent for perimenopausal women

- ⚠ Contraindications
  - Undiagnosed uterine bleeding
  - Pregnancy
- May cause vasomotor symptoms
- Lupron
  - 3.75 mg IM depot monthly for 3–6 months *or*
  - 11.25 mg IM for 1 month (lasts 3 months)
- Decapeptyl: 3.75 mg IM depot monthly for 3–6 months
- Zoladex: 3.6 mg SC monthly for 3–6 months
- Synarel
  - 200 mg BID
  - Given intranasally in alternating nostrils for morning and evening doses
- GnRH antagonists
- Mifepristone
- ⏱ Endometrial ablation
- ⏱ Myomectomy
  - Excision of fibroid(s)
  - Retains fertility
  - Uterine scarring may require cesarean section in subsequent childbirth
  - Approaches
    - Hysteroscopic
    - Laparoscopic
    - Abdominal
- ⏱ Uterine artery embolization or occlusion
- ⏱ Hysterectomy
  - Indications
    - Grossly enlarged uterus
    - Degenerative fibroids
    - Potential or suspected malignancy
    - Severe menorrhagia
    - Client preference
  - Methods
    - Abdominal
    - Vaginal
    - Laparoscopic

Providing Treatment: Complementary and Alternative Measures to Consider

- Dietary sources of iron replacement (see "Food Sources of Iron")

- Iron supplementation as indicated
  - Ferro-Sequels: 1–2 PO daily
  - Niferex: 150 1–2 PO daily
  - Ferrous gluconate: 1–2 PO daily
  - Floradix iron supplement
- Herbs (Romm, 2010)
  - Barberry
  - Green tea
  - Chasteberry
  - Red raspberry leaf
  - Vitex tea, tincture, or capsules
- Weight management
- Exercise
  - Yoga
  - Kegel exercises
  - Walking
- Dietary antioxidants
  - Vitamins A, C, and E
  - Zinc and selenium

Providing Support: Education and Support Measures to Consider

- Discussion about the following topics:
  - Clinical findings
  - Recommended testing
  - Planned follow-up
  - Medications recommended
    - Indications
    - Side effects
    - Anticipated results
- ⚠ Warning signs
  - Excessive bleeding
  - Pain
  - Change in bowel or bladder function
- Active listening
  - Client concerns
  - Family/personal support
  - Coping mechanisms
- Provide information and support if surgery is indicated
  - Preoperative testing
  - Anticipated hospital stay
  - Self-care after discharge

- 🌐 Allow grieving
  - Loss of fertility/body part
  - Body image changes with surgery
  - Potential perceived loss of femininity

Follow-up Care: Follow-up Measures to Consider

- Document
  - Findings
  - Diagnostic test results
  - Discussions with the client
  - Management plan
- Return for care
  - Reevaluation of uterine size
    - Annual examination
    - Serial ultrasound sizing
    - Change in bleeding pattern
    - Progression of symptoms
  - Assess for uterine malignancy: Women with documented myoma and intact uterus
  - Preoperative history and physical, as needed
  - Informed consent as indicated for
    - Lupron or other GnRH agonist or antagonist
    - Operative procedures

Multidisciplinary Practice: Consider Consultation, Collaboration, or Referral

- OB/GYN services
  - Grossly enlarged uterus
  - Severe or progressive symptoms
  - Evidence or suspicion of malignancy
  - Client preference
- Social services support, as needed
- For diagnosis or treatment outside the midwife's scope of practice

CARE OF THE WOMAN WITH GONORRHEA

Key Clinical Information

Gonorrhea is a bacterial infection caused by the organism *Neisseria gonorrhoeae*, which can infect the eyes, mouth, anus, and joints as well as the reproductive tract. Significant effects of gonococcal infections include infertility, premature rupture of membranes, preterm labor, and infection of the newborn's eyes resulting in blindness if left untreated. Gonorrhea, like other STIs, increases the transmission risk of those exposed to HIV. Fluoroquinolone-resistant gonorrhea is now widespread throughout the United States, prompting the CDC to change its recommendations for use of this class of antimicrobials for the treatment of gonorrhea (King & Brucker, 2011). Co-infection with *Chlamydia trachomatis* is common, so treatment for both is recommended when either infection is diagnosed. Treatment of the patient includes treatment of recent sex partners to prevent reinfection and further transmission (CDC, 2010).

Client History and Chart Review: Components of the History to Consider

- Age
- Reproductive history
  - GP TPAL, LMP
    - Potential for pregnancy
    - Birth control method
  - Review previous history
    - Pap smear
    - STI testing
    - STI treatments
  - Sexual history
    - Number of partners for self or partner(s)
    - Vaginal, oral, or anal intercourse
    - Condom use
      - Male condom
      - Female condom
- Problem-focused history
  - Onset, duration, and severity of symptoms
  - Last unprotected intercourse
  - Symptom profile for gonorrhea
    - May be asymptomatic
    - Urinary frequency and dysuria
    - Urethritis
    - Vaginal discharge
    - Anal discharge
    - Sore throat
    - ♂ Urethral discharge
    - Pelvic inflammatory disease (PID)
      - Pain with intercourse
      - Genital pain and discharge
      - Fever
      - Lower abdominal pain
      - Intermenstrual bleeding
      - Painful bowel movements
- Medical/surgical history
  - Allergies
  - Medications
  - Chronic health conditions
- Social history
  - Behavioral risk factors
  - Alcohol or drug use
  - Exposure to more than five sexual partners
  - Male partner who is bisexual
  - Social support
  - Access to health care
- Review of systems

Physical Examination: Components of the Physical Exam to Consider

- Vital signs, including temperature: Temperature greater than 38°C is suspicious for PID
- Pelvic examination (Varney, Kriebs, & Gegor, 2004)
  - Bartholin's glands, urethra, and Skene's glands (BUS)
    - Discharge
    - Inflammation
  - Vaginal, cervical, or anal discharge: Yellow or mucopurulent
  - Evidence of PID
    - Pain on cervical motion
    - Adnexal or uterine tenderness
    - Lower abdominal pain

Clinical Impression: Differential Diagnoses to Consider

(ICD9data.com, 2012)

- Gonorrhea
- Chlamydia

- PID
- Endometriosis
- Ectopic pregnancy
- Ovarian cyst
- Cervicitis
- Cervical malignancy

Diagnostic Testing: Diagnostic Tests and Procedures to Consider

- Gonorrhea testing (CDC, 2010)
  - Gram stain
    - ♂ Diagnostic for male urethral specimen only
    - Gram-negative intracellular diplococci *plus*
    - Polymorphonuclear leukocytes
  - Culture test types
    - DNA probe
    - Enzyme-linked immunosorbent assay (antigen specific)
    - Nucleic acid amplification tests
  - Culture specimen sites
    - Oropharyngeal
    - Urine
    - Rectal
    - Endocervical
    - ♂ Urethral
- Chlamydia testing
- Syphilis testing
- Wet preparation
- Pelvic ultrasound: Presence of inflammatory mass
- CBC with sedimentation rate: Sedimentation rate greater than 15 mm/hr is suspicious
- HIV counseling and testing
- ⚠ Note: Visual inspection of the vaginal discharge is nonspecific and cannot be used alone for diagnosis. Multiple pathogens may be present. Perform additional testing as required for accurate diagnosis.

Providing Treatment: Therapeutic Measures to Consider

(FitzMaurice et al., 2011; Hatcher et al., 2011)

- Begin treatment based on symptoms

- CDC recommendations for uncomplicated gonorrhea (CDC, 2010)
  - One-time dosing
    - Provided on site
    - Compliance ensured by direct observation
  - Ceftriaxone 250 mg IM (Pregnancy Category B)
    - 1% lidocaine as a diluent to reduce the injection pain
    - If not an option, use the following alternatives
  - Cefixime: 400 mg PO (Pregnancy Category B)
  - Other single-dose injectable regimens
    - Ceftizoxime 500 mg IM *or*
    - Cefoxitin 2 g IM, administered with probenecid 1 g orally, *or*
    - Cefotaxime 500 mg IM
  - *Plus* treatment for chlamydia, if this infection has not been ruled out
- If chlamydia has not been ruled out, add:
  - Azithromycin 1 g PO (Pregnancy Category B) *or*
  - Doxycycline 100 mg PO BID for 7 days (Pregnancy Category D)
- Pharyngeal infection: Ceftriaxone 250 mg IM (Pregnancy Category B)
  - 1% lidocaine used as a diluent to reduce the injection pain
  - *Plus* treatment for chlamydia, if this infection has not been ruled out
- Consider patient-delivered partner treatment (PDPT)

Providing Treatment: Complementary and Alternative Measures to Consider

- ⚠ Alternative therapies are not a substitute for medical treatment
- Supportive measures to promote healing
  - Adequate rest
  - Sitz baths with comfrey leaf tea or Epsom salts
  - Nutritional support
    - Live culture yogurt
    - Blue-green algae
    - Vitamins C and E

- Herbal support formulas (Soule, 1995)
  - Adjunct to medical therapy
  - Use two to three times daily
  - Prepare as a tea or tincture
    - Red clover: 2 parts
    - Calendula: 2 parts
    - Yarrow: 1 part
    - Dandelion root: 1 part
- Acidophilus capsules orally or per vagina to prevent yeast overgrowth

Providing Support: Education and Support Measures to Consider

- Diagnosis
  - Potential sequelae of STI
  - Treatment recommendations
  - Partner notification and referral for treatment
    - PDPT can be considered
    - Give prescription and written materials
    - **www** Legal regulations vary; check www.cdc.gov/std/ept
  - State reporting requirements
  - Symptoms of acute PID
- Treatment instructions: Avoidance of sexual relations
  - Until treatment is completed
  - Until symptoms have resolved
  - Until partner treatment is completed
- When and how to access care
- STI transmission and prevention: Emphasize use of condoms

Follow-up Care: Follow-up Measures to Consider

- Document
  - Confirmation of diagnosis
  - Medication administration
  - Epidemiologic reporting
- Indications to return for care (CDC, 2010)
  - Symptoms of acute PID
  - Persistent symptoms
  - Reinfection

- Drug-resistant organism
- Noninfectious process
- Repeat testing only in the following circumstances:
  - Persistent symptoms
  - New partner for self or for partner
  - Pregnant women
- Offer HIV and other STI counseling and testing

Multidisciplinary Practice: Consider Consultation, Collaboration, or Referral

- OB/GYN services or STI clinic
  - Signs and symptoms of PID
  - Client requiring hospitalization
  - Gonorrhea infection with the following:
    - Symptoms of meningitis
    - Disseminated infection
- Social services
- For diagnosis or treatment outside the midwife's scope of practice

CARE OF THE WOMAN WITH HEPATITIS

Key Clinical Information

Hepatitis is an inflammation of the liver, most often caused by viral infection (CDC, 2010). There are five primary hepatitis viruses: A, B, C, D, and E. Hepatitis A and E are usually acquired through ingestion of contaminated food or water. Hepatitis B, C, and D typically result from parenteral contact with infected bodily fluids. Hepatitis B and C are the forms most frequently seen in women's health practice. Hepatitis B is 100 times more infectious than HIV, with both hepatitis B and C occurring concurrently with HIV infection in some women and complicating management of these disorders (Khalili, 2006). Approximately 10% of all infected adults develop chronic hepatitis B infection, which may lead to permanent liver damage, liver failure, or liver cancer (AIDS Education and Training Centers [AETC], 2007b). Noninfectious hepatitis may be caused by autoimmune dysfunction, alcohol abuse, or drug-related liver injury, especially as a result of combined alcohol and acetaminophen use.

Client History and Chart Review: Components of the History to Consider

(CDC, 2010)

- Age
- Medical/surgical history
  - Allergies
  - Medications: Acetaminophen-based products
  - Chronic illnesses
    - Organ transplant
    - Anemia
    - HIV/AIDS
- Social history
  - Drug and/or alcohol use
  - Emigration, travel, or adoption from endemic areas
    - Asia
    - Africa
    - Pacific Islands (including Hawaii)
    - South or Central America and Mexico
- Presence, onset, duration, and severity of symptoms
  - May be asymptomatic
  - Malaise and lethargy
  - Fever and chills
  - Right upper quadrant pain
  - Jaundice
  - Nausea and vomiting
  - Dark urine
  - Pale-colored stools
- Risk factors for hepatitis exposure
  - IV drug use and needle sharing
  - Sexual contacts
  - Tattoos or body piercings
  - Healthcare workers
  - Ingestion of raw shellfish
  - Children born to women with viral hepatitis
  - Partner with tattoos or body piercing
  - Hemodialysis patients
  - Blood or organ recipient before 1992
- Indications for hepatitis A vaccine (CDC, 2010)
  - Children at ages 12–23 months

- People traveling to any area of the world for longer than 12 months except the United States, Canada, Western Europe, Japan, New Zealand, and Australia
  - Illegal drug users, both oral and injecting
  - People who have blood clotting disorders
  - People who work with hepatitis A–infected primates or hepatitis A in a research laboratory setting
  - Any person who wishes to be immune to hepatitis A
- Indications for hepatitis B vaccine (CDC, 2010)
  - Universal immunization
    - Infants
    - Adolescents
    - Adults
  - Immunization of at-risk individuals
    - Adolescents before sexual activity
    - Diagnosis of STI, including HIV
    - Travel to areas in which hepatitis B is endemic
    - Occupational risk
    - Multiple sexual partners
    - IV drug use
  - Client preference
- Contraindications to hepatitis B vaccine: Allergy to yeast
- Review of systems

Physical Examination: Components of the Physical Exam to Consider

(AETC, 2007a)

- Vital signs, including weight: Watch for evidence of portal hypertension
- Skin
  - Evidence of jaundice
    - Mucous membranes
    - Sclera
  - Petechiae
  - Bruising
- Chest
  - Cardiac rate and rhythm
  - Lung fields

- Abdomen
  - Right upper quadrant pain
  - Liver margins
  - Splenomegaly
  - Abdominal ascites
  - Abdominal girth
- Extremities: Edema
- Neurologic system
  - Mental status
  - Coordination

Clinical Impression: Differential Diagnoses to Consider

(ICD9data.com, 2012)

- Hepatitis A, B, or C
- Jaundice
- Nausea and vomiting
- Hepatitis, nonviral
- Hepatitis, viral
- Biliary disease
- Cholelithiasis
- Other liver disorders

Diagnostic Testing: Diagnostic Tests and Procedures to Consider

(King & Brucker, 2011)

- Hepatitis workup
  - Anti-HAV-IgM (immunoglobulin M class antibody to the hepatitis A virus)
  - HBsAg (hepatitis B surface antigen)
  - Anti-HBs (total antibody to hepatitis B surface antigen)
  - Anti-HCV (antibody to hepatitis C virus antigens)
  - Alanine aminotransferase (ALT) elevated with liver inflammation
- Jaundice present
  - International Normalized Ratio (INR) and prothrombin time
  - ⚠ 🕐 Elevated levels indicate fulminant infection

- Hepatitis A
  - Anti-HAV-IgM
    - Negative: Infection is ruled out
    - Positive: Acute infection
- Hepatitis B
  - HBsAg
    - Detected 1–12 weeks post infection
    - Positive: Infection with hepatitis B
    - Negative: Susceptibility to hepatitis B
  - HBsAb or anti-HBs
    - Positive: Immunity
    - Negative: Infection
  - HBcAb (hepatitis core antibody) or anti-HBc
    - Indicates past or present infection
    - May be present in those chronically infected
      - False positive is possible
      - Positive HBsAb: Recovery
      - Positive HBsAg: Chronic infection
  - IgM antibody to hepatitis B core antigen (IgM anti-HBc)
    - Positive: Acute infection
    - Marker appears 6–14 weeks after infection
    - Will disappear within 6 months of acute disease
  - Hepatitis Be antigen (HBeAg)
    - Positive: Acute infection
    - Marker appears 4–12 weeks after infection
- Hepatitis C
  - Anti-HCV
    - Test reliable: 5–6 weeks post infection
    - Negative: Infection unlikely
      - Repeat in 1–2 months if there is no other etiology for the symptoms
      - Immunocompromised client: Consider HCV-RNA testing
    - Positive: Acute or chronic infection
      - Consider HCV-RNA testing
- Liver function tests (LFTs)
  - Aspartate aminotransferase (AST)
  - Alanine aminotransferase (ALT)
  - Lactate dehydrogenase (LDH)

- Bilirubin
  - ◆ During acute phase
  - ◆ 📞 Elevated levels indicate a need for specialist care
- HIV testing
- Ultrasound, right upper quadrant: Gallbladder

Providing Treatment: Therapeutic Measures to Consider

(CDC, 2010; King & Brucker, 2011)

- Hepatitis A vaccine
  - Inactivated virus vaccine
  - Two doses, 6 months apart
- Hepatitis B vaccines: Recombinant vaccines
  - Age-related doses differ by manufacturer
  - Series of immunizations (three doses)
  - Given with hepatitis B immune globulin (HBIG) immediately after exposure
- Hepatitis B immune globulin
  - Given as soon as possible after exposure (up to 7 days)
  - One or two doses
- Hepatitis B infection
  - Treatment is based on interrupting the viral life cycle, similar to the approach used by HIV treatment
  - Six drugs are currently approved for treatment of hepatitis B infection
- ⚠️ 🌐 Midwives and other birth care providers are at risk for occupational exposure to hepatitis B: Guidelines for post-exposure prophylaxis are available at http://www.cdc.gov/hepatitis/HBV/PEP.htm
- Hepatitis C infection
  - Treatment is based on stimulating the appropriate antiviral immunologic response
  - Two drugs are currently approved for treatment of hepatitis C infection

Providing Treatment: Complementary and Alternative Measures to Consider

- Supportive care

  - Whole-foods diet containing a minimum of toxins
  - Adequate rest
- Immunomodulating herbs commonly used in viral infections (Romm, 2010)
  - Astragalus
  - Atractylodes
  - Condonopsis
  - Eluthero
  - Licorice
  - Lingustrum
  - Reishi
  - Shitake mushroom

Providing Support: Education and Support Measures to Consider

- Provide information about hepatitis
  - Types
  - Route(s) of transmission
    - ◆ Fecal–oral, or contaminated food or water (hepatitis A)
    - ◆ Blood or body fluids (hepatitis B)
    - ◆ Blood (hepatitis C)
  - Prevention measures (CDC, 2010)
    - ◆ Avoid contact with blood or body fluids
    - ◆ Wash hands before eating and after toileting
    - ◆ Use safe sexual practices
    - ◆ Avoid undercooked food in endemic areas
    - ◆ Avoid sharing needles or razors
- Acetaminophen use
  - Abstain from alcohol when taking acetaminophen
  - Do not exceed the recommended dose
  - Be aware that over-the-counter medications may contain acetaminophen
- 🔻 Discussion about the following topics:
  - Hepatitis A and B immunizations
  - Options for treatment and supportive care, as needed
  - Potential effects of illness
  - Medications
  - Criteria for referral

Follow-up Care: Follow-up Measures to Consider

- Document
  - Symptoms
  - Risk factors
  - Test results
  - Discussions with the client
  - Follow-up plan
- Retesting (CDC, 2010)
  - Post immunization
  - After illness or exposure
    - Incubation lasts 1–4 months
    - It may take up to 6 months to make a determination:
      - Whether the client has recovered *or*
      - Whether the client remains chronically infected (hepatitis B)
- Return for care
  - Weekly during the acute phase of infection
  - Periodic liver function tests
  - STI testing, as needed

Multidisciplinary Practice: Consider Consultation, Collaboration, or Referral

- Medical services
  - Diagnosis of hepatitis for detailed evaluation and treatment
  - Evidence of the following conditions:
    - Liver failure
    - Ascites
    - Acetaminophen overdose
- Social services
  - Addiction treatment
  - Clean needle programs
- For diagnosis or treatment outside the midwife's scope of practice

CARE OF THE WOMAN WITH HERPES SIMPLEX VIRUS

Key Clinical Information

Herpes simplex virus (HSV) is a chronic lifelong infection caused by the HSV-1 or HSV-2 organism.

These common viruses can be sexually transmitted and frequently cause significant discomfort to those with active genital lesions. Approximately 75% of Americans with herpes infections are infected with HSV-1 and 25% with HSV-2, although many individuals are unaware that they harbor the viruses (Romm, 2010). The goal of therapy is to encourage the virus to become dormant and to support the immune system so that it stays quiescent and the client remains asymptomatic. Unfortunately, it is possible to spread herpes infection without a noticeable lesion.

Herpes infection in the HIV-positive client increases the likelihood of transmission of HIV (CDC, 2010). Infants who are exposed to HSV during the labor and birth process and during early infancy can acquire systemic infection, resulting in serious illness or death. For this reason, cesarean birth may be offered to pregnant women with a history of recurrent HSV outbreaks during pregnancy. Cesarean birth is recommended for pregnant women with an active HSV lesion during late pregnancy; see "Care of the Pregnant Woman with Herpes Simplex Virus" in Chapter 3. However, with suppressive HSV therapy in the last month of pregnancy, most women with HSV can anticipate a vaginal birth.

Client History and Chart Review: Components of the History to Consider

(CDC, 2010)

- Age
- Reproductive history
  - LMP
  - Current method of birth control
  - Sexual orientation
  - Sexual practices
    - Oral–genital sex
    - Anal sex
    - Safe sex practices
  - Last examination and testing results
    - HSV and other STI testing
    - HIV status
    - Pap smear results

- Problem-oriented history (CDC, 2010)
  - Previous history of genital or oral lesions
  - Partner with oral or genital HSV
  - Current symptoms
    - Onset, duration, and severity
    - Presence and location of lesions
      - Vesicular lesions
      - Ulcerative lesions
    - Pain, tingling, and dysuria
    - Other associated symptoms
      - Prodrome
      - Itching
    - Precipitating factors
      - Stress
      - Fever or infection
      - Menses
      - Sun exposure
- Review of systems
- Medical/surgical history
  - Allergies
  - Medications
  - Chronic illnesses
  - Immunosuppression
    - HIV/AIDS
    - Cancer
    - Burns
    - Organ transplant
    - Steroid use
- Psychosocial assessment
  - Impact of symptoms
  - Emotional response to new diagnosis
  - Relationship status with sexual partner(s)
  - Socioeconomic status: Ability to pay for medication
- Primary HSV infection associated with the following conditions (CDC, 2010):
  - Fever
  - Headache
  - Malaise
  - Local lesions at site of infection
  - Lymphadenopathy
  - ⚠ Herpes meningitis
  - ⚠ Increased risk of perinatal transmission at term

- ⏷ Risk factors for HSV infection (CDC, 2010; Romm, 2010)
  - 🌐 Race
    - African Americans are more likely to test positive for HSV
    - Mexican Americans are more likely to test positive for HSV
    - White individuals are more likely to have active symptoms
    - White teens are the fastest-growing HSV-positive population
  - Compromised immune system
  - Multiple sex partners
  - Increasing age
  - Less education
  - Lower socioeconomic status
  - Cocaine use
- History for a pregnant woman with HSV, upon presentation in labor
  - Taking suppressive therapy
  - Presence of active lesions
  - Prodromal symptoms

Physical Examination: Components of the Physical Exam to Consider

- Vital signs, including temperature
- Palpation of inguinal lymph nodes
- External genital examination
  - Characteristic lesions
    - Vesicles
    - Shallow ulcers
  - Lesions on the following areas:
    - Vulva
    - Urethra
    - Vagina
    - Cervix
    - Thighs
    - Anus
    - Buttocks
- Speculum examination: Vaginal or cervical discharge
- ⚠ Visual inspection of external genitalia, vagina, and cervix
  - For pregnant women with a history of HSV
  - Upon presentation for labor

- Bimanual examination: Cervical or uterine motion tenderness
- Neurologic examination
  - Neck tenderness
  - Light sensitivity

Clinical Impression: Differential Diagnoses to Consider

(ICD9data.com, 2012)

- Genital herpes
- Herpetic vulvovaginitis
- Herpes gestationis
- Herpetic meningoencephalitis
- Chancre
- Contact dermatitis

Diagnostic Testing: Diagnostic Tests and Procedures to Consider

(CDC, 2010)

- Culture lesions using viral media for HSV
  - Poor sensitivity
  - Negative does not mean no HSV
  - Positive results: Should type the HSV isolate
- Polymerase chain reaction (PCR) test
  - Tests for HSV DNA
  - Negative does not mean no HSV
- Serologic type-specific glycoprotein G (IgG)–based assay
  - For clients who have recurrent genital symptoms with negative cultures
  - For clients with a clinical diagnosis of HSV but no laboratory confirmation
  - Partner with genital herpes
- IgM testing is not useful; it is not type specific
- Syphilis serology
- Additional STI testing as indicated

Providing Treatment: Therapeutic Measures to Consider

(CDC, 2010)

- First clinical episode of genital herpes
  - Zovirax (acyclovir): 400 mg PO TID for 7–10 days *or*

- Zovirax: 200 mg PO 5 times a day for 7–10 days *or*
  - Famciclovir: 250 mg PO TID for 7–10 days *or*
  - Valacyclovir 1 g PO BID for 7–10 days
  - Treatment can be extended if healing is incomplete after 10 days of therapy
- Episodic therapy for recurrent genital herpes infection
  - Zovirax (acyclovir): 400 mg PO TID for 5 days *or*
  - Zovirax: 800 mg PO BID for 5 days *or*
  - Zovirax: 800 mg PO TID for 2 days *or*
  - Famciclovir: 125 mg PO BID for 5 days *or*
  - Famciclovir: 1000 mg PO BID for 1 day *or*
  - Famciclovir: 500 mg once, followed by 250 mg PO BID for 2 days, *or*
  - Valacyclovir: 500 mg PO BID for 3 days *or*
  - Valacyclovir: 1 g PO QD for 5 days
- Suppressive therapy for recurrent genital herpes infection
  - Zovirax (acyclovir): 400 mg PO BID *or*
  - Famciclovir: 250 mg PO BID *or*
  - Valacyclovir: 500 mg PO QD *or*
  - Valacyclovir: 1 g PO QD
  - Consider suppressive therapy in the uninfected partner of an HSV-positive individual
- Treatment of genital herpes in pregnancy
  - A primary herpes outbreak poses the most risk to the fetus and neonate
  - Zovirax (acyclovir): 400 mg PO BID at 36 weeks' gestation
    - For history of HSV in pregnant woman
    - Available data are reassuring regarding this regimen's lack of teratogenicity
- Acetaminophen or ibuprofen for pain relief

Providing Treatment: Complementary and Alternative Measures to Consider

(Romm, 2010)

- Nutritional supplements
  - L-Lysine
    - 1 g QD for prevention
    - 1 g TID for outbreak

- Vitamin C: 250–500 mg
  - BID with prodrome
  - Up to 5 g daily for 3 days with outbreak
  - Dose less than 4 g for the pregnant woman
  - Combine with acidophilus: 1 capsule with meals
- Zinc 25 mg daily for 6 weeks
  - Take with vitamin C
  - Not recommended in the pregnant woman
- Vitamin E oil: Topical use 2 to 4 times daily
- Herbal support
  - Lemon balm, tea, or topical application
  - Tea tree oil topical application
  - Echinacea tea, tincture, tablets, or capsules TID for 2 weeks
  - Aloe vera ointment or cream
  - Sitz bath or salve made with the following herbals:
    - Lemon balm
    - Calendula
    - Peppermint or geranium oil

Providing Support: Education and Support Measures to Consider

- Diet (Romm, 2010)
  - Avoid foods high in arginine: Chocolate, cola, peanuts, cashews, pecans, almonds, sunflower and sesame seeds, peas, corn, coconut, and gelatin
  - Include foods high in lysine: Margarine, yogurt, cheese, milk, brewer's yeast, potatoes, fish, chicken, eggs
- Rest and comfort measures
- Discuss and provide written information about the following topics:
  - Nutritional support
  - Herpes management (CDC, 2010)
    - Medications
      - Episodic
      - Suppressive therapy
    - Abstinence during outbreaks

- Potential for transmission with no lesions
  - Partner notification
  - Condom use
- Washing hands after lesion contact
- Avoidance of handling infants during a period with active lesions
- Effects on the following aspects of life:
  - Sexuality
  - HIV susceptibility
  - Childbearing
  - Self-image
- Warning signs and symptoms
  - Meningitis
  - Secondary infection
  - Depression
- www Client resources: American Social Health Association

Follow-up Care: Follow-up Measures to Consider

- Document location, size, and appearance of lesions
- Return for care
  - Symptoms persisting for more than 10 days
  - Worsening symptoms
    - Stiff neck
    - Unremitting fever
    - Inability to urinate
  - Ineffective coping
- Pregnancy (CDC, 2010) (see "Care of the Pregnant Woman with Herpes Simplex Virus")

Multidisciplinary Practice: Consider Consultation, Collaboration, or Referral

- OB/GYN services
  - Symptoms of herpes meningitis
  - Symptoms of systemic infection
  - Symptoms of ocular herpes
  - Pregnancy
    - Initial outbreak during pregnancy
    - Cesarean birth during active genital outbreak
- For diagnosis or treatment outside the midwife's scope of practice

CARE OF THE WOMAN WITH HUMAN IMMUNODEFICIENCY VIRUS

Key Clinical Information

Human immunodeficiency virus (HIV) attacks the immune system by destroying CD4$^+$ T cells. Decreased numbers of these cells leave individuals open to opportunistic infections, as well as other infections, diseases, and complications, leading to acquired immunodeficiency syndrome (AIDS). Untreated HIV leads to AIDS at a variable progression depending on viral, host, and environmental factors; treatment of HIV prolongs life expectancy (National Institute of Allergy and Infectious Diseases [NIAID], 2011). Although HIV/AIDS affects women of all ages, races, and backgrounds, a greater percentage of African American and Hispanic women have these conditions (CDC, 2010). HIV may be transmitted to women during penetrative intercourse, via oral–genital, or digital–genital contact with an infected sexual partner, and through HIV-contaminated needles during IV drug use. Most women contract HIV infection through heterosexual contact, whether consensual or involuntary (CDC, 2010; NIAID, 2011). Transmission is enhanced when the HIV-exposed woman is menstruating or has breaks in the skin or mucous membrane, such as occurs with ulcerative STIs or trauma.

A lack of access to early diagnosis and adequate treatment, including during pregnancy, further contributes to increases in HIV progression among women and infection in newborns (NIAID, 2011). By comparison, prompt treatment with antiretroviral therapies improves survival rates considerably. As HIV screening rates in the United States are currently unacceptably low, the CDC recommends routine HIV screening of *all* patients ages 13–64 and *all* pregnant women (CDC, 2010). This agency endorses an opt-out testing process with a streamlined consenting process in all healthcare settings, including STI clinics (CDC, 2010).

Promising new research is being directed toward prevention efforts involving vaginal topical microbicides, which disrupt attachment of the virus to the vaginal wall (NIAID, 2011). Effective topical microbicides provide women with a means to protect themselves from exposure by offering a measure that does not rely on partner participation, knowledge, or acceptance. A variety of vaccination strategies and use of prophylactic antiretroviral medications for high-risk but uninfected individuals is currently undergoing clinical trials (NIAID, 2011). The rate of maternal-to-child transmission (MTCT) in pregnant HIV-positive women is reduced to 2% with use of antiretroviral regimens and other interventions, such as elective cesarean section at 38 weeks' gestation and avoidance of breastfeeding (CDC, 2010).

Midwives have a role in education, screening, and prevention of HIV in women and their partners. They also have a role in providing care to HIV-infected women within comprehensive, multidisciplinary programs that address the complex medical, emotional, and social needs of women who are HIV positive or who have AIDS (ACNM, 2007).

Client History and Chart Review: Components of the History to Consider

(CDC, 2011; NIAID, 2011)

- Age
- Pregnancy, gynecologic, and sexual history
  - LMP and contraception method
  - Pregnancy status
  - Previous diagnosis and/or treatment
    - STIs
    - Abnormal cervical cytology
  - HIV risk assessment
    - HIV knowledge and perception of risk
    - Current HIV prevention behaviors
    - Previous HIV screening
  - Risk factors for HIV infection (CDC, 2011; NIAID, 2011)
    - Younger age (15–39)
    - African American or Hispanic American ethnicity
    - Lack of awareness of the partner's risk factors

- Substance abuse or IV drug abuse
- Sexual inequality resulting in the following:
  - Nonconsensual sex
  - Lack of condom use
- Sex with incarcerated male(s)
- Risk factors for HIV-1 infection
  - Client or partner with more than five sexual partners
  - Diagnosis or symptoms of any STI
  - IV drug use: Self or partner
  - Exposure to blood or body fluids
- Risk factors for HIV-2 infection
  - Travel or residence in areas where HIV-2 is endemic
    - West Africa
    - Angola
    - France
    - Mozambique
    - Portugal
  - Clinical evidence of HIV infection with negative HIV-1 test
- Medical/surgical history
  - Allergies
  - Medications
  - Chronic diseases or disorders
  - HIV-associated illnesses
    - Herpes zoster
    - Oral hairy-cell leukoplakia
    - Candidiasis
      - Oral
      - Persistent vaginal
    - Idiopathic thrombocytopenic puerpera
    - Listeriosis
    - Tuberculosis
- Social history
  - Support systems
    - Living situation
    - Economic factors
    - Access to services
  - Substance abuse
  - Mental health issues

- Signs and symptoms of acute retroviral syndrome (CDC, 2010)
  - Fever
  - Lymphadenopathy
  - Pharyngitis
  - Rash
  - Maculopapular lesions
  - Mucocutaneous ulceration
  - Myalgia or arthralgia
- Signs and symptoms of active HIV infection
  - Abnormal cytology: CIN grade 2 or 3
  - PID
  - Constitutional symptoms for more than 1 month
    - Fever
    - Weight loss
    - Diarrhea
    - Peripheral neuropathy
- Review of systems

Physical Examination: Components of the Physical Exam to Consider

- Vital signs, including temperature
  - Weight loss: Compare current weight with previous weight
- Skin
  - Rash
  - Erythematous maculopapular rash
  - Mucocutaneous ulceration
  - Lesions
  - Herpes zoster
- Head, eyes, ears, nose, and throat (HEENT)
  - Cervical lymph nodes
  - Oral candidiasis or ulcerative lesions
  - Pharyngeal erythema
- Chest
  - Cardiac assessment
  - Lung sounds
  - Presence of cough
- Abdomen: Enlargement of liver or spleen
- Extremities
  - Range of motion
  - Joint tenderness or swelling

- Femoral lymph nodes
- Muscle wasting
- Pelvic examination
  - Lesions
  - Mucocutaneous ulceration of genitals
  - Discharge
    - Mucopurulent cervicitis
    - Bacterial vaginosis (BV)
    - Vulvovaginal candidiasis (VVC)
  - Cervical lesions
    - Cervicitis
    - Friability
    - Masses
  - Uterine motion tenderness
  - Adnexal mass or pain
- Neurologic examination
  - Peripheral neuropathy
  - Facial palsy
  - Mental health status
  - Cognitive impairment

Clinical Impression: Differential Diagnoses to Consider

(ICD9data.com, 2012)

- HIV infection, asymptomatic
- IV drug abuse or addiction
- Acute retroviral syndrome
- AIDS
- Opportunistic infection
- Kaposi's sarcoma
- Candidiasis
- Tuberculosis
- Cervical cancer
- Viral hepatitis

Diagnostic Testing: Diagnostic Tests and Procedures to Consider

- HIV screening (CDC, 2010)
  - Screen women aged 13–64
  - Screen all pregnant women
  - Screen all patients, male and female, presenting to STI clinics

- Screen high-risk women annually
- "Opt-out" testing is recommended
  - Client-advised testing is routine
  - Testing is done unless the client declines it
- An antibody screen becomes positive more than 2–14 weeks post infection
- HIV-1 antibody testing
  - Rapid HIV-1 testing (CDC, 2009, 2010)
    - Oral, blood, or plasma
    - False-positive results may occur
    - Testing may occur at the point of care
      - STI clinic
      - Labor and delivery
    - A reactive test result requires confirmatory testing
      - Western blot *or*
      - Immunofluorescent assay (IFA) *and*
      - Retest with a blood specimen in 4 weeks
  - Indications for rapid HIV testing in labor and delivery (Lampe et al., 2004)
    - Unknown HIV status
    - Little or no prenatal care
  - Screening enzyme immunoassay (EIA)
    - Venous sample (tiger-top tube)
    - Detects antibodies
    - False-positive results may occur
    - A positive test result requires confirmatory testing
- Confirmatory testing
  - Western blot test
  - Polymerase chain reaction (PCR) test
- Other laboratory testing
  - Gonorrhea and chlamydia testing
  - Pap smear
  - Wet preparation
  - Hepatitis A, B, and C serology
  - Syphilis serology
- HIV infection strongly suspected
  - CBC
  - Chemistry profile
  - Blood urea nitrogen and creatinine
  - Toxoplasmosis antibody test
  - Tuberculosis testing

- ◆ Mantoux skin test
- ◆ Chest x-ray
- Monitoring of HIV treatment response and viral load
  - Viral RNA and p24 antigen
  - Nucleic acid amplification (NAT)

Providing Treatment: Therapeutic Measures to Consider

(King & Brucker, 2011)

- Highly active antiretroviral therapy (HAART)
  - Can delay the onset of HIV-related complications
  - Currently 31 antiretroviral drugs are approved for HIV treatment (NIAID, 2011)
  - Classes of HIV drugs
    - ◆ Reverse transcriptase inhibitors
    - ◆ Protease inhibitors
    - ◆ Fusion/entry inhibitors
    - ◆ Integrase inhibitors
    - ◆ Multidrug combination therapies
  - Side effects are significant
- Prevent maternal-to-child transmission (MTCT)
  - The biggest burden of MTCT occurs in developing countries
- Midwives and other birth care providers are at risk for occupational exposure to HIV
  - Follow the guidelines for post-exposure prophylaxis

Providing Treatment: Complementary and Alternative Measures to Consider

(Romm, 2010)

- Alternative therapies are not a substitute for medical treatment
- Chronic disease is a positive predictor for use of complementary and alternative medicine (CAM): CAM is often used to treat the side effects of conventional therapies
- Immunomodulating herbs commonly used in HIV/AIDS

- Astragalus
- Atractylodes
- Condonopsis
- Eluthero
- Licorice
- Lingustrum
- Reishi
- Shitake mushroom
- HIV immune support
  - Adequate rest
  - Stress reduction
  - Balanced diet
    - ◆ Fresh fruits and vegetables
    - ◆ Limit nonorganic meat and dairy
    - ◆ Antioxidant foods
    - ◆ Fish oil (omega-3 fatty acids)

Providing Support: Education and Support Measures to Consider

- HIV-1 antibody testing
  - An antibody screen becomes positive more than 2–14 weeks post infection
  - Pretest counseling
    - ◆ Opt-out choice
    - ◆ Routes of transmission
    - ◆ Prevention measures
- Information about testing
  - Specimen collection technique
  - Confidentiality
  - Test interpretation
  - Timing of results
  - Partner notification
- HIV risk-reduction practices
  - Abstaining from intercourse
  - Selecting low-risk partners
  - Negotiating partner monogamy
  - Condom use
- Client resources: American Social Health Association
- Encourage creative and supportive measures
  - Meditation or spiritual practices
  - Art therapy
  - Dance

- Support groups
- Religious involvement
- Community involvement
- Participation in HIV prevention programs

Follow-up Care: Follow-up Measures to Consider

- Document
  - Results
  - Post-test counseling
  - Plan for continued care
- HIV-negative client
  - Provide HIV prevention education
  - Perform HIV risk assessment at return visits
- HIV-positive client: Arrange case management
- Provide ongoing reproductive health care as appropriate
- Labor care for women with HIV (AECT, 2007a)
  - Vaginal birth
    - Appropriate for women taking antiretroviral therapy (ART)
    - Appropriate for women with a viral HIV-RNA load less than 1000 copies/mL
    - Avoid fetal exposure to maternal blood and body fluids
      - ➤ Prolonged rupture of membranes: Active management of labor
      - ➤ External fetal heart rate monitoring: ⚠ Do not use an internal fetal scalp electrode
      - ➤ No invasive intrauterine monitoring
      - ➤ Maintain an intact perineum
  - Cesarean section at 38 weeks' gestation
    - Indicated in HIV-positive women who are not currently taking ART
    - Indicated in women with a viral HIV-RNA load greater than 1000 copies/mL
    - Per client preference
- Breastfeeding is contraindicated

Multidisciplinary Practice: Consider Consultation, Collaboration, or Referral

- HIV/infectious disease specialist
  - Women with previously diagnosed HIV

- Medical evaluation
- Treatment plan
- Coordination of case management with current HIV-care provider
  - Women with a new HIV diagnosis: Refer for case management and medical care
    - Reproductive health counseling
    - Medical evaluation and treatment
- Psychosocial services
  - Psychosocial evaluation
  - Mental health
  - Crisis counseling
  - Substance abuse services
  - Housing and financial support services
- Behavioral health services: Risk-reduction measures
  - HIV-negative status with HIV behavioral risk factors
  - HIV-positive status with behavioral risk factors
    - Affecting potential for:
      - ➤ Coinfection with other STIs
      - ➤ Spread of infection
    - Affecting ART and/or medical treatment compliance
- Perinatology services
  - Maternal HAART
  - Prevention of perinatal HIV transmission
  - Consultation for labor and birth care
- Pediatric services: For follow-up monitoring and care of neonate
- For diagnosis or treatment outside the midwife's scope of practice

CARE OF THE WOMAN WITH HUMAN PAPILLOMAVIRUS

Key Clinical Information

More than 40 types of human papillomavirus (HPV) affect the genital tract, but only a few types are considered to pose a high risk for the development of cervical cancer. Types 16, 18, 31, 33, and 35 are associated with cervical dysplasia and can contribute to the development of anal, cervical, penile, and vulvar cancers. Other types can cause visible genital warts. The overall prevalence of HPV in American women is 27%; the highest prevalence (45%) is found among women aged 20–24 (Dunne, Unger, Sternberg, McQuillan, Patel, & Markowitz, 2007). In individuals with an intact immune system and healthy immune response, more than 90% of HPV infections resolve within 2 years (ACS, 2007). Recently developed HPV vaccines—Gardasil and Cervarix—are important preventive strategies for young women and young men to guard against these infections. Screening tests for HPV can indicate the presence or absence of one or more high-risk types of HPV and are used to guide clinical management of women infected with HPV (CDC, 2011).

Client History and Chart Review: Components of the History to Consider

(ACS, 2007)

- Age
- Reproductive history
  - LMP, GP TPAL
  - Current method of birth control
  - Previous tests
    - ◆ HPV testing
    - ◆ Abnormal cervical cytology
- Sexual practices
  - Condom use
  - Number of sexual partners
  - Uncircumcised partner
  - Anal sex with penetration
- Onset, duration, and severity of current symptoms
  - Location of lesions
  - Other associated symptoms
- Medical/surgical history
  - Allergies
  - Medications: Long-term use of OCPs
  - Chronic illnesses
  - STIs
  - HIV/AIDS
- Social history
  - Tobacco use: Increases risk of progression
  - Drug and/or alcohol use: Associated with higher-risk behaviors

- Risk factors for HPV infection
  - Previous or current STIs
  - Diminished immune response
  - Unprotected sexual activity
  - More than five lifetime sexual partners for self or partner(s)
- Review of systems

Physical Examination: Components of the Physical Exam to Consider

- HEENT
  - Conjunctival warts
  - Nasal warts
  - Oral/pharyngeal warts
- External genitalia
  - Genital warts
  - Friable lesions
  - Anogenital warts
- Speculum examination: Cervical or vaginal lesions
- Bimanual examination: Palpate for abnormality of cervix or vagina
  - Contour
  - Consistency
  - Mass
- Consider colposcopy
  - External genitalia
  - Vagina
  - Cervix
- Consider application of topical solutions
  - 5% acetic acid (white vinegar)
    - ◆ HPV lesions turn acetowhite
  - Lugol's solution (strong iodine)
    - ◆ Normal squamous cells stain mahogany brown
    - ◆ HPV lesions and columnar cells remain unstained

Clinical Impression: Differential Diagnoses to Consider

(ICD9data.com, 2012)

- Genital warts
- *Condyloma acuminatum*

- Syphilitic *condyloma latum*
- *Musculosum contagiosum*
- Dysplasia
  - Vulvar
  - Vaginal

Diagnostic Testing: Diagnostic Tests and Procedures to Consider

- HPV testing
  - Cervicovaginal
  - Anal
- Other STI testing, as indicated
  - Gonorrhea/chlamydia nucleic acid amplification tests
  - Rapid plasma reagin (RPR)
  - HIV counseling and testing
- Cytology
  - Specimen source
    - Cervicovaginal
    - Anal
  - Specimen collection
    - Slide: Most cost-effective for screening
    - Liquid-based cytology
      - ➤ Allows for reflex HPV testing
      - ➤ Preferred method for post-treatment follow-up of HSIL/CIN grades 2 and 3
- HCG as indicated, before treatment
- Stool for occult blood

Providing Treatment: Therapeutic Measures to Consider

(CDC, 2010)

- HPV vaccines
  - Gardasil: HPV types 6, 11, 16, and 18
    - Recommended age of vaccination: 11–12 years
    - Range: 9–26 years for both females and males
    - Dose: 0.5 mL IM at 0, 2, and 6 months
  - Cervarix: HPV types 16 and 18
    - Recommended age of vaccination: 11–12 years

- Range: 10–25 years for females
- Dose: 0.5 mL IM at 0, 1, and 6 months
- Vitamin therapy
  - Vitamin E: 400 IU daily
  - Vitamin C: 500–1000 mg daily
- Client-applied therapy for visible warts
  - Imiquimod cream 5%
    - Apply every night three times a week until clear
    - Wash off after 6–10 hours
    - Can weaken latex barrier methods of contraception
    - Not for use during pregnancy
  - Podofilox 0.5% solution or gel
    - Apply BID for 3 days
    - No treatment for 4 days
    - Repeat up to four cycles
    - Not for use in pregnancy
- Provider applied therapy for visible warts
  - Cryotherapy
  - Podophyllin resin
    - Apply weekly to warts
    - Wash off in 1–4 hours
    - Not for use in pregnancy
  - Trichloroacetic acid or bichloracetic acid
    - Apply weekly to lesions
    - Protect normal tissue with petrolatum
  - Surgical removal
    - For large numbers of warts
    - Nonresponsive to other methods
- Alternate treatment
  - Intralesional interferon injection (Yang, Yu-guo, Zhong-ming, Zhi-jian, & Qi-wen, 2009)
  - Laser ablation

Providing Treatment: Complementary and Alternative Measures to Consider

- Forgo medical therapies and wait for spontaneous resolution of warts (Rubano, 2010)
  - Warts may remain stable, decrease, increase, or resolve
  - Approximately 75% will resolve within 2 years
  - Preferred strategy in pregnant women

- Antioxidant foods
  - Blueberries
  - Red peppers
  - Plums
  - Pumpkin
  - Tomatoes
- Herbal remedies (Romm, 2010)
  - Tea tree oil
  - Echinacea tea or tincture daily to boost immune response
  - Lemon balm
  - Astragalus
- Stress management
- Visualization of the area as healed and whole

Providing Support: Education and Support Measures to Consider

- Age- and culturally appropriate information
  - Male and female condoms provide limited protection; uncovered areas are not protected
  - The wart virus is not curable but may become dormant
    - Regression is most likely in adolescents
    - The virus can be transmitted even when no warts are visible
  - Oral, pharyngeal, or anal warts can occur with exposure
  - Screen for depression and anxiety as needed
  - Partner evaluation and treatment as needed
- Treatment recommendations
  - Medication/remedy use
  - Anticipated response to treatment
  - Signs or symptoms indicating the need to return for care
- Risk of cervical dysplasia
  - Increased risk for abnormal Pap smear results
  - Emphasize need for annual Pap smears
  - Smoking increases the risk of progression
  - The immune response affects regression or progression
- Encourage smoking cessation

Follow-up Care: Follow-up Measures to Consider

- Document
  - Location, number, and size of lesions
  - Treatment method
  - Anticipated follow-up
- Return for care
  - As necessary for treatment chosen
  - For HPV screening results and interpretation
  - As indicated by:
    - Clinical response to treatment
    - Cytology results (see "Care of the Woman with an Abnormal Pap Smear")
    - HPV test results (see "Care of the Woman with an Abnormal Pap Smear")

Multidisciplinary Practice: Consider Consultation, Collaboration, or Referral

- OB/GYN services
  - Ablative therapy
    - Cryotherapy
    - Laser
  - Interferon injection of lesions
  - Extensive lesions
  - Anal lesions
- Behavior risk modification
  - Safe sex practices
  - Drug and alcohol rehabilitation
  - Smoking cessation
- For diagnosis or treatment outside the midwife's scope of practice

CARE OF THE WOMAN WITH NIPPLE DISCHARGE

Key Clinical Information

Nipple discharge in the absence of pregnancy and lactation occurs in 10% to 15% of women with benign breast conditions. It may represent a physiologic variation of normal or, alternatively, it may be the presenting symptom of a pathologic process. Regular and frequent stimulation of the nipples and breasts, such as nursing a baby with a Lactaid device or engaging in frequent sexual foreplay, may result in milk production. Bilateral galactorrhea is associated with hypothyroidism, with amenorrheic syndromes such as occur with pituitary adenoma, and with pharmacologic causes (Breast Expert Workgroup, 2005). Fortunately, many pituitary tumors are benign and grow exceedingly slowly. However, without treatment, enlarging tumors may cause pressure on optic nerves, resulting in permanent visual loss or blindness.

Unilateral spontaneous nipple discharge that is clear, serous, or bloody requires prompt evaluation for underlying malignancy. Spontaneous discharge is suspected when a woman notes staining on her clothing or bedding. Spontaneous discharge from a single duct or that associated with a proximate underlying mass is of particular concern (Aliotta & Schaefer, 2006; Breast Expert Workgroup, 2005).

Client History and Chart Review: Components of the History to Consider

- Age
- Reproductive history
  - GP TPAL, LMP
  - Usual menstrual patterns
  - Current method of birth control
  - Infertility
- Breast history
  - Lactation, duration, and most recent dates
  - Self-breast examination practices
  - Breast disorders
    - Mastitis
    - Breast abscess
    - Fibrocystic breast disorder
    - Breast cancer
  - Breast stimulation or trauma
- Onset and duration of symptoms
  - Nature of discharge
    - Bloody, serous, greenish, or milky
    - Unilateral or bilateral
    - Spontaneous or expressed
    - Recent breast changes
  - Associated symptoms
    - Breast pain, tenderness, or masses
    - Fever

- ⚠ Headache
- ⚠ Visual changes
- Presence of menstrual dysfunction
  - Amenorrhea
  - Irregular or scanty menses
- Change in libido
- Causes of nipple discharge (Thompson, 2004)
  - Pregnancy and lactation
  - Breast manipulation
  - Medications
  - Endocrine disorders
  - Malignancy
- Medical/surgical history
  - Medications that may cause nipple discharge (Thompson, 2004)
    - Phenothiazine
    - Cimetidine
    - Methyldopa
    - Metoclopramide
    - Oral contraceptives
    - Reserpine
    - Tricyclic antidepressants
    - Verapamil
  - Health conditions
    - Hypothyroidism
    - Family history
      - Breast disease
      - Endocrine disorder
- Review of systems

Physical Examination: Components of the Physical Exam to Consider

- Breast examination (Breast Expert Workgroup, 2005)
  - Sitting and supine
  - Presence of spontaneous nipple discharge: Crusting of discharge on nipple
  - Breast asymmetry or retraction
  - Venous patterns
  - Masses
    - Size
    - Proximity to nipple
    - Characteristics

- Breast skin changes
  - Thickening or coarseness
  - Edema
  - Scaling
  - Redness and/or heat
  - "Orange peel" sign
  - Lymph nodes
    - Axillary
    - Clavicular
- Hirsutism
- Thyroid palpation

Clinical Impression: Differential Diagnoses to Consider

(ICD9data.com, 2012; Kapenhas-Vades, Feldman, Cohen, & Boobol, 2008)

- Nipple discharge
- Intraductal papilloma
- Atypical ductal hyperplasia
- Atypical lobular hyperplasia
- Ductal ectasia
- Galactorrhea
- Hyperprolactinemia
- Hypothyroidism, acquired

Diagnostic Testing: Diagnostic Tests and Procedures to Consider

(Kapenhas-Vades et al., 2008; Leung & Pacaud, 2004)

- Pregnancy testing
- Purulent discharge
  - Culture of discharge
  - Ultrasound for fluctuant mass
- ⚠ Spontaneous bloody, serous, or clear discharge (Breast Expert Workgroup, 2005; Kapenhas-Vades et al., 2008)
  - Mammogram
  - 🕐 Mammary ductoscopy
  - 🕐 Breast biopsy
- Milky discharge
  - Thyroid testing: TSH
  - Prolactin level
    - Nonpregnant: Less than 0–20 ng/mL

- Pregnant: 10–300 ng/mL
- Prolactinoma: more than 200 ng/mL
  - Head CT for prolactinoma
  - MRI for abnormalities of the pituitary or sella turcica

Providing Treatment: Therapeutic Measures to Consider

(Leung & Pacaud, 2004)

- Treatment is based on the cause of the discharge
- Idiopathic galactorrhea, normal prolactin levels
  - Eliminate the cause, if it has been determined
  - No treatment required
- Pharmacologic cause
  - Change the medication, if appropriate
  - No treatment required
- 🕐 Pituitary tumor or elevated prolactin levels: Refer the client for evaluation and treatment
  - Bromocriptine
    - To normalize prolactin levels
    - To shrink a pituitary tumor
  - Large or bromocriptine-resistant tumors: Surgical removal
- 🕐 Hypothyroidism: Thyroid replacement therapy
- Breast infection (see "Care of the Mother with Mastitis")
- Ductal ectasia
  - Observation
  - 🕐 Surgical repair of the affected duct(s)
- Intraductal papilloma
  - Observation
  - 🕐 Surgical removal
- 🕐 Malignancy: Surgical treatment

Providing Treatment: Complementary and Alternative Measures to Consider

- Emotional support
- Comfort measures
  - Warm castor oil packs to the breasts
  - Bach flower remedies to balance the client's emotional state
- Immune support formulas

Providing Support: Education and Support Measures to Consider

- Provide information
  - Diagnosis
  - Recommendations for evaluation
  - Treatment options
  - Breast pads to absorb discharge
- Teach or review self-breast examination
- Offer active listening
- Address the client's fears and concerns

Follow-up Care: Follow-up Measures to Consider

- Document
  - Characteristics of the discharge
  - Presence or absence of a mass
  - Diagnostic testing and results
  - Discussions with the client
  - Plan for continued care
  - Referrals
- Pregnancy (see "Diagnosis of Pregnancy")
- Galactorrhea, negative diagnostic imaging, pharmacologic or physiologic cause
  - Observation
  - Periodic prolactin levels to assess stability
  - 🕐 Persistent galactorrhea: Refer the client to an endocrinologist
  - Assess for recurrence after treatment
- Galactorrhea, pathologic: Return for care after evaluation and medical or surgical treatment
  - Response evaluated with:
    - Serum prolactin levels
    - MRI of any tumor
  - Assess for:
    - Symptom recurrence
    - Prolactinoma tumor regrowth
    - Contralateral breast disease
- Spontaneous unilateral nipple discharge (Breast Expert Workgroup, 2005)
  - Negative testing: Reevaluate in 3 months
  - 🕐 Persistent discharge: Refer to breast specialist
- Routine well-woman care

Multidisciplinary Practice: Consider Consultation, Collaboration, or Referral

- Breast care specialist
  - Ductal ectasia
  - Intraductal papilloma
  - Breast cancer
- Endocrinology services
  - Pituitary adenoma
  - Hypothyroidism
  - Persistent galactorrhea
- For diagnosis or treatment outside the midwife's scope of practice

CARE OF THE WOMAN WITH PARASITIC INFESTATION

Key Clinical Information

Lice and scabies are two common parasites that can be particularly challenging in midwifery practice. An infestation of lice can be difficult to eradicate, and because they are mobile, lice may affect the office environment and housekeeping practices after a client has been diagnosed. Lice and scabies live on human blood and may contribute to the spread of impetigo. Head lice prefer the nape of the neck, whereas body lice inhabit seams of clothing or bedding and move onto the host to feed. Pubic or crab lice live in the genital region but may be found on any hairy aspect of the body. The scabies mite burrows under the skin. Persistent itching may result from reinfestation, allergic dermatitis, or secondary skin infection (CDC, 2010).

There has been an increase in pediculosis in recent years, as populations of lice have developed resistance to certain overused treatments. Additionally, concern about the use of neurotoxic insecticides to treat parasitic infestations has led to investigation of the effectiveness of alternative therapies (Burgess, 2009).

Client History and Chart Review: Components of the History to Consider

- LMP, pregnancy status

- Symptoms
  - Onset, duration, and location
    - Itching
    - Presence of nits (lice)
    - Presence of skin tracks (scabies)
  - Other associated symptoms
    - Joint aches
    - Rash or skin changes
    - Headache
    - Fever
- Medical/surgical history
  - Allergies
  - Medications
  - Health conditions: Asthma
- Social history
  - Exposure to lice, nits, or scabies
    - Environmental exposure
      - Shared personal items
      - Infested clothes or bedding
    - Interpersonal exposure
      - Intimate contacts
      - Household contacts
      - Public contacts
        - School or day care
        - International travel
  - Sexual partner or family member symptoms
  - General hygiene and housekeeping habits
- Review of systems

Physical Examination: Components of the Physical Exam to Consider

(Burgess, 2009; CDC, 2010)

- Observe for signs of parasites
  - Anogenital region
  - Extremities
  - Nape of the neck
- Presence of the following:
  - Lice (1-mm crablike organism)
  - Nits (small, white teardrop-shaped orb attached to a hair shaft)
  - Skin tracks from scabies burrows
  - Tick or other insect(s) or bites

- Secondary signs
  - Redness and erythema
  - Rash
  - Blisters
  - Scabbing
  - Crusting
- Pelvic examination as indicated: STI symptoms
- Lymph nodes for enlargement

Clinical Impression: Differential Diagnoses to Consider

(CDC, 2010; ICD9data.com, 2012)

- Pediculosis
- Pediculosis pubis
- Scabies
- Crusted scabies
- Anogenital eczema
- Allergic dermatitis
- Impetigo
- Viral exanthem, unspecified

Diagnostic Testing: Diagnostic Tests and Procedures to Consider

- Visual inspection with an illuminating magnifier
- Microscopic examination of the parasites
- Culture of skin lesions
- Vaginal wet preparation
- STI testing
- Additional testing as needed
  - Lyme titer
  - Viral tests

Providing Treatment: Therapeutic Measures to Consider

(Burgess, 2009; CDC, 2010)

- Pediculosis
  - Permethrin 1% cream rinse: Pregnancy Category B
  - Pyrethrin with piperonyl butoxide: Pregnancy Category C
  - Instructions

- ◆ Apply to the affected area(s)
- ◆ Wash off after 10 minutes
- ◆ Avoid pyrethrin or permethrin in clients with the following conditions:
  - ➤ Asthma
  - ➤ Ragweed allergy
- ■ Alternative options
  - ◆ Malathion 0.5% lotion: Pregnancy Category B
    - ➤ Apply to the affected area(s)
    - ➤ Wash off after 8–12 hours
  - ◆ Ivermectin
    - ➤ Dose: 250 mg/kg PO, repeat in 2 weeks
    - ➤ Avoid in pregnancy or lactation
- • Scabies treatment
  - ■ Permethrin cream 5%
    - ◆ Apply to all areas of the body from the neck down
    - ◆ Wash off after 8–14 hours
  - ■ Ivermectin: 200 mg/kg PO, repeat in 2 weeks
  - ■ Alternative regimen: Lindane 1%
    - ◆ 1 oz. of lotion or 30 g of cream
    - ◆ Apply in a thin layer to the body from the neck down
    - ◆ Thoroughly wash off after 8 hours
    - ◆ ⚠ May cause a severe neurotoxic reaction
    - ◆ ⚠ Do not use in the following situations:
      - ➤ Immediately after a bath or shower
      - ➤ In persons with extensive dermatitis
      - ➤ In women who are pregnant or lactating
      - ➤ In children younger than 2 years
- • Impetigo: Superficial *Staphylococcus* or *Streptococcus* infection
  - ■ Antibacterial soap or cleanser
  - ■ Topical antibiotic such as Bactroban
  - ■ Oral antibiotic therapy

Providing Treatment: Complementary and Alternative Measures to Consider

- • [www] Lice R Gone Shampoo: Safe Solutions, Inc., (888) 443-8738, www.safesolutionsinc.com

- • Head or pubic lice
  - ■ Coat the affected area with olive oil
  - ■ Comb with a fine-toothed comb
  - ■ Wash with soap or shampoo
  - ■ Apply a cream rinse
  - ■ Comb again
  - ■ Apply a vinegar rinse
    - ◆ Use caution, as this treatment may cause burning of the eyes and genitals
- • Salt scrub to the affected area
  - ■ Mix coarse salt with oil
  - ■ Follow with a soap wash
- • Wash of herbal painted daisy infusion
  - ■ Source of pyrethrins
  - ■ Use the wash on the affected area TID
- • Shave the affected area
- • Physically remove nits (nit pick)

Providing Support: Education and Support Measures to Consider

- • Provide written medication instructions
- • Recommend treatment for all contacts
- • Avoid sexual contact until treatment is complete
- • Review the transmission mechanisms
- • Cleanse bedding and clothing
  - ■ Hot water wash with bleach
  - ■ Hot dryer
- • Vacuum the living quarters
- • Wash throw rugs

Follow-up Care: Follow-up Measures to Consider

- • Document
  - ■ Presence of parasites
  - ■ Medication recommendations and instructions
- • Return for care
  - ■ One week if symptoms are not eliminated
  - ■ Reinfestation
  - ■ Secondary infection
  - ■ Medication side effects

Multidisciplinary Practice: Consider Consultation, Collaboration, or Referral

- Infection control department: Evidence or risk of an epidemic
- Laboratory: Identification of an unusual parasite
- Emergency department or medical services: Symptoms of neurotoxicity with lindane
- For diagnosis or treatment outside the midwife's scope of practice

CARE OF THE WOMAN WITH PELVIC INFLAMMATORY DISEASE

Key Clinical Information

Pelvic inflammatory disease (PID) is one of the most common and serious complications of STIs. PID is caused when bacteria ascend from the vagina into the upper genital tract, which most often occurs during menses (Fogel, 2013). The most common causative bacteria are *Neisseria gonorrhoeae* and *Chlamydia trachomatis*; however, the normal flora of the gastrointestinal and genital tracts can also cause PID.

Diagnosis of PID is based on clinical presentation, which can be vague. It is essential that the sexual partner(s) of women with suspected PID be treated before resumption of sexual activity. PID can result in significant scarring in the fallopian tubes as well as in the pelvis. Scarring can contribute to infertility, chronic pelvic pain, and other related disorders. Women with HIV are more likely to require hospitalization with PID (CDC, 2010).

Client History and Chart Review: Components of the History to Consider

(CDC, 2010; Fogel, 2013)

- Age: PID is most common in adolescents
- Reproductive history
  - LMP, GP TPAL
    - ◆ Menstrual/pregnancy status
    - ◆ Current method of contraception
  - Most recent Pap smear and STI testing
  - Sexual orientation and practices

- New sexual partner for self or for partner
- Recent procedure, delivery, or termination of pregnancy
- Risk factors for PID
  - Active infection with chlamydia or gonorrhea
  - Previous infection with STI
  - Sexually active adolescent
  - IUD insertion
  - Multiple sexual partners
  - Douching
- Symptom profile
  - Location, onset, duration, and severity of symptoms
  - Triad of symptoms for empiric treatment (CDC, 2010)
    - ◆ Lower abdominal pain
    - ◆ No other apparent cause of illness *and*
      - ➤ Cervical motion tenderness *or*
      - ➤ Uterine tenderness *or*
      - ➤ Adnexal tenderness
    - ◆ Additional diagnostic criteria
      - ➤ Fever > 101°F (38.3°C)
      - ➤ Mucopurulent vaginal or cervical discharge
      - ➤ Many white blood cells on saline wet preparation
      - ➤ Elevated erythrocyte sedimentation rate
      - ➤ Elevated C-reactive protein
      - ➤ Positive CT or GC results
  - Other associated symptoms
    - ◆ Dyspareunia
    - ◆ Referred pain
    - ◆ Menstrual irregularities
    - ◆ Malaise
- Medical/surgical history
  - Allergies
  - Medications
  - Chronic illnesses
  - Previous surgery
- Social history
  - Drug or alcohol use
  - Living situation
- Review of systems

Physical Examination: Components of the Physical Exam to Consider

- Vital signs, including temperature
- Abdominal examination
  - Lower abdominal tenderness
    - Guarding
    - Distention
    - Rebound tenderness
  - Presence or absence of bowel sounds
- Pelvic examination
  - Speculum examination
    - Mucopurulent cervical discharge
    - Collection of cervical cultures
  - Bimanual examination
    - Cervical motion tenderness
    - Uterine enlargement or tenderness
    - Adnexal mass or tenderness

Clinical Impression: Differential Diagnoses to Consider

(ICD9data.com, 2012)

- Pelvic inflammatory disease
- Ectopic pregnancy
- Ovarian cyst
- Septic abortion
- Endometritis
- Endometriosis
- Cystitis
- Appendicitis
- Reproductive tract malignancy

Diagnostic Testing: Diagnostic Tests and Procedures to Consider

(CDC, 2010)

- Urinalysis
- Serum or urine HCG
- STI testing, including HIV
- CBC with differential
- Erythrocyte sedimentation rate
- C-reactive protein
- Gram stain and culture of cervical discharge

- Presence of gram-negative intracellular diplococci
- 10 white blood cells per high-power field
- Pelvic ultrasound or MRI
  - Thickened fluid-filled tubes
  - Free fluid in pelvis
  - Tubo-ovarian abscess
- Diagnostic laparoscopy

Providing Treatment: Therapeutic Measures to Consider

(CDC, 2010)

- Choice and location of treatment varies
  - With severity of illness
  - With anticipated client concordance with plan of care
- Outpatient treatment for mild to moderately severe PID
  - Option 1
    - Ceftriaxone: 250 mg IM in a single dose *plus*
    - Doxycycline: 100 mg PO BID for 14 days *with or without*
    - Metronidazole: 500 mg PO BID for 14 days
  - Option 2
    - Cefoxitin: 2 g IM in a single dose *with*
    - Probenecid: 1 g PO in a single dose *plus*
    - Doxycycline: 100 mg PO BID for 14 days *with or without*
    - Metronidazole: 500 mg PO BID for 14 days
  - Other parenteral third-generation cephalosporins
    - Ceftizoxime or cefotaxime *plus*
    - Doxycycline: 100 mg PO BID for 14 days *with or without*
    - Metronidazole: 500 mg PO BID for 14 days
  - Alternative regimens for PID
    - Appropriate when there is low community prevalence of gonorrhea
    - Appropriate when there is low individual risk of gonorrhea

- ◆ Fluoroquinolones
  - ➤ Levofloxacin: 500 mg orally once daily *or*
  - ➤ Ofloxacin: 400 mg PO BID for 14 days *with or without*
  - ➤ Metronidazole: 500 mg orally twice a day for 14 days
- 📞 Hospital-based treatment
  - ■ Criteria for considering hospital-based treatment
    - ◆ An acute abdominal cause such as appendicitis cannot be excluded
    - ◆ Pregnant women
    - ◆ Oral antimicrobial therapy is ineffective or inappropriate
    - ◆ PID accompanied by the following symptoms:
      - ➤ Nausea and vomiting
      - ➤ High fever
      - ➤ Tubo-ovarian abscess
  - ■ Transition to oral treatment 24–48 hours after clinical improvement
  - ■ Oral antibiotics are given to provide 14 total days of coverage
  - ■ Parenteral regimen A
    - ◆ Cefotetan: 2 g IV every 12 hours *or*
    - ◆ Cefoxitin: 2 g IV every 6 hours *plus*
    - ◆ Doxycycline: 100 mg PO or IV every 12 hours
  - ■ Parenteral regimen B
    - ◆ Clindamycin: 900 mg IV every 8 hours *plus*
    - ◆ Gentamicin
      - ➤ Loading dose, IV or IM: 2 mg/kg of body weight
      - ➤ Maintenance dose: 1.5 mg/kg every 8 hours
      - ➤ Single daily dosing may be substituted
  - ■ Alternative parenteral regimen
    - ◆ Ampicillin/sulbactam: 3 g IV every 6 hours *plus*
    - ◆ Doxycycline: 100 mg PO or IV every 12 hours

Providing Treatment: Complementary and Alternative Measures to Consider

- ⚠ Alternative therapies are not a substitute for prompt medical care
- Comfort measures
  - ■ Warm heat to the abdomen
  - ■ Adequate rest
- Remedies for healing and immune support
  - ■ Balanced nutrition
  - ■ Echinacea
  - ■ Rescue remedy
  - ■ Visualization

Providing Support: Education and Support Measures to Consider

- Provide information
  - ■ Diagnosis
  - ■ Need to evaluate and/or treat partner(s)
  - ■ Treatment recommendations
    - ◆ Need to complete all medications
    - ◆ Avoidance of intercourse
      - ➤ Until medications completed + 7 days
      - ➤ Until partner treated + 7 days
  - ■ Mandatory STI reporting
  - ■ Test of cure as indicated
  - ■ Potential complications
    - ◆ Pelvic abscess
    - ◆ Infertility
    - ◆ Ectopic pregnancy
    - ◆ Chronic pelvic pain
- Provide written materials
  - ■ Medication instructions
  - ■ Transmission of infection
  - ■ Warning signs
  - ■ When to return for care
- Prevention of recurrence
  - ■ Abstinence
  - ■ Condom use
  - ■ Mutual monogamy
  - ■ Regular STI screening

Follow-up Care: Follow-up Measures to Consider

- Document
  - Criteria used for diagnosis
  - Treatment regimen
  - Medication administration
  - Client education
  - Mandatory reporting
  - Plan for continued care
  - Criteria for consultation or referral
- Outpatient therapy
  - Client contact within 24–48 hours
  - Hospitalization if only limited improvement occurs within 72 hours (CDC, 2010)
- Test of cure 4–6 weeks with diagnosis of either chlamydia or gonorrhea
- HIV testing if not done as part of the initial workup

Multidisciplinary Practice: Consider Consultation, Collaboration, or Referral

- OB/GYN services
  - Acutely ill women requiring hospitalization
  - Pregnant women with PID
  - Clients who do not improve within 24–72 hours of outpatient treatment
- Emergency care: Other nonreproductive-related acute abdomen
- For diagnosis or treatment outside the midwife's scope of practice

CARE OF THE WOMAN WITH PELVIC PAIN

Key Clinical Information

The symptom of pelvic pain can be classified into acute and chronic pelvic pain. Acute pelvic pain is defined as moderate to severe pain of less than 7 days' duration (Sauerland et al., 2006). It requires timely evaluation and accurate diagnosis to institute the appropriate corrective action. On occasion, the ability to differentiate between acute and nonacute pain can be challenging. A careful workup is essential to determine whether prompt referral for emergency care is indicated.

Chronic pelvic pain is a common finding in women's health and may be related to reproductive functioning, the bladder or bowel, or residual effects of abdominal infection or surgery (Schuiling & Gasiewicz, 2013). Many women with chronic pelvic pain are ultimately diagnosed with endometriosis (Schorge et al., 2008). Low-grade pelvic pain can occur in women who have been subject to sexual assault or molestation, whereas ovarian malignancy or digestive tract pathology often present with vague pelvic symptoms.

Client involvement and support during investigation of chronic pelvic pain is essential. Validation of the client's discomfort and concerns is as critical to evaluation and treatment of this challenging problem as a skillfully obtained history, review of systems, and thorough physical examination. The evaluation of chronic pelvic pain often takes place over many visits.

Client History and Chart Review: Components of the History to Consider

- Age
- Reproductive history
  - LMP, GP TPAL
    - Potential for pregnancy: Current method of contraception
    - Method of birth control
    - Menstrual patterns
    - Vaginal and/or cesarean births
  - Most recent examination, Pap smear, and STI testing
  - History of gynecologic issues
    - STIs or PID
    - Endometriosis
    - Ectopic pregnancy
    - Premenstrual dysphoric disorder
  - Current sexual practices
    - Change in sexual partner for self or for partner
    - Number of lifetime sexual partners

- [www] Pain profile
  - Location: Local or radiating
  - Onset: Sudden, gradual, or cyclic
  - Timing/correlation
    - Menstrual cycle
    - Pelvic infection
    - Sexual violence
    - Abortion
  - Duration of pain: Intermittent or constant
  - Severity and quality of pain
    - Cramping
    - Aching
    - Knifelike
  - Precipitating or exacerbating factors
    - Menses
    - Intercourse
    - Bowel or bladder function
  - Associated symptoms
    - Fever and chills
    - Shoulder pain
    - Nausea and vomiting
    - Diarrhea, constipation, or obstipation
    - Cervicovaginal discharge
      - Bloody
      - Mucopurulent
    - Painful urination
    - Change in bowel or bladder function
    - Weight loss
    - Dyspareunia
  - Relief measures used and client response
- Potential causes of acute pelvic pain (see the "Clinical Impression" section)
- Medical/surgical history
  - Medications
  - Allergies
  - Health conditions
    - Diverticular disease
    - Appendicitis
    - Renal calculi
    - Previous abdominal surgery
- Family history
  - Endometriosis
  - Dysmenorrhea
  - Ovarian cancer
  - Diverticular disease
  - Colon cancer
- Psychosocial history and status
  - Physical or sexual violence
  - Drug or alcohol use
  - Living situation
- Mental health status
  - Client affect and presentation
  - [icon] Client's interpretation of pain
  - Coping ability
- Review of systems

Physical Examination: Components of the Physical Exam to Consider

- Vital signs, including temperature: Orthostatic hypotension
- Abdominal examination
  - Distention
  - Masses
  - Pain on superficial or deep palpation
  - Rebound tenderness
  - Guarding
  - Presence or absence of bowel sounds
- Costovertebral angle tenderness
- Pelvic examination
  - External genitalia
    - Urethra
    - Labia
    - Bartholin's and Skene's glands
    - Vaginal muscular tone: Cystocele
  - Speculum examination
    - Presence of cervical discharge
    - Chadwick's sign
    - Bleeding
    - Lesions
  - Bimanual examination
    - Cervical motion tenderness
      - Mild
      - Moderate
    - Uterus
      - Size, shape and position
      - Pain or tenderness
      - Prolapse

- ◆ Palpation
  - ➤ Adnexa: Size, masses, or pain
  - ➤ Fornices
- Rectal examination
  - Pain
  - Masses
  - Rectocele or fistula

Clinical Impression: Differential Diagnoses to Consider

(ICD9data.com, 2012)

- Potential diagnoses featuring pelvic pain include the following (Kripke, 2007; Sauerland et al., 2006; Swanton, Iyer, & Reginald, 2006):
- Reproductive pelvic disorders
  - Endometriosis
  - Pelvic congestion
  - Uterine fibroids
  - Pelvic inflammatory disease
  - Chronic pelvic pain post-PID
  - Ovarian mass or cancer
  - Ectopic pregnancy
  - Mucopurulent cervicitis
  - Septic abortion
  - Spontaneous abortion or miscarriage
  - Ovarian cyst
  - Torsion of ovary
- Nongynecologic pelvic disorders
  - Peritoneal adhesions
  - Interstitial cystitis
- Gastrointestinal system disorders
  - Acute appendicitis
  - Diverticulitis
  - Ulcerative colitis
  - Bowel obstruction
  - Incarcerated inguinal hernia
- Lower abdominal trauma
- Physiologic causes
  - Mid-cycle pain
  - Pelvic relaxation
- Infections
  - Chlamydia
  - Gonorrhea

- Low-grade PID
- Urinary tract infection
- Psychogenic pain

Diagnostic Testing: Diagnostic Tests and Procedures to Consider

- Urinalysis
- Serum or urine HCG
- CBC with differential
- Erythrocyte sedimentation rate
- Pap smear
- STI testing
- Stool for occult blood
- Cancer antigen (CA-125) (postmenopausal clients)
  - Nonspecific: Elevated in ovarian cancer
  - A level of 35 m/mL is considered suspicious
  - May be falsely elevated in premenopausal women
- Carcinoembryonic antigen (CEA): Elevated in the presence of some cancers
- Pelvic ultrasound or CT (American Roentgen Ray Society, 2006)
  - Transvaginal
  - Abdominal
- Diagnostic laparoscopy
- Colonoscopy

Providing Treatment: Therapeutic Measures to Consider

- Prompt medical care is indicated for acute abdominal or pelvic pain
  - For severe acute pain, the client should receive nothing by mouth until a definitive diagnosis is made
  - Provide adequate analgesia during diagnostic studies (Kripke, 2007)
    - ◆ NSAIDs
      - ➤ Ibuprofen: 600 mg TID for 5–7 days
      - ➤ Naproxen sodium: 500 mg BID for 7–10 days
    - ◆ Opioids
- Additional treatment is based on definitive diagnosis

Providing Treatment: Complementary and Alternative Measures to Consider

- Symptomatic treatment while test results are pending
  - Rest
  - Local heat
  - Positioning
  - Physical activity
- Dietary support
  - Well-balanced diet
  - Maintain optimal bowel and bladder function
    - ◆ Limit intake of fatty foods, caffeine, and alcohol
    - ◆ Adequate fiber and fluid intake
- Stress management
  - Acupuncture
  - Expressive therapy
    - ◆ Visualization
    - ◆ Acceptance
  - Coping skills for living with chronic pain
- Active listening to client's concerns

Providing Support: Education and Support Measures to Consider

- 🌀 Encourage client participation in the evaluation process
  - Pain mapping: Symptom diary and menstrual record (Swanton et al., 2006)
  - Provide reassurance, comfort, and active listening
  - Teach coping skills for living with chronic pain
  - Review danger signs (e.g., fever, acute pain, syncope)
- Information and discussion
  - Working diagnosis/differential diagnosis
  - Plan for evaluation
  - Treatment options
  - Community resources
  - Support groups
  - Access to care if the client's condition worsens
  - Indications for consultation and/or referral

- 🌀 Acute pain with referral
  - Anticipate hospital admission
  - Nothing by mouth
  - Medical or surgical treatment

Follow-up Care: Follow-up Measures to Consider

- Document
  - Symptom profile
  - Clinical findings
  - Criteria used for diagnosis
  - Client instructions
  - Consultation and/or referral
  - Plan for continued care
- Nonacute presentation
  - Reevaluate within 24–48 hours
  - Phone or face-to-face contact
- Return for care
  - Worsening symptoms
  - Persistent symptoms
  - As indicated by testing
  - At frequent intervals until the diagnosis is confirmed
  - For continued support
- 🌀 Consider laparoscopic evaluation for diagnosis

Multidisciplinary Practice: Consider Consultation, Collaboration, or Referral

- OB/GYN services
  - Suspected or confirmed obstetric/gynecologic cause
    - ◆ Pelvic abscess
    - ◆ Ectopic pregnancy
    - ◆ Endometriosis
    - ◆ Septic abortion
    - ◆ Uterine/pelvic prolapse
  - Uncertain diagnosis
  - Persistent pain or pain that is unresponsive to treatment
- Medical/surgical or emergency services
  - Nongynecologic surgical emergency
  - Uncertain diagnosis
  - Temperature greater than 102°F with rebound tenderness or guarding

- Mental health services
  - Pain with apparent psychogenic basis after workup
  - Ineffective coping ability
  - Diagnosis of a chronic disorder
- Pain management clinic
- For diagnosis or treatment outside the midwife's scope of practice

CARE OF THE WOMAN WITH POLYCYSTIC OVARIAN SYNDROME

Key Clinical Information

Polycystic ovary syndrome (PCOS) is an endocrine disorder characterized by chronic anovulation and hyperandrogenism (Fritz & Speroff, 2011). PCOS is the most common endocrine disease in childbearing women, affecting 5% to 10% of this population. PCOS can present with hirsutism, infertility, menstrual irregularities, and biochemical abnormalities. Several professional groups have proposed diagnostic criteria for PCOS, based on the presence of ovulatory dysfunction, hyperandrogenism, and polycystic ovaries, and the exclusion of other disorders, in varying combinations. Table 7-2 outlines the criteria for diagnosis of PCOS.

Management strategies for PCOS depend on whether the woman desires pregnancy and include therapies such as lifestyle modification, use of oral contraceptives, progestins, and insulin sensitizers. Management must also take into account the potential health risks that these women face, such as cardiovascular disease, type 2 diabetes mellitus, and lipid abnormalities. In addition to the physical manifestations of PCOS, women with PCOS are at increased risk of depression, anxiety, low self-esteem, and psychosexual dysfunction (King, 2006).

Client History and Chart Review: Components of the History to Consider

(Costello, 2005; Hart, Hickey, & Franks, 2004; Richardson, 2003; Schroeder, 2003; Sheehan, 2003)

- Age
- Menstrual history
  - Age at menarche
  - Menstrual pattern
  - Last normal menstrual period
- Gynecologic history
  - Presence of secondary sex characteristics
  - Gynecologic surgery
  - Sexual history/activity

Table 7-2   Criteria for PCOS Diagnosis

ROTTERDAM CRITERIA	NATIONAL INSTITUTE OF HEALTH CONSENSUS CRITERIA	ANDROGEN EXCESS SOCIETY CRITERIA
1. Oligo-anovulation and/or anovulation	1. Menstrual irregularity due to oligo-anovulation or anovulation	1. Androgen excess (clinical and/or biochemical)
2. Clinical and/or biochemical signs of hyperandrogenism	2. Evidence of hyperandrogenism whether clinical (hirsutism, acne, male pattern balding) or biochemical	2. Ovarian dysfunction (oligo-anovulation and/or polycystic ovarian morphology)
3. Polycystic ovaries (Diagnosed by transvaginal ultrasound: 12 or more follicles in each ovary measuring 2–9 mm in diameter and/or increased ovarian volume (> 10 mL)	3. Exclusion of other causes of hyperandrogensim and menstrual irregularity, such as congenital hyperplasia, androgen-secreting tumors, and hyperprolactinemia	3. Exclusion of other androgen excess or ovulatory disorders

Source: Adapted from American College of Obstetricians and Gynecologists, 2002; Sheehan, 2003.

- Contraceptive history
  - Depo-Provera
  - Mirena/Paragard
  - Continuous oral contraceptives
  - Implanon or Norplant
  - NuvaRing
- Pregnancy and breastfeeding history
  - Pregnancy terminations
  - Infertility
  - Abortions: Spontaneous or elective
  - Length of breastfeeding
- Medical and surgical history
  - Thyroid disorders
  - Weight changes: Loss or gain
  - Systemic illness
- Medications that may contribute to anovulation or hyperandrogenism
  - Oral contraceptives
  - Non-oral contraceptives
    - Depo-Provera
    - Mirena (IUD)
    - Implanon
  - Danazol and androgenic progestins
- Family history
  - Polycystic ovary syndrome
  - Obesity
  - Thyroid disease
  - Infertility/miscarriage
  - Diabetes
  - Cardiovascular disease
  - Dyslipidemia
- Psychosocial assessment
  - Stressors
  - Nutrition patterns
    - Adequacy of diet
    - Eating disorders
  - Physical activity level, including participation in competitive sports
  - Effects of PCOS on self-image: Symptoms of depression and/or anxiety
  - Support systems and coping strategies
- Review of systems
  - Constitutional: Increase in weight, fatigue or anxiety, or temperature intolerance
  - Skin and hair: Male pattern baldness, facial hair growth, acne, hyperpigmentation, dry skin, or brittle hair and nails
  - Neck: Change in neck size; noticing that shirt collars feel tighter
  - Breasts: Decrease in breast size, galactorrhea
  - Cardiovascular: Chest pain, shortness of breath, exertional dyspnea, exercise intolerance, ankle swelling
  - Endocrine: Polydipsia, polyphagia, polyuria
  - Neurological: Headache, visual disturbances

Physical Examination: Components of the Physical Exam to Consider

(American College of Obstetricians and Gynecologists [ACOG], 2002; Costello, 2005; Schroeder, 2003)

- Vital signs
- Height/weight
  - Body mass index
    - 25–30 = overweight
    - > 30 = obese
  - Weight changes
  - Weight distribution: Waist-to-hip ratio > 0.72 is considered abnormal
  - Ratio of muscle to adipose tissue
- Thyroid examination
  - Enlargement
  - Nodularity
  - Physical findings consistent with thyroid disorders
- Skin/hair
  - Acne
  - Hirsutism
  - Androgenic alopecia (male pattern baldness)
  - Acanthosis nigricans in the axillae, nape of the neck, under the breasts, or skin flexures (signs of insulin resistance)
- Breast exam: Assess for decrease in breast size
- Cardiovascular
  - Hypertension
  - Abnormal heart sounds
  - Decreased peripheral pulses
  - Lower-extremity edema

- Abdominal exam
  - Striae (Cushing's syndrome)
  - Enlargement
  - Masses
- Pelvic/bimanual exam
  - Loss of vaginal rugae
  - Clitoromegaly
  - Enlarged uterus or ovaries
- Neurological exam: Visual impairment (pituitary tumor)
- Psychological exam: Depression screen

Clinical Impression: Differential Diagnoses to Consider

(ACOG, 2002; ICD9data.com, 2012; Schroeder, 2003; Sheehan, 2003)

- Polycystic ovarian syndrome
- Hypogonadotropic hypogonadism (nutrition, excessive exercise, chronic disease)
- Hyperprolactinemia
- Pituitary tumor
- Acromegaly
- Primary ovarian failure
- Exogenous androgens
- Thyroid disease
- Androgen-secreting tumor
- Congenital adrenal hyperplasia
- Ovarian and adrenal tumors
- Cushing's syndrome

Diagnostic Testing: Diagnostic Tests and Procedures to Consider

- Lab tests
  - Human chorionic gonadotropin (HCG): Evaluate for intrauterine pregnancy
  - Follicle-stimulating hormone (FSH)
    - Evaluate for menopause
    - Level is typically slightly decreased or normal in clients with PCOS
  - Luteinizing hormone (LH)
    - Evaluate for ovarian tumors
    - Level is elevated in 50–60% of clients with PCOS

- Decreased levels raise suspicion for ovarian tumor
- LH/FSH ratio
  - Evaluate for premature primary ovarian failure
  - Ratio is greater than 2 in PCOS
- Prolactin
  - Evaluate for pituitary tumors and Cushing's syndrome
  - Level is slightly elevated in some women with PCOS
- 24-hour urine free cortisol
  - Evaluate for Cushing's syndrome
  - Mild elevations are seen in PCOS
  - If more than 2 times the upper limit of normal, the result is more consistent with Cushing's syndrome
- Thyroid-stimulating hormone (TSH)
  - Evaluate for thyroid dysfunction
  - Level is typically normal with PCOS
- Estradiol (E_2)
  - Evaluate for premature ovarian failure or prolactinoma
  - Level is typically slightly decreased with PCOS
- Androgens: Dehydroepiandrosterone sulfate (DHEA-S)
  - Evaluate for Cushing's syndrome, ovarian tumor, or menopause
  - Level is typically normal or slightly elevated with PCOS
  - Moderate elevations or decreased levels are cause for concern
- Total testosterone
  - Evaluate for adrenal disorders or tumors
  - Level is typically normal or slightly elevated with PCOS
  - Moderate elevations are suspicious for tumor
- Sex hormone binding globulin (SHBG)
  - Evaluate for tumors
  - Level is typically suppressed with PCOS
  - Elevations are suspicious for tumor

- Free androgen index (FAI): Typically elevated with PCOS
- 17-Hydroxyprogesterone
  - Evaluate for adrenal tumor or ovarian cancer
  - Level is decreased with PCOS
  - Elevated levels are cause for concern
- 2-hour 75 g oral glucose tolerance test (OGTT) if BMI > 28: Evaluate for glucose intolerance or diabetes mellitus
- Fasting lipid profile (FLP): Evaluate for hyperlipidemia secondary to hyperandrogenism
- C-reactive protein (CRP)
  - May be elevated
  - PCOS patients have higher incidence of pro-inflammatory and atherogenic markers
- Screening tests
  - Depression
  - Anxiety
  - Impaired quality of life
  - Eating disorders
- Diagnostic procedures
  - Pelvic ultrasound (preferably transvaginal ultrasound)
    - Frequently shows ovaries of increased size due to either a greater number of follicles/cysts or an increased ovarian volume
    - Findings may be nonspecific
  - Endometrial biopsy
    - Unopposed estrogen from chronic anovulation puts PCOS patients at higher risk for endometrial hyperplasia and cancer

Providing Treatment: Therapeutic Measures to Consider

(ACOG, 2002; Costello, 2005; Sheehan, 2003)

- Combined oral contraceptives (COC)
  - Appropriate for first-line and long-term management

- Non-androgenic third-generation progestins
  - Norgestimate
  - Desogestrel
  - Drospirenon
- Medroxyprogesterone acetate: 10 mg for 7–10 days every 1–3 months
  - To induce menses
  - To reduce endometrial hyperplasia
  - To restore menstrual regularity
- Insulin sensitizers: Metformin
  - Improves hyperinsulinemia, hyperandrogenism, and menstrual cyclicity, and facilitates ovulation
  - Lower incidence of first-trimester pregnancy loss with metformin use
  - Improves cardiovascular risk factors
  - Improves pregnancy outcomes
- Thiazolidinediones (TZDs): Pioglitazone and rosiglitazone
  - Improve hyperandrogenism and cause ovulatory cycles
  - Can cause an increase in BMI and waist-to-hip ratio
- Antiandrogens
  - For treatment of hirsutism
  - Indicated if COC use is contraindicated
  - Birth control is needed, as all antiandrogens have teratogenic potential
  - Options
    - Spironolactone: 50–200 mg/day
    - Flutamide: 250 mg/day
    - Finasteride: 2.5–5 mg/day
- Topical agent for hirsutism: Eflornithine
  - Slows hair growth
  - Does not remove hair
- Ovulation inducers: Clomiphene citrate
  - 50–100 mg/day for 5 days at the beginning of the menstrual cycle
  - Restores menstrual regularity, prevents endometrial hyperplasia, and induces ovulation by stimulating the release of pituitary gonadotropins
  - When combined with metformin, is more effective than either agent used alone

- Tamoxifen
  - 5–40 mg/day for 4 days at the beginning of the menstrual cycle
  - Not FDA approved for ovulation induction
- Exogenous gonadotropins: Urinary follicle stimulating hormone (uFSH) (Metrodin) and recombinant FSH (rFSH) (Gonal F and Puregon)
  - Induce ovulation in women who are resistant to clomiphene
  - Carry the risk of multiple follicle development, multiple-fetus pregnancies, and ovarian hyperstimulation syndrome
- Human menopausal gonadotropin (HMG)
  - Contains FSH, LH, and large quantities of potentially allergenic urinary proteins
  - Carries an increased risk of ovarian hyperstimulation syndrome
- Lipid-lowering medications: Statins, fibrates, niacin, ezetimibe
- Blood-pressure-lowering medications and aspirin: Reduce cardiovascular risk
- Surgical laparoscopic ovarian drilling/electrocautery: To induce ovulation

Providing Treatment: Complementary and Alternative Measures to Consider

- Lifestyle modification
  - Diet: Reduced fat intake and increased fiber
  - Exercise: To achieve weight control
  - Weight loss
  - Smoking cessation
- Cosmetic therapies for hirsutism
  - Bleaching
  - Plucking
  - Shaving
  - Waxing
  - Electrolysis
  - Laser therapy

Providing Support: Education and Support Measures to Consider

(ACOG, 2002; Costello, 2005; Schroeder, 2003)

- Provide age-appropriate information
  - Explain diagnosis
    - Much of pathophysiology is not fully understood
- Potential for associated conditions
  - Increased cardiovascular risk
    - Hypertension
    - Elevated serum lipids
    - Decreased antioxidant capacity
    - Blood vessel dysfunction
    - Abnormal coagulation
  - Type 2 diabetes
    - Risk in women with PCOS is 5–10 times the risk in the general population
    - Onset occurs as early as the third or fourth decade of life
    - Approximately 30% of women with PCOS have impaired glucose intolerance
  - Cancer: Higher risk for endometrial, breast, and ovarian cancer
  - Pregnancy-related risks
    - Infertility
    - Miscarriage
    - Gestational diabetes
  - Depression and anxiety: Negative cosmetic effects
- Plan for testing and results
- Expectation of treatment
  - Return of menses and fertility
  - Absence of hirsutism
  - Prevention of complications

Follow-up Care: Follow-up Measures to Consider

(ACOG, 2002; Schroeder, 2003; Sheehan, 2003)

- Documentation
  - Working diagnosis
  - Plan for continued care
- Office follow-up
  - Regular follow-up every 6 months to monitor weight, blood pressure, and fasting glucose and lipids
  - Breast exam, Pap smear, and mammogram as recommended for all women
  - Antiandrogen therapy: Every 3–6 months initially

- Progestin therapy for anovulatory dysfunctional uterine bleeding: Every 3–6 months initially
- In women trying to conceive, if no pregnancy occurs after 6 months, return for additional infertility evaluations

Multidisciplinary Practice: Consider Consultation, Collaboration, or Referral

- OB/GYN or gynecologic endocrinologist
  - Abnormal unexplained vaginal bleeding or very heavy bleeding
  - Anovulatory dysfunctional bleeding not responding to medications
  - Suspicion of other hyperandrogen disorders needing exclusion
  - Severe hyperlipidemia
  - Recurrent miscarriages
  - Infertility management
  - Treatment failure
- Mental health services: Signs of depression or anxiety
- For diagnosis or treatment outside the midwife's scope of practice

CARE OF THE WOMAN WITH PREMENSTRUAL SYMPTOMS, SYNDROME (PMS), OR DYSPHORIC DISORDER (PMDD)

Key Clinical Information

Since ancient times, women's menstrual cycles have been linked to lunar phases; many negative and magical effects were ascribed to menstrual blood, such as turning wine sour, killing hives of bees, and driving dogs mad (Fritz & Speroff, 2011). Today, negative stereotypes persist through the characterization of premenstrual symptoms as solely psychoemotional in nature. Midwives provide a real service to women by listening to women speak about their menstrual experiences and educating women in what is known about normal menstruation, its variations, and its complications.

While premenstrual symptoms are very common, affecting 75% to 90% of women at some time in their lives, most women take these symptoms in stride. Using prospective symptom charting, it is estimated that premenstrual syndrome (PMS) affects 20% to 30% of women, whereas premenstrual dysphoric disorder (PMDD) affects 2% to 8% of women (Fritz & Speroff, 2011). PMS is recognized as a gynecologic diagnosis, while PMDD is an acknowledged psychiatric diagnosis. Both include physical and emotional symptomatology and are thought to result from a complex pathologic interaction between ovarian hormones, central nervous system neurotransmitters, and other neurohormonal systems. Serotonin dysregulation has been implicated as the basis of many of the psychological features of PMS and PMDD (Hatcher et al., 2011).

Treatment is aimed at finding relief measures or medical treatments that are acceptable to the individual woman and that support her within the context of her life. Attention to lifestyle, diet, home life, and other life choices is an integral part of the assessment and treatment for PMS and PMDD.

Client History and Chart Review: Components of the History to Consider

- Age
- Pregnancy history
  - GP TPAL
  - Current stage of reproductive life
- Menstrual history
  - LMP
  - Age at menarche
  - Years of menstruation
  - Normal cyclic pattern
  - Method of contraception
- Symptom profile
  - Timing of symptoms in cycle
  - Age at onset of symptoms
  - Onset, duration, and severity of symptoms
  - Symptom clusters (Taylor, Schuiling, & Sharp, 2013)
    - Turmoil
      - Hostility
      - Aggression

- ➤ Mood swings
- ➤ Anxiety
- ➤ Depression
- ➤ Sadness
- ➤ Guilt
- ➤ Tearfulness
- ➤ Desire to be alone
- ◆ Fluid retention
  - ➤ Weight gain
  - ➤ Abdominal bloating
  - ➤ Painful breasts
  - ➤ Swelling of hands and feet
  - ➤ Skin disorders
- ◆ Hyperarousal
  - ➤ Bursts of energy or activity
  - ➤ Carbohydrate cravings and binge eating
  - ➤ Increased sense of well-being
  - ➤ Increased libido
  - ➤ Impulsiveness
- ◆ Somatic symptoms
  - ➤ Aches and pains
  - ➤ Migraine and tension headaches
  - ➤ Nausea
  - ➤ Decreased libido
  - ➤ Lethargy
  - ➤ Abdominal pain
  - ➤ Decreased appetite
- Effects of symptoms on daily living
  - Self-image
  - Relationships
  - Employment
- Ability to effectively self-treat symptoms: Relief measures used and rate of success
- Medical/surgical history
  - Allergies
  - Medications
  - Health conditions
    - ◆ Endocrine disorders
    - ◆ Heart disease and hypertension
    - ◆ Mental health disorders
  - Other medical conditions
- Psychosocial history and status

- Potential contributing factors
  - ◆ Life stressors
  - ◆ Ineffective stress response
  - ◆ Sexual abuse
  - ◆ Cultural beliefs regarding menstruation
  - ◆ Self-beliefs regarding menstruation
- Drug, alcohol, and tobacco use
- Usual physical activity
- Diet review
- Social and family support
- Stressors
- Review of systems

Physical Examination: Components of the Physical Exam to Consider

Conduct an age-appropriate physical examination:

- If none has occurred within the previous 6–12 months
- With new onset of symptoms
- To update pertinent systems data

Clinical Impression: Differential Diagnoses to Consider

(ICD9data.com, 2012)

- Premenstrual syndrome
- Premenstrual dysphoric disorder: Comorbid with mood, anxiety, or another mental health disorder
- Perimenopausal changes
- Endocrine disorder
  - Hypothyroidism
  - Hyperthyroidism
- Mental health disorder

Diagnostic Testing: Diagnostic Tests and Procedures to Consider

(Fritz & Speroff, 2011; Hatcher et al., 2011; Schorge et al., 2008)

- Prospective charting of symptoms for 2–3 menstrual cycles
  - Premenstrual symptoms screening tool

- ▪ www Daily record of symptoms and self-assessment of problem severity
- • PMS diagnosis
  - ▪ Cyclic appearance of at least one affective and one somatic symptom during the luteal phase
  - ▪ Symptoms begin 5–7 days before menses
  - ▪ Symptoms remit within 4 days of menses onset
  - ▪ Confirmation of symptoms for at least two consecutive cycles
- • PMDD diagnosis
  - ▪ Cyclic appearance of at least five symptoms during the luteal phase
  - ▪ Symptoms begin 5–7 days before menses
  - ▪ Symptoms remit within 4 days of menses onset
  - ▪ Confirmation of symptoms for at least two consecutive cycles
  - ▪ Does not require somatic symptoms for diagnosis
  - ▪ Must be differentiated from alternate or concomitant psychiatric disorders
  - ▪ Of the five symptoms, at least one must be from the core symptoms
    - ◆ Core symptoms
      - ➤ Markedly depressed mood
      - ➤ Marked anxiety and tension, being on edge
      - ➤ Sudden feelings of sadness and rejection
      - ➤ Persistent and marked irritability
    - ◆ Other symptoms
      - ➤ Decreased interest in usual activities
      - ➤ Lack of energy, fatigue, or lethargy
      - ➤ Insomnia or hypersomnia
      - ➤ Physical symptoms such as bloating and breast tenderness
      - ➤ Difficulty concentrating
      - ➤ Marked change in appetite
      - ➤ Feeling overwhelmed
- • Thyroid panel
- • Depression screening tool (see "Assessment of the Woman with Mental Health Symptoms")

Providing Treatment: Therapeutic Measures to Consider

(Hatcher et al., 2011; Schorge et al., 2008; Taylor, Schuiling, & Sharp, 2013)

- • Regular aerobic exercise
- • Vitamin and mineral supplementation
  - ▪ Calcium: 400 mg QID
  - ▪ Magnesium: 200–400 mg/day
  - ▪ Vitamin E: 400 IU/day
  - ▪ Vitamin B_6, taken in B complex
- • Selective serotonin reuptake inhibitors (SSRI)
  - ▪ Effective in reducing psychological symptoms
  - ▪ Continuous dosing strategy with coexisting depression
  - ▪ Intermittent dosing strategy with cyclic symptoms
    - ◆ Fluoxetine (Sarafem): 20 mg
      - ➤ Daily *or*
      - ➤ 14 days prior to menses through first day of menses
      - ➤ Pregnancy Category C
    - ◆ Sertraline (Zoloft): 50–150 mg
      - ➤ Daily *or*
      - ➤ 14 days prior to menses through first day of menses
      - ➤ Pregnancy Category C
- • Hormonal treatment, such as combined oral contraceptives
  - ▪ Use if symptoms are primarily physical
  - ▪ Drospirenone-containing pills show promise for PMS/PMDD
  - ▪ Cycle suppression or control should reduce cyclic symptoms
- • Anxiolytic medications
  - ▪ Short-term use only
  - ▪ May exacerbate symptoms
  - ▪ Options
    - ◆ Alprazolam
    - ◆ Diazepam
    - ◆ Lorazepam
    - ◆ Buspirone

- Diuretic
  - Aldactone: 25–100 mg
  - Use daily during the luteal phase
- NSAIDs
  - Prostaglandin inhibitors
  - Use during the luteal phase
  - Mefenamic acid (Ponstel)
  - Naproxen sodium (Anaprox or Aleve)
- Treatment for women with coexisting dysmenorrhea (see "Care of the Woman with Dysmenorrhea")

Providing Treatment: Complementary and Alternative Measures to Consider

(Romm, 2010; Taylor, Schuiling, & Sharp, 2013)

- Light therapy
- Tryptophan-containing foods
  - Chocolate
  - Cheddar cheese
  - Salmon
  - Oats
  - Chick peas
  - Sunflower and pumpkin seeds
  - Bananas, mangos, and dates
  - Peanut and sesame butter
  - Red meats and turkey
- Evening primrose oil
- Herbal balancing formula
  - Mix equal parts
    - Chamomile
    - Red raspberry leaf
    - Chasteberry (Vitex)
  - Prepare as a tea or tincture
  - Use daily
- Diuretic formula for luteal phase of the menstrual cycle
  - Dandelion leaf or root: 2 parts
  - Stinging nettle: 2 parts
  - Peppermint: 1 part
  - Black cohosh: 1 part
  - Mix and prepare as a tincture (preferable) or tea

- Use 10–30 gtts tincture TID or tea in the morning and at night
- Premenstrual depression
  - St. John's wort: may alter the effectiveness of hormonal birth control

Providing Support: Education and Support Measures to Consider

- Review of the menstrual cycle and its function
  - Prospective menstrual charting
  - Daily symptom charting
    - Onset
    - Duration
    - Relation to cycle
    - www Use a validated tool
- Reinforce the benefits of the following:
  - Excellent and balanced nutrition
  - Regular daily exercise
  - Personal time
- Discuss potential lifestyle changes
  - Stress reduction techniques
    - Music or art therapy
    - Dance
    - Yoga
    - Prayer/meditation
  - Foster self-image and autonomy
  - Encourage family and friends to help
  - Allow for personal time
  - Shared responsibility
- Explore fertility/sexuality/relationship issues

Follow-up Care: Follow-up Measures to Consider

- Document
  - Symptom profile
  - Criteria used for diagnosis
  - Treatment plan
    - Behavioral
    - Pharmacologic
    - Nutritional supplements

- Differentiate between PMDD and depression
  - The client should keep a prospective symptom diary for two or more cycles
  - Review the symptoms
  - Plot them on a menstrual calendar
- Return for continued care
  - In 2–3 months for symptom diary review
  - For persistent or worsening symptoms
  - For medication follow-up
  - For well-woman care

Multidisciplinary Practice: Consider Consultation, Collaboration, or Referral

- OB/GYN or medical services: For underlying medical or gynecologic problem
- Mental health services
  - For mental health issues unrelated to PMS
  - Severe premenstrual dysphoric disorder
  - Client who is a danger to self or to others
- Support groups and community resources
  - Women's groups
  - PMS support group
- For diagnosis or treatment outside the midwife's scope of practice

CARE OF THE WOMAN WITH SYPHILIS

Key Clinical Information

Syphilis is a complex systemic sexually transmitted bacterial disease caused by the spirochete *Treponema pallidum*. It is infectious only when mucocutaneous lesions are present, although testing and treatment are recommended for any exposure (CDC, 2010). Syphilis infection includes the following possible stages: primary infection (ulcer or chancre at the infection site), secondary infection (rash, mucocutaneous lesions, and lymphadenopathy), and latent stage (asymptomatic) and tertiary infection (cardiac, neurologic, ophthalmic, auditory, or gummatous lesions). Early latent syphilis is defined as infection acquired within 1 year, whereas late latent syphilis is infection acquired more than 1 year previously, yet still in the latent stage. Treatment is most successful when the disease is diagnosed in the primary or secondary stage. Prevention of perinatal transmission of *T. pallidum* and development of congenital syphilis in the newborn depend on routine serologic screening of the pregnant woman at the first prenatal visit (CDC, 2010).

Client History and Chart Review: Components of the History to Consider

(CDC, 2010)

- Age
- Reproductive history
  - LMP, GP TPAL
    - Perinatal losses
    - Current method of contraception
  - Last examination, Pap smear, and STI screen
  - Previous diagnosis or treatment of STIs
  - Sexual activity
    - Number of lifetime partners
    - New partner for self or for partner
- Duration, onset, and severity of symptoms
- Signs and symptoms of syphilis
  - Primary syphilis
    - Chancre at the site of infection
    - Develops 10–90 days post exposure
    - Single painless sore
    - Raised edges
    - Lasts 1–5 weeks
    - Infection persists after the chancre heals
  - Secondary syphilis
    - Symptoms develop 2–28 weeks post exposure
    - Symmetric, macular, papular, non-itchy rash
    - *Condylomata lata*
    - Mucous membrane lesions
    - Alopecia
    - Symptoms of systemic illness
      - Generalized malaise
      - Fever
  - Latent phase
    - No clinical manifestations
    - Lasts 2–30 years after infection
    - Testing is essential for diagnosis

- Tertiary syphilis
  - Gumma (a soft rubbery granuloma) development
  - Neurologic symptoms
    - Headache
    - Symptoms of central nervous system involvement
    - Auditory or visual symptoms
    - Paralysis
    - Mental illness
    - Cardiopulmonary symptoms
      - Shortness of breath
      - Hypertension
- Medical/surgical history
  - Allergies
  - Medications
  - Chronic or acute health conditions
  - HIV status, if known
- Social history
  - Drug or alcohol abuse
  - Exchange of sex for money or drugs
  - 🌐 Residence in a developing country where syphilis is endemic
- Review of systems

Physical Examination: Components of the Physical Exam to Consider

(King & Brucker, 2011)

- Vital signs, including blood pressure and temperature
- Observe skin and soft tissue for signs of primary infection
  - Alopecia
  - Generalized lymphadenopathy
  - Rash
    - Palms and soles
    - Neck and head
    - Torso
  - Mucous membrane ulcers
- Cardiopulmonary assessment
  - Presence of murmur
  - Lung sounds

- Neurologic assessment
  - Cranial nerve abnormalities
  - Diminished reflexes
  - Change in personality
- Pelvic examination
  - Primary chancre: Characteristic painless, firm ulcer
  - *Condylomata lata*
  - Evaluation for signs of other STIs
  - Collection of specimens for testing

Clinical Impression: Differential Diagnoses to Consider

(ICD9data.com, 2012)

- Syphilis
  - Primary
  - Secondary
  - Latent (early or late)
  - Tertiary
- Acute bacterial infection
- Viral infections
- Mononucleosis
- Hansen's disease
- HPV-related condyloma

Diagnostic Testing: Diagnostic Tests and Procedures to Consider

(CDC, 2010; King & Brucker, 2011)

- Rapid plasma reagin (RPR) or Venereal Disease Research Laboratory (VDRL) titers
  - Signs or symptoms
  - Exposure
  - Diagnosis of any STI
  - Pregnancy
    - Initial prenatal visit
    - With a stillborn child at greater than 20 weeks' gestation
    - Repeat for high-risk population
      - At 28–32 weeks' gestation
      - On admission for labor or birth
  - Positive VDRL or RPR 1–4 weeks after chancre

- ◆ False positive may occur in the following circumstances:
  - ➤ Acute infection
  - ➤ Autoimmune disorders
  - ➤ Older age
  - ➤ Pregnancy
  - ➤ Injection drug use
- ◆ Tests to confirm results: Fluorescent treponemal antibody absorbed (FTA-ABS) or microhemagglutination assay for antibody to *T. pallidum* (MHA-TP)
- Wet preparation
- Chlamydia and gonorrhea testing
- HCG testing
- Hepatitis screen
- HIV counseling and testing

Providing Treatment: Therapeutic Measures to Consider

(CDC, 2010)

- Parenteral penicillin G is the treatment of choice
- Primary and secondary syphilis and early latent syphilis: Benzathine penicillin G
  - 2.4 million units IM as a one-time dose
  - In pregnant women, may repeat the dose in 7 days for the following conditions:
    - ◆ Primary syphilis
    - ◆ Secondary syphilis
    - ◆ Early latent syphilis
    - ◆ Ultrasound for signs of fetal or placental syphilis
- Penicillin allergy: Primary or secondary
  - Desensitization to penicillin is recommended
  - Doxycycline: 100 mg PO BID for 14 days (Pregnancy Category D)
  - Tetracycline: 500 mg PO QID for 14 days (Pregnancy Category D)
- Indications for 3-week series
  - Late latent syphilis
  - Syphilis of unknown duration
  - Treatment failure in the absence of tertiary disease

- Benzathine penicillin G: 7.2 million units total dose
  - ◆ Give IM weekly for three doses
  - ◆ 2.4 million units

Providing Treatment: Complementary and Alternative Measures to Consider

(Herbs2000.com, 2011)

- ⚠ Alternative measures are not a substitute for prompt antibiotic treatment
- General measures to promote healing
  - Probiotic supplement
  - Avoid tryptophan-containing foods or supplements
- Herbal support
  - Astragalus—capsules or tincture
  - Butcher's broom—capsules
  - Rooibos tea

Providing Support: Education and Support Measures to Consider

(American Social Health Association, 2011; CDC, 2010)

- Reinforce the need for sex partners to be tested
  - A partner who was exposed to syphilis within 90 days of the test can be infected yet seronegative
  - A partner who was exposed to syphilis more than 90 days prior to the test should be treated presumptively while awaiting serology results
- Selected time frames before treatment are used for identifying at-risk partners
  - More than 3 months' duration of symptoms for primary syphilis
  - More than 6 months' duration of symptoms for secondary syphilis
  - Twelve months' duration for early latent syphilis
- Provide written information
  - Prevention education materials
  - Medication information and instructions

- ⚠️ Jarisch-Herxheimer reaction may occur with the first 24 hours after treatment
  - ➤ Acute febrile reaction with headache and myalgia
  - ➤ Can result in preterm labor or fetal distress in pregnant women
  - ➤ Should not delay treatment
  - ▪ STI reporting and contact follow-up: Notification of the Public Health Department
  - ▪ Return visit and follow-up testing
- Active listening
- Discussion of strategies
  - ▪ Informing partner(s)
  - ▪ Behavioral change

Follow-up Care: Follow-up Measures to Consider

(American Social Health Association, 2011; CDC, 2010)

- Document
  - ▪ Method of infection confirmation
  - ▪ Changes in titers
  - ▪ Treatment plan
  - ▪ Follow-up protocol
  - ▪ Required case reporting
    - ◆ Disease diagnosis and treatment
    - ◆ Sexual contacts
- Return for continued care
  - ▪ As indicated during pregnancy
  - ▪ Reevaluate and retest
    - ◆ Primary or secondary syphilis: 6 and 12 months
    - ◆ Latent syphilis: 6, 12, and 24 months
    - ◆ HIV-positive client: Every 3 months for 2 years
  - ▪ Retreatment
    - ◆ Persistent symptoms
    - ◆ Failure to have fourfold decline in nontreponemal test titers
  - ▪ HIV testing for treatment failures
  - ▪ Development of Jarisch-Herxheimer reaction
    - ◆ Antipyretics if used
    - ◆ Observation in labor unit

Multidisciplinary Practice: Consider Consultation, Collaboration, or Referral

- OB/GYN services
  - ▪ For acute illness with primary infection
  - ▪ Pregnancy complicated by syphilis
  - ▪ Jarisch-Herxheimer reaction
  - ▪ Treatment failures
- Medical services: For tertiary or neurosyphilis
- Pediatric services: Infants at risk for congenital syphilis
- For diagnosis or treatment outside the midwife's scope of practice

CARE OF THE WOMAN WITH TRICHOMONIASIS

Key Clinical Information

Trichomoniasis is the term for an infection caused by the motile flagellate parasitic protozoan *Trichomonas vaginalis*. This highly contagious STI affects both men and women, with approximately 180 million women developing this disease worldwide each year (Romm, 2010). Trichomoniasis is characterized by malodorous, frothy, yellow-green vaginal discharge and petechiae on the cervix. These objective signs may be accompanied by vaginal pruritus and irritation, dyspareunia, and dysuria. The effects of *T. vaginalis* infection range from simple discomfort in the woman, to increased morbidity and mortality for her fetus secondary to preterm labor, rupture of membranes or delivery, and low birth weight (CDC, 2010). Because infection with *T. vaginalis* can enhance HIV transmission, all women with trichomonal infections, as well as their sex partners, should be treated promptly. Treatment of asymptomatic trichomoniasis infections with metronidazole during pregnancy may actually increase the risk of preterm labor and does not improve perinatal outcomes (King & Brucker, 2011). The CDC (2010) continues to recommend treating symptomatic *T. vaginalis* infections in pregnancy.

Client History and Chart Review: Components of the History to Consider

(CDC, 2010)

- Age
- Reproductive history
  - GP TPAL, LMP
    - ◆ Potential for pregnancy
    - ◆ Method of birth control
    - ◆ Symptoms of pregnancy
    - ◆ Gestational age, if pregnant
  - Pregnancy history
    - ◆ Preterm labor and birth
    - ◆ Premature rupture of membranes
    - ◆ Low birth weight infant
  - Sexual history and practices
    - ◆ Use of condoms
    - ◆ Previous diagnosis of STI
    - ◆ Risk factors for PID
    - ◆ New sexual partner for self or for partner
    - ◆ Multiple partners for self or for partner
    - ◆ Heterosexual relationship
    - ◆ Same-sex relationship
    - ◆ Use of sex toys
- Symptom history
  - Pain
    - ◆ Location
    - ◆ Severity
    - ◆ Precipitating factors
  - Vulvovaginal symptoms
    - ◆ Itching
    - ◆ Irritation
    - ◆ Burning
    - ◆ Dyspareunia
    - ◆ Dysuria
  - Presence of discharge
    - ◆ Frothy
    - ◆ Yellow-green
    - ◆ Malodorous, described as foul or fishy smelling
  - Treatments used and results
  - Aggravating and alleviating factors
  - Signs or symptoms of PID

- Medical/surgical history
  - Allergies
  - Medications
  - Chronic health problems
- Social history
- Alcohol or drug use
- Sexual, physical, or emotional abuse

Physical Examination: Components of the Physical Exam to Consider

(CDC, 2010)

- Vital signs
- Abdominal palpation for signs of PID
  - Rebound tenderness
  - Guarding
- Pelvic examination
  - External genitalia
    - ◆ Frothy discharge at introitus
    - ◆ Vulvar irritation
    - ◆ Foul or fishy-smelling odor
  - Speculum examination
    - ◆ Vaginal discharge
    - ◆ Vaginal walls may appear erythematous
    - ◆ "Strawberry spots" (tiny petechiae) on cervix and/or vaginal wall
    - ◆ Friable cervix
  - Bimanual examination
    - ◆ Cervical motion tenderness
    - ◆ Uterine enlargement or tenderness
    - ◆ Painful adnexal mass
- ⚠ Note: Visual inspection of the vaginal discharge is nonspecific and cannot be used alone for diagnosis. Multiple pathogens may be present. Perform additional testing as required for a complete diagnosis.

Clinical Impression: Differential Diagnoses to Consider

(ICD9data.com, 2012)

- Trichomoniasis
- BV

- Candida vulvovaginitis
- Chlamydia
- Gonorrhea
- PID
- Ectopic pregnancy

Diagnostic Testing: Diagnostic Tests and Procedures to Consider

(CDC, 2010)

- Wet preparation for motile trichomonads: Sensitivity 60–70%
- Rapid point-of-service tests: Sensitivity up to 83%
  - OSOM Trichomonas Rapid Test
  - Affirm VP III
- Liquid-based Pap smear (CDC, 2010): Sensitivity up to 98%
- Culture of discharge: Gold standard
  - Standard culture
  - InPouch TV culture system

Providing Treatment: Therapeutic Measures to Consider

(CDC, 2010; FitzMaurice et al., 2011; Hatcher et al., 2011)

- Recommended regimen
  - Metronidazole 2 g PO one time or
  - Tinidazole 2 g PO one time
- Alternative regimen: Metronidazole 500 mg PO BID for 7 days
- Regimen for pregnant women: Metronidazole 2 g PO one time
- Regimen for nursing mothers
  - Refrain from breastfeeding the infant during treatment
  - Pump and discard breastmilk
    - Metronidazole: From onset of treatment until 24 hours after the last dose
    - Tinidazole: From onset of treatment until 3 days after the last dose
- Consider patient-delivered partner treatment (PDPT)

Providing Treatment: Complementary and Alternative Measures to Consider

- ⚠ Alternative measures are not a substitute for antibiotic therapy
- Nutritional support to offset effects of antibiotics on the gut
  - Yogurt
  - Applesauce
  - Acidophilus or probiotics
- Remedies with antimicrobial properties
  - Echinacea
  - Licorice root
- Garlic clove, peeled and raw
  - Tie dental floss to it or place in gauze
  - Per vaginum at night for 7 nights

Providing Support: Education and Support Measures to Consider

- Provide information
  - Infection cause and transmission: Almost exclusively acquired through sexual contact
  - Effects on reproductive organs and future fertility
  - Potential effect on pregnancy
    - Premature rupture of membranes
    - Preterm labor
    - Preterm birth
    - Low birth weight infant
  - ♂ Partner notification and referral for treatment
    - PDPT can be considered
    - Give prescription and written materials
    - www Legal regulations vary; check www.cdc.gov/std/ept
  - Treatment plan
- Medication instructions
  - Reinforce the importance of taking the medication as prescribed
  - Avoid alcohol during treatment
    - Metronidazole: 24 hours after last dose
    - Tinidazole: 72 hours after last dose
  - Maintain abstinence
    - Until the treatment is complete
    - Until symptoms resolve in both partners

- Prevention measures
  - Safe sexual practices
  - Reduction of high-risk behaviors
  - Condom use for prevention of STIs
  - Return for care if there is a potential for STIs

Follow-up Care: Follow-up Measures to Consider

- Document
  - Criteria for diagnosis
  - Treatment regimen
  - Discussion and instructions
  - Plan for continued care
- Follow-up testing is not indicated in the following scenarios:
  - The client is asymptomatic at diagnosis
  - Symptom resolution occurs with treatment
- Return to the provider's office with persistent symptoms (CDC, 2010)
  - HIV testing
  - Treatment failure with metronidazole 2 g
    - Reinfection excluded
    - Tinidazole: 2 g PO one time *or*
    - Metronidazole: 500 mg PO BID for 7 days
  - Persistent treatment failure
    - Metronidazole: 2 g PO for 5 days *or*
    - Tinidazole: 2 g PO for 5 days
  - Continued treatment failure
    - CDC consultation [(404) 718-4141; http://www.cdc.gov/std] and
    - *T. vaginalis* susceptibility testing

Multidisciplinary Practice: Consider Consultation, Collaboration, or Referral

- OB/GYN services
  - Persistent symptoms
  - Antibiotic-resistant trichomoniasis
  - Pelvic infection (PID)
  - Positive HIV or hepatitis B status
  - Persistent pelvic pain
  - Ectopic pregnancy
- Pediatric services
  - Delivery of an infant to an infected mother
  - Infant shows signs of fever and/or abnormal vaginal discharge

- For diagnosis or treatment outside the midwife's scope of practice

CARE OF THE WOMAN WITH VULVOVAGINAL CANDIDIASIS

Key Clinical Information

Vulvovaginal candidiasis (VVC) is so common that many women assume that every form of vaginitis is a "yeast infection." As many as 75% of women will develop a VVC infection at least once in their lives, and 5% will experience recurrent vulvovaginal candidiasis (RVVC) infection (King & Brucker, 2011).

Candida yeasts are part of the normal vaginal flora. Changes to the balance of the vaginal environment that affect the acidity or hormonal balance often result in overgrowth of *Candida*, however (Romm, 2010). VVC has many different appearances, ranging from curdy white vaginal discharge in the uncomplicated case to severely excoriated skin creases in the complicated case; the latter presentation is more common in the woman with poorly controlled diabetes. Careful attention to the microscopic evaluation of the wet preparation with KOH is necessary to determine the presence of *Candida*; other components of the microscopic examination of vaginal discharge are done to confirm the absence of other types of vaginal infection.

Client History and Chart Review: Components of the History to Consider

- Age
- Reproductive health history
  - GP TPAL, LMP
  - Current method of birth control
  - Gestational age, if pregnant
  - Douching/genital hygiene
- Problem history
  - Symptoms
    - Onset, location, and duration
    - Common description (CDC, 2010)
      - Intense itching
      - Abnormal discharge
      - Vaginal soreness

> ➤ Burning with urination
> ➤ Pain with intercourse
> ➤ Bread-like yeasty odor
- Treatments tried and efficacy
- Medical/surgical history
  - Allergies
  - Medications
    - ◆ Antibiotic use
    - ◆ Steroid use
  - Chronic illness as a contributing factor
    - ◆ Diabetes or gestational diabetes
    - ◆ Immunocompromised condition
      - ➤ HIV/AIDS
      - ➤ Cancer
- Social history
  - Tight or damp clothing
  - Underwear made from synthetic fabrics
  - Stress
  - Diet high in concentrated sugar

Physical Examination: Components of the Physical Exam to Consider

- Pelvic examination
  - Red, excoriated external genitalia
  - Vulvar fissures
  - Vulvar edema
  - White, adherent, curdy discharge within the vagina
  - Collect a vaginal discharge specimen for provider-performed microscopy
- Assess for signs of monilia
  - On skin folds
  - Cutaneous infection
  - Oral cavity
- Observe for signs or symptoms of concomitant vaginitis or STIs

Clinical Impression: Differential Diagnoses to Consider

(ICD9data.com, 2012)

- Vulvovaginal candidiasis
- Oral candidiasis (thrush)
- Intertriginous candidiasis

- Vulvovaginitis, unspecified
- Bacterial vaginosis
- Trichomoniasis
- Vulvar vestibulitis or vulvodynia
- Chlamydia
- Gonorrhea
- Chronic cervicitis
- Foreign body, vaginal
- Impetigo

Diagnostic Testing: Diagnostic Tests and Procedures to Consider

- Wet preparation; provider-performed microscopy (CDC, 2010)
  - Saline
    - ◆ Mycelia
    - ◆ Branching hyphae
    - ◆ White blood cells
    - ◆ 10× and 40× magnification
  - A KOH slide is most useful to diagnose VVC
    - ◆ Negative whiff test
    - ◆ Budding yeast
    - ◆ Branching hyphae
    - ◆ 10× magnification
- Vaginal pH testing is not useful for diagnosing VVC (CDC, 2010)
  - pH less than 4.5 = normal
  - VVC does not alter the vaginal pH
- Gram stain of vaginal discharge
- Culture of vaginal discharge
- Severe or recurrent infection
  - Fasting blood sugar
  - HIV testing
  - Culture of skin exudate
- Other STI testing as indicated by the client's history

Providing Treatment: Therapeutic Measures to Consider

- Oral agents: Diflucan
  - 150 mg PO for one or two doses
  - Not recommended for use in pregnancy (CDC, 2010)
- Vaginal creams, suppositories, and topical agents

Vaginally Delivered Medications

These agents are oil based and can weaken the latex commonly used in condoms and diaphragms.

- Terconazole: 3- or 7-day therapy (Pregnancy Category C)
- Nystatin vaginal tablets: 1 tablet per vagina for 14 days (Pregnancy Category A)
- Monistat Derm for cutaneous symptoms
- Over-the-counter antifungals
  - Tioconazole (Vagistat)
  - Miconazole (Monistat)
  - Clotrimazole (Gyne-Lotrimin, Mycelex)
  - Butoconazole (Femstat)

Providing Treatment: Complementary and Alternative Measures to Consider

(Romm, 2010)

- Dietary support
  - Cranberries or cranberry juice
  - Yogurt or acidophilus capsules
  - Probiotics: 4–8 billion units/day
- Tub bath with 1 cup vinegar in water
- Vaginal treatments
  - Acidophilus capsules: 1 per vagina at bedtime for 5–7 days
  - Boric acid capsules: 1 per vagina at bedtime for 5–7 days
    - ⚠ Boric acid is poisonous if taken orally
  - Herbal sitz bath or peri-wash two times a day
    - 1 tablespoon tea tree oil
    - 2 tablespoons cider vinegar
    - 2 cups warm water
  - Black walnut tincture
  - Sage
  - Oregano
  - Olive leaf

Providing Support: Education and Support Measures to Consider

- Medication instructions

  - Take the complete course of medication
  - Avoid intercourse while using the medication
- General hygiene
  - Wipe front to back after toileting
  - Promptly change out of damp clothing or swimsuits
  - Wear loose, well-ventilated clothing
- After bathing
  - Dry the genital region thoroughly before dressing (use a blow dryer on the cool setting)
  - Wear cotton panties and loose clothing (boxer shorts are a good choice)
- Avoid the following:
  - Excessive sugar or alcohol in the diet
  - Douching
  - Products containing perfume or deodorant
    - Bubble bath
    - Feminine hygiene sprays
    - Tampons or sanitary pads
    - Toilet paper

Follow-up Care: Follow-up Measures to Consider

- Document: Wet preparation and pH findings
- No follow-up visit is needed if the client's symptoms resolve
- Return for care
  - If symptoms have not improved within 5–7 days
  - For additional testing: Consider vaginal culture
  - As indicated by other test results

Multidisciplinary Practice: Consider Consultation, Collaboration, or Referral

- OB/GYN services: Recurrent or unresponsive infection
- Medical services
  - For fasting glucose > 126 g/dL (diagnostic of diabetes)
  - Positive HIV titer
  - Evidence of immunocompromise
- For diagnosis or treatment outside the midwife's scope of practice

WEB RESOURCES FOR CLINICIANS

RESOURCE	URL
American Social Health Association: Sexual health information for clients	http://www.ashastd.org/
American Society of Colposcopy and Cervical Pathology: Consensus guidelines	http://www.asccp.org/ConsensusGuidelines/ConsensusGuidelinesOverview/tabid/5956/Default.aspx
Association of Reproductive Health Professionals: Managing premenstrual symptoms	http://www.arhp.org/Publications-and-Resources/Quick-Reference-Guide-for-Clinicians/PMS/Appendix-B
Breast Cancer Risk Assessment Tool	http://www.cancer.gov/bcrisktool/
California Department of Health: Breast algorithms	http://qap.sdsu.edu/screening/breastcancer/bda/flowcharts/risk_ago1.html
Centers for Disease Control and Prevention: 2010 sexually transmitted diseases treatment guidelines	http://www.cdc.gov/std/treatment/2010/default.htm
Centers for Disease Control and Prevention: Division of Viral Hepatitis	http://www.cdc.gov/ncidod/diseases/hepatitis/
Centers for Disease Control and Prevention: Division of HIV/AIDS Prevention	www.cdc.gov/hiv/dhap.htm
Centers for Disease Control and Prevention: Parasites	http://www.cdc.gov/parasites/
Centers for Disease Control and Prevention: STI fact sheets	http://www.cdc.gov/std/healthcomm/fact_sheets.htm
Daily record of severity of problems: For diagnosis of PMS/PMDD	http://pmdd.factsforhealth.org/have/dailyrecord.asp
Endometriosis Association	http://www.endometriosisassn.org/physician_resources.html
Expedited Partner Therapy	www.cdc.gov/std/ept
HIV: WHO Guidelines to prevent maternal-to-child-transmission	http://www.who.int/hiv/pub/mtct/pmtct/en/
HIV: Post-exposure guidelines for healthcare workers	http://www.aidsinfo.nih.gov/Guidelines/GuidelineDetail.aspx?GuidelineID=10
Pelvic Pain Assessment Form	http://www.pelvicpain.org/pdf/History_and_Physical_Form/IPPS-H&PformR-MSW.pdf
Vermont Department of Health: Tanner stages	http://healthvermont.gov/family/toolkit/tools%5CJ-1%20CARD%20Tanner%20Stages.pdf
World Health Organization: Colposcopy manual	http://screening.iarc.fr

REFERENCES

Adamson, G. D., & Pasta, D. J. (2010). Endometrial fertility index: The new validated endometriosis staging system. *Fertility and Sterility, 94*, 1609–1615. Retrieved from http://www.endometriosiszone.org/content/PDF/EFI-Endometriosis-FNS-Fertil-Steril-Article.pdf

AIDS Education and Training Centers (AETC). (2007a). Clinical manual for management of the HIV-infected adult. Retrieved from http://www.aidsetc.org/aidsetc?page=cm-00-00

AIDS Education and Training Centers (AETC). (2007b). Hepatitis B infection. Retrieved from http://www.aidsetc.org/aidsetc?page=cm-511_hepb

Aliotta, H. M., & Schaeffer, N. J. (2013). Breast conditions. In K. D. Schuiling & F. E. Likis (Eds.), *Women's gynecologic health* (2nd ed., pp. 375–403). Burlington, MA: Jones & Bartlett Learning.

American Cancer Society (ACS). (2006a). Detailed guide: Endometrial cancer: What are the risk factors for endometrial cancer? Retrieved from http://www.cancer.org/docroot/CRI/CRI_2_3x.asp?dt=11

American Cancer Society (ACS). (2006b). What are the risk factors for cervical cancer? Retrieved from http://www.cancer.org/docroot/CRI/CRI_2_3x.asp?rnav=cridg&dt=8

American Cancer Society (ACS). (2007). ACS recommendations for HPV vaccine use to prevent cervical cancer and pre-cancers. Retrieved from http://www.cancer.org/docroot/CRI/content/CRI_2_6X_ACS_Recommendations_for_HPV_Vaccine_Use_to_Prevent_Cervical_Cancer_and_PreCancers_8.asp?sitearea=&level=

American Cancer Society (ACS). (2010). Breast cancer. Retrieved from http://www.cancer.org/acs/groups/content/@nho/documents/document/breastcancerpdf.pdf

American College of Nurse–Midwives (ACNM). (2007). *Human immunodeficiency virus and acquired immunodeficiency disease. Position statement.* Silver Spring, MD: Author.

American College of Nurse–Midwives (ACNM). (2011). *Definition of midwifery and scope of practice of Certified Nurse–Midwives and Certified Midwives.* Silver Spring, MD: Author.

American College of Obstetricians and Gynecologists (ACOG). (2002). ACOG Practice Bulletin. Polycystic ovary syndrome. *International Journal of Gynaecology & Obstetrics, 80*(3), 335–348.

American Roentgen Ray Society. (2006). CT and ultrasound are equally valuable in diagnosing pelvic pain in women. *Women's Health Law Weekly, 18.* Retrieved from http://www.newsrx.com/newsletters/Womens-Health-Law-Weekly/2006-05-28/052520063331098WH.html

American Social Health Association. (2011). Learn about STIs/STDs. Syphilis: Fast facts. Retrieved from http://www.ashastd.org/learn/learn_syphilis_facts.cfm

American Society for Colposcopy and Cervical Pathology. (2011). Consensus guidelines. Retrieved from http://www.asccp.org/ConsensusGuidelines/ConsensusGuidelinesOverview/tabid/5956/Default.aspx

Bickley, L. S., & Szilagyi, P. S. (2009). *Bates' guide to physical examination and history taking* (10th ed.). Philadelphia, PA: Wolters Kluwer.

Bond, S. (2009). Caring for women with abnormal Papanicolaou tests during pregnancy. *Journal of Midwifery & Women's Health, 54*, 201–210. doi: 10.1016/j.jmwh.2009.01.004

Breast Expert Workgroup. (2005). *Breast cancer diagnostic algorithms for primary care providers* (3rd ed.). California Department of Health Services. Retrieved from http://qap.sdsu.edu/screening/breastcancer/bda/algo_booklet/download.html

Burgess, I. (2009). Current treatments for pediculosis capitis. *Current Opinion in Infectious Diseases, 22*, 131–136. doi: 10.1097/QCO.0b013e328322a019

Centers for Disease Control and Prevention (CDC). (2009). Rapid HIV testing. Retrieved from http://www.cdc.gov/hiv/topics/testing/rapid/

Centers for Disease Control and Prevention (CDC). (2010). 2010 sexually transmitted diseases treatment guidelines. Retrieved from http://www.cdc.gov/std/treatment/2010/default.htm

Centers for Disease Control and Prevention (CDC). (2011). Division of HIV/AIDS Prevention. Retrieved from www.cdc.gov/hiv/dhap.htm

Cochran, S. (2011). Lesbian and bisexual health fact sheet. Retrieved from http://www.womenshealth.gov/publications/our-publications/fact-sheet/lesbian-bisexual-health.cfm#c

Costello, M. (2005). Polycystic ovary syndrome: A management update. *Australian Family Physician, 34*(3), 127–133.

Dennehy, C. (2006) The use of herbs and dietary supplements in gynecology: An evidence-based review. *Journal of Midwifery & Women's Health, 51*(6), 402–409.

Dunne, E., Unger, E., Sternberg, M., McQuillan, G., Patel, S., & Markowitz, L. (2007). Prevalence of HPV infection among females in the United States. *Journal of the American Medical Association, 297*(8), 813–819.

Faucher, M. A., & Schuiling, K. D. (2013). Normal and abnormal uterine bleeding. In K. D. Schuiling &

F. E. Likis (Eds.), *Women's gynecologic health* (2nd ed., pp. 609–642). Burlington, MA: Jones & Bartlett Learning.

FitzMaurice, E., Keller, E., Trebbin, J., & Wilson, J. (2011). Strategies for partner management when treating sexually transmitted infection. *Journal of Midwifery & Women's Health, 56*, 608–614. doi: 10.1111/j.1542-2011.2011.00087.x

Fogel, C. I. (2013). Sexually transmitted infection. In K. D. Schuiling & F. E. Likis (Eds.), *Women's gynecologic health* (2nd ed., pp. 485–530). Burlington, MA: Jones & Bartlett Learning.

Foulkes, H. B., Pettigrew, M. M., Livingston, K. A., & Niccolai, L. M. (2009). Comparison of sexual partnership characteristics and associations with inconsistent condom use among a sample of adolescents and adult women diagnosed with chlamydia trachomatis. *Journal of Women's Health, 18*(3), 393–399.

Frank, J. E. (2008). The colposcopic examination. *Journal of Midwifery & Women's Health, 53*, 447–452. doi: 10.1016/j.jmwh.2008.04.001

Fritz, M. A., & Speroff, L. (2011). *Clinical gynecologic endocrinology and infertility.* Philadelphia, PA: Williams & Wilkins.

Galaal, K. A., Deane, K., Sangal, S., & Lopes, A. D. (2007). Interventions for reducing anxiety in women undergoing colposcopy. *Cochrane Database of Systematic Reviews, 3*, CD006013.

Grube, W., & McCool, W. (2004). Endometrial biopsy. In H. Varney, J. M. Kriebs, & C. L. Gegor (Eds.), *Varney's midwifery* (4th ed.). Sudbury, MA: Jones and Bartlett.

Hart, R., Hickey, M., & Franks, S. (2004). Definitions, prevalence and symptoms of polycystic ovaries and polycystic ovary syndrome. *Best Practice and Research: Clinical Obstetrics & Gynaecology, 18*(5), 671–683.

Hatcher, R. A., Trussell, J., Stewart, F., Nelson, A. L., Cates, W., Kowal, D., & Policar, M. S. (2011). *Contraceptive technology* (20th ed.). New York, NY: Ardent Media.

Herbs2000.com. (2011). Syphilis. Retrieved from http://www.herbs2000.com/disorders/syphilis.htm

Hudson, T. (2008). *Women's encyclopedia of natural medicine.* McGraw-Hill. Retrieved from http://www.scribd.com/doc/25163597/Womens-Encyclopedia-of-Natural-Medicine

ICD9Data.com. (2012). The web's 2012 free medical coding source. Retrieved from http://www.icd9data.com/

Kapenhas-Vades, E., Feldman, S. M., Cohen, J. M., & Boobol, S. K. (2008). Mammary ductoscopy for evaluation of nipple discharge. *Annals of Surgical Oncology, 15*, 2720–2727. doi: 10.1245/s10434-008-0012-1

Kearney, A. J., & Murray, M. (2009). Breast cancer screening recommendations: Is mammogram the only answer? *Journal of Midwifery & Women's Health, 5*, 393–400. doi: 10.1016/j.jmwh.2008.12.010

Khalili, M. (2006). Coinfection with hepatitis viruses and HIV. *HIV InSite.* Retrieved from http://hivinsite.ucsf.edu/InSite?page=kb-05-03-04

King, J. (2006). Polycystic ovary syndrome. *Journal of Midwifery & Women's Health, 51*(6), 415–422.

King, J. (2011). Noncontraceptive uses of hormonal contraception. *Journal of Midwifery & Women's Health, 56*, 628–635. doi: 10.1111/j.1542-2011.2011.00118.x

King, T., & Brucker, M. (Eds.). (2011). *Pharmacology in women's health.* Sudbury, MA: Jones and Bartlett.

Klein, S. (2005). Evaluation of palpable breast masses. *American Family Physician, 71*, 1731–1738.

Kripke, C. (2007). Opioid analgesia during evaluation of acute abdominal pain. *American Family Physician, 76*, 971. Retrieved from http://www.aafp.org/afp/20071001/cochrane.html#c2

Lampe, M., Branson, B., Paul, S., Burr, C., Gross, E., Eicher, C., . . . Fowler, M. G. (2004). Rapid HIV-1 antibody testing during labor and delivery for women of unknown HIV status: A practical guide and model protocol. Retrieved from http://www.cdc.gov/hiv/topics/testing/resources/guidelines/pdf/Labor&DeliveryRapidTesting.pdf

Leung, A. K., & Pacaud, D. (2004). Diagnosis and management of galactorrhea. *American Family Physician.* Retrieved from http://www.aafp.org/afp/20040801/543.html

Madigan Army Medical Center. (2006). *Breast mass.* Tacoma, WA: Author. Retrieved from http://www.mamc.amedd.army.mil/referral/guidelines/gensurg_breastmass.htm

McFarlin, B. L. (2006). Ultrasound assessment of the endometrium for irregular vaginal bleeding. *Journal of Midwifery & Women's Health, 51*, 440–449.

MedlinePlus. (2006). Secondary amenorrhea. In U.S. National Library of Medicine, National Institutes of Health, *Medical encyclopedia.* Retrieved from http://www.nlm.nih.gov/medlineplus/ency/article/001219.htm

Meyers, D., Wolff, T., Gregory, K., Marion, L., Moyer, V., Nelson, H., . . . Sawaya, G. F. (2008). USPSTF Recommendations for STI screening. *American Family Physician, 77*(6), 819–824.

Mortensen, G. L., & Adeler, A. L. (2010). Qualitative study of women's anxiety and information needs after a diagnosis of cervical dysplasia. *Journal of Public Health, 18*, 473–482.

Moses, S. (2007). Colposcopy. In *Family practice notebook.* Retrieved from http://www.fpnotebook.com/GYN153.htm

National Cancer Institute. (2011). A snapshot of breast cancer. Retrieved from http://www.cancer.gov/aboutnci/servingpeople/snapshots/breast.pdf

National Institute of Allergy and Infectious Diseases (NIAID). (2011). HIV/AIDS. Retrieved from http://www.niaid.nih.gov/topics/hivaids/Pages/Default.aspx

Patel, M. (2005). *Endometrial biopsy and uterine evacuation.* Birmingham, AL: University of Alabama. Retrieved from http://www.obgyn.uab.edu/medicalstudents/obgyn/uasom/documents/EMBx.pdf

Pavlin, N. L., Parker, R. M., Piggin, A. K., Hopkins, C. A., Temple-Smith, M. J., Fairley, C. K., . . . Chen, M. Y. (2010). Better than nothing? Patient-delivered partner therapy and partner notification for chlamydia: The views of Australian general practitioners. *BMC Infectious Diseases, 10,* 274–280. doi: 10.1186/1471-2334-10-274

Ribaldone, R., Capuano, A., & Di Oto, A. (2010). Role of HPV testing in the follow-up of women treated for cervical dysplasia. *Archives of Gynecology and Obstetrics, 282,* 193–197.

Richardson, M. (2003). Current perspectives in polycystic ovary syndrome. *American Family Physician, 68*(4), 697–704.

Romm, A. (2010). *Botanical medicine for women's health.* St. Louis, MO: Churchill Livingstone.

Ross, J., Judlin, P., & Nilas, L. (2007). European guideline for the management of pelvic inflammatory disease. *International Journal of STD & AIDS, 18*(10), 662–666.

Rubano, E. (2010). Genital warts in emergency medicine treatment and management. Retrieved from http://emedicine.medscape.com/article/763014-treatment#a1129

Sauerland, S., Agresta, F., Bergamaschi, R., Borzellino, G., Budzynski, A., Champault, G., . . . Neugebauer, E. A. (2006). Laparoscopy for abdominal emergencies: Evidence-based guidelines of the European Association for Endoscopic Surgery. *Surgical Endoscopy, 20,* 14–29.

Schorge, J. O., Schaffer, J. I., Halvorson, L. M., Hoffman, B. L., Bradshaw, K. D., & Cunningham, F. G. (2008). *Williams gynecology.* New York, NY: McGraw-Hill Medical.

Schroeder, B. (2003). ACOG releases guidelines on diagnosis and management of polycystic ovary syndrome. *American Family Physician, 67*(6), 1619–1620.

Schuiling, K. D., & Gasiewizc, N. (2013). Pelvic pain. In K. D. Schuiling & F. E. Likis (Eds.), *Women's gynecologic health* (2nd ed., pp. 669–699). Burlington, MA: Jones & Bartlett Learning.

Schuiling, K. D., & Likis, F. E. (Eds.). (2013). *Women's gynecologic health* (2nd ed.). Burlington, MA: Jones & Bartlett Learning.

Sellors, J. W., & Sankaranarayanan, R. (2003). Colposcopy and treatment of cervical intraepithelial neoplasia: A beginner's manual. Retrieved from http://screening.iarc.fr/colpochap.php?lang=1&chap=5

Sheehan, M. (2003). Polycystic ovarian syndrome: Diagnosis and management. *Clinical Medicine & Research, 2*(1), 13–27.

Swanton, A., Iyer, L., & Reginald, P. W. (2006). Diagnosis, treatment and follow up of women undergoing conscious pain mapping for chronic pelvic pain: A prospective cohort study. *British Journal of Obstetrics and Gynaecology, 113*(7), 792–796.

Taylor, D., Schuiling, K. D., & Sharp, B. A. C. (2013). Menstrual cycle pain and discomforts. In K. D. Schuiling & F. E. Likis (Eds.), *Women's gynecologic health* (2nd ed., pp. 609–642). Burlington, MA: Jones & Bartlett Learning.

Thompson, S. R. (2004). Nipple discharge. In National Institutes of Health, *MedlinePlus medical encyclopedia.* Retrieved from http://www.nlm.nih.gov/medlineplus/ency/article/003154.htm

Ulery, M., Carter, L., McFarlin, B. L., & Giurgescu, C. (2009). Pregnancy-associated breast cancer: Significance of early detection. *Journal of Midwifery & Women's Health, 54,* 357–363. doi: 10.1016/j.jmwh.2008.12.007

Varney, H., Kriebs, J. M., & Gegor, C. L. (Eds.). (2004). *Varney's midwifery* (4th ed.). Sudbury, MA: Jones and Bartlett.

Verga, C. A. (2013). Benign gynecologic conditions. In K. D. Schuiling & F. E. Likis (Eds.), *Women's gynecologic health* (2nd ed., pp. 669–699). Burlington, MA: Jones & Bartlett Learning.

Vermont Public Health Department. (n.d.). *The Tanner stages.* Retrieved from http://healthvermont.gov/family/toolkit/tools%5CJ-1%20CARD%20Tanner%20Stages.pdf

Wright, T. C. Jr., Massad, L. S., Dunton, C. J., Spitzer, M., Wilkinson, E. J., & Solomon, D. (2007a). 2006 consensus guidelines for the management of women with abnormal cervical screening tests. *Journal of Lower Genital Tract Disease, 11,* 201–222.

Wright, T. C. Jr., Massad, L. S., Dunton, C. J., Spitzer, M., Wilkinson, E. J., & Solomon, D. (2007b). 2006 consensus guidelines for the management of women with cervical intraepithelial neoplasia or adenocarcinoma in situ. *Journal of Lower Genital Tract Disease, 11,* 223–239.

Yang, J., Yu-guo, P., Zhong-ming, Z., Zhi-jian, Y., & Qi-wen, D. (2009). Interferon for the treatment of genital warts: A systematic review. *BMC Infectious Diseases, 9,* 156–164.

8

Primary Care in Women's Health

Primary health care for women encompasses health promotion, disease prevention, diagnosis and treatment of common health problems and can be provided with compassion and expertise by midwives. Primary care is defined as the "provision of integrated, accessible health care services by clinicians who are accountable for addressing a large majority of personal health care needs, developing a sustained partnership with patients, and practicing in the context of family and community" (Donaldson, Yordy, & Vaneselow, 1994, p. 31). Many midwives now include primary care within their scope of practice. Skill in assessment and diagnosis of common primary care health problems enhances midwifery care, even when the midwife refers the client for treatment. The practice guidelines in this section provide an overview of selected primary care health conditions.

The nature and scope of women's health care provided by midwives in the United States has expanded in recent years (Farley, Tharpe, Miller, & Ruxer, 2006). Women use healthcare services more often than men, and women typically make healthcare decisions for the family. Historically, midwives have assumed a role as healthcare providers offering services to childbearing women and their newborns. Over the years, however, the services midwives offer have evolved to include women's health care for a wider range of clients. The inclusion of primary care health services within midwifery practice opens opportunities for midwives to provide care, education, and support for women to make positive health choices beyond the childbearing year.

Following the healthcare reforms of the early 1990s, the American College of Nurse–Midwives in 1997 developed a formal position statement that defines midwives as primary care providers for women from adolescence to senescence and includes providing primary care for newborns. In the contemporary healthcare system, projections are that an additional 45,000 primary care providers will be needed to meet the demand generated when the Patient Protection and Affordable Care Act (PPACA) becomes fully implemented in 2014 (U.S. Department of Health and Human Services, 2012). An estimated 32 million people who are currently uninsured will be eligible for healthcare coverage. Midwives can be valuable contributors to meet this need. And midwives continue to provide primary care services to those vulnerable women who "fall through the cracks" in the current healthcare system.

Recommendations have been made to reshape healthcare regulations across the nation to remove barriers that preclude healthcare providers from practicing to the full extent of their education, training, and competence (Institute of Medicine, 2010). These recommendations are indicative of a shift in national perspective that recognizes the need to engage a wide range of health practitioners so as to meet the healthcare needs of the diverse populations of the United States. Other recommendations consistent with midwifery practice and philosophy include refining healthcare delivery systems to include individualization of planning and delivery of services, access to a "medical home" and "maternity home" that is acceptable and accessible to the client, and provision of an opportunity to develop supportive long-term stable healthcare relationships within a multidisciplinary team setting (Oni-Orisa, Hiersteine, & Swett, 2010). These changes open a window of opportunity for midwives to take a larger role in providing healthcare services in our country.

Women tend to live longer than men and have a high incidence of chronic disease, particularly in vulnerable and underserved populations. Ensuring access to adequate care can be attained through education of increasing numbers of multidisciplinary healthcare providers, such as midwives, who are skilled in providing a wide range of essential health services. Such services are most effective when offered with an attitude of mutual respect fostered by clear and consistent communication, and seek to promote personal autonomy and empowerment of women within the context of their lives.

Expansion of midwifery practice to include primary care services requires the midwife to seek out collaborative practice and educational opportunities in which to attain skill and knowledge of current primary care practices and development of a broad-based multidisciplinary network of consultants. Clients value a midwife's ability to assess a wide range of health concerns, provide information for informed decision making, and following discussion, provide a problem-oriented referral to the healthcare provider who is best able to meet the clients' health needs. This process honors each woman's autonomy and fosters development of a trusting relationship.

Midwives can expand their primary care scope of practice through professional continuing education programs and mentored clinical experience. Formal continuing education, self-study, and an experienced colleague with whom to consult provide a safe basis for learning and optimal care for the midwifery client. Ultimately, each midwife is responsible for caring for women with conditions that are within her or his scope of practice based on licensure, education, skill, and the clinical practice setting.

ASSESSMENT OF THE WOMAN WITH CARDIOVASCULAR SYMPTOMS

Key Clinical Information

Cardiovascular disease (CVD) is the most common cause of death in women in the United States. Although most research about the prevention and treatment of heart disease has been performed using male subjects, the American Heart Association noted that more women than men die of heart disease every year (Mosca et al., 2007). CVD is caused by atherosclerosis, which narrows blood vessels supplying the heart, thereby reducing blood flow. The average lifetime risk for CVD in women approaches one in two, making prevention and detection of this disease essential during routine healthcare encounters.

The risk of cardiovascular disease increases significantly after the onset of menopause (Mosca et al., 2007). Many women may be unaware of a problem until significant symptoms develop. Symptoms of menopause such as fatigue, headache, palpitations, anxiety, depression, and sleep disturbances are also symptoms of hypertension (Maas & Franke, 2009), a major clinical indicator of cardiovascular disease. Symptoms can be noticeable, or they can be absent even when disease is present.

Risk factors include obesity, sedentary lifestyle, diet, diabetes, and hypertension. Ethnic background is associated with risk for CVD; for example, African American women have higher rates of cardiovascular disease than other women. Modifiable risk factors such as weight, activity level, smoking, and diet are key components of preventive and therapeutic care. Midwives must keep in mind the risk factors, signs, and symptoms of cardiovascular disease in women.

Client History and Chart Review: Components of the History to Consider

(AHA, 2007; National Heart, Lung, and Blood Institute [NHLBI], 2003)

- Age
- GP TPAL
- LMP
  - Menstrual status/life stage
  - Current method of contraception
- Medical/surgical history
  - Allergies
  - Medications
    - Contraceptive hormones
    - Hormone replacement therapy
- Depression screening
- Maternity history: Preeclampsia and eclampsia significantly increase CVD risk later in life
- Health conditions
  - Diabetes
  - Dyslipidemia
  - Hypertension
  - Valvular heart disease
  - Coronary or peripheral vascular disease
  - Rheumatic fever
  - Collagen vascular disease
  - Kidney disease
  - Cushing's syndrome
  - Thyroid or parathyroid disease
  - Sleep disorders
  - Congenital heart disorders
- Family history
  - Coronary artery disease
    - Myocardial infarction

- Cerebrovascular accident
- Conduction disorders
- Tachyarrhythmias
- Sudden death
  - Hypertension
  - Diabetes
- Social history
  - Drugs and alcohol
    - Alcohol use
    - Ephedra (formerly included in over-the-counter weight loss supplements, now prohibited by the FDA)
    - Cocaine
    - Amphetamines
  - Tobacco use (cigarettes, snuff, chewing tobacco)
  - Employment stress (physical and emotional)
  - Life stressors
  - Usual coping methods
  - Support systems
  - Physical activity and exercise patterns
  - Dietary habits and patterns
    - Meal patterns
    - High-fat foods
    - Salt use and high-sodium foods
- Ethnicity: Elevated coronary vascular disease risk (AHA, 2004)
  - African American: Hypertension/stroke
  - Hispanic American: Stroke
  - Mexican American: Labile hypertension
  - Native American: Labile hypertension
- Symptoms related to cardiovascular disorders
  - Women may be asymptomatic with progressive disease
  - Inability to perform normal daily tasks without resting
  - Type, severity, and duration of symptoms
    - Headache
    - Visual or cognitive changes
    - Numbness or weakness
    - Chest pain or sensation of tightness (angina)
    - Palpitations
    - Shortness of breath with or without exertion

- ◆ Unexplained dizziness and or syncope
- ◆ Peripheral and/or dependent edema
- ◆ Nocturnal dyspnea
- ◆ Nocturia
- ◆ Cough
- Review of systems

Physical Examination: Components of the Physical Exam to Consider

(AHA, 2007; NHLBI, 2003)

- General inspection
  - Abdominal girth and body habitus
    - ◆ Apple body shape
      - ➤ Body fat stored around the abdomen and chest and surrounding the internal organs
      - ➤ Associated with coronary heart disease, diabetes, and high blood pressure
    - ◆ Pear body shape: Body fat stored around the hips and thighs
  - Signs of prior stroke or cerebrovascular accident
- Height, weight, and body mass index (BMI) determination
- Blood pressure (NHLBI, 2003): Measure supine and standing
- Skin and soft tissue
  - Color
    - ◆ Pallor
    - ◆ Cyanosis
    - ◆ Blanching
  - Adipose tissue
    - ◆ Amount
    - ◆ Distribution
- Pulse
  - Rate and rhythm
  - Atrial fibrillation
  - Bruits
  - Decreased pulses in carotid arteries or extremities

- Eyes: Fundoscopic examination
- Neck
  - Thyroid palpation
  - Carotid pulse
  - Auscultation for carotid bruit
- Chest
  - Contour
  - Respiratory rate and effort
    - ◆ Auscultate breath sounds
    - ◆ Use of accessory muscles
  - Cardiac evaluation
    - ◆ Auscultation of heart
    - ◆ Rate and rhythm
    - ◆ Presence or absence of the following:
      - ➤ Murmur
      - ➤ Thrills
  - Percussion of chest
- Abdomen
  - Masses
  - Auscultation for bruits
- Extremities
  - Color and temperature
  - Pulses
  - Capillary refill
  - Evaluation for nonhealing wounds and ulcers
  - Edema
  - Auscultation for femoral bruits
- Neurologic examination
  - Speech patterns
  - Gait
  - Focal deficits

Clinical Impression: Differential Diagnoses to Consider

(ICD9Data.com, 2012)

- Hypertension
- Dyslipidemia
- Coronary artery disease
- Valvular heart disease
- Diabetes mellitus
- Metabolic syndrome
- Chronic obstructive pulmonary disease

Diagnostic Testing: Diagnostic Tests and Procedures to Consider

(Mosca et al., 2007; Wyner, Marfell, Karsnitz, & Rousseau, 2007)

- Complete blood count
- Urinalysis
- Fasting serum lipid profile
  - Total cholesterol
  - High-density lipoprotein (HDL) cholesterol
  - Low-density lipoprotein (LDL) cholesterol
  - Triglycerides
- Chemistry profile
  - Blood urea nitrogen (BUN)
  - Creatinine
  - Fasting blood glucose
  - Renal and hepatic function profiles
- Serum electrolytes
  - Calcium
  - Magnesium
- Serum uric acid
- Thyroid-stimulating hormone (TSH)
- Electrocardiogram: 12 lead
- Chest x-ray
- Cardiac stress test
- Echocardiogram
- Holter monitoring
- Pulmonary function testing
- Sleep evaluation

Providing Treatment: Therapeutic Measures to Consider

(Mosca et al., 2007; Wyner et al., 2007)

- Lifestyle modifications
  - Smoking cessation
    - Behavioral counseling
    - Nicotine replacement therapy
  - Alcohol moderation: One or fewer drinks per day
- [www] Dietary Approaches to Stop Hypertension (DASH) diet
- Exercise or physical activity
  - At least 10 minutes daily

- Increase as tolerated to 30–60 minutes per session (NHLBI, 2003)
- Resistance training twice a week
- Vaccination against influenza
- Initiation of medical therapies (see relevant clinical practice guidelines)
  - By primary care practitioner or referral specialist
  - As indicated by client condition
  - Per scope of practice or practice setting
- Aspirin (Agency for Healthcare Research and Quality [AHRQ], 2009): Routine preventive use in healthy women younger than age 55 is not recommended

Providing Treatment: Complementary and Alternative Measures to Consider

⚠ Alternative measures are not a substitute for medical treatment in a client who does not have a favorable response with lifestyle changes.

- Herbal supplements
  - Antioxidants
    - Black chokeberry
    - Blueberries
  - Sea vegetables for minerals
  - Vitamin C
- Stress-reduction activities
- Review personal life goals

Providing Support: Education and Support Measures to Consider

(AHA, 2007; NHLBI, 2003)

- Review Joint National Commission 7 (JNC-7) and AHA recommendation
- DASH diet instructions
- Physical activity instructions
- Weight management instructions
  - If BMI is greater than 25, encourage weight loss of 10% from baseline
  - Waist circumference should be 35 inches or less
- Tobacco cessation instructions

- Medication information
  - Correct dosing
  - Anticipated benefits
  - Side effects
  - Need for long-term treatment and follow-up
- Provide information as applicable
  - Diabetes management
  - Treatment of chronic atrial fibrillation
  - Personal cardiac risk assessment
  - Potential cardiac risks of hormone use
- Criteria for the following:
  - Emergency care
  - Prompt care
  - Referral
  - Return office visit

Follow-up Care: Follow-up Measures to Consider

- Document
  - Risk factors
  - Diagnosis
  - Discussions with the client
  - Treatment plan
- Return for continued care
  - As indicated by laboratory results
  - Evaluation of lifestyle changes
  - Blood pressure (BP) monitoring
  - Evaluation of medication side effects
  - Reproductive health care
  - Support during the following programs:
    - Smoking cessation
    - Dietary and lifestyle changes
- Coronary heart disease risk assessment (AHA, 2007)
  - Begin assessment at age 20
  - Update coronary heart disease family history annually
  - At each visit, assess the following:
    - Tobacco use
    - Physical activity
    - Nutritional status
    - Alcohol intake

- Every 2 years (minimum), assess the following:
  - BP
  - Pulse
  - BMI
  - Waist circumference
- Every 2–5 years, based on the client's risk profile, assess the following (AHA, 2007):
  - Fasting serum lipids
  - Fasting blood glucose
- Make 10-year coronary heart disease risk estimation
  - **www** Use an online risk calculator
  - Risk stratification
    - High risk: > 20%
    - Intermediate risk: 10–20%
    - Low risk: < 10%

Multidisciplinary Practice: Consider Consultation, Collaboration, or Referral

- Emergency services
  - Systolic BP > 200 mm Hg or diastolic BP > 120 mm Hg
  - Signs or symptoms suspicious for stroke or myocardial infarction
- Medical services
  - Suspected cardiovascular dysfunction
  - Elevated lipid levels consistent with dyslipidemia
  - Hypertension
  - Metabolic syndrome
  - Diabetes
- Behavior modification programs
- For diagnosis or treatment outside the midwife's scope of practice

CARE OF THE WOMAN WITH HYPERTENSION

Key Clinical Information

Hypertension is a major risk factor for cardiovascular disease and contributes significantly to morbidity and mortality in women (Pimenta, Amodeo, & Oparil,

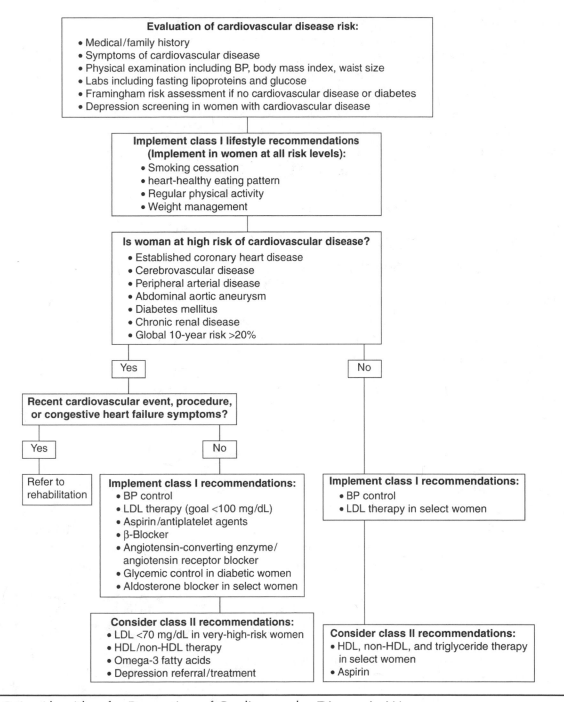

Figure 8-1 Algorithm for Prevention of Cardiovascular Disease in Women

Source: From Mosca, L., et al. (2007). Evidence based guidelines for cardiovascular disease prevention in women: 2007 Update. *Circulation, 115,* 1481–1501.

2008). As women age, hypertension becomes more common, affecting nearly half of women by their sixth decade of life (AHA, 2011). Black American women develop hypertension earlier in life, have higher blood pressure readings, and have an overall higher incidence of hypertension than white American women. The Centers for Disease Control and Prevention (CDC, 2010a) estimates that 44% of all black American women older than age 20 have hypertension. Black American women also have higher rates of morbidity and mortality due to hypertension and cardiovascular disease.

The onset of menopause significantly increases risk for hypertension in women. More than 50% of women over age 60 develop hypertension (Maas & Franke, 2009). Hypertension is a direct contributor to the significant increase in stroke, heart attack, heart failure, and renal failure in postmenopausal women (Lobo, 2009). Blood pressure should be kept below 140/90 mm Hg to prevent these conditions. It was once thought that hormone replacement therapy (HRT) would provide a protective effect on heart health in postmenopausal women. However, the Women's Health Initiative (WHI) research project demonstrated that the risks of long-term HRT outweigh any benefit to cardiac health (National Institutes of Health [NIH], 2010).

Pharmacologic treatments are appropriate for women at high risk of hypertension and to avert immediate health threats. Lifestyle issues such as weight management, diet, and physical activity help correct the underlying causes of hypertension, and are the mainstays in reducing hypertension risk and associated diseases.

Client History and Chart Review: Components of the History to Consider

- Age
- Ethnicity
- Gravida, para, LMP
  - Menstrual status/life stage
  - Current method of contraception
  - Prior maternity history of preeclampsia or eclampsia

- Medical/surgical history
- Current medication history
  - Contraceptive hormones
  - Hormone replacement therapy
  - Supplements
  - Medications for other medical conditions
- Depression screening
- Family history
- Presence, onset, and duration of any symptoms related to hypertension
  - Confusion
  - Tinnitus
  - Fatigue
  - Palpitations
  - Epistaxis
  - Vision change
  - Most women are asymptomatic
- Review of systems

Physical Examination: Components of the Physical Exam to Consider

- Height and weight
- BMI
- Blood pressure
  - Take with appropriate-sized cuff
  - Allow several minutes rest before taking and between readings
  - Obtain with the patient sitting and standing
  - Obtain from both the right and left arms
  - Retake after a rest period

Table 8-1   Classification of Blood Pressure for Adults

BLOOD PRESSURE CLASSIFICATION	SYSTOLIC BP (MM HG)	DIASTOLIC BP (MM HG)
Normal	< 120	**and** < 80
Prehypertension*	120–139	**or** 80–90
Stage 1 hypertension	140–159	**or** 90–99
Stage 2 hypertension	≥ 160	≥ 100

*Prehypertension is not a disease state but a predictor of future hypertension.

- Fundoscopic exam
- Heart exam
- Thyroid exam
- Assess for pedal edema
- Assessment for bruits
  - Carotid arteries
  - Abdomen
- [www] Risk calculation of CVD

Clinical Impression: Differential Diagnoses to Consider

(ICD9Data.com, 2012)

Consider the following classifications of hypertension:

- Benign essential hypertension
- Unspecified essential hypertension
- Hypertensive heart disease
  - Benign hypertensive heart disease
  - Unspecified hypertensive heart disease

Diagnostic Testing: Diagnostic Tests and Procedures to Consider

- Complete blood count
- Urinalysis
- Fasting serum lipid profile
- Fasting glucose
- Chemistry profile
  - Blood urea nitrogen
  - Creatinine
  - Fasting blood glucose
  - Renal and hepatic function profiles
- Serum electrolytes
- Serum uric acid
- Thyroid-stimulating hormone

Providing Treatment: Therapeutic Measures to Consider

- [www] Review the JNC-7 and AHA recommendations
- Lifestyle and diet modification for all women
- Weight management
  - If BMI is greater than 25, encourage weight loss of 10% from baseline

- Waist circumference should be 35 inches or less
- Physical activity of moderate intensity at least 30 minutes on most days of the week
  - Brisk walking
  - Aerobic activity
  - Resistance training
- Tobacco cessation
  - Behavioral counseling
  - Nicotine replacement therapy
- Low-fat, heart-healthy DASH diet
  - Whole grains
  - Fruits and vegetables
  - Legumes and nuts
  - Lean meat
  - Low-fat or nonfat dairy
  - Reduce trans fat consumption to as low as possible
  - Reduce saturated fat to less than 10% of calories
  - Limit alcoholic beverages to one per day or less
  - Limit daily salt intake to 2.3 grams (½ tsp) or less
- Omega-3 fatty acids (EPA and DHA): 800–1000 mg supplement daily or consumption of fish with high omega-3 content twice per week
- BP control medications depending on risk factors and clinical condition (King & Brucker, 2011)
  - Thiazide diuretics
  - Angiotensin-converting enzyme (ACE) inhibitors
  - Angiotensin-receptor blockers (ARBs)
  - Calcium-channel blockers (CCBs)
- Avoid estrogen supplements in women with hypertension
- Aspirin (AHRQ, 2009)
  - Routine preventive use in healthy women younger than age 55 is not recommended
  - Use low-dose (baby) aspirin 81 mg/day in women (Mosca et al., 2007)
    - In women aged 55–79 if BP is controlled
    - If 10-year risk per Framingham score is 6–10% or greater)

- Stress-reduction activities
  - Adequate rest and sleep
  - Biofeedback
  - Tai Chi
  - Relaxation techniques
  - Meditation or yoga
  - Support groups
  - Dedicated personal time

Providing Treatment: Complementary and Alternative Measures to Consider

- Dietary or herbal supplements
  - Pomegranate juice
  - Cayenne
  - Parsley
  - Red wine or grape-skin products
- ⚠ The following cardiotonic herbs are used in combination for mild hypertension and should not be used if cardioactive drugs are also taken (Romm, 2010):
  - Black cohosh
  - Garlic
  - Coleus
  - Cramp bark
- Review all herbal supplements taken for potential interactions with cardiac medications or cardiac conditions

Providing Support: Education and Support Measures to Consider

(AHA, 2007; NHLBI, 2006)
- DASH diet instructions
- Physical activity instructions
- Weight management instructions
- Tobacco cessation instructions
- Self-monitoring of BP
- ▽ Medication information
  - Correct dosing
  - Anticipated benefits
  - Side effects
  - Need for long-term treatment and follow-up
- Provide information as applicable
  - Personal cardiac risk assessment
  - Potential cardiac risks of hormone use

- Criteria for the following:
  - Emergency care
  - Prompt care
  - Referral
  - Return office visit

Follow-up Care: Follow-up Measures to Consider

- Document
  - Risk factors
  - Diagnosis
  - Discussions with the client
  - Treatment plan
- Return for continued care
  - As indicated by laboratory results
  - Evaluation of lifestyle changes
  - BP monitoring
  - Evaluation of medication side effects
  - Reproductive health care
- Support during the following programs:
  - Smoking cessation
  - Dietary and lifestyle changes

Multidisciplinary Practice: Consider Consultation, Collaboration, or Referral

- Emergency services
  - Systolic BP > 200 mm Hg or diastolic BP > 120 mm Hg
  - Signs or symptoms suspicious for stroke or myocardial infarction
- Medical services
  - Suspected cardiovascular dysfunction
  - Metabolic syndrome
  - Diabetes
  - Hypertension unresponsive to medication and lifestyle change
- Lifestyle modification programs
  - Smoking cessation
  - Drug and/or alcohol reduction
  - Weight management
  - Stress management
  - Heart healthy cooking
- For diagnosis or treatment outside the midwife's scope of practice

CARE OF THE WOMAN WITH HYPERLIPIDEMIA

Key Clinical Information

Hyperlipidemia is a disorder of lipid metabolism that results in abnormally high levels of cholesterol, triglycerides, and/or lipoproteins in the blood. Hyperlipidemia is a major risk factor for CVD and is often underreported in women (Mosca et al., 2007). Hyperlipidemia disorders can be familial or acquired through lifestyle patterns.

Screening for dyslipidemia is recommended to begin at age 45 in women with no risk factors, and after age 20 for those with risk factors. Risk factors that prompt early screening include women with diabetes, hypertension, a family history of heart disease in a close male relative younger than age 50 or a close female relative younger than age 60, a personal history of heart disease, obesity, and smoking. Serial laboratory evaluation is recommended every 5 years for women with normal values (United States Preventive Services Task Force [USPSTF], 2008).

In most patients with moderate hyperlipidemia, nonpharmacologic treatment methods are initiated first. These include specific modifications in diet, regular exercise, and smoking cessation. The National Cholesterol Education Panel (NCEP) issues guidelines on treating hyperlipidemia (NHLBI, 2004). The most recent NCEP III report recommends tailoring treatment goals to an individual's overall risk for CVD. Thus a comprehensive physical exam and medical history are performed, and risk assessment for dyslipidemias according to Framingham criteria is determined.

Client History and Chart Review: Components of the History to Consider

- Medical history
  - Hypothyroidism
  - Liver disease
  - Peripheral vascular disease
  - Renal disease
  - Cardiac disease
  - Liver disease
  - Diabetes
- Family history
  - Familial hyperlipidemia
  - Early CVD
  - Liver disease
- Medication history
  - Diuretics
  - Beta blockers
  - Anabolic steroids
  - Glucocorticosteroids
  - Estrogens and androgens
  - Retinoids
  - Cyclosporine
  - Protease inhibitors
- Lifestyle habits
  - Dietary habits and patterns
  - Alcohol use
  - Tobacco use
  - Review of systems

Physical Examination: Components of the Physical Exam to Consider

- Height and weight
- BMI
- Blood pressure
- [www.] Risk calculation of CVD
- Heart examination
- Thyroid
- Hip-to-waist ratio: Risk increases proportionally with a ratio greater than 1
- Presence of xanthomas
  - Elbows
  - Knees
  - Achilles tendons
  - Metacarpal joints
  - Eyelids
- Signs of atherosclerosis: Assess for bruits
  - Carotid arteries
  - Abdomen
  - Femoral arteries

Clinical Impression: Differential Diagnoses to Consider

(ICD9Data.com, 2012)

Consider the following types of dyslipidemia:

- Hypercholesterolemia
- Mixed hyperlipidemia
- Other and unspecified hyperlipidemia

Diagnostic Testing: Diagnostic Tests and Procedures to Consider

- Complete blood count
- Urinalysis
- Fasting glucose
- Fasting serum lipid profile

Table 8-2   Lipid Profile Interpretation

	CATEGORY
Total Cholesterol	
< 200	Normal
200–239 mg/dL	Borderline high
240 mg/dL and above	High
LDL Cholesterol	
< 100 mg/dL	Optimal
100–129 mg/dL	Near optimal
130–159 mg/dL	Borderline high
160–189 mg/dL	High
190 and above	Very high
HDL Cholesterol	
60 mg/dL and above	Optimal: low risk for CVD
< 50 mg/dL (women)	Low: risk factor for CVD
Triglycerides	
< 150 mg/dL	Optimal
150–199 mg/dL	Borderline high
200–499 mg/dL	High
500 mg/dL and above	Very high

Providing Treatment: Therapeutic Measures to Consider

(NHLBI, 2004)

- Attention to lifestyle and diet for all women
  - Weight management
  - Smoking cessation
  - Aerobic exercise
    - 30 minutes per day on most days of the week
    - At least 120 minutes per week or more
- Dietary modifications
  - Decrease saturated fat to less than 7% of calories
  - Eliminate trans fats from diet
    - Hydrogenated vegetable oils
    - Found in commercially prepared baked goods
  - Increase intake of soluble fiber
  - [www] Follow Mediterranean diet
    - Lower consumption of meats, eggs, and dairy
    - Higher consumption of fish and vegetables
    - Higher consumption of monounsaturated fats (avocado, olives, and almonds)
    - Lower consumption of saturated fats (palm oil and coconut oil)
- Omega-3 fatty acids (EPA and DHA): 800–1000 mg supplement daily or consumption of fish with high omega-3 content twice per week
- Pharmacologic treatment depending on risk factors and clinical condition (King & Brucker, 2011)
  - Statins
    - Reduce cholesterol production
    - Lipitor or Crestor (most potent)
    - Lescol (least potent)
    - ⚠ Watch for drug–drug interactions
  - Niacin (nicotinic acid)
    - Niacor
    - Reduces cholesterol and LDL production

- Bile acid–binding resins
  - ◆ Increases conversion of cholesterol into bile salts in the liver
  - ◆ Questran
- Fibrates
  - ◆ Reduce triglyceride production
  - ◆ Triglide
- Cholesterol absorption inhibitors
  - ◆ Inhibit intestinal absorption of cholesterol
  - ◆ Zetia

Providing Treatment: Complementary and Alternative Measures to Consider

- Dietary supplements
  - Nuts
  - Safflower oil
  - Oat bran
  - Plant sterols
    - ◆ Found in certain foods such as nuts, fruits, vegetables, and enriched margarine
    - ◆ Lower LDL cholesterol
- Herbal supplements (Romm, 2010)
  - Garlic
  - Guggul
  - Globe artichoke
  - Salvia
  - Fenugreek

Providing Support: Education and Support Measures to Consider

- Diet modification instructions
- Physical activity instructions
- Weight management instructions
- Tobacco cessation instructions
- Medication information
  - Correct dosing
  - Anticipated benefits
  - Side effects
  - Need for long-term treatment and follow-up

- Provide information as applicable
  - Personal cardiac risk assessment
  - Potential cardiac risks of hormone use
- Criteria for the following:
  - Prompt care
  - Referral
  - Return office visit

Follow-up Care: Follow-up Measures to Consider

- Document
  - Risk factors
  - Diagnosis
  - Discussions with the client
  - Treatment plan
- Return for continued care
  - For repeat testing after 6–8 weeks of diet and lifestyle modification as instructed (NHLBI, 2004)
  - As indicated by laboratory results
  - Evaluation of lifestyle changes
  - Medication monitoring
  - Reproductive health care
  - Support during the following programs:
    - ◆ Smoking cessation
    - ◆ Dietary and lifestyle changes

Multidisciplinary Practice: Consider Consultation, Collaboration, or Referral

- Medical services
  - Suspected cardiovascular dysfunction
  - Hypertension
  - Metabolic syndrome
  - Diabetes
- Lifestyle modification programs
  - Smoking cessation
  - Weight management
  - Diet management
- For diagnosis or treatment outside the midwife's scope of practice

ASSESSMENT OF THE WOMAN WITH DERMATOLOGIC SYMPTOMS

Key Clinical Information

The skin is the largest organ of the body, functioning as a protective barrier and thermoregulatory organ. As the body's first line of defense against the environment, the skin is subject to injury, infection, pigment changes, burns, stings, tumors, rashes, and other conditions. Many systemic illnesses and conditions produce dermatologic signs. Although skin lesions can represent localized conditions, they can also be a cutaneous manifestation of a systemic condition, such as the rash associated with rubella virus infection or an allergic response. Many disorders can be accurately diagnosed by careful evaluation of lesion appearance. A comprehensive dermatologic text with color plates is a useful tool when evaluating dermatologic conditions; online color images are also available. To be most effective, examination of the skin should include areas inaccessible to self-examination, because this may yield additional information necessary to make an accurate diagnosis.

People of all races and ethnicities have differences in skin pigmentation and hair primarily due to genetic variations. Endogenous and exogenous environmental factors, such as exposure to the elements, hormonal influences, medications, and immune response, also influence skin thickness and color, and hair distribution and quality, and must be taken into account when assessing skin conditions.

Many common dermatologic problems are treated with topical medications, such as corticosteroids and antifungal agents. Many formulations and brands are readily available. Selection of an appropriate therapeutic agent requires integration of several factors: the lesion or rash location and skin characteristics, the clinical state of the lesion (e.g., dry, oozing, pruritic), and the base in which the active medication is delivered (e.g., cream, ointment, solution). Only a small selection of medications available for the condition described are included within each guideline here; many other medications may be appropriate and available.

Client History and Chart Review: Components of the History to Consider

- Age
- Medical/surgical history
  - Allergies and sensitivities
  - Current medications (especially recent onset of use)
  - Chronic and acute conditions
  - Previous surgery
  - Previous skin conditions
- Sunscreen use
- Skin type
  - Tanning ability
  - Sensitivities
- Family history
  - Melanoma and other skin cancers
  - Psoriasis
  - Skin sensitivities
- Dermatologic symptom profile
  - Onset, duration, and severity of symptoms
    - Associated event or injury
    - Rapid or gradual onset
    - Effect of symptoms related to severity
  - Location and distribution of lesions/changes
    - Local
    - Diffuse
  - Characteristics of skin lesion(s)
    - Color changes
      - Red
      - White
      - Black or brown
      - Blue
    - Texture
      - Raised or flat
      - Scaly or coarse
      - Crusted or oozing
      - Blistered
    - Borders
      - Geographic
      - Clearly demarcated
      - Gradual or diffuse
    - Exudate or discharge
      - Clear or serous

- ➤ Purulent
- ➤ Bloody
- ◆ Presence of inflammation
  - ➤ Redness
  - ➤ Heat
  - ➤ Pain
- ■ Associated factors and additional symptoms
  - ◆ Itching
  - ◆ Fever or chills
  - ◆ Nausea and vomiting
  - ◆ Pain
  - ◆ Swelling
  - ◆ Hair loss
- ■ Remedies used and their effects
- • Potential exposures
  - ■ Infections
  - ■ Infestations
  - ■ Bites and stings
    - ◆ Animals
    - ◆ Insects
    - ◆ Snakes
    - ◆ Spiders
    - ◆ Jellyfish
  - ■ Sun exposure
  - ■ Chemicals, toxins, and skin products: Recent change in laundry detergent or body soap /lotion
- • Review of systems

Physical Examination: Components of the Physical Exam to Consider

(Rousseau, 2007)

- • General physical examination, with focus on the presenting concern
- • Vital signs, including temperature
- • Thyroid
- • Lymph nodes
- • Signs of systemic disease
- • Observation and palpation of the lesion(s)
  - ■ Location and distribution of lesion(s)
  - ■ Size and number of lesion(s)
  - ■ Symmetry of lesion(s)

- ■ Surface contour of lesions
  - ◆ Flat
  - ◆ Raised
  - ◆ Macular
  - ◆ Papular
  - ◆ Bullous
  - ◆ Annular
- ■ Margin characteristics
  - ◆ Geographic, irregular
  - ◆ Clear, smooth, linear
  - ◆ Blended
  - ◆ Raised
  - ◆ Rolled
  - ◆ Varied
- ■ Coloration of lesion(s)
  - ◆ Pigment color(s)
  - ◆ Patchy
  - ◆ Confluent
- ■ Appearance of lesion(s)
  - ◆ Scaling
  - ◆ Crusting
  - ◆ Ulceration
  - ◆ Erosion
  - ◆ Presence of exudate

Clinical Impression: Differential Diagnoses to Consider

(ICD9Data.com, 2012)

- • Symptoms involving skin and other integumentary tissue, such as
  - ■ Hair-related lesions
  - ■ Nodular lesions
  - ■ Papular lesions
  - ■ Pigmented lesions
  - ■ Ulcerated lesions

Diagnostic Testing: Diagnostic Tests and Procedures to Consider

- • Wet preparation of exudate
- • Culture of lesions
  - ■ Fungal
    - ◆ Dermatophyte test medium
    - ◆ Useful in treatment-resistant cases

- Bacterial: Routine culture; consider Gram stain
- Herpes: Viral culture medium
- Skin biopsy
  - Punch biopsy
  - Excisional biopsy
  - Skin scraping
- Serology and titers
  - Rubella
  - Rapid plasma reagin (RPR)
  - HIV
- Testing for systemic disorders
  - Thyroid disorder (TSH)
  - Antinuclear antibody (lupus)
  - Lyme titer

Providing Treatment: Therapeutic Measures to Consider

- General relief measures
  - Acetaminophen
  - Ibuprofen
  - Benadryl
  - Topical aloe vera with lidocaine
- See the specific condition practice guideline

Providing Treatment: Complementary and Alternative Measures to Consider

- Measures to promote healing and foster immune response
  - Well-balanced diet
  - Limit alcohol, spicy foods, and hot drinks: Cause vasodilation
  - Adequate rest
  - Exposure to light and air (unless contraindicated by medication use)
  - Limit occlusive skin coverings unless indicated
- Symptomatic relief: Itching
  - Cool colloidal oatmeal baths
  - Herbal wash
    - Chamomile
    - Calendula
    - Aloe
    - Marshmallow herb

Providing Support: Education and Support Measures to Consider

Provide information on the following topics:
- Working diagnosis
  - Testing recommendations
  - Relief measures
  - Skin care
  - Care of contacts, as applicable
- Treatment plan options
  - Medication instructions
  - Prevention methods
  - Warning signs and symptoms
- Instructions to return for care
  - As indicated by diagnosis
  - If condition worsens or recurs

Follow-up Care: Follow-up Measures to Consider

- Document
  - Lesion(s)
    - Location(s)
    - Appearance
    - Size and spread
    - Margins
  - Discussions with the client
  - Criteria for diagnosis
  - Treatment and follow-up plan
- Return for continued care
  - Persistent or worsening symptoms
  - Medication reaction(s)
  - Routine follow-up

Multidisciplinary Practice: Consider Consultation, Collaboration, or Referral

- Dermatology services
  - Severe or worsening symptoms
  - No improvement with treatment
- Medical services: When dermatologic symptoms are associated with other concerning findings
- For diagnosis or treatment outside the midwife's scope of practice

CARE OF THE WOMAN WITH ACNE

Key Clinical Information

Acne is an inflammatory skin condition that can develop when skin pores become clogged due to excess oil production, allowing comedones (blackheads), pustules (whiteheads), and cysts to form. These lesions can form on the back, neck, chest, and, most commonly, face. Acne is common in adolescence, when the increase in testosterone production in both males and females leads to increased sebaceous gland activity. Acne also occurs in adulthood. Exacerbations can be triggered by hormonal changes at various times in the menstrual cycle, oral contraceptives, heavy use of cosmetics, certain medications (such as steroids), and high levels of humidity and sweating. Acne can result in emotional stress, embarrassment, and poor self-image, especially during the adolescent years. Treatment varies with the severity of the condition and underlying contributing factors; in general, early and aggressive treatment is advocated.

Client History and Chart Review: Components of the History to Consider

- Age
- Overall diet quality
- Onset and severity of condition
  - Duration
  - Frequency and relationship to menses
  - Signs or symptoms of associated infection
  - Effect on well-being and mental health
- Hormonal use, including contraception
- Routine skin care habits
- Prior treatments and efficacy

Physical Examination: Components of the Physical Exam to Consider

- Overall skin condition
- General hygiene, body habitus, and health
- Presence, location, and distribution of the following:
  - Comedones, open or closed
  - Inflammatory papules and pustules
  - Cysts
  - Acne pitting and scarring
- Signs of secondary infection

Clinical Impression: Differential Diagnoses to Consider

(ICD9Data.com, 2012)

- Acne
- Rosacea
- Erythematous skin reactions
- Contact dermatitis
- Other local infections of the skin and subcutaneous tissue

Diagnostic Testing: Diagnostic Tests and Procedures to Consider

Diagnosis is made with visual inspection and exclusion of other causes (see Table 8-3).

Providing Treatment: Therapeutic Measures to Consider

(Romm, 2010; Strauss et al., 2007)

- Topical agents for mild acne
  - Tretinoin: 0.025% cream or 0.01% gel; increase strength as tolerated and indicated
  - Benzoyl peroxide gel or wash: 2.5–10%
  - Erythromycin gel, ointment, or solution
  - Clindamycin phosphate gel, lotion, and solution
  - Tetracycline cream (Topicycline)
  - Isotrexin: Combination of isotretinoin and erythromycin
    - Use of tretinoin in the evening and topical antibiotic in the morning leads to synergistic treatment effects
  - Azelaic acid cream (Azelex)
  - Retinoids
    - Adapalene gel 1% (Differin)
    - Tazarotene (Tazorac)
  - Salicylic acid: Over-the-counter products in strengths from 0.2% to 5%

Table 8-3 Differential Diagnosis of Acne Vulgaris

DIAGNOSIS	AGE OF ONSET	IMPORTANT FACTORS	COMMON LOCATION	CLINICAL PRESENTATION
Acne rosacea	Most often ages 30–50	Slow onset aggravated by cold, alcohol, hot foods, stress, or an unknown etiology	Central face	Central facial flushing, telangiectasias; can present with inflammatory papulopustular eruptions; stinging and burning often reported
Perioral dermatitis	Primarily adults	Often associated with use of high-potency topical steroids	Chin, perioral, and nasolabial folds	Papules and pustules, similar to eczema
Gram-negative folliculitis	Later teen years or any age	Associated with long-term antibiotic therapy, resistant acne, and sometimes hot tub immersion	Nose including nasal passages; mouth areas; and neck	Pustular and cystic lesions; large nodules
Acneiform eruptions	Teenage to adult years	Often associated with oral medications such as corticosteroids, contact dye, and testosterone	Chest, upper arms, and scalp	Small papules, pustules, or closed comedones

- Oral agents for moderate to severe acne
  - Minocycline (Minocin)
    - Category D: Do not use in pregnancy
    - Can cause hyperpigmentation
  - Doxycycline (Doryx)
    - Category D: Do not use in pregnancy
    - Can cause photosensitivity
  - Tetracycline
    - Category D: Do not use in pregnancy
    - Can lead to *Candida albicans* vaginitis
  - Erythromycin
    - Safe in pregnancy
    - Can cause gastrointestinal (GI) upset
- Oral contraceptives (OCs)
  - Some OCs reduce the amount of sebum produced by the skin
  - Ortho-TriCyclen
  - Estrostep
  - Yaz

- For acne flares related to menses
  - Oral antibiotics for 3 days at ovulation, then for 5 days during menses
  - Daily topical tretinoin and antibiotics

Providing Treatment: Complementary and Alternative Measures to Consider

(Romm, 2010)
- Anti-inflammatory herbs
  - Witch hazel cream
  - Tea tree oil 5% lotion
  - Burdock root oral tincture
  - Chamomile topical cream
  - Calendula topical wash: Contains flavinoids and retinoids
- Facial steam: Opens pores
- Zinc: 25 mg twice daily for 2 weeks, then once daily for 2 months
- Vitamin B_6: 50 mg daily

Providing Support: Education and Support Measures to Consider

- Provide support and affirmation
- Instruct in use of medication: Most topical treatments, including OTC products, can cause dry, red skin with mild peeling
- Instruct in facial hygiene
  - Do not squeeze, pick, or scratch pimples: Can lead to infection
  - Wash skin at least twice daily
    - Non-drying soap such as Cetaphil or Neutrogena *or*
    - 5% benzoyl peroxide wash
  - Wash skin after exercise
  - Use only water-based cosmetics
- Dietary recommendations (Cordain, 2002)
  - Diet high in omega-3 fatty acid: Anti-inflammatory agent
  - Limit refined carbohydrates and high glycemic load (Ferdowsian & Levin, 2010): Cause insulin surge and increased sebum production
  - Limited data on diet and acne are available
- Avoid sun exposure

Follow-up Care: Follow-up Measures to Consider

- Document
  - Clinical findings and diagnosis
  - Discussions with the client on medication use
  - Treatment plan
- Return for continued care: To assess treatment effectiveness

Multidisciplinary Practice: Consider Consultation, Collaboration, or Referral

- Dermatology services
  - Severe or cystic acne
  - Treatment of resistant acne with isotretinoin
  - Acne with scarring
  - Dermabrasion, photodynamic therapy, or other treatments
  - No improvement with treatment

- For diagnosis or treatment outside the midwife's scope of practice

CARE OF THE WOMAN WITH BACTERIAL SKIN INFECTIONS

Key Clinical Information

Bacterial skin infections can take several forms. Cellulitis is a diffuse skin infection of the tissues under the skin, often brought on when a cut or injury allows bacteria to enter the skin. Skin that is swollen, or dry and flaky, can be more prone to becoming an entry point for bacteria. While cellulitis can occur anywhere on the body, the legs are more commonly affected (Pye, 2010). The infection can spread throughout nearby tissues to the lymph nodes and into the bloodstream. if left untreated, cellulitis can quickly become a serious health condition. The incidence of cellulitis secondary to methicillin-resistant *Staphylococcus aureus* (MRSA), a life-threatening infection, is increasing. Therefore, prompt attention to signs and symptoms of cellulitis is essential.

Impetigo is a contagious skin infection most commonly seen in infants and children. In adults, it is usually the result of injury to the skin. Typical organisms involved are S. *aureus* and *Streptococcus pyogenes*. This condition is usually self-limiting and clears within 2 to 3 weeks, although treatment is necessary to prevent the post-streptococcal glomerulonephritis that can occur with some strains of S. *pyogenes* (Butarro, Trybulski, Bailey, & Sandberg-Cook, 2007).

Client History and Chart Review: Components of the History to Consider

- Age
- BMI
- Onset of symptoms
- Recent skin injury
  - Cuts or scrapes
  - Insect bite
  - Surgery

- Tattoo
- Animal bite
- Exposure to other infected individuals
- Presence of signs and symptoms
    - Itching
    - Pain
    - Fever and chills
    - Tenderness
    - Swelling
    - Redness
- Participation in contact sports (wrestling)
- Diabetes
- Use of intravenous drugs

Physical Examination: Components of the Physical Exam to Consider

- Vital signs, including temperature
- Assessment of the skin
    - Localized areas of erythema
    - Color and texture: Redness, induration
    - Integrity: Wounds, scratches, cracking
    - Sensation: Pain, itching
- Presence of systemic symptoms, such as chills
- Cellulitis
    - Acute rapidly spreading lesion
    - Red, hot, tender skin and subcutaneous tissue
    - Irregular and raised borders, due to edema
- Abscesses
    - Furuncles, folliculitis, or carbuncles
    - Characterized by the following:
        - Local cellulitis
        - Regional lymphadenopathy
        - Formation of a fluctuant mass
- Impetigo
    - Acute purulent infection
    - Painless, itchy, fluid-filled blisters
    - Characterized by 1- to 3-cm red sores surrounded by a honey-colored crust
    - Erythematous halo suggests strep infection
    - Large confluent lesions may occur

- Common around the nose and mouth, or trunk and buttocks in children
- Can occur on breasts, legs, or other areas secondary to scratching

Clinical Impression: Differential Diagnoses to Consider

(ICD9Data.com, 2012)

- Cellulitis and abscess
- Impetigo

Diagnostic Testing: Diagnostic Tests and Procedures to Consider

- Diagnosis is primarily by clinical assessment
- Culture of lesion(s) or exudate
- Gram stain of exudate
- CBC and differential

Providing Treatment: Therapeutic Measures to Consider

- ⚠ Cellulitis
    - Requires prompt antibiotic therapy for 7–10 days
    - Dicloxacillin 250–500 mg PO every 6 hours, or intravenous antibiotics
    - Incision and drainage (I&D) of abscess, if present
    - Debridement of necrotic or devitalized tissue
- Impetigo
    - Topical or systemic antibiotics
    - Topical antibiotic mupirocin (Bactroban)
    - Oral therapy: 7–10 days
        - Dicloxacillin: 500 mg PO QID
        - Ciprofloxin: 500 mg PO BID
        - Sulfa-trimethoprim: DS 1 PO BID
    - Scrub with soap and water or chlorhexidine gluconate solution
    - Wash affected area TID; apply antibiotic ointment
    - To avoid spreading the infection, apply a dressing

Providing Treatment: Complementary and Alternative Measures to Consider

- For impetigo, soak the affected area in a vinegar solution (1 Tbs to 16 oz water) for 20 minutes
- Dry thoroughly after bathing
- Expose skin to sunlight and air
- Avoid close-fitting clothing

Providing Support: Education and Support Measures to Consider

- Impetigo
  - Instruction about the condition and medication use
  - Do not share bedding, towels, or clothing with an infected person
  - Avoid scratching or touching sores to prevent spread to other areas
  - Wash the infected person's bedding, linens, towels, and clothes daily
  - Wash hands frequently
- Cellulitis
  - Instruction about condition and medication use
  - ⚠ Signs and symptoms of worsening infection
    - Fever or chills
    - Increased areas of redness
    - Increased pain
    - Drainage
  - Use a skin moisturizer daily: Prevents cracking and peeling of skin
  - Protect the hands and feet
  - Promptly treat superficial skin infections

Follow-up Care: Follow-up Measures to Consider

- Document
  - Clinical findings and diagnosis
  - Discussions with the client on medication use
  - Treatment plan

- Return for continued care
  - Recheck of cellulitis in 1–3 days
  - If the condition is not responsive to treatment

Multidisciplinary Practice: Consider Consultation, Collaboration, or Referral

- Medical services: Skin lesions accompanied by fever, malaise, or other constitutional symptoms
- For diagnosis or treatment outside the midwife's scope of practice

CARE OF THE WOMAN WITH DERMATITIS

Key Clinical Information

Dermatitis is a general term that describes skin inflammation. There are several common causes of dermatitis, most of which are associated with similar symptoms of swelling, dryness, redness, and itching. A generalized body rash can occur in response to ingestion of a food, medication, or other substance that causes an allergic response. Mangos, seafood, peanuts, and eggs are examples of foods known to cause allergic reactions in some individuals. Allergic symptoms can range from very mild to severe, with rash frequently being an early symptom (Medline Plus, 2009).

Contact dermatitis is often caused by a hypersensitivity reaction to an irritant in the environment. This condition is localized to the skin following contact with the offending substance and will often resolve within several days. Common plant irritants include poison ivy, poison oak, and poison sumac. Common chemical irritants include soaps, cleaning products, and cosmetic supplies (Frosch & John, 2011). Contact dermatitis is not contagious from one person to another, or from one body part to another.

Atopic dermatitis, also known as eczema, is a chronic skin disorder that is thought to be caused by an abnormal immune reaction in the skin, leading to long-term inflammation. It is most commonly seen in childhood; however, many individuals experience recurrent bouts throughout life. Eczema affects women more often than men and is thought to have a genetic component (Butarro et al., 2007). Women with eczema often have a family history of other allergic conditions, such as asthma or hay fever. Eczema comes in various forms, some of which are caused by environmental allergens, changes in temperature, or contact with substances such as soap or sweat. The most common symptoms are dry, red, scaly skin that itches or burns. Eczema is a chronic condition that, with appropriate self-care and treatment, can be managed effectively.

Client History and Chart Review: Components of the History to Consider

- Age
- Onset, duration, and characteristics of symptoms
  - Pruritus
  - Traveling or static rash
- Associated symptoms
  - Swelling
    - Facial or throat area
    - Difficulty breathing
  - Change in consciousness
  - Feeling of panic or anxiety
- Current medication history
- Recent dietary history: Food allergies
- Recent activity around potential irritants
  - Outdoor activities (plants)
  - Cleaning
  - Occupational history
- Family and personal history of other atopic disease such as asthma or allergies
- Usual skin care regimen: Change in laundry detergents or body soap/lotions
- Current relief measures used and efficacy
- Review of systems

Physical Examination: Components of the Physical Exam to Consider

- Food- or medication-induced dermatitis
  - Red, raised rash
  - Travels over time
  - Hives that coalesce
    - May have associated symptoms
      - Facial and throat swelling
      - Intense pruritus
- Contact dermatitis
  - Scale and plaque formation
  - Desquamation
  - Moist epidermis and lacy border
  - Associated symptoms
    - Pruritus
    - Burning
    - Stinging
- Eczema: Atopic dermatitis
  - Intensely itching skin lesions with the following characteristics:
    - Erythema
    - Scaling
    - Excoriations
    - Itching often is first, with rash following its appearance
  - Common locations
    - Hands and feet
    - Creases of elbows and knees
    - Behind the ears
  - Moist epidermis and lacy border
  - Associated symptoms
    - Pruritus
    - Burning
    - Stinging
  - Lichenification (thick, leather-like area) can occur with long-term irritation

Clinical Impression: Differential Diagnoses to Consider

(ICD9Data.com, 2012)

- Acute allergic reaction
- Atopic dermatitis
- Contact dermatitis and eczema
- Dermatitis to substances taken internally

Diagnostic Testing: Diagnostic Tests and Procedures to Consider

- Diagnosis is primarily by clinical assessment and exclusion of other causes

- Skin biopsy
- Allergic reaction "patch testing"

Providing Treatment: Therapeutic Measures to Consider

(King & Brucker, 2011)

- Food- or medication-induced dermatitis
  - Topical corticosteroid preparations have limited value
  - Oral course of steroids for those with no symptom resolution in several days: Consult with medical or dermatologic services
  - Antihistamine for itching
    - Cetirizine (Zyrtec)
    - Diphenhydramine (Benadryl)
    - Hydroxyzine (Atarax)
- Contact dermatitis and eczema
  - Topical corticosteroid preparation selection depends on severity (see Table 8-4)
    - Use the lowest effective potency

- Long-term use of high-strength corticosteroids can weaken the skin and worsen the condition
- Do not cover with an occlusive dressing
- Once-daily use has similar efficacy to more frequent dosing
- Use several times daily for acute flare-ups
- Use once or twice weekly for maintenance
  - Topical immunomodulators
    - Pimecrolimus cream (Elidil)
    - Tacrolimus ointment (Protopic)
  - Oral antihistamines for pruritus as needed

Providing Treatment: Complementary and Alternative Measures to Consider

- Contact dermatitis
  - Oatmeal baths
  - Cool compresses
  - Burow's solution (Domeboro) compresses
  - Calamine lotion
  - Aloe lotion

Table 8-4 Potencies of Selected Brands of Topical Corticosteroids

BRAND NAME	GENERIC NAME
Class 1: Superpotent	
Clobex Lotion/Spray/Shampoo, 0.05%	Clobetasol propionate
Cormax Cream/Solution, 0.05%	Clobetasol propionate
Diprolene Ointment, 0.05%	Betamethasone dipropionate
Olux E Foam, 0.05%	Clobetasol propionate
Olux Foam, 0.05%	Clobetasol propionate
Temovate Cream/Ointment/Solution, 0.05%	Clobetasol propionate
Ultravate Cream/Ointment, 0.05%	Halobetasol propionate
Vanos Cream, 0.1%	Fluocinonide
Psorcon Ointment, 0.05%	Diflorasone diacetate
Psorcon E Ointment, 0.05%	Diflorasone diacetate
Class 2: High Potency	
Diprolene Cream AF, 0.05%	Betamethasone dipropionate
Elocon Ointment, 0.1%	Mometasone furoate
Florone Ointment, 0.05%	Diflorasone diacetate
Halog Ointment/Cream, 0.1%	Halcinonide
Lidex Cream/Gel/Ointment, 0.05%	Fluocinonide

(continues)

Table 8-4 Potencies of Selected Brands of Topical Corticosteroids (continued)

BRAND NAME	GENERIC NAME
Psorcon Cream, 0.05%	Diflorasone diacetate
Topicort Cream/Ointment, 0.25%	Desoximetasone
Topicort Gel, 0.05%	Desoximetasone
Class 3: Medium–High Potency	
Cutivate Ointment, 0.005%	Fluticasone propionate
Lidex-E Cream, 0.05%	Fluocinonide
Luxiq Foam, 0.12%	Betamethasone valerate
Topicort LP Cream, 0.05%	Desoximetasone
Class 4: Medium Potency	
Cordran Ointment, 0.05%	Flurandrenolide
Elocon Cream, 0.1%	Mometasone furoate
Kenalog Cream/Spray, 0.1%	Triamcinolone acetonide
Synalar Ointment, 0.03%	Fluocinolone acetonide
Westcort Ointment, 0.2%	Hydrocortisone valerate
Class 5: Mild Potency	
Capex Shampoo, 0.01%	Fluocinolone acetonide
Cordran Cream/Lotion/Tape, 0.05%	Flurandrenolide
Cutivate Cream/Lotion, 0.05%	Fluticasone propionate
DermAtop Cream, 0.1%	Prednicarbate
DesOwen Lotion, 0.05%	Desonide
Locoid Cream/Lotion/Ointment/Solution, 0.1%	Hydrocortisone
Pandel Cream, 0.1%	Hydrocortisone
Synalar Cream, 0.03%/0.01%	Fluocinolone acetonide
Westcort Cream, 0.2%	Hydrocortisone valerate
Class 6: Low Potency	
Aclovate Cream/Ointment, 0.05%	Alclometasone dipropionate
Derma-Smoothe/FS Oil, 0.01%	Fluocinolone acetonide
Desonate Gel, 0.05%	Desonide
Synalar Cream/Solution, 0.01%	Fluocinolone acetonide
Verdeso Foam, 0.05%	Desonide
Class 7: Lowest Potency	
Cetacort Lotion, 0.5%/1%	Hydrocortisone
Cortaid Cream/Spray/Ointment	Hydrocortisone
Hytone Cream/Lotion, 1%/2.5%	Hydrocortisone
Micort-HC Cream, 2%/2.5%	Hydrocortisone
Nutracort Lotion, 1%/2.5%	Hydrocortisone
Synacort Cream, 1%/2.5%	Hydrocortisone

- Eczema
  - Stress reduction
  - Cool compresses with olive oil when itching symptoms start

Providing Support: Education and Support Measures to Consider

- Provide information
  - Working diagnosis
    - Relief measures
    - Skin care
  - Treatment plan options
    - Medication instructions
    - Prevention methods
    - Warning signs and symptoms
- Contact dermatitis
  - Reassurance of self-limiting nature
  - Limit contact with known irritants
- Eczema: A chronic condition that can be managed
  - Skin care
    - Use one recommended mild soap (e.g., Neutrogena) and skin moisturizer
    - Apply a heavy moisturizer (e.g., Cutemol OTC) to the affected area TID
    - Apply a skin moisturizer after bathing while the skin is damp
    - Relieve itching with cold compresses
    - Avoid scratching, which exacerbates eczema
  - Reduce episodes
    - Avoid long showers and baths
    - Use lukewarm water for showers and baths
    - Limit contact with known irritants
    - Use a home humidifier
    - Wear protective gloves for activities requiring hand submersion in water
    - Maintain cool temperatures and avoid overheating and sweating

Follow-up Care: Follow-up Measures to Consider

- Document
  - Clinical findings and diagnosis
  - Discussions with the client on medication use
  - Treatment plan

- Return for continued care: To assess treatment effectiveness

Multidisciplinary Practice: Consider Consultation, Collaboration, or Referral

- Medical/allergy services
  - Diagnostic testing
  - Food- or medication-induced dermatitis that does not respond to treatment
- Dermatology services
  - Eczema that does not respond to treatment
  - Eczema requiring the highest-potency corticosteroids
  - Eczema requiring topical immune modulator medications (tacrolimus)
  - Phototherapy
- For diagnosis or treatment outside the midwife's scope of practice

CARE OF THE WOMAN WITH DERMATOLOGIC INFESTATIONS

Key Clinical Information

Pediculosis is a bodily infestation of lice. Lice are blood-sucking insects that live in hair-bearing regions of the body (head lice and pubic lice); they may also live in the seams of clothing (body lice). Pediculosis is spread by having contact with an infested person, or his or her clothing, bedding, or personal care items such as brushes. Each year, 6 to 12 million people in the United States are infested with head lice; infestation is most common in school-age children (CDC, 2010b).

Pubic lice are commonly seen in the teenage population and are usually spread by sexual contact. While pubic lice infestations can be spread by contact with infected clothing, bedding, and toilet seats, this route of transfer is uncommon. Risk factors for pubic lice include multiple sexual partners, sexual contact with an infested person, and sharing bedding or clothing with an infested person. Intense itching is the primary symptom of a lice infestation, due to the parasite biting the skin. The itching tends to be worse during the night. Symptoms may occur anywhere from 1 day after exposure to 2 to 4 weeks after exposure, and lice can live up to 30 days on humans (Haisley-Royster, 2011).

Body lice do not live on the skin but rather in the seams of clothing; they move from this location to the body to feed. Those areas where clothing seams are right next to the body, such as waistbands or bra strap areas, are often involved and may be excoriated from scratching. Infestations of body lice can be problems in communities with poverty and overcrowding. Reused mattresses and communal beds are risk factors.

Scabies mites are arthropods that burrow into the skin and deposit their eggs, forming visible linear or wavy marks as they move just beneath the skin. Eggs mature in approximately 3 weeks. The itchy rash is an allergic response to the mite. The hands and the areas between the fingers are common places for mites to colonize, as well as the abdomen, genitals, and wrists (Haisley-Royster, 2011). Similar to lice, scabies is contagious and spreads with direct contact with an infested person; transfer of mites via personal articles or bedding is much less common.

Outbreaks of lice or scabies can occur in areas where people congregate, such as in nursing homes, child care centers, and schools. These pathogens are found in people of all ages, races, and ethnic groups and across all socioeconomic strata.

Client History and Chart Review: Components of the History to Consider

- Age
- Location of symptoms
- Onset, duration, and characteristics of symptoms
  - Capitis (head lice): Pruritus of the scalp is the primary symptom
  - Corporis (body lice): Pruritus of the shoulders and abdomen is common
  - Pubis (pubic lice): Pruritus of the pubic area is the primary symptom
  - Scabies: Pruritus of the affected area is the primary symptom
  - Pruritus becomes worse at night

- Recent exposure to potential infestations
  - School-age children
  - Sexual contact history
  - Use of others' bedding, hats, scarves, or personal care items

Physical Examination: Components of the Physical Exam to Consider

- Pediculosis inspection
  - Visible moving lice, nits (white egg sacs), rash, and bites in the affected area(s)
  - Use bright lights and a magnifying glass
  - Part the client's hair to the scalp in small sections
  - Pubic lice bites may leave bluish color lesions
- Scabies inspection
  - Gray or skin-colored lesions
  - Linear or wavy ridges ending in minute vesicles or papules

Clinical Impression: Differential Diagnoses to Consider

(ICD9Data.com, 2012)

- Pediculosis
- Scabies

Diagnostic Testing: Diagnostic Tests and Procedures to Consider

- Diagnosis is primarily made by clinical assessment

Providing Treatment: Therapeutic Measures to Consider

- Head lice (pediculosis capitus)
  - Permethrin 1% shampoo (Nix) used as directed: Kills only lice, not nits
  - Piperonyl butoxide (RID)
  - Remove eggs with a nit comb
    - Metal combs are more effective than plastic combs
    - Apply a small amount of olive oil to the hair to make removal easier
    - Repeat combing in 7–19 days after permethrin treatment

- Lindane 1% shampoo: Used only as a last-resort medication for repeated infestations
  - ◆ Neurotoxic pediculocide with potentially severe side effects
    - ➤ Allergic reaction
    - ➤ Seizures
  - ◆ Use only if the client's weight is more than 110 lb
  - ◆ Use only as directed
- Pubic lice (pediculosis pubis)
  - Permethrin 1% shampoo (Nix) used as directed
  - Benadryl for itching
- Body lice (pediculosis corporis)
  - Throw away affected clothing
  - Anti-lice medications are not needed if clothing and bedding are properly washed
  - Benadryl for itching
- Scabies
  - Permethrin 5% cream (Elimite)
  - Diphenhydramine (Benadryl) or cetirizine (Zyrtec) for itching
- All medications are Pregnancy Category B

Providing Treatment: Complementary and Alternative Measures to Consider

- Hair: Clean 1-2-3 (anise oil, coconut oil, or ylang ylang oil in an alcohol base) (Ogg & Cochran, 2006)
- Vinegar (5% acetic acid) hair rinse loosens nits (eggs)
  - Apply at full strength to affected areas, avoiding the eyes and mucous membranes
  - Rinse well with plain water
  - Comb out nits

Providing Support: Education and Support Measures to Consider

For all types of infestations, provide information on the following topics:

- Diagnosis
- Treatment plan options: Medication instructions

- Head and pubic lice
  - Vacuum carpets and upholstered furniture
  - Wash bedding, clothes, towels, and sleepwear in hot water
  - For items that cannot be laundered:
    - ◆ Dry cleaning *or*
    - ◆ Store in a sealed plastic bag for 2 weeks *or*
    - ◆ Place in a hot dryer (140 °F) *or*
    - ◆ Place in a freezer
  - Follow the complete treatment regimen to completely eradicate the infestation
  - Disinfect combs and brushes in alcohol or hot water at more than 131 °F (head lice)
- Prevention methods
  - Do not share combs, hats, scarves, hair pieces, bedding, or clothing (head lice)
  - Abstain from sexual activity until both partners have been treated (pubic lice)
  - Do not accept used mattresses (body lice)
- Treatment failure due to repeated exposure or lack of complete treatment regimen

Follow-up Care: Follow-up Measures to Consider

- Document
  - Clinical findings and diagnosis
  - Discussions with the client on medication use
  - Treatment plan
  - Signs and symptoms of secondary infection due to scratching

Multidisciplinary Practice: Consider Consultation, Collaboration, or Referral

- Medical services: Usually not needed
- For diagnosis or treatment outside the midwife's scope of practice

CARE OF THE WOMAN WITH FUNGAL INFECTIONS

Key Clinical Information

Superficial fungus infections of the skin are common in all age groups. Dermatophytes are fungi that invade and infect the skin, hair, and nails. These infections are commonly known as ringworm (though no worm is involved), athlete's foot, and jock itch. Dermatophyte skin infections are considered contagious. These infections can be spread between individuals if direct skin-to-skin contact is made with the rash or if skin contact is made with the hands of an individual who has been scratching the fungal skin rash. Direct contact with a contaminated item can also spread the fungus. While athlete's foot can be passed from person to person, it is not always contagious. Athlete's foot may present as a rash on one or both feet and can involve the hands. A "two feet and one palm" presentation is a very common presentation of athlete's foot, especially in men (Butarro et al., 2007). Nail fungus can be transmitted from person to person but is more often spread by shared use of contaminated nail care tools.

Tinea versicolor is a common fungal infection that often affects adolescents and young adults. With this condition, the skin changes color, becoming either lighter or darker than the surrounding skin. The areas most commonly affected are the shoulders, back, and chest (Butarro et al., 2007).

For some individuals, dermatophyte skin and nail infections are quite persistent. Poor response is often a result of the challenges inherent in adherence to long-term therapy; fungal infections in commonly covered areas, such as the feet, are also more resistant to cure. Women should be instructed in the importance of consistent and complete therapy to eradicate skin fungal infections.

Client History and Chart Review: Components of the History to Consider

- Age
- Location of symptoms
- Onset, duration, and characteristics of symptoms
  - Pruritus
  - Rash
  - Fissures
  - Scaling
- Risk factors associated with dermatophyte infestation
  - Compromised immune system

- Use of communal gym or pool facilities
- Contact with individuals with fungal infection
- Contact with infected farm or stray animals

Physical Examination: Components of the Physical Exam to Consider

- Tinea pedis
  - Examine the feet and between the toes
  - Look for scaling, fissures, and maceration
- Tinea manuum
  - Usually affects the dominant hand
  - Scaling, papules, and clustered vesicles
  - When the hand is affected, feet are usually affected
- Tinea corporis
  - Examine the trunk and extremities
  - Well-defined round lesions
  - Red, raised lesions with occasional blisters
  - Lesions may coalesce
- Tinea capitis
  - Loss of hair
  - Flaking and scaling on the scalp
- Tinea unguium
  - Spreads under the nails
  - Brown or yellowish discoloration of nails
  - Nail thickening
- Tinea versicolor
  - Trunk, arms, and neck
  - Scaly hypo- or hyper-pigmented areas

Clinical Impression: Differential Diagnoses to Consider

(ICD9Data.com, 2012)

- Dermatophytosis
- Unspecified local infection of skin and subcutaneous tissue

Diagnostic Testing: Diagnostic Tests and Procedures to Consider

- Diagnosis is primarily by clinical assessment
- To confirm diagnosis
  - KOH exam
  - Woods lamp

- Skin biopsy
- Skin culture

Providing Treatment: Therapeutic Measures to Consider

(Medline Plus, 2011)

- Tinea pedis
  - OTC antifungal cream
    - Clotrimazole (Lotrimin)
    - Miconazole (Donistat-Derm)
    - Ketoconazole (Nizoral cream)
    - Terbinafine (Lamisil)
  - Terbinafine spray (Lamisil AT)
  - OTC medicated foot powder
  - Oral griseofulvin or fluconazole for resistant cases: 4- to 8-week course for foot infections
- Tinea manuum
  - OTC antifungal cream
    - Clotrimazole (Lotrimin)
    - Miconazole (Donistat-Derm)
    - Ketoconazole (Nizoral cream)
    - Terbinafine (Lamisil)
  - Terbinafine spray (Lamisil AT)
  - Oral griseofulvin or fluconazole for resistant cases: 2- to 4-week course for skin infections
- Tinea corporis
  - OTC antifungal cream
    - Clotrimazole (Lotrimin)
    - Miconazole (Donistat-Derm)
    - Ketoconazole (Nizoral cream)
    - Terbinafine (Lamisil)
  - Terbinafine spray (Lamisil AT): Use for at least 2 weeks
  - Oral griseofulvin, ketoconazole, or fluconazole for resistant cases: Use for at least 2 weeks
- Tinea capitis
  - Oral griseofulvin (Fulvin PG): 4- to 6-week course for scalp infections
  - Medicated shampoo
- Tinea unguium
  - Topical preparations are not effective

- Oral antifungals are the mainstay of therapy: Terbinafine (Lamisil) 250 mg once daily
  - 6- to 8-week course for fingernail fungus
  - 12 weeks for toenail fungus
- Tinea versicolor
  - OTC body wash or cream with ketoconazole (Nizoral): BID for 10–14 days
  - Topical application of 1% selenium sulfide shampoo (Selsun Blue): Twice weekly for 15 minutes for 2–4 weeks
  - Oral ketoconazole (Nizoral): 200 mg single-dose treatment

Providing Treatment: Complementary and Alternative Measures to Consider

For tinea pedis, tinea manuum, and tinea versicolor, use the following treatments:

- Vinegar soak: 1 part vinegar to 1 part water
- Bleach bath: Add ¼ cup bleach to bath
- Burow's solution soak (Domeboro)

Providing Support: Education and Support Measures to Consider

- Discussions with client
  - Some forms of fungus reoccur easily
  - Tinea corporis can form scarring that lasts up to a year
  - Treatment plan
    - Medication use and length of therapy
    - Wash sheets and nightclothes for tinea corporis
- Preventive measures
  - Keep the skin and feet clean and dry
  - Wear sandals or shoes at gyms, lockers, and pools
  - Avoid touching pets with bald spots
  - Do not share personal care items such as brushes, razors, towels, and headgear

Follow-up Care: Follow-up Measures to Consider

- Document
  - Clinical findings and diagnosis

- Discussions with the client on diagnosis and medication use
- Treatment plan
- Return for continued care: To assess treatment effectiveness

Multidisciplinary Practice: Consider Consultation, Collaboration, or Referral

- Dermatology services
  - Severe infections resistant to treatment
  - Infections resistant to treatment
- For diagnosis or treatment outside the midwife's scope of practice

CARE OF THE WOMAN WITH LYME DISEASE

Key Clinical Information

Lyme disease is caused by a bacterium carried by certain types of ticks. Deer ticks can be so small that they are difficult to see, and most people with Lyme disease never see a tick on their body. Symptoms of early Lyme disease mimic those of the flu; consequently, they may not be recognized. Symptoms can wax and wane over time, and if untreated, Lyme disease can spread to the brain, heart, and joints. The initial symptom, seen in approximately 70% to 80% of persons infected with the bacterium, is a circular red rash (erythema migrans) with a white center that looks like a "bull's eye" (Bhate & Schwartz, 2011). The rash appears, on average, in 7 days at the site of a tick bite but can appear anytime within 3 to 30 days of exposure. Lyme disease acquired during pregnancy presents a small, yet serious risk of transplacental infection resulting in possible stillbirth; however, when the mother receives appropriate early antibiotic treatment, excellent perinatal outcomes are obtained (CDC, 2011b). Rapid and full recovery is expected in those persons treated with antibiotics in the early stages of Lyme disease. Approximately 10% to 20% of patients, particularly those who were diagnosed with Stage II disease, may have persistent or recurrent symptoms after antibiotic therapy and are considered to have "post-treatment Lyme disease syndrome" (PTLDS) (Bhate & Schwartz, 2011).

Client History and Chart Review: Components of the History to Consider

(University of Maryland Medical Center, 2011b)

- Age
- Recent activities with potential tick exposure
  - Gardening
  - Hiking
  - Walking in high grasses
  - Contact with animals
- Geographic distribution
  - Northeastern states
  - Upper Midwestern states
- Onset and duration of symptoms
  - Rash presents 3–30 days after a tick bite
  - Rash expands over a period of several days
- Symptoms in Stage I: Primary Lyme disease
  - Flu-like symptoms
  - Fever or chills
  - General malaise
  - Headache
  - Muscle pain
  - Stiff neck
- Symptoms in Stage II: Secondary Lyme disease
  - May occur days to weeks after the tick bite
  - Severe fatigue and malaise
  - Additional erythema migrans lesions may appear
  - Dizziness
  - Palpitations
  - Muscle and joint pain
  - Headache
  - Stiff neck
- Symptoms in Stage III: Tertiary Lyme disease
  - May occur months to years after the tick bite
  - Symptoms of Stage II as noted previously
  - Additional symptoms
    - Muscle weakness
    - Numbness and tingling
    - Joint swelling
    - Facial paralysis
    - Pain

◆ Speech difficulty

◆ Cognitive decline

◆ Unusual or strange behavior

◆ Visual problems

◆ Sleep disorders

Physical Examination: Components of the Physical Exam to Consider

- Circumscribed erythema migrans: "Bull's eye" lesion of 3–15 cm at the site of the tick bite
  - Flat or slightly raised red spot
  - May have a clear area in the center
  - Additional lesions may appear on the body as the disease progresses
- Presence of Bell's palsy
- Assessment of neck and joints
  - Swelling
  - Pain
  - Range of motion
- Neurologic assessment

Clinical Impression: Differential Diagnoses to Consider

(ICD9Data.com, 2012)

- Lyme disease

Diagnostic Testing: Diagnostic Tests and Procedures to Consider

- Two-tiered testing is recommended (see Figure 8-2).

Providing Treatment: Therapeutic Measures to Consider

With an early diagnosis of Lyme disease, the following treatments are used:

- Amoxicillin: 500 mg PO TID for 14–21 days (full 21 days for pregnancy)
- Doxycycline: 100 mg PO BID for 10–21 days (not for use in pregnancy)
- Cefuroxime axetil: 500 mg PO BID for 14–21 days

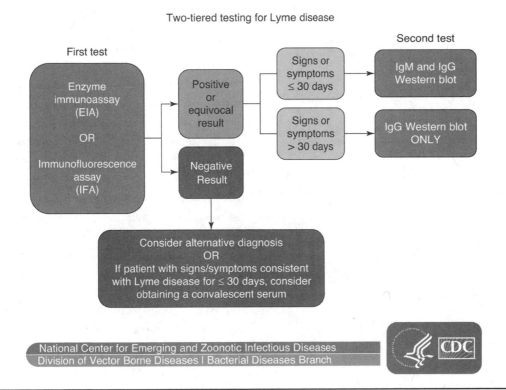

Figure 8-2 Two-Tiered Testing for Lyme Disease

Source: Centers for Disease Control and Prevention.

Providing Treatment: Complementary and Alternative Measures to Consider

(University of Maryland, 2011b)

⚠️ Complementary therapies are used as an adjunct to medical therapy to treat symptoms and prevent adverse effects of medical therapy.

- Probiotic therapy to counteract the effects of antibiotics on the gut
- Herbs
  - Cat's claw for anti-inflammatory and antibacterial effects
  - Green tea for antioxidant and anti-inflammatory effects
  - Garlic for antibacterial effects and immune support
- Homeopathy based on constitutional symptoms

Providing Support: Education and Support Measures to Consider

- Discussions with the client
  - Diagnosis: Reassure the client of the likelihood of full recovery with antibiotic treatment
  - Treatment plan: Medication regimen
- Prevention
  - Visual inspection of the skin after outdoor activity
  - Protective clothing
    - Long-sleeved shirt
    - Long pants tucked into socks
    - Light-colored clothes to contrast with ticks
  - Tick and insect repellants
    - DEET
    - Repellants for pets
  - Tick removal with fine-tipped tweezers; disinfect the site with alcohol

Follow-up Care: Follow-up Measures to Consider

- Document
  - Clinical findings and diagnosis
  - Discussions with the client on medication use
  - Treatment plan

- Return for continued care: To assess treatment effectiveness

Multidisciplinary Practice: Consider Consultation, Collaboration, or Referral

- Refer for evaluation and treatment
  - Neurologic symptoms present
  - Evidence of Stage II or III disease
  - Diagnostic uncertainty
- For diagnosis or treatment outside the midwife's scope of practice

CARE OF THE WOMAN WITH PSORIASIS

Key Clinical Information

Psoriasis is a chronic immune-mediated skin disorder that causes skin redness, scaling, and irritation. Psoriasis can show up anywhere—on the eyelids, ears, mouth and lips, skin folds, hands and feet, or nails. The skin at each of these sites is different and often requires different treatment. Approximately 80% of those persons presenting with psoriasis have mild to moderate psoriasis, with the plaque type being the most common form (National Psoriasis Foundation, 2012). Many cases of mild psoriasis can be managed successfully with intermittent or long-term use of topical agents. Some women see an improvement in the severity of their psoriasis during pregnancy, whereas others report their psoriasis gets worse during this period. Treatment of mild psoriasis during pregnancy with low-strength topical corticosteroids is considered acceptable, although all corticosteroid medications are classified into Pregnancy Category C and should be used only if necessary.

The etiology of this disorder is thought to involve a combination of genetic factors and exposure to external triggers, which vary from person to person. Stress is considered to be a common trigger. The condition comes and goes in cycles of remissions and flare-ups over a lifetime. As many as 30% of people with psoriasis also develop psoriatic arthritis, which causes pain, stiffness, and swelling in and around the joints (National Psoriasis Foundation, 2012). Psoriasis is an uncomfortable and at times disfiguring skin disease, which can be difficult and frustrating to treat.

Client History and Chart Review: Components of the History to Consider

- Age
- Family history of psoriasis
- Onset and duration of symptoms
  - Severe pruritus
  - Dry, flaking skin
  - Severe dandruff
  - Associated symptoms
    - Joint pain
    - Joint swelling
- Location of symptoms
- Medication history
  - Lithium
  - Antimalaria drugs
  - Inderal
  - Quinidine
  - Indomethacin
- Recent illness: May trigger guttate psoriasis
- Recent stress
- Recent skin injury: Vaccinations, sunburn, or scratches
  - Can trigger Koebner phenomena, which is the formation of psoriasis plaques along a site of injury
- Effect of condition on mental health and self-image

Physical Examination: Components of the Physical Exam to Consider

- Vital signs, including BMI
- Affect, posture, and evidence of self-care
- Plaque type (most common)
  - Red, raised, inflamed lesions
  - May have overlying loose, silver-colored scale
  - May crack and bleed
  - Typically found on the knees, elbows, scalp, back, hands, and feet
- Guttate (Latin for "teardrop")
  - Small red papules (1–2 cm)

- Primarily seen on the trunk
- Can occur suddenly
- Erythrodermic
  - Generalized intense erythema
  - Affects most of the body surface
- Pustular
  - Sterile white blister pustules (2–3 mm)
  - Pustules coalesce, then desquamate
- Evaluation of joints
  - Warmth, redness, pain, and swelling
  - Distal joints are most often affected

Clinical Impression: Differential Diagnoses to Consider

(ICD9Data.com, 2012)

- Psoriasis

Diagnostic Testing: Diagnostic Tests and Procedures to Consider

The diagnosis is made by clinical assessment and exclusion of other causes.

Providing Treatment: Therapeutic Measures to Consider

(Menter et al., 2009)

- Treatment depends on the type and severity of disease
- Mild psoriasis
  - Less than 3% of the body is affected
  - Topical corticosteroids of the lowest to medium potency (see Table 8-4)
    - Applied 1–2 times daily for 2–4 weeks
    - Taper to maintenance dosing once or twice a week
  - OTC salicylic acid cream
    - Reduces scaling
    - Do not use concurrently with systemic salicylic acid
- Moderate psoriasis
  - 3–10% of the body is affected
  - Topical corticosteroids
  - Phototherapy

- Severe psoriasis
  - More than 10% of the body is affected
  - Oral medications per dermatology

Providing Treatment: Complementary and Alternative Measures to Consider

- Omega-3 fish oil supplements: 300–1000 mg daily
- Stress reduction techniques
  - Can be very effective in reducing outbreaks
  - Yoga, medication, biofeedback, and deep breathing
  - Avoid consumption of members of the nightshade family (e.g., tomatoes, potatoes, eggplant)
  - Eliminate red meats, processed foods, and refined carbohydrates from the diet
- Medical nutrition therapy (Brown et al., 2004)
  - Diet high in fresh fruits and vegetables, as well as whole grains
  - Scant fish, fowl, and dairy consumption
  - Olive oil
  - Nuts

Providing Support: Education and Support Measures to Consider

- Provide information
  - Working diagnosis: Recommended relief measures
  - Treatment plan options
    - Medication instructions
    - Strategies to prevent flare-ups
    - Signs and symptoms of worsening disease
- Skin care
  - Heavy moisturizer (e.g., Cutemol) applied several times daily
  - Avoid use of skin products with alcohol, deodorant soaps, and strong detergents
  - Wear soft clothing to reduce skin irritation
  - Avoid scratching and picking
- Daily baths for symptom relief
  - Colloidal oatmeal
  - Epsom or Dead Sea salt
  - Soak for 15 minutes

- Moderate ultraviolet light exposure
  - 2–3 times per week
  - Sun or artificial light
  - Use sunscreen in nonaffected areas
- Avoid triggers
  - Smoking
  - Alcohol
  - Stress

Follow-up Care: Follow-up Measures to Consider

- Document
  - Clinical findings
  - Discussions with the client
    - Diagnosis
    - Skin care
    - Preventive measures
- Return for continued care to assess efficacy

Multidisciplinary Practice: Consider Consultation, Collaboration, or Referral

- Dermatology services
  - Treatment of moderate to severe psoriasis
  - Arthritic symptoms
  - Mild psoriasis that does not respond to treatment
- Stress management
- For diagnosis or treatment outside the midwife's scope of practice

CARE OF THE WOMAN WITH ROSACEA

Key Clinical Information

Rosacea is a common skin disorder, sometimes called "adult acne," that is characterized by red facial patches with small pimples, typically occurring around the nose, cheeks, mouth, and forehead. Small blood vessels called telangiectasias may also appear in the affected areas. Rosacea can cause increased skin sensitivity and burning with application of creams or sunscreen. The etiology of this disorder is not known, but it can be exacerbated by things that cause vasodilatation, such as sun and wind exposure, hot weather, stress, and alcohol. Rosacea is a chronic condition that can lead to permanent changes in facial appearance and can cause an individual stress and embarrassment in social situations. It can be successfully managed by medications and lifestyle changes to avoid known triggers, which vary from person to person (Goldgar, Keahey, & Houchins, 2009).

Client History and Chart Review: Components of the History to Consider

- Age
- Onset and duration of symptoms
  - Blush easily
  - Skin sensitivity
  - Pimples
  - Eye irritation
    - Dryness
    - Gritty feeling
    - Unable to tolerate contact lenses
- Family history of rosacea
- Personal history of migraines: Vasodilation may be a common link (F. Powell, 2005)

Physical Examination: Components of the Physical Exam to Consider

- Red rash on the face
  - Butterfly pattern across the nose and cheeks
  - Small, thin blood vessels
  - Red pimples
- Assessment of eyes
  - Eyelid swelling
  - Redness
  - Tearing

Clinical Impression: Differential Diagnoses to Consider

(ICD9Data.com, 2012)

- Rosacea

Diagnostic Testing: Diagnostic Tests and Procedures to Consider

Diagnosis is made by clinical assessment and exclusion of other causes.

Providing Treatment: Therapeutic Measures to Consider

- For symptoms that include flushing and telangiectasias: Topical ointment or cream antibiotics applied 1–2 times daily
  - Metronidazole (Metrocream)
  - Tretinoin (Renova)
  - Benzoyl peroxide and azelaic acid (Azelex)
  - Alternating antibiotic therapies may improve the client's condition
- For symptoms that include small pimples and pustules
  - Topical ointment or cream antibiotics
  - Oral antibiotics
    - Tetracyline
    - Minocycline
    - Erythromycin
    - Doxycycline: Low-dose Oracea 40 mg once daily
- Eye symptoms: Artificial tears and lubricants QID
- Widespread or severe rosacea
  - Photodynamic therapy
  - Isotretinoin

Providing Treatment: Complementary and Alternative Measures to Consider

- Dilute vinegar soaks daily
  - 1 part vinegar to 6 parts water
  - Natural disinfectant
- Green tea facial soak: Reduces inflammation
- Stress reduction techniques

Providing Support: Education and Support Measures to Consider

- Prevention of flare-ups
  - Keep a log of those conditions that cause flare-ups
  - Avoid known triggers
    - Sun and wind
    - Hot and cold temperatures
    - Stress
    - Spicy foods
    - Alcohol

- ◆ Hot beverages
- ◆ Exercise
- ◆ Skin care products
- Skin care
  - ▪ Wash with a gentle soap (such as Cetaphil)
  - ▪ Avoid facial products containing alcohol
  - ▪ Use products labeled "non-comedogenic"
  - ▪ Protect the face in the winter with a scarf or ski mask
  - ▪ Use a mild sunscreen daily (SPF product 30 or greater)

Follow-up Care: Follow-up Measures to Consider

- Document
  - ▪ Clinical findings
  - ▪ Discussions with the client
    - ◆ Diagnosis
    - ◆ Skin care
    - ◆ Preventive measures
- Return for continued care as needed

Multidisciplinary Practice: Consider Consultation, Collaboration, or Referral

- Dermatology services
  - ▪ Treatment requiring isotretinoin
  - ▪ Severe ocular rosacea symptoms
  - ▪ Rosacea that does not respond to treatment
- For diagnosis or treatment outside the midwife's scope of practice

CARE OF THE WOMAN AT RISK FOR SKIN CANCER

Key Clinical Information

Skin cancer is the most common form of cancer in the United States. Its incidence is increasing in all age groups, including children. Sun exposure is the major cause of skin cancer.

Common forms of skin cancer include basal cell, squamous cell, and melanoma (National Cancer Institute, 2011). Basal and squamous cell cancers are relatively easy to treat. In contrast, malignant melanoma, especially in its later stages, is a serious systemic malignancy that is difficult to treat.

The most common precursor to skin cancer is actinic keratosis (AK), found on areas of the skin receiving the most sun exposure. There are often several AK lesions present at one time. They develop slowly over time and are sometimes felt as rough bumps on the skin surface before they are visible. Women should be instructed to do a full body self-examination for signs and symptoms of potential skin cancer every month and to use strategies to prevent skin cancer, such as use of sunscreen and reducing skin exposure to direct sun (Skin Cancer Foundation, 2011).

Client History and Chart Review: Components of the History to Consider

(American Academy of Dermatology, 2011)

- Age
- Race and ethnicity: Darker skin provides a protective effect
- Fair complexion: Increases the risk of skin cancer
  - ▪ Fair skin that freckles
  - ▪ Sunburns easily
  - ▪ Blue- or green-colored eyes
  - ▪ Red or blond hair
- Use of sun lamps or tanning beds
- Presence of several large or many small skin moles
- Family history of unusual moles
- Family history of melanoma
- Medical history
  - ▪ Prior history of actinic keratosis
  - ▪ Radiation
  - ▪ Weakened immune system
- Recent history
  - ▪ Change in a mole or skin lesion
  - ▪ Slow-healing lesion

Physical Examination: Components of the Physical Exam to Consider

(American Academy of Dermatology, 2011)

- Actinic keratosis (potentially precancerous lesions)
  - ▪ Superficial pink or red scaly patches

- May appear on the face, lips, ears, back of hands, forearms, or neck
- May burn or itch
- Size of a pinhead to a quarter
- Basel cell carcinoma
  - Flat lesion or dome-shaped bump
  - May be covered by small superficial blood vessels
  - Texture may be shiny and translucent
  - Found in body areas with high sun exposure, such as the face, arms, neck, or back of hands
- Squamous cell carcinoma
  - Flat, red, scaly patches
  - Often form a crust
- Melanoma
  - Pigmented lesions
  - Can evolve from a preexisting mole or freckle
  - Color variations: Blue, black, brown, variegated
  - Diameter larger than 6 mm
  - Asymmetry of lesion

Clinical Impression: Differential Diagnoses to Consider

(ICD9Data.com, 2012)

- Skin cancers
- Seborrheic keratosis

Diagnostic Testing: Diagnostic Tests and Procedures to Consider

- Skin biopsy

Providing Treatment: Therapeutic Measures to Consider

- Actinic keratosis
  - Cryotherapy
  - Photodynamic therapy
  - Medication
    - Fluorourical
    - Imiquimod
    - Diclofenac gel

- Cancerous lesions
  - Curettage and desiccation
  - Surgical excision
  - Cryosurgery
  - Radiation

Providing Treatment: Complementary and Alternative Measures to Consider

- None

Providing Support: Education and Support Measures to Consider

(American Academy of Dermatology, 2011)

- Prevention
  - Limit sun exposure, especially from 10 A.M. to 4 P.M.
  - Wear protective clothing such as a long-sleeved shirt and a wide-brimmed hat
  - Use sunscreen daily all year, even when it is cloudy: SPF of 30 or more; higher SPF when outdoors for longer periods
  - Avoid or limit use of tanning beds
  - Investigate asymmetric lesions
- ⚠ ABCDE rules: Signs to report
  - **A**symmetry: One side of mole does not match the other
  - **B**order irregularity: Ragged or notched edges
  - **C**olor: Pigmentation of a mole is not uniform; various shades of brown or black, with red, white, or blue
  - **D**iameter: Larger than 6 mm or the size of a pencil eraser
  - **E**volution
    - Change in size, shape, or color
    - New onset of itching or tenderness
    - New onset of bleeding

Follow-up Care: Follow-up Measures to Consider

- Document
  - Clinical findings
  - Discussions with the client
    - Preventive measures
    - Referral
- Return for continued care as needed

Definitions of Common Dermatologic Terms

Abscess: a lesion that contains pus and extends into the dermis or subcutis

Atrophy: a thinning of the epidermis or dermis

Bulla: a blister

Crust: an accumulation of dried serum, blood, or purulent exudate

Cyst: a sac containing liquid or semisolid material usually in the dermis

Erosion: a loss of epidermis above the basal layer leaving a denuded surface

Excoriation: linear crusts and erosions due to scratching

Keloid: tough, irregularly shaped scar tissue that progressively enlarges

Lichenification: thickening of the epidermis marked by the presence of fine papules

Macule: a circumscribed change in skin color without elevation or depression

Nodule: a palpable solid lesion, greater than 0.5 cm and less than 2 cm in diameter

Papule: a solid elevated lesion usually 0.5 cm or less in diameter

Plaque: a raised lesion that has greater surface area than elevation

Purpura: a nonblanching red or violet color from extravasation of blood into tissue

Pustule: a circumscribed elevated lesion that contains pus

Scale: a heaping up of stratum corneum or keratin

Scar: fibrous tissue replacing normal skin in areas of healing

Sclerosis: a hardening or induration of skin

Telangiectasia: dilated superficial blood vessels

Ulcer: a loss of epidermis and part or all of the dermis, leaving a depressed, moist lesion

Vesicle: an elevated lesion that contains free fluid, 0.5 cm or less in diameter

Wheal (hive): a rounded or flat-topped elevated lesion formed by local dermal edema

Source: Adapted from Drugge, R. J. (1996). Electronic textbook of dermatology. Retrieved from http://telemedicine.org/terms.htm

Multidisciplinary Practice: Consider Consultation, Collaboration, or Referral

- Dermatology for evaluation and treatment
- For diagnosis or treatment outside the midwife's scope of practice

ASSESSMENT OF THE WOMAN WITH ENDOCRINE SYMPTOMS

Key Clinical Information

The endocrine system regulates and affects nearly all body systems. Disruption within the endocrine system may cause a multitude of symptoms that may initially appear to be unrelated. Women are more likely than men to be affected by endocrine disorders; for this reason, the endocrine system and its function must be considered during evaluation of women's health problems. The primary endocrine disorders affecting women are diabetes mellitus and thyroid conditions (Avery & Baum, 2007). Menstrual dysfunction is often the primary presenting complaint that alerts the midwife of an increased likelihood of an endocrine disorder. Additionally, a woman who complains of depression should be evaluated for organic causes, such as thyroid disorders. Other evidence of endocrine disorders includes such changes as unusual hair loss, weight gain or loss, pronounced thirst, an enlarged thyroid, or skin changes. Identification of endocrine disorders typically prompts consultation or referral to an endocrine specialist for definitive diagnosis, formulation of the treatment plan, and, when appropriate, collaborative care (Avery & Baum, 2007).

Client History and Chart Review: Components of the History to Consider

(Avery & Baum, 2007)

- Age
- Menstrual and reproductive history
  - LMP, GP TPAL
    - Potential for pregnancy
    - Method of birth control
    - History of infertility
  - Usual menstrual pattern
    - Cyclic versus noncyclic
    - Prolonged versus brief
    - Heavy versus light or absent
    - Presence of mittelschmerz
    - Change in menses
      - Duration
      - Type of change
      - Associated symptoms
        - Weight gain
        - Hirsutism
        - Galactorrhea
- Recent symptoms
  - Onset, duration, and severity
  - Description
  - Contributing or mitigating factors
  - Self-help measures used and results
  - Effects of the symptoms on the client
- Medical/surgical history
  - Allergies
  - Current medications, especially drugs affecting thyroid function or TSH levels
    - Glucocorticoids
    - Dopamine and dopamine antagonists
    - Phenytoin
    - Octreotide
    - Amiodarone
  - Chronic conditions
  - Surgeries
  - Illness or disorders
- Family history
  - Chronic and acute conditions
  - Diabetes or other endocrine disorders
- Social history
  - Nutrition and activity patterns
    - Use of iodized salt
    - Changes in energy level
    - Sleep patterns
  - Life stresses
    - Living situation
    - Drug or alcohol use
    - Domestic violence
- Symptoms of endocrine disorders
  - Hypothyroidism
    - Lethargy and malaise
    - Cold intolerance
    - Menorrhagia or amenorrhea
    - Depression, irritability, and apathy
  - Hyperthyroidism
    - Nervousness
    - Anxiety
    - Heat intolerance
    - Diplopia
    - Shortness of breath
    - Weakness
    - Oligomenorrhea
  - Hyperparathyroidism
    - Asymptomatic *or*
    - Vague generalized symptoms
      - Fatigue
      - Anorexia
      - Weakness
      - Arthralgia
      - Polyuria
      - Constipation
      - Nausea and vomiting
      - Mental disturbance

- Hypoparathyroidism
  - Paresthesia of hands, feet, and circumoral area
  - Notable alterations in of mental and emotional status
  - Lethargy
- Hypopituitarism
  - Failure to lactate
  - Symptoms associated with the following problems:
    - Luteinizing hormone (LH) deficiency
    - Follicle-stimulating hormone (FSH) deficiency
    - Thyroid-stimulating hormone (TSH) deficiency
    - Adrenocorticotropic hormone (ACTH) deficiency
- Hyperpituitarism
  - Amenorrhea
  - Galactorrhea
  - Infertility, decreased libido, or vaginal dryness
  - Tumor impingement
    - Headache
    - Visual field changes
- Diabetes mellitus
  - Polydipsia
  - Polyuria
  - Polyphagia
  - Blurred vision
  - Paresthesias
  - Fatigue
  - May be asymptomatic
- Hypofunction of adrenal cortex
  - Fatigue and weakness
  - Anorexia, nausea, and vomiting
  - Abdominal pain, constipation, and diarrhea
  - Salt craving
  - Syncope
  - Personality changes and irritability
- Review of systems

Physical Examination: Components of the Physical Exam to Consider

(Avery & Baum, 2007)

- Complete physical examination, including vital signs
- Hypothyroidism
  - Signs may be subtle
  - Skin changes: Cool, pale, tough, dry skin
  - Head, eyes, ears, nose, and throat (HEENT)
    - Thinning, brittle hair
    - Hoarse, husky voice
    - Thyroid enlargement
  - Circulatory
    - Bradycardia
    - Cardiomyopathy
    - Pericardial effusion
    - Anemia
  - Neurologic: Cerebellar ataxia
- Hyperthyroidism
  - General
    - Tremors
    - Weight loss
    - Brisk reflexes
    - Increased perspiration
  - Skin changes: Warm, moist skin
  - HEENT
    - Exophthalmos
    - Lid lag
    - Thyroid
      - Enlargement: Diffuse and/or nodular
      - Mass
  - Circulatory
    - Thyroid bruit
    - Palpitations
    - Tachycardia
    - Atrial fibrillation
- Hyperparathyroidism
  - Musculoskeletal
    - Arthralgia
    - Osteoporosis
  - Genitourinary
    - Polyuria
    - Renal calculi

- Hypoparathyroidism
  - Typically results from damage to or excision of the parathyroid gland
  - HEENT: Cataract development
  - Neurologic: Increased neuromuscular excitability
    - Muscle cramps
    - Tetany
  - Abnormalities of the skin, hair, teeth, and nails
- Diabetes mellitus
  - General: Obesity or recent weight loss
  - Skin
    - Striae
    - Fungal infections
      - Intertriginous candida
      - Vulvovaginitis
  - Circulatory
    - Diminished peripheral circulation
    - Poor wound healing
  - Elevated blood glucose/inadequate insulin: Fruity odor to the breath (ketoacidosis)
- Hypofunction of the adrenal cortex
  - General
    - Weight loss
    - Personality changes and irritability
  - Skin: Cutaneous and mucosal hyperpigmentation
  - Circulatory
    - Hypotension
    - Syncope
- Hyperfunction of the adrenal cortex
  - General
    - Thick body, thin extremities, and round face
    - Cervicodorsal and supraclavicular fat pads
  - Skin changes
    - Thin fragile skin, easy bruising, and poor wound healing
    - Acne and hirsutism
  - Circulatory: Hypertension
  - Endocrine: Hyperglycemia

Clinical Impression: Differential Diagnoses to Consider

(ICD-9Data.com, 2012)

- Diabetes mellitus
- Menstrual dysfunction
- Thyroid disorders
  - Enlarged thyroid
  - Thyroid nodule or mass
  - Hypothyroidism
  - Hyperthyroidism
- Polycystic ovarian syndrome
- Hypothalamic dysfunction
- Pituitary dysfunction
- Adrenal dysfunction

Diagnostic Testing: Diagnostic Tests and Procedures to Consider

- General testing
  - Urinalysis
  - Chemistry profile
  - Lipid profile
- Thyroid testing: Normal ranges (verify ranges with the laboratory)
  - TSH: 0.45–4.5 mIU/L
  - Free T_4: 0.8–2.0 ng/dL
- For diabetes testing, see "Care of the Woman with Diabetes Mellitus"
- For hyperthyroidism testing, see "Care of the Woman with Hyperthyroidism"
- For hypothyroidism testing, see "Care of the Woman with Hypothyroidism"
- Pituitary insufficiency
  - TSH: Normal or low
  - Free T_4: Low
  - Free T_3: Low or normal
- Parathyroid disorders
  - Abnormal serum calcium, usually found incidentally on chemistry screening
  - Hyperparathyroidism
    - Serum calcium elevated (greater than 10.5 mg/dL)
    - Serum phosphate low (less than 2.5 mg/dL)

◆ Elevated serum parathyroid hormone levels confirm the diagnosis
- Hypoparathyroidism
  ◆ Serum calcium low (less than 8.8 mg/dL)
  ◆ Serum phosphate elevated (greater than 4.5 mg/dL)
  ◆ Low or absent parathyroid hormone levels confirm the diagnosis
- Evaluation of adrenal function: Consider referral for testing and evaluation

Providing Treatment: Therapeutic Measures to Consider

- 📞 Initiation of medical therapies based on the diagnosis
- Maintenance treatment by the midwife in consultation
  - Balanced nutrition
    ◆ Avoid simple carbohydrates
    ◆ Maintain an optimal BMI
  - Adequate rest
  - Regular physical activity
    ◆ Balance activity with nutritional intake
    ◆ Helps regulate blood glucose
- For diabetes, see "Care of the Woman with Diabetes Mellitus"
- For hyperthyroidism, see "Care of the Woman with Hyperthyroidism"
- For hypothyroidism, see "Care of the Woman with Hypothyroidism"

Providing Treatment: Complementary and Alternative Measures to Consider

⚠ Alternative measures may help to restore balance but are not a substitute for medical evaluation and treatment.

- General measures to promote well-being include the following:
  - Emotional support
  - Stress reduction
  - Sea vegetables
    ◆ Trace minerals
    ◆ Iodine

Providing Support: Education and Support Measures to Consider

- Provide information about the diagnosis
  - Potential effects
    ◆ On the client and her family
    ◆ On the client's reproductive capacity
  - Testing recommendations
  - Signs and symptoms indicating a need to return for care
  - Recommended follow-up
  - Local resources
- Listen to and address the client's concerns

Follow-up Care: Follow-up Measures to Consider

- Document
  - Diagnosis
  - Criteria for consultation
  - Individualized plan of care
    ◆ Follow-up testing: Type and frequency
    ◆ Medications: Type, dose, and titration parameters
    ◆ Physician notification parameters
- Return for continued care as indicated
  - Support
  - Reproductive or women's health care
  - Ongoing surveillance of endocrine disorders
  - Care of selected problems in a medically stable client

Multidisciplinary Practice: Consider Consultation, Collaboration, or Referral

- Medical or endocrinology services
  - Clients with evidence of endocrine dysfunction
    ◆ Relevant workup
    ◆ Initiation of treatment
      ➤ Develop management recommendations
      ➤ 🔖 Delineate individualized best care parameters through a clear management plan
      ➤ Delegate ongoing and follow-up care

- ◆ Collaborative care of endocrine disorders
- ◆ Ongoing care of endocrine disorders
  - ▪ Clients with a confusing presentation
- Reproductive endocrinology services: Endocrine-related infertility
- Social support services: Support groups
  - ▪ Diabetes
  - ▪ Infertility
- For diagnosis or treatment outside the midwife's scope of practice

CARE OF THE WOMAN WITH DIABETES MELLITUS

Key Clinical Information

Diabetes refers to a group of metabolic disorders resulting in hyperglycemia from inadequate insulin production and secretion, inadequate response to insulin, or a combination of these mechanisms (American Diabetes Association [ADA], 2011a). The four types of diabetes are classified based on their etiology:

- *Type 1 diabetes* is characterized by an autoimmune destruction of the pancreatic beta cells resulting in an inability to produce or secrete insulin and affects 5% to 10% of individuals with diabetes.
- *Type 2 diabetes* pathology includes insulin resistance and a relative lack of insulin and affects 90–95% of those with diabetes.
- *"Other"* includes specific types of diabetes that are not classified as type 1 or type 2; these types result from genetic disorders, infections, drugs, and chemicals. This category represents an uncommon but important subset of individuals diagnosed with diabetes.
- *Gestational diabetes.* (See "Care of the Pregnant Woman with Gestational Diabetes.")

Midwives play a role in the diagnosis and referral of women for management of diabetes. Midwives may also be involved in pregnancy and childbirth care, women's primary health care and screening, and contraceptive management of diabetic women.

Client History and Chart Review: Components of the History to Consider

(ADA, 2011b; Avery & Baum, 2007)

- Age
- Menstrual and reproductive history
  - ▪ LMP, GP TPAL
  - ▪ Potential for pregnancy
  - ▪ Method of birth control
  - ▪ History of infertility
  - ▪ Usual menstrual pattern
  - ▪ Associated symptoms
  - ▪ Weight gain
- Symptoms of diabetes mellitus
  - ▪ Polydipsia
  - ▪ Polyuria
  - ▪ Polyphagia
  - ▪ Weight loss
  - ▪ Blurred vision
  - ▪ Paresthesias
  - ▪ Fatigue
  - ▪ May be asymptomatic
- Medical/surgical history
  - ▪ Allergies
  - ▪ Current medications
  - ▪ Chronic conditions
  - ▪ Surgeries
  - ▪ Illness or disorders
- History of diabetes, if previously diagnosed
  - ▪ Self-management and response
  - ▪ Awareness of hyperglycemic and hypoglycemic episodes
- Family history
  - ▪ Chronic and acute conditions
  - ▪ Diabetes and other endocrine disorders
- Social history
  - ▪ Eating patterns
  - ▪ Physical activity patterns
  - ▪ Changes in energy level
  - ▪ Sleep patterns
  - ▪ Life stresses
  - ▪ Living situation
  - ▪ Drug or alcohol use
  - ▪ Domestic violence

- Women at risk for type 2 diabetes
  - Overweight/obesity (BMI greater than or equal to 25) with one or more additional risk factors
  - Physical inactivity
  - First-degree relative with diabetes
  - High-risk race/ethnicity
    - African American
    - Latino
    - Native American
    - Asian American
    - Pacific Islander
  - Hypertension (greater than or equal to 140/90 mm Hg) or on hypertensive medications
  - HDL cholesterol less than or equal to 35 mg/dL (0.90 mmol/L)
  - Triglyceride greater than or equal to 250 mg/dL (2.82 mmol/L)
  - Hemoglobin A_{1c} greater than or equal to 5.7% on previous testing
  - Impaired glucose tolerance (IGT) or impaired fasting glucose on previous testing
  - History of giving birth to a baby weighing more than 9 lb
  - History of gestational diabetes mellitus (GDM)
  - Polycystic ovarian syndrome (PCOS)
  - Age 45 or older
- Review of systems

Physical Examination: Components of the Physical Exam to Consider

(ADA, 2011b)

- Signs of diabetes mellitus
  - General
    - Obesity or recent weight loss
    - Fruity odor to the breath (ketoacidosis)
  - Skin
    - Striae
    - Fungal infections
    - Intertriginous candida

  - Circulatory
    - Diminished peripheral circulation
    - Poor wound healing
  - Vulvovaginitis, including frequent candiasis
- Physical examination for the woman with diabetes, including vital signs
  - Height, weight, and BMI
  - Blood pressure
  - Fundoscopic examination
  - Thyroid palpation
  - Skin inspection
    - For acanthosis nigricans
    - Insulin injection sites
  - Comprehensive foot examination
    - Inspection
    - Palpation of dorsalis pedis and posterior tibial pulses
    - Patellar and Achilles reflexes
    - Sensation and proprioception

Diagnostic Testing: Diagnostic Tests and Procedures to Consider

Screening and diagnostic testing are essentially the same in diabetes; see Table 8-5 (ADA, 2011b). Laboratory evaluation for the diabetic woman includes the following tests:

- Hemoglobin A_{1c}, every 3 months
- Fasting lipid profile

Table 8-5 Diagnostic Criteria for Diabetes

LABORATORY TEST	CRITICAL VALUE
Hemoglobin A_{1c}	Greater than or equal to 6.5%
Fasting plasma glucose (FPG)	Greater than or equal to 126 mg/dL (7.0 mmol/L)
Two-hour plasma glucose in a 75-g oral glucose tolerance test	Greater than or equal to 200 mg/dL (11.1 mmol/L)
Random plasma glucose	Greater than or equal to 200 mg/dL (11.1 mmol/L)

Source: ADA, 2011b.

- Liver function tests
- Urine albumin-to-creatinine ratio
- Serum creatinine and calculated glomerular filtration rate
- Thyroid-stimulating hormone

Clinical Impression: Differential Diagnoses to Consider

(ICD-9Data.com, 2012)

- Diabetes mellitus—specify by type

Providing Treatment: Therapeutic Measures to Consider

- Initiation of medical therapies based on the diagnosis by the consultant medical service
- Maintenance by the midwife in consultation
  - Balanced nutrition
    - Avoid simple carbohydrates
    - Maintain an optimal BMI
  - Adequate rest
  - Regular physical activity
    - Balance activity with nutritional intake
    - Helps regulate blood glucose
- Type 2 diabetes (ADA, 2011b; King & Brucker, 2011)
  - Individual and group diet and exercise therapy
  - Oral drug therapy (King & Brucker, 2011)
    - Sulfonylureas, such as glyburide (Micronase)
    - Biguanides, such as metformin (Glucophage)
    - Alpha-glucosidase inhibitors, such as acarbose (Precose)
    - Meglitinides, such as nateglinide (Starlix)
    - Thiazolidinediones, such as pioglitazone (Actos)
    - DPP-4 inhibitors, such as sitaglipin phosphate (Januvia)
  - Injectable drug therapy
    - Incretin mimetics, such as exanatide (Byetta)
    - Insulin therapy

Providing Treatment: Complementary and Alternative Measures to Consider

⚠ Alternative measures may help to restore balance but are not a substitute for medical evaluation and treatment.

- Dietary supplements include the following options:
  - Bilberry
    - Lowers blood sugar
    - Lowers blood pressure
    - Improves microcirculation
  - Blue-green algae
  - Chromium
  - Cinnamon ¼–½ tsp daily (Hlebowicz, Darwiche, Björgell, & Almér, 2007)
    - Delays gastric emptying
    - Lowers blood glucose

Providing Support: Education and Support Measures to Consider

- Provide information about the diagnosis
  - Potential effects
    - On the client and her family
    - Family planning concerns
  - Testing recommendations: Glycemic goals; see Table 8-6
  - Signs and symptoms indicating a need to return for care
  - Recommended follow-up
  - Local resources

Table 8-6 Glycemic Goals for Most Nonpregnant Adults with Diabetes

LABORATORY TEST	CRITICAL VALUE
Hemoglobin A$_{1c}$	Less than 7.0%
Preprandial capillary plasma glucose	70–130 mg/dL (3.9–7.2 mmol/L)
Peak postprandial capillary plasma glucose	Less than 180 mg/dL (10.0 mmol/L)

Source: ADA, 2011b.

- Discuss and arrange referrals to various providers; see the "Multidisciplinary Practice" section
- Review the importance of diet and exercise
- Review the importance of self-monitoring of blood glucose
- Listen to and address the client's concerns

Follow-up Care: Follow-up Measures to Consider

- Document
  - Diagnosis
  - Criteria for consultation
  - Individualized plan of care
    - ◆ Follow-up testing: Type and frequency
    - ◆ Medications: Type, dose, and titration parameters
    - ◆ Physician notification parameters
- Return for continued care as indicated
  - Support
  - Reproductive health care or women's health care: Need for preconception care when pregnancy is planned
  - Ongoing surveillance of endocrine disorders
  - Care of selected problems in the medically stable client

Multidisciplinary Practice: Consider Consultation, Collaboration, or Referral

Care of women with diabetes is best formulated through a therapeutic alliance of the healthcare team.

- Medical or endocrinology services
  - Clients with a new diagnosis of diabetes
    - ◆ Relevant workup
    - ◆ Initiation of treatment
      - ➤ Develop management recommendations
      - ➤ Delineate individualized best care parameters
      - ➤ Delegate ongoing and follow-up care
    - ◆ Collaborative care of diabetes and other aspects of health care
  - Clients for ongoing management of diabetes

- Registered dietician for medical nutrition therapy (MNT)
- Diabetes educator for diabetes self-management education
- Dental examination
- Ophthalmology: Annual dilated eye exam
- Mental health services as needed
- Social support services
  - Diabetic support group
  - Weight-loss support group
- For diagnosis or treatment outside the midwife's scope of practice

CARE OF THE WOMAN WITH HYPERTHYROIDISM

Key Clinical Information

Hyperthyroidism refers to a group of disorders that result in elevations of free thyroxine (T_4), triiodothyronine (T_3), or both, and abnormally low levels of thyroid-stimulating hormone (TSH). Hyperthyroidism is twice as likely to occur in women as in men, with a prevalence of 2% in women. The most common disorder leading to hyperthyroidism is Graves' disease, an autoimmune disorder also known as diffuse toxic goiter. Graves' disease accounts for 60% to 80% of individuals with hyperthyroidism. Hyperthyroidism can be overt, subclinical, or transient. Of particular interest to midwives are two pregnancy-related hyperthyroid conditions: transient hyperthyroidism of hyperemesis gravidarum (THHG) and postpartum hyperthyroidism. Both of these conditions are usually mild and often self-limiting without specific treatment. Thyrotoxicosis or thyroid storm is a hypermetabolic state resulting from extreme increases in thyroid hormone levels and constitutes a medical emergency. Women with a new diagnosis of hyperthyroidism should be referred to an endocrinologist for evaluation and management (Avery & Baum, 2007).

Client History and Chart Review: Components of the History to Consider

(Avery & Baum, 2007)

- Age
- Menstrual and reproductive history
  - LMP, GP TPAL
    - Potential for pregnancy
    - Method of birth control
    - History of infertility
  - Usual menstrual pattern
    - Cyclic versus noncyclic
    - Prolonged versus brief
    - Heavy versus light or absent
    - Presence of mittelschmerz
    - Change in menses
      - ➤ Duration
      - ➤ Type of change
      - ➤ Associated symptoms
        - ◗ Weight gain
        - ◗ Hirsutism
        - ◗ Galactorrhea
- Recent symptoms
  - Onset, duration, and severity
  - Description
  - Contributing or mitigating factors
  - Self-help measures used and their results
  - Effects of symptoms on the client
- Medical/surgical history
  - Allergies
  - Current medications
  - Drugs affecting thyroid function or TSH levels
    - Glucocorticoids
    - Dopamine and dopamine antagonists
    - Phenytoin
    - Octreotide
    - Amiodarone
  - Chronic conditions
  - Surgeries
  - Illness or disorders
- Family history
  - Chronic and acute conditions
  - Endocrine disorders
- Social history
  - Nutrition and activity patterns
    - Use of iodized salt
    - Changes in energy level

- Sleep patterns
  - Life stresses
    - Living situation
    - Drug or alcohol use
    - Domestic violence
- Signs and symptoms of hyperthyroidism
  - Nervousness
  - Anxiety
  - Heat intolerance
  - Diplopia
  - Shortness of breath
  - Weakness
  - Oligomenorrhea
- Review of systems

Physical Examination: Components of the Physical Exam to Consider

- Complete physical examination, including vital signs
- Hyperthyroidism
  - General
    - Tremors
    - Weight loss
    - Brisk reflexes
    - Increased perspiration
  - Skin changes: Warm, moist skin
  - HEENT
    - Exophthalmos
    - Lid lag
  - Thyroid
    - Enlargement: Diffuse and/or nodular
    - Mass
  - Circulatory
    - Thyroid bruit
    - Palpitations
    - Tachycardia
    - Atrial fibrillation

Clinical Impression: Differential Diagnoses to Consider

(ICD-9Data.com, 2012)

- Thyroid disorders: Hyperthyroidism

Diagnostic Testing: Diagnostic Tests and Procedures to Consider

- General testing
  - Urinalysis
  - Chemistry profile
  - Lipid profile
- Thyroid testing
  - Normal ranges (verify ranges with the laboratory)
    - TSH: 0.45–4.5 mIU/L
    - Free T_4: 0.8–2.0 ng/dL
  - Hyperthyroid
    - TSH: Low
    - Free T_4: High to normal
    - T_3: High
  - Additional thyroid tests
    - Thyroid-binding globulin
    - Thyroid antibodies for autoimmune disorders affecting the thyroid
    - Thyroid scan
      - Iodine uptake
      - Radioactive uptake
      - Evaluates for the presence of nodules
      - Indicates the likelihood of malignancy
    - Ultrasound
    - Fine-needle biopsy

Providing Treatment: Therapeutic Measures to Consider

- Initiation of medical therapies based on the diagnosis
- Maintenance by the midwife in consultation
- Hyperthyroid treatments (King & Brucker, 2011)
  - Radioactive iodine
  - Thionamides: Initial doses, titrate to euthyroid
  - Propylthiouracil: 100–150 mg/day PO divided q 8 hr
  - Methimazole: 5–15 mg PO QD
- Surgery
- Symptomatic relief: Beta-adrenergic antagonists, such as atenolol

Providing Treatment: Complementary and Alternative Measures to Consider

⚠ Alternative measures may help to restore balance but are not a substitute for medical evaluation and treatment.

- General measures to promote well-being include the following:
- Emotional support
- Stress reduction
- Sea vegetables
  - Trace minerals
  - Iodine

Providing Support: Education and Support Measures to Consider

- Provide information about the diagnosis
  - Potential effects
    - On the client and her family
    - On the client's reproductive capacity
  - Testing recommendations
  - Signs and symptoms indicating a need to return for care
  - Recommended follow-up
  - Local resources
- Listen to and address the client's concerns

Follow-up Care: Follow-up Measures to Consider

- Document
  - Diagnosis
  - Criteria for consultation
  - Individualized plan of care
    - Follow-up testing: Type and frequency
    - Medications: Type, dose, and titration parameters
    - Physician notification parameters
- Return for continued care as indicated
  - Support
  - Reproductive health care
  - Ongoing surveillance of endocrine disorders
  - Care of selected problems in a medically stable client

Multidisciplinary Practice: Consider Consultation, Collaboration, or Referral

- Medical or endocrinology services
  - Clients with evidence of endocrine dysfunction
    - ◆ Relevant workup
    - ◆ Initiation of treatment
      - ➤ Develop management recommendations
      - ➤ Delineate individualized best care parameters
      - ➤ Delegate ongoing and follow-up care
    - ◆ Collaborative care of endocrine disorders
    - ◆ Ongoing care of endocrine disorders
  - Clients with a confusing presentation
- For diagnosis or treatment outside the midwife's scope of practice

CARE OF THE WOMAN WITH HYPOTHYROIDISM

Key Clinical Information

Hypothyroidism refers to a group of disorders resulting in laboratory findings of low serum free T_4 and elevated thyroid-stimulating hormones. Overt disease is less common but more easily recognized by the clinician (Avery & Baum, 2007). Because the thyroid hormones influence the metabolic processes throughout the body, effects of hypothyroidism are multisystemic and profound; they include significant cardiovascular and neuromuscular risks. Subclinical hypothyroidism (SCH) and/or the presence of thyroid peroxidase antibodies (TPOAb) can be associated with subfertility, infertility, spontaneous abortion, postpartum thyroid dysfunction, depression including postpartum depression, and impaired cognitive and psychomotor child development (Wier & Farley, 2006). The prevalence of hypothyroidism in the United States ranges from 4% to 10% in the adult female population.

Client History and Chart Review: Components of the History to Consider

(Avery & Baum, 2007)

- Age
- Menstrual and reproductive history
  - LMP, GP TPAL
    - ◆ Potential for pregnancy
    - ◆ Method of birth control
    - ◆ History of infertility
  - Usual menstrual pattern
    - ◆ Cyclic versus noncyclic
    - ◆ Prolonged versus brief
    - ◆ Heavy versus light or absent
    - ◆ Presence of mittelschmerz
    - ◆ Change in menses
      - ➤ Duration
      - ➤ Type of change
      - ➤ Associated symptoms
        - ❯ Weight gain
        - ❯ Hirsutism
      - ➤ Galactorrhea
- Recent symptoms
  - Onset, duration, and severity
  - Description
  - Contributing or mitigating factors
  - Self-help measures used and results
  - Effects of symptoms on the client
- Medical/surgical history
  - Allergies
  - Current medications: Drugs affecting thyroid function or TSH levels
    - ◆ Glucocorticoids
    - ◆ Dopamine and dopamine antagonists
    - ◆ Phenytoin
    - ◆ Octreotide
    - ◆ Amiodarone
  - Chronic conditions
  - Surgeries
  - Illness or disorders
- Family history
  - Chronic and acute conditions
  - Endocrine disorders

- Social history
  - Nutrition and activity patterns
    - Use of iodized salt
    - Changes in energy level
    - Sleep patterns
  - Life stresses
    - Living situation
    - Drug or alcohol use
    - Domestic violence
- ▼ Signs and symptoms of hypothyroidism
  - Lethargy and malaise
  - Cold intolerance
  - Weight gain
  - Menorrhagia or amenorrhea
  - Depression, irritability, and apathy
- Review of systems

Physical Examination: Components of the Physical Exam to Consider

- Complete physical examination, including vital signs
- Hypothyroid signs may be subtle
  - Skin changes
    - Cool, pale, tough, dry skin
    - Thinning, brittle hair
  - Head, eyes, ears, nose, and throat
    - Hoarse, husky voice
    - Thyroid enlargement
    - Periorbital edema
  - Cardiovascular system
    - Bradycardia
    - Mild hypertension
    - Narrowed pulse pressure
    - Anemia
  - Neuromuscular
    - Cerebellar ataxia
    - Decline in memory function
    - Visuospatial impairment
    - Carpal tunnel syndrome

Clinical Impression: Differential Diagnoses to Consider

(ICD-9Data.com, 2012)

- Thyroid disorders:
  - Enlarged thyroid
  - Hypothyroid

Diagnostic Testing: Diagnostic Tests and Procedures to Consider

Thyroid testing includes the following measures:

- Normal ranges (verify ranges with the laboratory)
  - TSH: 0.45–4.5 mIU/L
  - Free T_4: 0.8–2.0 ng/dL
- Hypothyroidism: TSH high (greater than 4.5 mIU/L)
  - Repeat in 2 weeks *with*
  - Free T_4 low (less than 0.8 ng/dL)
- Subclinical hypothyroidism
  - Elevated TSH
  - Normal free T_4
- Additional thyroid tests
  - Thyroid-binding globulin
  - Thyroid antibodies for autoimmune disorders of the thyroid
  - Thyroid scan
    - Iodine uptake
    - Radioactive uptake
    - Evaluates for the presence of nodules
    - Indicates the likelihood of malignancy
  - Ultrasound
  - Fine-needle biopsy

Providing Treatment: Therapeutic Measures to Consider

- Initiation of medical therapies based on the diagnosis
- Maintenance by the midwife in consultation
- Hypothyroidism
  - Levothyroxine sodium (Synthroid): 25–50 mg PO daily
  - Titrate to euthyroid based on:
    - Clinical profile
    - Laboratory testing 4 weeks after any dose change

Providing Treatment: Complementary and Alternative Measures to Consider

⚠ Alternative measures may help to restore balance but are not a substitute for medical evaluation and treatment.

- General measures to promote well-being
- Dietary supplements
  - Blue-green algae
  - Sea vegetables
    - Trace minerals
    - Iodine

Providing Support: Education and Support Measures to Consider

- Provide information about the diagnosis
  - Potential effects
    - On the client and her family
    - On the client's reproductive capacity
  - Testing recommendations
  - Signs and symptoms indicating a need to return for care
  - Recommended follow-up
  - Local resources
- Listen to and address the client's concerns

Follow-up Care: Follow-up Measures to Consider

- Document
  - Diagnosis
  - Criteria for consultation
  - Individualized plan of care
    - Follow-up testing: Type and frequency
    - Medications: Type, dose, and titration parameters
    - Physician notification parameters
- Return for continued care as indicated
  - Support
  - Reproductive health care
  - Ongoing surveillance of endocrine disorders
  - Care of selected problems in the medically stable client

Multidisciplinary Practice: Consider Consultation, Collaboration, or Referral

- Medical or endocrinology services
  - Clients with evidence of endocrine dysfunction
    - Relevant workup
    - Initiation of treatment
      - Develop management recommendations
      - Delineate individualized best care parameters
      - Delegate ongoing and follow-up care
    - Collaborative care of endocrine disorders
    - Ongoing care of endocrine disorders
  - Clients with a confusing presentation
- Reproductive endocrinology: Endocrine-related infertility
- Social support services
  - Support groups
  - Infertility
- For diagnosis or treatment outside the midwife's scope of practice

ASSESSMENT OF THE WOMAN WITH GASTROINTESTINAL SYMPTOMS

Key Clinical Information

Problems of the gastrointestinal (GI) tract can range from simple nausea to the presence of obstructing colon cancer. The GI tract plays a role in the immune system, and as such holds a prominent part in women's health and wellness. Inquiry into usual bowel function is an essential component of the client history. GI symptoms can present as a signal of a GI disorder or may be a sign or symptom of an infectious process or of an endocrine, reproductive, or nervous system disorder. Many women react to stress with somatic GI symptoms such as nausea or diarrhea. A woman's social history may reveal psychosocial factors that contribute to her GI disorder. Validation of the woman's concerns is a first step in addressing this very real problem.

Evaluation of the GI system begins with the oral cavity and ends with the anus. Multiple factors, such as poor dentition, poor dietary habits, and alcohol and drug abuse, can contribute to the primary presenting condition. The practice guidelines in this section are divided among the common GI symptoms for which women may present for care.

Client History and Chart Review: Components of the History to Consider

(Angelini, Hodgman, & McConaughey, 2007)

- Age: Reproductive history
  - LMP, GP TPAL
  - Menstrual status
  - Potential for pregnancy
  - Method of birth control
  - Last examination, Pap smear, and sexually transmitted infection testing, as applicable
- Medical history
  - Allergies
  - Current medications
    - Aspirin
    - Nonsteroidal anti-inflammatory drugs (NSAIDs)
    - Oral contraceptive pills
    - Antibiotics
    - Laxatives, fiber, and stool softeners
    - Antidiarrheals
    - Narcotics
    - Cardiac medications
  - Chronic and acute conditions
    - Diverticulitis
    - Gallbladder disease
    - Peptic ulcer disease
    - Diabetes
    - Migraine
    - Hyperthyroidism
- Surgical history
  - Cholecystectomy
  - Oophorectomy
  - Appendectomy
- Symptom profile
  - Type of symptoms
    - Onset, duration, and location
    - Severity and character
    - Timing in relation to meals
    - Associated symptoms
  - Changes in GI/genitourinary function
  - Effects of symptoms on daily living
  - Exacerbating or alleviating factors
  - Self-help measures used and their effectiveness
  - Common GI symptoms
    - Abdominal pain or cramping
    - Bloating
    - Bloody stool or vomitus
    - Constipation
    - Diarrhea
    - Flatus
    - Heartburn or dyspepsia
    - Nausea and vomiting
    - Weight gain or loss
- GI history
  - Usual diet: Recent dietary changes
  - Eating patterns
  - Elimination patterns
  - Pica or food cravings
- Family history
  - Diabetes mellitus
  - Diverticular disease
  - Duodenal ulcers
  - Gallbladder disease: Increased risk in Native Americans
  - Gastroesophageal reflux disorder
  - Colon cancer
- Social history
  - Living situation
  - Food preferences (i.e., spicy, rich, fatty, low fiber)
  - Dietary habits (i.e., timing and amount of meals, social setting for meals)
  - Travel to or habitation in areas with intestinal parasites
  - Use of folk remedies
  - Stressors
  - Drug, alcohol, and tobacco use
  - Support systems
- Review of systems

Physical Examination: Components of the Physical Exam to Consider

(Angelini et al., 2007)

- Vital signs, including height, weight, and BMI
- General physical examination with the focus directed by the client's history
  - Current level of discomfort
  - Observe for evidence of the following conditions:
    - Dehydration
    - Ketoacidosis
    - Malnutrition
    - Alcohol or drug abuse
    - Endocrine dysfunction
- Head, eyes, ears, nose, and throat
  - Examination of mouth and throat
    - Presence and condition of teeth
    - Presence and size of tonsils
    - Ability to swallow
  - Lymph nodes
  - Palpation of thyroid
- Thorax and chest
  - Auscultation of heart and lungs
  - Costovertebral angle tenderness (CVAT)
- Abdominal examination
  - Inspection for shape, symmetry, and pulsations
  - Auscultation for bowel sounds and bruits
  - Percussion
    - Organ margins
    - Masses
    - Ascites
  - Palpation, light and deep
    - Pain
    - Rigidity
    - Involuntary guarding
    - Rebound tenderness
    - Masses
- Bimanual abdominopelvic examination
  - Pain
  - Masses
- Rectal examination
  - Rectovaginal wall

- Appendiceal inflammation
- Anal sphincter tone and patency
- Hemorrhoids
- Masses

Clinical Impression: Differential Diagnoses to Consider

(ICD9Data.com, 2012)

- Gastrointestinal symptoms
  - Abnormal bowel sounds
  - Diarrhea
  - Difficulty swallowing
  - Heartburn
  - Nausea and vomiting
- Upper GI disorders
  - Dyspepsia
  - Gallbladder disease
  - Gastroesophageal reflux disorder
  - Gastroenteritis
  - Hiatal hernia
  - *Helicobacter pylori* infection
  - Lactose intolerance
  - Pancreatitis
  - Peptic ulcer disease
  - Pica
- Lower GI disorders
  - Bowel obstruction
  - Constipation
  - Colitis
  - Diarrhea, functional
  - Diverticular disease
  - Hemorrhoids
  - Hernia, obstructing
  - Intestinal parasites
  - Irritable bowel syndrome
  - Rectal bleeding
- Pregnancy and gynecologic disorders
  - Ectopic pregnancy
  - Endometriosis
  - Ovarian cyst
  - Pelvic inflammatory disease
  - Pregnancy, diagnosis
  - Pregnancy, nausea and vomiting

- Other disorders with GI symptoms
  - Dehydration
  - Endocrine dysfunction
  - Hepatitis
  - GI malfunction from mental factors
  - Malignancy
  - Pyelonephritis
  - Renal calculi
- Abdominal pain, unknown etiology

Diagnostic Testing: Diagnostic Tests and Procedures to Consider

- Testing based on history and examination findings
- Human chorionic gonadotropin (HCG)
- Urinalysis or urine culture
- Wet prep
- Chlamydia and/or gonorrhea cultures
- Complete blood count with peripheral smear
- Erythrocyte sedimentation rate (ESR)
- *H. pylori* testing
- Stool testing
  - Occult blood
  - Ova and parasites
  - Culture
- Liver function testing
- Hepatitis screen
- Amylase and lipase levels
- CA-125/CEA
- Endoscopy
  - Upper endoscopy
  - Sigmoidoscopy
  - Colonoscopy
- Ultrasound
  - Pelvic
  - Gallbladder and pancreas
- Computed tomography or magnetic resonance imaging of the abdomen

Providing Treatment: Therapeutic Measures to Consider

- Treatment is based on the differential diagnosis
- For constipation, see "Care of the Woman with Constipation"

- For diarrhea, see "Care of the Woman with Diarrhea"
- For nausea and vomiting, see "Care of the Woman with Nausea and Vomiting"
- For heartburn, see "Care of the Woman with Heartburn"

Providing Treatment: Alternative Measures to Consider

⚠ Alternative therapies are not a substitute for medical evaluation and treatment of acute symptoms.

- For constipation, see "Care of the Woman with Constipation"
- For diarrhea, see "Care of the Woman with Diarrhea"
- For nausea and vomiting, see "Care of the Woman with Nausea and Vomiting"
- For heartburn, see "Care of the Woman with Heartburn"

Providing Support: Education and Support Measures to Consider

- Dietary recommendations
  - Drink ample fluids
  - Limit caffeine and alcohol intake
  - In case of lactose intolerance:
    - Limit all dairy products
    - Check labels for dairy in packaged products
  - Adequate fiber intake; high-fiber foods
    - Peas, beans, and lentils
    - Fresh and dried fruits
    - Uncooked vegetables
    - Whole-grain breads and cereals
- Physical activity: 20–60 minutes daily
  - Increases endorphins
  - Improves blood flow to the gut
  - Improves bowel function
- Provide information
  - Working diagnosis
  - Testing recommendations
  - Recommended medications and treatment
  - Anticipated results

- Side effects
- Warning signs and symptoms
- Referral criteria and mechanism

Follow-up Care: Follow-up Measures to Consider

- Document
  - Criteria for diagnosis
  - Treatment and follow-up plan
  - Indications for specialty care or consultation
  - Discussion of recommendations with the client
- Return for continued care
  - As indicated by test results
  - For follow-up of chronic problems
  - Five to 10 days with no improvement *or*
  - Sooner with worsening signs or symptoms

Multidisciplinary Practice: Consider Consultation, Collaboration, or Referral

- Emergency services
  - Acute abdomen
  - Intestinal obstruction
- Medical/surgical services: If the following conditions are confirmed or suspected
  - Gallbladder disease
  - Colorectal malignancy
  - GI bleeding
  - For a nonacute GI problem unresponsive to therapy within 7–21 days
- OB/GYN services
  - Ectopic pregnancy
  - Reproductive malignancy
  - Hyperemesis gravidarum
  - Hydatidiform mole
- For diagnosis or treatment outside the midwife's scope of practice

CARE OF THE WOMAN WITH CONSTIPATION

Key Clinical Information

Constipation is defined as the infrequent or difficult evacuation of stool. Straining, incomplete evacuation of stool, abdominal fullness or bloating, and a sensation of obstruction may be present (Angelini et al., 2007; King & Brucker, 2011). The Bristol Stool Scale can be helpful in eliciting a description of the shape and consistency of the stool from the client (Rao et al., 2011). Constipation is more common in women and nonwhite populations. It can range from a transitory symptom that recurs occasionally to an intractable condition associated with severe disease. American diets tend to be deficient in fiber, which is essential to healthy bowel function; fiber deficiency can, in turn, promote constipation.

Client History and Chart Review: Components of the History to Consider

(Angelini et al., 2007)

- Menstrual status
- Pregnancy: See "Care of the Pregnant Woman with Constipation"
- Medical/surgical history
  - Allergies
  - Medications that can affect GI motility
    - Iron supplements
    - NSAIDs
    - Laxatives, fiber, and stool softeners
    - Narcotics
  - Chronic and acute conditions
- Past surgical history: Hysterectomy
- Constipation symptom profile
  - Frequency of stool passage
  - Difficulty with stool passage
  - Characteristics of stool
  - Timing of change in GI/genitourinary function
  - Effects of symptoms on daily living
  - Exacerbating or alleviating factors
  - Self-help measures used and their effectiveness
  - Common symptoms associated with constipation
    - Abdominal pain or cramping
    - Bloating
    - Bloody stool
    - Flatus

- GI history
  - Usual diet
    - Recent dietary changes
    - Fiber content in the diet
    - Intake of fluids
  - Eating patterns
  - Elimination patterns
  - Pica or food cravings
- Review of systems

Bristol Stool Scale: Indication of Gut Transit Time

- Type 1: separate hard lumps (hard to pass)
- Type 2: sausage-shaped, but lumpy
- Type 3: like a sausage, but with cracks on its surface
- Type 4: like a sausage or a snake, smooth and soft
- Type 5: soft blobs with clear-cut edges (passed easily)
- Type 6: fluffy pieces with ragged edges, a mushy stool
- Type 7: watery, no solid pieces, entirely liquid

Source: Rao et al., 2011.

Physical Examination: Components of the Physical Exam to Consider

(Angelini et al., 2007)
- Vital signs, including weight and BMI
- Abdominal examination
  - Inspection for shape, symmetry, and pulsations
  - Auscultation for bowel sounds and bruits
  - Palpation, light and deep
    - Masses, pain
    - Presence of lumpy, hard stools in the bowel
- Rectovaginal examination
  - Rectocele
  - Presence of hard stool in the lower bowel

- Rectal examination
  - Anal reflex "wink" test
  - Tone of sphincter during squeeze and expulsion
  - Hemorrhoids
  - Masses

Clinical Impression: Differential Diagnoses to Consider

(ICD9Data.com, 2012)

- Constipation
- Bowel obstruction
- Diverticular disease
- Hemorrhoids
- Hernia, obstructing
- Rectal bleeding

Diagnostic Testing: Diagnostic Tests and Procedures to Consider

- Complete blood count with peripheral smear
- Serum electrolytes
- Serum calcium
- Thyroid-stimulating hormone
- Stool testing: Occult blood
- Endoscopy
  - Sigmoidoscopy
  - Colonoscopy

Providing Treatment: Therapeutic Measures to Consider

(Angelini et al., 2007; King & Brucker, 2011)
The choice of therapy is based on the underlying cause of the constipation.

- Restoration of intestinal flora
  - Probiotics, such as Florastor
  - Prebiotics, such as oligosaccharides
- Bulk-forming agents: Metamucil, Fiberall, Perdiem
- Non-absorbable sugars: Lactulose
- Emollients: Docusate products, Colace, Pericolace

- Lubricants: Mineral and olive oil products
- Saline laxatives: Magnesium, sodium, or potassium salts
- Stimulants: Aloe, cascara sagrada, danthron, senna
- Hyperosmotics: Glycerin suppositories
- Enemas

Providing Treatment: Alternative Measures to Consider

⚠ Alternative therapies are not a substitute for medical evaluation of acute symptoms.

- Increase consumption of fiber and fluids through the diet
- Cascara sagrada: 10 gtts fluid extract; stimulates bowel function
- Flaxseed meal
  - Increases bulk of the stool
  - Source of omega-3 fatty acids
- Omega-3 supplements
- Senna: Use sparingly; very effective but may cause cramping

Providing Support: Education and Support Measures to Consider

- Dietary recommendations
  - Hydration
  - Drink ample fluid: Limit caffeine and alcohol intake
  - In case of lactose intolerance:
    - ◆ Limit all dairy products
    - ◆ Check labels for dairy in packaged products
  - Fiber intake; high-fiber foods
    - ◆ Peas, beans, and lentils
    - ◆ Fresh and dried fruits
    - ◆ Uncooked vegetables
    - ◆ Whole-grain breads and cereals
- Physical activity: 20–60 minutes daily
  - Increases endorphins
  - Improves blood flow to the gut
  - Improves bowel function

- Bowel retraining
  - Plan time for elimination
  - Most effective after physical activity
  - Consistent time each day

Follow-up Care: Follow-up Measures to Consider

- Document
  - Criteria for diagnosis
  - Treatment and follow-up plan
- Return for continued care
  - Seven to 10 days with no improvement *or*
  - Sooner with worsening signs or symptoms

Multidisciplinary Practice: Consider Consultation, Collaboration, or Referral

- Emergency services
  - Acute abdomen
  - Intestinal obstruction
- Medical/surgical services, when the following conditions are confirmed or suspected:
  - Colorectal malignancy
  - GI bleeding
  - For nonacute GI problem unresponsive to therapy within 7–21 days
- For diagnosis or treatment outside the midwife's scope of practice

CARE OF THE WOMAN WITH DIARRHEA

Key Clinical Information

Diarrhea is the passage of frequent unformed stools of a liquid consistency. It is considered mild if no alterations in daily activities occur, moderate if accommodations in lifestyle are needed, and severe when confinement to home or bed is necessary (Angelini et al., 2007). In approximately 90% of cases, diarrhea is related to a self-limited viral or bacterial infectious process lasting 3 to 5 days. When diarrhea is prolonged over several weeks, the index of suspicion for other disorders, such as celiac disease, lactase disorders, or alcoholism, should be raised (King & Brucker, 2011).

Client History and Chart Review: Components of the History to Consider

(Angelini et al., 2007)

- Medical/surgical history
  - Allergies
  - Current medications
    - NSAIDs
    - Antibiotics
    - Laxative use or abuse
    - Cardiac medications
  - Chronic and acute conditions
    - Celiac disease
    - Lactase disorders
    - Alcoholism
    - Diabetes
    - Inflammatory bowel syndrome
    - Hyperthyroidism
- Diarrhea symptom profile
  - Frequency of stools
  - Onset and duration
  - Severity and character
  - Associated symptoms
  - Effects of symptoms on daily living
  - Self-help measures used and their effectiveness
- Common symptoms associated with diarrhea include
  - Abdominal pain or cramping
  - Bloating
  - Bloody stool
  - Flatus
  - Fever
  - Nausea and vomiting
  - Weight loss
- Dietary history
  - Fluid intake
  - Recent ingestion of potentially contaminated food or water
- Social history
  - Recent exposure to someone with GI illness
  - Drug, alcohol, and tobacco use
  - Recent travel to areas with possible food or water contamination
- Review of systems

Physical Examination: Components of the Physical Exam to Consider

(Angelini et al., 2007)

- Vital signs, including recent weight changes and BMI
- General physical examination with the focus directed by the client's history
  - Current level of discomfort/distress
  - Observe for evidence of the following conditions:
    - Dehydration
    - Weight loss
    - Ketoacidosis
    - Alcohol or drug abuse
    - Endocrine dysfunction
- Abdominal examination
  - Auscultation for bowel sounds and bruits
  - Palpation, light and deep
  - Pain

Clinical Impression: Differential Diagnoses to Consider

(ICD9Data.com, 2012)

- Diarrhea
- Abnormal bowel sounds
- Gastroenteritis
- Lactose intolerance
- Pancreatitis
- Colitis
- Diarrhea, functional
- Irritable bowel syndrome
- Rectal bleeding
- Dehydration
- Endocrine dysfunction

Diagnostic Testing: Diagnostic Tests and Procedures to Consider

- Laboratory testing is not needed for self-limiting diarrhea of 24–48 hours' duration
- Stool testing
  - Occult blood
  - Ova and parasites
  - Culture

Providing Treatment: Therapeutic Measures to Consider

(Angelini et al., 2007; King & Brucker, 2011)

- Diarrhea: Symptomatic treatment
  - Opiates: Paregoric, codeine
  - Absorbents: Polycarbophil
  - Antiperistaltics: Loperamide, diphenoxylate, bismuth subsalicylate
- Traveler's diarrhea: After stool culture results
  - Metronidazole
  - Tinidazole
  - Ciprofloxin
  - Azithromycin
  - Noroxcin
  - Levaquin
  - Floxin
  - Xifaxan
- Irritable bowel syndrome
  - Diarrhea: Imodium or Lotronex
  - Constipation: Fiber supplements, lactulose
  - GI spasm: Tricyclic antidepressants or Zelnorm
  - Depression/anxiety: Antidepressants or anxiolytics
  - Probiotics to restore normal GI flora

Providing Treatment: Complementary and Alternative Measures to Consider

⚠ Alternative therapies are not a substitute for medical evaluation and treatment of acute symptoms.

- Increase dietary fiber to regulate fluid balance in the stool
- Herbs
  - Peppermint
  - Slippery elm
  - Bilberry
- Elimination diets
  - Gluten-free diet
  - Lactose-free diet
  - Food allergies

Providing Support: Education and Support Measures to Consider

- Dietary recommendations: Acute diarrhea
  - Repletion of fluids and electrolytes
    - Drink ample fluids
    - Eat broths, saltines, and bananas
    - Drink sports drinks or electrolyte replacement liquids
    - Limit caffeine and alcohol intake
  - Apple sauce (pectin)
  - Cultured foods (live bacteria)
  - Lactose intolerance and during diarrheal episode
    - Limit all dairy products
    - Check labels for dairy in packaged products
- ▽ Provide information
  - Working diagnosis
  - Recommended medications and treatment
    - Anticipated results
    - Side effects
  - Warning signs and symptoms

Follow-up Care: Follow-up Measures to Consider

- Document
  - Criteria for diagnosis
  - Treatment and follow-up plan
- Return for the following conditions:
  - Dehydration with inability to orally replace fluids
  - Pus or blood in the stool

Multidisciplinary Practice: Consider Consultation, Collaboration, or Referral

- Emergency services
  - Acute abdomen
  - Severe dehydration
- Medical/surgical services: For chronic diarrhea unresponsive to therapy within 7–21 days
- Dietician
  - Gluten intolerance
  - Lactose intolerance
  - Food allergies

- For diagnosis or treatment outside the midwife's scope of practice

CARE OF THE WOMAN WITH HEARTBURN

Key Clinical Information

Heartburn, also referred to as pyrosis or dyspepsia, is a burning sensation in the upper GI system that results from reflux of gastric contents, known as *chyme*. Heartburn is an occasional occurrence for many people; an estimated 60 million Americans experience heartburn at least once a month (Angelini et al., 2007). Heartburn occurs more often in the presence of gastric fullness and conditions that affect the functioning of the lower esophageal sphincter of the stomach. Pregnant women and older adults are most likely to have daily heartburn and to seek treatment for this distressing symptom. Heartburn is associated with a number of chronic disorders that can be considered in the differential diagnosis when a client presents with heartburn.

Client History and Chart Review: Components of the History to Consider

(Angelini et al., 2007; King & Brucker, 2011)

- Age
- Pregnancy: See "Care of the Pregnant Woman with Heartburn"
- Medical history
  - Allergies
  - Current medications
    - NSAIDs
    - Estrogen
  - Chronic and acute conditions
    - Gallbladder disease
    - Peptic ulcer disease
    - Diabetes
- Surgical history: Cholecystectomy
- Heartburn symptom profile
  - Onset, duration, and location
  - Severity and character
  - Associated symptoms

- Changes in GI function
- Effect of symptoms on daily living
- Exacerbating or alleviating factors
- Self-help measures used and effectiveness
- Common symptoms associated with heartburn
  - Abdominal pain or cramping
  - Bloating
  - Early satiety
  - Postprandial fullness
  - Nausea
  - Anorexia
  - Burping or belching
- Dietary history
  - Usual diet
  - Heartburn triggers
    - Fatty foods
    - Fried foods
    - Coffee
    - Chocolate
    - Peppermint
    - Alcohol
    - Rapid eating
    - Overeating
    - Lying flat after meals
- Family history
  - Duodenal ulcers
  - Gastroesophageal reflux disorder
- Social history
  - Stressors
  - Drug, alcohol, and tobacco use
- Review of systems

Physical Examination: Components of the Physical Exam to Consider

(Angelini et al., 2007)

- Vital signs, including weight and BMI
- General physical examination with the focus directed by the client's history and current level of discomfort
- Head, eyes, ears, nose, and throat
  - Examination of mouth and throat
  - Presence and condition of teeth
  - Ability to swallow

- Abdominal palpation and auscultation
  - Gastric fullness
  - Pain or referred pain
  - Rebound tenderness
  - Distension

Clinical Impression: Differential Diagnoses to Consider

(ICD9Data.com, 2012)

- Heartburn
- Gastroesophageal reflux disorder
- Hiatal hernia
- *Helicobacter pylori* infection
- Difficulty swallowing
- Dyspepsia
- Gastroenteritis
- Lactose intolerance
- Pancreatitis
- Peptic ulcer disease

Diagnostic Testing: Diagnostic Tests and Procedures to Consider

- Testing based on history and examination findings
- Complete blood count with peripheral smear
- Erythrocyte sedimentation rate (ESR)
- *H. pylori* testing
- Liver function testing
- Endoscopy
- Upper endoscopy
- Ultrasound
- Gallbladder and pancreas

Providing Treatment: Therapeutic Measures to Consider

(Angelini et al., 2007; King & Brucker, 2011)

- Treatment is based on the differential diagnosis
- Heartburn
  - Antacids
    - Calcium carbonate (Tums)
    - Aluminum hydroxide (Amphogel)
    - Magnesium hydroxide (milk of magnesia)
    - Magnesium/aluminum combination (Mylanta, Maalox, Gelusil)
    - Sodium bicarbonate
    - Simethicon (Mylicon)
  - H_2 receptor antagonists
    - Cimetidine (Tagamet): 400 mg BID or 800 mg at bedtime
    - Ranitidine (Zantac): 150 mg BID or 300 mg at bedtime
    - Famotidine (Pepcid): 20 mg BID or 40 mg at bedtime
    - Nizatidine (Axid): 150 mg BID
  - Proton pump inhibitors (PPIs)
    - Esomeprazole (Nexium)
    - Lansoprazole (Prevacid)
    - Omeprazole (Prilosec)
    - Pantoprazole (Protonix)
    - Rabeprazole (Aciphex)
- Antimicrobial treatment for *H. pylori* infection (King & Brucker, 2011)
  - The most effective treatment regimens include the following medications:
    - Proton pump inhibitors plus
    - Clarithromycin *and*
    - Amoxicillin *or*
    - Metronidazole
  - Duration of treatment ranges from 7 to 14 days
  - Shorter treatment improves compliance
  - Failed short-term therapy requires 14-day retreatment
    - Three-drug regimens
      - Clarithromycin + metronidazole + PPI
      - Amoxicillin + metronidazole + PPI
      - Tetracycline + metronidazole + sucralfate
    - Four-drug regimens
      - Bismuth + metronidazole + clarithromycin + PPI
      - Bismuth + metronidazole + tetracycline + PPI
      - Bismuth + metronidazole + tetracycline + H_2 blocker
      - H_2 blocker needs to be taken for 4–6 weeks
    - Combination product: Helidac (H_2 blocker)

Providing Treatment: Complementary and Alternative Measures to Consider

⚠️ Alternative therapies are not a substitute for medical evaluation and treatment of acute symptoms.

- For gastroesophageal reflux disease, consider the following adjunct therapies:
  - Chamomile tea
  - Slippery elm
  - Papaya enzyme tablets with meals and at bedtime
  - Hazelnuts with meals and at bedtime

Providing Support: Education and Support Measures to Consider

- Dietary recommendations
  - Avoid heartburn dietary triggers
    - Separate ingestion of solids and liquids by 30 minutes
    - Limit caffeine and alcohol intake
    - Avoid overeating
  - Eat small, frequent meals
  - Wear loose-waisted clothing
- Posture
  - Remain upright for 1 hour after eating
  - Sleep with elevated head and shoulders
- Smoking cessation
- Provide information
  - Working diagnosis
  - Recommended medications and treatment
    - Anticipated results
    - Side effects
  - Warning signs and symptoms

Follow-up Care: Follow-up Measures to Consider

- Document
  - Criteria for diagnosis
  - Treatment and follow-up plan
- Return for continued care
  - Five to 10 days with no improvement *or*
  - Sooner with worsening signs or symptoms

Multidisciplinary Practice: Consider Consultation, Collaboration, or Referral

- Medical/surgical services
  - Confirmed or suspected conditions:
    - Gallbladder disease
    - GI bleeding
  - For nonacute GI problem that does not respond to therapy within 7–21 days
- For diagnosis or treatment outside the midwife's scope of practice

CARE OF THE WOMAN WITH NAUSEA AND VOMITING

Key Clinical Information

Treatment of nausea and vomiting in the pregnant woman is very familiar to midwives. These symptoms are associated with a wide variety of conditions in nonpregnant women, such as a response to an ingested chemical or toxin, physical or sexual assault, or a viral infection; or a primary disorder of the GI tract, or the central nervous system.

Client History and Chart Review: Components of the History to Consider

(Angelini et al., 2007)

- LMP, GP TPAL
- Reproductive status, potential for pregnancy
- Pregnancy: See "Care of the Pregnant Woman with Nausea and Vomiting"
- Medical history
  - Allergies
  - Current medications
    - Many medications have nausea and vomiting as a side effect
    - Oral contraceptive pills
    - Estrogen
  - Chronic and acute conditions
    - Gallbladder disease
    - Peptic ulcer disease
    - Pancreatitis
    - Appendicitis
    - Migraine headaches

- Surgical history
  - Cholecystectomy
  - Oophorectomy
  - Appendectomy
- Nausea and vomiting symptom profile
  - Onset, duration, and frequency
  - Severity and character
  - Effects of symptoms on daily living
  - Exacerbating or alleviating factors
  - Self-help measures used and their effectiveness
  - Common symptoms associated with nausea and vomiting
    - Retching or dry heaves
    - Abdominal pain or cramping
    - Hypersalivation
    - Tachycardia
    - Abdominal muscle contractions
    - Weight gain or loss
    - Fever
    - Chills
    - Body aches
    - Abdominal pain
    - Changes in GI function
- Dietary history
  - Ability to ingest and retain food
  - Ability to ingest and retain liquids
  - Foods attempted
- Family history: Gallbladder disease
- Social history
  - Exposure to others with nausea and vomiting
  - Stressors
  - Drug, alcohol, and tobacco use
- Review of systems

Physical Examination: Components of the Physical Exam to Consider

(Angelini et al., 2007)

- Vital signs, including temperature, weight, and BMI
- General physical examination with the focus directed by the client's history
  - Current level of discomfort

- Observe for evidence
  - Illness
  - Dehydration
  - Alcohol or drug abuse
- Head, eyes, ears, nose, and throat
  - Examination of mouth and throat
  - Presence and condition of teeth
  - Ability to swallow
  - Lymph nodes
- Abdominal examination
  - Inspection for shape, symmetry, and pulsations
  - Auscultation for bowel sounds and bruits
  - Percussion
    - Organ margins
    - Masses
    - Ascites
  - Palpation, light and deep
    - Pain
    - Rigidity
    - Involuntary guarding
    - Rebound tenderness
    - Masses

Clinical Impression: Differential Diagnoses to Consider

(ICD9Data.com, 2012)

- Nausea and vomiting
- Difficulty swallowing
- Gallbladder disease
- Gastroenteritis
- Crohn's disease
- Pregnancy, nausea and vomiting
- Dehydration
- Endocrine dysfunction

Diagnostic Testing: Diagnostic Tests and Procedures to Consider

- Testing based on history and examination findings
- Human chorionic gonadotropin (HCG)
- Hepatitis screen
- Ultrasound: Gallbladder and pancreas

Providing Treatment: Therapeutic Measures to Consider

(Angelini et al., 2007; King & Brucker, 2011)

Treatment is based on the differential diagnosis and the severity of the client's symptoms.

- Antihistamines: Diphenhydrazine, dimenhydrinate, doxylamine, meclizine
- Phenothiazines: Prochlorperazine, promazine, thiethylperazine
- Nonphenothiazine antiemetic: Trimethobenzamine
- Serotonin antagonists: Ondansetron, dolasetron
- Butyrophenones: Droperidol
- Anticholinergics: Scopolamine
- Benzamides: Metoclopramide
- Benzodiazapines: Lorazepam, alprazolam
- Fluid and electrolyte replacement
- Vitamin B_6 or B complex
- Intravenous hydration

Providing Treatment: Alternative Measures to Consider

Alternative therapies are not a substitute for medical evaluation and treatment of acute symptoms.

- Acupuncture or acupressure
- Ginger—tea, candied, gingersnaps, or raw

Providing Support: Education and Support Measures to Consider

- Dietary recommendations
  - Nothing by mouth to rest the gut
  - Await cessation of nausea and vomiting or return of appetite
    - Progressive diet; start with small amounts
    - Bland easily digested foods
    - Liquids with electrolytes or sugars
    - Carbonated drinks such as cola or ginger ale
- Provide information and support
  - Discuss condition or cause of nausea and vomiting
  - Working diagnosis

- Recommended medications and treatments
  - Anticipated results
  - Side effects
- Warning signs and symptoms

Follow-up Care: Follow-up Measures to Consider

- Document
  - Criteria for diagnosis
  - Treatment and follow-up plan
- Return for continued care
  - Inability to keep anything down for 24 hours
  - Five to 7 days with no improvement *or*
  - Sooner based on severity of signs or symptoms
  - If a medication side effect is suspected, consider a trial of an alternative medication, if available

Multidisciplinary Practice: Consider Consultation, Collaboration, or Referral

- Emergency services
  - Acute abdomen
  - Intestinal obstruction
- Medical/surgical services
  - Gallbladder disease
  - For non-acute GI problem that does not respond to therapy within 7–21 days
- OB/GYN services
  - Hyperemesis gravidarum
  - Hydatidiform mole
- Mental health or psychiatric services
  - Post-traumatic reaction
- For diagnosis or treatment outside the midwife's scope of practice

ASSESSMENT OF THE WOMAN WITH MENTAL HEALTH SYMPTOMS

Key Clinical Information

Mental health is a state of psychological and emotional well-being that allows individuals to form satisfying relationships, effectively resolve conflicts, and successfully adapt to changing circumstances. Approximately one in four adults in America suffers from a diagnosable mental health disorder in a given year (National Institute of Mental Health [NIMH], 2007). Patterns of mental illness vary by gender, with women being more likely than men to suffer from depression, anxiety, somatic complaints, and post-traumatic stress syndrome (World Health Organization [WHO], 2004). Caregiver stress affects women disproportionately and is on the rise as the U.S. population ages (NIMH, 2007).

Mood and anxiety disorders disturb sleep, diminish attention, and can result in impaired cognitive function. The development of mood and anxiety disorders can be affected by heritability and genetic factors, early life experiences, psychiatric or medical comorbidities, and adult stress and trauma. The resilient individual has sufficient physical and emotional reserves, as well as social support, to cope with ordinary life challenges. Midwives, however, commonly encounter women who have lived through major life-altering experiences such as serious poverty, immigration, loss of family, partner violence, sexual abuse, and assault. When such life experiences are shared during care, the midwife should be sensitive to the potential for mood and anxiety disorders and conduct a thorough symptom review with the woman.

Midwifery assessment and care include assessment, diagnosis, and provision, or arranging for the provision, of treatment of mental health disorders. Active listening is a crucial part of the midwifery assessment process, and it places the midwife in a prime position to evaluate the mental well-being of each woman who presents for care. Emotional distress can be expressed through somatic complaints, requiring the midwife to consider both pathophysiologic and psychologic origins of presenting conditions or symptom complexes. As with other health issues, a strong network of referral options is beneficial in directing women to the type of care that best meets their needs. Women with mental health issues or severe psychiatric problems can be referred to a mental health professional for further evaluation and coordination of treatment.

Client History and Chart Review: Components of the History to Consider

(American Psychiatric Association [APA], 2006)

- Report of symptoms documented using the client's own words
- History of current problem
  - Symptoms: Emotional and physical
    - Onset, duration, and cycles
    - Precipitating factors or events
    - Treatments used and their efficacy
    - Changes in the following:
      - Weight
      - Appetite
      - Sleep patterns
      - Social activities
      - Relationships
  - Client's feelings of danger to self or to others
  - Suicide attempts or ideation
  - Expectations for care
- Mental health status
  - Description and theme of mood
    - Effect on daily life
      - Appetite
      - Activities
      - Sleep patterns
    - Delusions
    - Paranoia
    - Suicidal ideation: Thoughts, plans, intent, and means
  - General cognitive status
    - Orientation
    - Memory
    - Attention
    - Abstract thinking and reasoning
    - Speech patterns
    - Alterations in thought processes or responses (e.g., emotional organization and content)
      - Persistent unwanted thoughts
      - Worry out of proportion to life events
      - Pessimistic thinking
      - Rage
      - Panic

- ➤ Guilt
- ➤ Worthlessness
- ➤ Hopelessness
- ➤ Agitation
- ➤ Alteration in short-term memory
- ➤ Sadness
- ➤ Indecision
- ➤ Inability to concentrate
- ➤ Irritability
- ➤ Anxiety
  - Previous mental health symptoms, diagnosis, or treatment
- Reproductive history
  - LMP, GP TPAL
  - Children at home
  - Reproductive losses or negative experiences and emotional sequelae
  - Sexual orientation and preferences
  - Current menstrual status
  - Current method of contraception
- Medical/surgical history
  - Allergies
  - Current medications
    - ◆ Hormones
    - ◆ Antidepressants
    - ◆ Analgesics
    - ◆ Other medications
    - ◆ Dietary supplements or herbal remedies
  - Medical conditions
    - ◆ Viral infection
    - ◆ Endocrine problems
    - ◆ Chronic pain
    - ◆ Chronic fatigue
    - ◆ Multiple sclerosis
    - ◆ Cancer
  - Previous surgery
  - Repeated visits to healthcare providers for vague symptoms
- Social history
  - 🌐 Cultural background
    - ◆ Effect on the primary symptoms
    - ◆ Social stigma related to seeking help
    - ◆ Cultural variations in symptoms presentation

- Nature of primary affiliate relationships: Partner, spouse, children
- Housing and occupant situation
- Extended family and community support systems
- Alcohol, drug, or tobacco abuse
- Emotional, sexual, or physical abuse
- Employment or financial status
- Life stresses, transitions, and coping techniques
- Related family history
  - Mental illness or disorders
  - Alcohol, drug abuse, or addiction
  - Chronic illness and caretaking requirements
  - Loss of family members or loved one(s)
- Usual diet and food choices
- Review of systems

Physical Examination: Components of the Physical Exam to Consider

(APA, 2006)

- Vital signs
- Weight, height, and BMI: Comparison with previous data
- 🌐 Mental status assessment
  - Posture
  - Mood
  - Body language and movements
  - Personal hygiene and dress
  - Cooperation, participation, and eye contact
  - Affect
  - Presence of disordered thinking
- Physical manifestations of mental health issues
  - Facial expression
  - Body language
  - Eye contact
  - Tics or agitation
  - Diminished affect
  - Slow speech or movements
  - Hyperactivity
  - Obsessive–compulsive behaviors
  - Auditory or visual hallucinations
  - Low BMI

- Evaluation for a physiologic basis of the symptoms
  - Thyroid
  - Cardiopulmonary status
  - Neurologic functioning
  - Reproductive (hormonal) systems

Clinical Impression: Differential Diagnoses to Consider

(ICD9Data.com, 2012)

> Consider the possibility of dual diagnosis—for example, a client with both an emotional or psychiatric problem and a substance abuse problem, chronic health issue, or somatic presentation.

- Affective disorders
- Anxiety disorders
- Post-traumatic stress disorder
- Eating disorders
  - Anorexia nervosa
  - Bulimia nervosa
- Personality disorders
- Psychosis or schizophrenia
- Alzheimer's disease
- Endocrine dysfunction (e.g., thyroid, diabetes, adrenal)
- Hormone-related disorders
  - Premenstrual tension syndromes
  - Menopausal/postmenopausal mood disorder
  - Postpartum depression (see "Care of the Mother: Perinatal Mood and Anxiety Disorders")
- Substance abuse
- Seizure disorders
- Caregiver stress

Diagnostic Testing: Diagnostic Tests and Procedures to Consider

- Evaluation for a physical disorder
  - History
  - Physical examination

- Laboratory values
  - Electrolytes
  - Toxicology
  - Thyroid-stimulating hormone (TSH)
  - Follicle-stimulating hormone (FSH)
  - Luteinizing hormone (LH)
- Evaluation for symptoms of mental/emotional disorders: Use appropriate screening tools
  - Age appropriate
  - Developmentally appropriate
  - Culturally appropriate

Providing Treatment: Therapeutic Measures to Consider

- Self-care
  - Well-balanced diet, adequate sleep, and daily routine
  - Stress-relieving activities, such as yoga, massage, or hobbies
  - Physical activity or exercise (Strohle, 2009)
    - Written prescription for the activity that the client finds most motivating
    - Three or more sessions of moderate activity per week
    - Sessions of 20–30 minutes or more
    - Duration and intensity positively influence affect
    - The greatest efficacy is realized when activity sessions are self-initiated
    - Keeping an activity journal is recommended
  - Identify issues and concerns; talk with friends; journal emotional changes
  - Seek and accept help
  - Develop a sense of community through volunteering, work, and social organizations
- Interactive psychotherapy
  - Individual or group counseling
  - Art therapy
  - Music therapy
  - Expressive therapy
  - Cognitive therapy
  - Behavioral therapy

- Consider a trial of hormone replacement therapy for new-onset mild mental health dysfunction in perimenopausal or menopausal women with no precipitating events (see "Care of the Woman on Hormone Replacement Therapy")
- Commonly prescribed medications have potentially serious side effects
  - Check the side-effect profile before prescribing and against the client's symptoms and presentation
  - When in doubt, consult with or refer the client to a mental health prescribing professional
- Medication type by diagnosis
  - Affective (mood) disorders
    - Depression
      - Antidepressants
        - Flat or depressed mood
        - Sleep dysfunction
        - Obsessive self-flagellation
      - Anxiolytics if anxiety is also present
    - Bipolar disorders and mania: Mood stabilizers (lithium and anticonvulsants)
  - Anxiety disorders
    - Anxiolytics for acute and chronic anxiety or panic
    - Antidepressants for panic attacks, phobias, or obsessive–compulsive disorder
  - Post-traumatic stress disorder
    - Antidepressants for depression or obsessive thoughts or behaviors
    - Anxiolytics for panic, general anxiety, or mild paranoia
    - Antipsychotics
      - Agitation
      - Anxiety if anxiolytics have poor response or are contraindicated
      - For persistent paranoid thinking
  - Eating disorders
    - Antidepressants for mood disorder and obsessive thinking
    - Anxiolytics if anxiety is present
    - Antipsychotics if thinking is delusional

- Psychoses (thought disorders): Neuroleptics (antipsychotics)
- Caregiver stress
  - Antidepressants for mood disorder
  - Anxiolytics if anxiety is present
  - Sleep induction medication if insomnia is present

Providing Treatment: Complementary and Alternative Measures to Consider

- Seek a warm, safe, caring environment
  - Supportive friends and family
  - Basic needs met: Food, shelter, safety, and respect
- Herbal and supplements for minor mood disorders
  - Alpha linolenic acid (ALA) and eicosapentaenoic acid (EPA) (Lucas et al., 2011)
    - No mood improvement in the absence of depression
    - Effective for depression, including during menopause
    - May diminish hot flashes in menopausal women
    - ALA: 2 g/day
    - EPA: 200 mg/day to 1 g/day
  - Red clover
  - Dong quai
  - Black cohosh
  - Evening primrose
- Support groups
  - Women's groups
  - Bereavement support
  - Related to other medical diagnosis (e.g., breast cancer support)
  - Religious/spiritual groups

Providing Support: Education and Support Measures to Consider

- Engage the client in self-care (U.S. Department of Health and Human Services, 2006)
  - Eat a well-balanced, varied diet

- Get regular rest and adequate sleep
- Set attainable goals
  - Set priorities
  - Break large tasks into smaller ones
  - Assume a tolerable amount of responsibility
- Be with other people when able
- Participate in activities that may improve mood
  - Physical activity or exercise
  - Engage in pleasurable activities such as going to a movie or a ball game
  - Participate in religious, social, or other community-based activities
- Expect mood to improve gradually
- Postpone important decisions until improvement occurs
- Practice positive thinking
- Ask for and accept help from family and friends
  - Child or elder care
  - Specific tangible tasks such as meals and laundry
  - Companionship
- Provide information related to community resources
  - Health education services
  - Support groups
  - Crisis hotline number(s)
  - Women with abusive partners: Provide information
    - Safety planning
    - How to access safe housing
    - Effects of medications on ability to be vigilant
  - Women with medical treatment and/or referral: Provide detailed information
    - Medication
    - Name
    - Dosing instructions
    - Indication
    - Desired effects
    - Potential side effects

- Interactions
- Pregnancy category (as needed)
  - Referral information and goal of referral
  - Midwifery plan for continued care and follow-up
- Signs and/or symptoms indicating need for the following care:
  - Return for care
  - Immediate care
  - Emergency care

Follow-up Care: Follow-up Measures to Consider

- Document
  - If the client is positive for suicide ideation, note the timely referral/crisis intervention
  - Verify client follow-up with the referral(s)
- Provide, as appropriate:
  - Support and education related to the diagnosis
  - Treatment
    - Counseling
    - Continued medication use
  - Routine women's health care
    - Annual women's health exam and screening as indicated
    - Contraception or prenatal care as needed

Multidisciplinary Practice: Consider Consultation, Collaboration, or Referral

- Mental health services
  - Psychiatric emergency
    - Suicidal or homicidal ideation
    - Psychosis
    - Need for hospitalization
  - Symptoms that suggest a complex psychiatric disorder
    - Personality disorder
    - Psychosis
    - Schizophrenia
    - Severe mood or anxiety disorder
  - Failure to respond to medication or prescribed treatment
  - Formal psychotherapy indicated or requested

- Emergency services: Potential life-threatening drug reaction
- Social services
  - Concomitant substance abuse
  - Persistent psychosocial problems
  - Counseling
  - Nontraditional therapy options
- For diagnosis or treatment outside the midwife's scope of practice

CARE OF THE WOMAN WITH AFFECTIVE (MOOD) DISORDER

Key Clinical Information

Affective disorders affect mood, and include depression and bipolar disorder. Women are twice as likely as men to be affected by depression (Hyde, Mezulis, & Abramso, 2008). These disorders have physiologic as well as socioemotional effects. For example, women with depression are more likely to have low HDL cholesterol, while women with bipolar disorder are more likely to have elevated triglycerides (Sagud, Mihaljevic-Peles, Pivac, Jakovljevic, &, Muck-Seler, 2009; Whang et al., 2009). Additionally, women with affective disorders more commonly engage in "emotional eating" and substance use, resulting in a correlation between depression and elevated BMI, and between depression and less healthy diet and lifestyle choices. Major depression is a predictor of elevated risk for onset of metabolic syndrome (Goldbacher, Bromberger, & Matthews, 2009).

Susceptibility to affective disorders varies among individuals and is influenced by both genetic factors and life events. Genetic factors can influence the onset of major depression by determining the individual's sensitivity to stressful life events. Depression results in enhanced sympathetic nervous system activation. Persistent environmental stressors ultimately cause changes in central nervous system (CNS) structure and function that are unique to the individual. The brain is wonderfully adaptable, however, allowing cognitive and behavioral therapies to remodel neural pathways, and thereby enabling individuals to develop greater emotional resilience and positive coping skills.

When screening for depression using a validated tool, keep in mind that cultural variations can affect the credibility of women's answers. Best care occurs through thoughtfully examining symptom meaning, display, and the extent of depression as it relates to ethnicity or cultural heritage. A positive screening result should lead to more in-depth evaluation prior to diagnosis. Somatic symptoms can be more reliable indicators of depression than a patient's apparent emotional state (Grant, Jack, Fitzpatrick, & Ernst, 2008).

Cognitive and behavioral therapies offer women with depression the best opportunity for change, and integrated therapy can include antidepressant medications. Unfortunately, these medications often have significant side-effect profiles and a nonresponse rate as low as 38%; moreover, only 46% of individuals treated achieve remission (Agency for Healthcare Research and Quality, 2007).

Serotonin and norepinephrine reuptake inhibitors may have neurobehavioral effects on the neonate. Thus, when caring for pregnant women with depression, the benefit of pharmacologic treatment must be weighed against the potential for harm to both mother and neonate from untreated depression.

Client History and Chart Review: Components of the History to Consider

- Mental health history
  - Onset, duration, and severity of symptoms
  - Previous diagnosis of depression
  - Current or past antidepressant use
  - Major life events or stressors
  - Thoughts of suicide
  - Lifestyle
    - Sleep patterns
    - Diet
    - Physical activity
    - Drug, alcohol, or tobacco use
- Family history of affective disorders

- Presence of comorbid conditions
  - Cancer
  - Chronic pain
  - Crohn's disease
  - Diabetes mellitus
  - Irregular menses
  - Infertility
  - Thyroid disorder
- 🔻 Risk factors for depression (Grant et al., 2008; Whang et al., 2009)
  - Poverty
  - Physical, emotional, or sexual abuse during childhood
  - Insecure or disrupted parental attachment
  - History of sexual violence and victimization
  - Homelessness
  - Acute and chronic illness
  - Critical and unsupportive partner
  - Devaluing and restricting environments
- Associated behaviors and conditions
  - Drug and alcohol abuse
  - Emotional eating, particularly sweet foods
  - Multiple health conditions or frequent accidents or injuries
  - Polycystic ovary syndrome (PCOS)
  - Abnormalities of lipid metabolism
  - Coronary heart disease
  - Metabolic syndrome
  - Self-silencing
    - Limits intimacy and autonomy
    - Reinforces negative self-perceptions
    - Lowers self-esteem
    - Results in feelings of a "loss of self"
    - Exhibited as internal pressure
      - Deferring to the needs of others
      - Censoring self-expression
      - Repressing anger
      - Judging the self against an ideal
      - Inhibition of self-directed action
  - Depression (Sanders, 2006)
    - Depressed mood
    - Diminished interest in all activities
    - Weight loss or gain

- Cardiac arrhythmias
- Insomnia or hypersomnia
- Psychomotor agitation or retardation
- Fatigue or loss of energy
- Feelings of worthlessness or guilt
- Inability to concentrate
- Recurrent thoughts of death: Suicidal ideation, plan, or intent
  - Mania
    - Decreased need for sleep
    - Rapid or "pressured" speech
    - Distractibility
    - Flight of ideas
    - Increased goal-directed activity
    - Inflated self-esteem or grandiosity
    - Engaging in risk-taking behaviors
  - Bipolar disorders
    - Symptoms of depression and mania
    - Alternating types of symptoms
    - Self-harm is more likely during the manic phase

Physical Examination: Components of the Physical Exam to Consider

(Goldbacher et al., 2009; Whang et al., 2009)

- Weight and BMI
- Blood pressure, heart rate, and heart rhythm
- Observe for characteristics of metabolic syndrome or PCOS
  - Central obesity
  - Hirsutism
- Palpate thyroid
- Observe for signs of affective disorder
  - Rapid weight change
  - Flat affect
  - Slow speech and motion
  - Agitation
  - Tearfulness
- Cardiac effects of antidepressant medications
  - Ventricular arrhythmias
  - Elevations in resting heart rate and blood pressure

- Changes in QT parameters on ECG
- Reduced heart rate variability

Clinical Impression: Differential Diagnoses to Consider (ICD9Data.com, 2012)

- Adjustment reaction
- Mood disorders
- Depressive disorder
- Drug or alcohol dependence

Diagnostic Testing: Diagnostic Tests and Procedures to Consider

- [www] Screening tools
  - Reynolds Adolescent Depression Scale
  - CES Depression Scale (CES-D)
  - Beck Depression Inventory (BDI)
  - Beck Depression Inventory PC (BDI-PC)
  - Edinburgh Postnatal Depression Scale
  - Zung Depression Rating Scale
  - Patient Health Questionnaire (PHQ-9)
- ECG
- Thyroid-stimulating hormone
- Blood glucose
- Lipid profile

Providing Treatment: Therapeutic Measures to Consider

- Therapy
  - Cognitive-behavioral therapy
  - Expressive therapy (art/music)
  - Movement therapy (dance)
  - Psychoanalytic therapy
- Antidepressants (AHRQ, 2007)
  - Selective serotonin reuptake inhibitors (SSRIs) (American College of Obstetrics and Gynecology [ACOG], 2006)
    - May cause decrease in libido.
    - Avoid in pregnancy or preconception (Louik, Lin, Werler, Hernandez-Diaz, & Mitchell, 2007)
      - Associated with an increased risk of persistent pulmonary hypertension in the newborn

  - To avoid withdrawal symptoms, wean down slowly (ACOG, 2007)
    - Citalopram: 20–60 mg daily (Pregnancy Category C)
    - Escitalopram: 5–20 mg daily (Pregnancy Category C)
    - Fluoxetine: 20–80 mg daily (Pregnancy Category C)
    - Fluvoxamine: 50–300 mg daily (Pregnancy Category C)
    - Paroxetine: 10–60 mg daily
      - Avoid use in pregnancy (ACOG, 2007)
      - Fetal echocardiography should be considered for women exposed in the first trimester of pregnancy
    - Sertraline: 50–200 mg daily (Pregnancy Category C)
  - Norepinephrine reuptake inhibitors
    - Duloxetine: 30–60 mg BID (Pregnancy Category C)
    - Venlafaxine: 37.5–150 mg BID (Pregnancy Category C)
  - Tricyclic antidepressants: Long history of use, multiple side effects
    - Amitriptyline: 25–100 mg daily (Pregnancy Category D)
    - Imipramine: 75–150 mg daily (Pregnancy Category D)
    - Nortriptyline: 25–100 mg daily in divided doses (Pregnancy Category D)
- Other antidepressants (Sanders, 2006)
  - Bupropion: 150–450 mg daily (Pregnancy Category C)
  - Mirtazapine: 15–60 mg daily (Pregnancy Category C)
  - Trazodone: 50–150 mg at bedtime (Pregnancy Category C)
  - Mirtazapine: 15–45 mg at bedtime (Pregnancy Category C)
- Electroconvulsive therapy for major depression refractory to medical therapy (Sackeim et al., 2009)

Providing Treatment: Complementary and Alternative Measures to Consider

(Boyce & Barriball, 2010; Deligiannidis & Freeman, 2010; Fava, 2010; Frank, Maggi, Miniati, & Benvenuti, 2009; Raiput, Sinha, Mathur, & Agrawal, 2011; Ravindran et al., 2009)

- Nutritional support
  - Well-balanced diet
  - Folate
  - Omega 3 fatty acids
  - SAMe (S-adenosylmethionine)
- Herbal support
  - *German* chamomile
  - St. John's wort
  - Saffron
  - Licorice
- Mind–body techniques
  - Acupuncture
  - Yoga
  - Meditation
  - Guided imagery
  - Massage therapy
- Light therapy
- Interpersonal social rhythm therapy
  - Consistent sleep–wake cycles
  - Regular physical activity
  - Predictable meal times
  - Regular work and social schedule

Providing Support: Education and Support Measures to Consider

- Medication instructions and information
  - Dosing
  - Expected result
  - Side effects
  - When to call or return for care
    - Severe adverse effects
    - Suicidal thoughts
    - Routine follow-up

Follow-up Care: Follow-up Measures to Consider

- Document recommendations for therapy
  - Cognitive-behavioral therapy

- Medications
- Support groups
- Criteria for consultation or referral
- Follow-up instructions
- Evaluate medication use and effects
  - Self-administration of recommended dosing
  - GI symptoms
    - Nausea and vomiting
    - Diarrhea
  - Weight gain or loss
  - Somnolence
  - Change in blood pressure or heart rate
  - Changes in libido
  - Suicidal thoughts
  - Seizures
  - Effect on perceived quality of life

Multidisciplinary Practice: Consider Consultation, Collaboration, or Referral

- Psychiatric health professional
  - Diagnostic uncertainty
  - Client requests to see a psychiatric specialist
  - Presence of suicidal ideation
  - Apparent risk of harm to self or to others
  - Psychotic symptoms
  - Acute manic symptoms
  - Symptoms of bipolar disorder
  - Women who have a poor result on antidepressant medications
  - Women with severe depression who refuse medication
  - Inpatient psychiatric care indicated
- Mental health professional
  - Cognitive-behavioral therapy
  - Interpersonal social rhythm therapy
  - Counseling
  - Art therapy
  - Play therapy
  - Behavioral therapy
  - Group therapy
- Complementary and alternative care modalities
  - Acupuncturist
  - Yoga, mindfulness, or meditation classes

- Massage therapist
- Nutritionist
- Lifestyle coach
- For diagnosis or treatment outside the midwife's scope of practice

CARE OF THE WOMAN WITH ANXIETY DISORDER

Key Clinical Information

Anxiety is the most common mental health disorder in women and is frequently undiagnosed in primary care practice. Women may exhibit anxiety in various ways, many of which are difficult to elicit during an abbreviated office encounter. Anxiety is characterized by feelings of tension, fear, and emotional hyper-arousal. The spectrum of anxiety disorders includes generalized anxiety disorder, acute stress disorder, obsessive–compulsive disorder, phobias, and post-traumatic stress disorder. Anxiety is often masked by coexisting depression. A genetic predisposition for anxiety disorders has been found to contribute to the incidence and susceptibility to anxiety in the presence of life stressors, while cognitive and behavioral therapies have been found to be effective in treating these disorders and having a protective effect (Hofmann & Smits, 2008; Tambs et al., 2009).

Client History and Chart Review: Components of the History to Consider

(Barry, Pietrzak, & Petry, 2008; D. L. Powell, 2005; Tambs et al., 2009; WHO, 2004)

- [www] Mental health assessment using a clinician-rated psychometrically sound tool or patient self-report
  - Primary Care Evaluation of Mental Disorders (Prime-MD)
  - Patient Health Questionnaire (PHQ)
- Factors associated with anxiety symptoms or disorders
  - Family history
  - Trauma
  - Elevated BMI (> 30)

- Chronic illness
- Comorbid conditions
  - Depression
  - Hypertension
  - Diabetes
  - Chronic obstructive pulmonary disease
- Physical inactivity
- Caffeine intake
- Alcohol or drug use
- Use of medications associated with anxiety
  - Stimulants
  - Opioids
  - Anabolic steroids
  - Antihypertensive medications
  - Sympathomimetics
  - Psychiatric medications
- Caregiver stress (U.S. Department of Health and Human Services, 2006)
  - Associated with providing for the daily needs of other(s)
    - Typically an older relative or spouse
    - Other demands on time, such as children, job, and housework
    - Presents with somatic symptoms, anxiety, and depression
- Generalized anxiety disorder
  - General feelings of anxiety about "everything"
  - Physiologic and emotional hyperarousal
    - Muscle tension
    - Fatigue
    - Emotional irritability
    - Restlessness
    - Disordered sleep
  - Altered cognitive functioning
    - Difficulty concentrating
    - Distorted view of situation
    - Persistent, invasive thoughts and worries
  - Ineffective coping skills
    - Avoidance
    - Procrastination
    - Difficulty problem solving
- Panic disorder
  - Subjective symptoms of panic attack

◆ Tightness in the chest or throat

◆ Difficulty breathing without evidence of obstruction

◆ Dry mouth

◆ Trembling

◆ Palpitations

■ Feelings of unreality

■ Nausea

■ Symptoms of irritable bowel syndrome

- Obsessive–compulsive disorder: Persistent recurrence of thoughts and behaviors

  ■ Intrusive thoughts (obsessions)

  ■ Ritualized behaviors (compulsions)

- Phobias

  ■ Irrational fear out of proportion to a stimulus

  ■ Situation specific

- Post-traumatic stress disorder

  ■ Development of symptoms after a significant traumatic event

  ■ Symptoms

    ◆ Flashbacks to the event (reexperiencing)

    ◆ Emotional numbing to external stimuli

    ◆ Avoidance of things associated with the event

    ◆ Emotional hyperarousal and physiologic response to triggers

    ◆ Autonomic, cognitive, and dysphoric symptoms

    ◆ Eating disorders (Mitchell & Bulik, 2006)

Physical Examination: Components of the Physical Exam to Consider

- Vital signs
- Body habitus and posture
- Cardiopulmonary assessment
- Physical symptoms associated with anxiety or panic attack

  ■ Elevated BP, tachycardia, or tachypnea

  ■ Restlessness, trembling, and exaggerated startle response

  ■ Pallor, sweating, erythema, and cold and clammy hands

  ■ Vomiting, or loss of bowel or bladder control

Clinical Impression: Differential Diagnoses to Consider

(ICD9Data.com, 2012)

- Anxiety disorders
- Acute reaction to stress
- Post-traumatic stress disorder

Diagnostic Testing: Diagnostic Tests and Procedures to Consider

- **WWW** Screening for depression or anxiety using a validated tool such as the Primary Care Evaluation of Mental Disorders (PRIME-MD)
- Blood glucose
- CBC
- ECG
- Holter monitor testing
- Thyroid screening
- Adrenal testing

Providing Treatment: Therapeutic Measures to Consider

- Cognitive and behavioral therapies

  ■ Cognitive therapy

    ◆ Examines thought patterns and behaviors

    ◆ Client learns to deliberately repattern thought processes and actions

      ➤ Avoid negative and nonproductive thinking

      ➤ Enhance positive and productive thoughts and interactions

  ■ Behavior therapy

    ◆ Relaxation and coping techniques

    ◆ Deliberate repatterning of behaviors in stressful situations

  ■ Group therapy

    ◆ Exposure to others with similar experiences, fears, or feelings

    ◆ Opportunity to remodel thoughts and behaviors with peer support

    ◆ Hear how individuals with similar issues cope

- Stress-reduction programs
- Lifestyle changes
  - Regular sustained physical activity
  - Limiting caffeine, nicotine, and alcohol
  - Maintaining a relatively regular schedule
    - Meals
    - Sleep
    - Daily activities
    - Social engagements
- Anxiolytics and hypnotics
  - Benzodiazepines
    - Alprazolam (Xanax): 0.5–6 mg daily, half-life 6–20 hours (Pregnancy Category D)
    - Clonazepam (Klonopin): 0.5–8 mg daily, half-life 18–50 hours (Pregnancy Category D)
    - Diazepam (Valium): 2–60 mg daily, half-life 30–100 hours (Pregnancy Category D)
    - Lorazepam (Ativan): 2–6 mg/day in divided doses (Pregnancy Category D)
  - Other
    - Buspirone hydrochloride (BuSpar): 10–30 mg daily (Pregnancy Category B)
    - Zolpidem tartrate (Ambien): 5–10 mg at bedtime (Pregnancy Category B)

Providing Treatment: Complementary and Alternative Measures to Consider

(van der Watt, Laugharne, & Janca, 2008)

- Acupuncture
- Aromatherapy
- Patterned physical activity
- Herbal support
  - Hops
  - Kava-kava
  - Passion flower
  - Reishi
  - Valarian
- Massage
- Mindfulness training
- Meditation

Providing Support: Education and Support Measures to Consider

(Sharkansky, 2010)

- Acknowledge and validate the client's feelings and emotional state
- For women with significant anxiety related to obtaining care:
  - Reduce the power differential between the midwife and the woman
  - Greet women while they are dressed before conducting an intimate exam
  - Engage clients in decision making and respect women's need for autonomy
  - Provide developmentally, culturally, and literacy appropriate health education materials
  - View the individual as an expert about herself
    - Ask what will help minimize her stress during the exam
    - Explore which parts of the exam are difficult for her
  - Explain the exam process in advance
    - Listen to concerns
    - Provide choices where possible
    - Schedule extra time for the exam
  - Check in throughout the exam
    - Observe for escalating anxiety
    - Explain the exam as it occurs
    - Ask for immediate feedback regarding pain versus pressure
    - Honor the woman's need to stop the exam
- If anxiety escalates during exam or office visit:
  - Maintain a calm, compassionate presence
  - Speak softly using a matter-of-fact voice
  - Avoid sudden movements or noise
  - If necessary or requested, stop the exam
  - Ask (or remind) the woman where she is
  - Offer comfort measures
  - Provide a change of environment
- Debrief with the client following the exam
- Schedule additional follow-up for processing as needed

Follow-up Care: Follow-up Measures to Consider

(D. L. Powell, 2005)

- Document
  - Response to the exam
  - Significant findings
  - Discussions for follow-up care
  - Mutually agreed-upon plan of care and goals
    - Treat the acute phase
    - Prevent relapse
    - Allow return to normal functioning
  - Discussion of any history of trauma or abuse
- Report abuse as required by state law
- Return for evaluation of medication efficacy
  - 2- to 6-week intervals until stable
  - Interval based on access to counseling, therapy, or other resources
  - Assess for relief of acute symptoms

Multidisciplinary Practice: Consider Consultation, Collaboration, or Referral

- Psychiatric or mental health professional
  - Diagnostic uncertainty
  - The client requests a psychiatric specialist
  - Acute stress reaction
  - Acute post-traumatic stress disorder
  - Counseling or psychotherapy
- Complementary and alternative care modalities
  - Acupuncturist
  - Yoga, mindfulness, or meditation classes
  - Massage therapist
  - Nutritionist
  - Lifestyle coach
- For diagnosis or treatment outside the midwife's scope of practice

CARE OF THE WOMAN WITH EATING DISORDERS

Key Clinical Information

Eating disorders encompass a spectrum of serious health conditions that affect an individual's physical and mental health, and are associated with distortion of self-image. The most common eating disorders include anorexia nervosa, bulimia nervosa, and binge-eating disorder. Anorexia is characterized by self-starvation coupled with weight loss, often resulting in profoundly low BMI and associated amenorrhea. Bulimia is characterized by binge eating followed by "purging," which includes self-induced vomiting, use of laxatives or enemas, diet medications, and excessive exercising to maintain body weight or shape. Binge-eating disorder is a form of compulsive overeating accompanied by feelings of shame or self-hatred, and occurs in women of all body weights (Academy for Eating Disorders, 2011). While not typically included under the heading "eating disorders," obesity can be a symptom of disordered eating and often includes psychosocial contributing factors. Weight management is a multifaceted issue for women across the life span.

Client History and Chart Review: Components of the History to Consider

(Academy for Eating Disorders, 2011)

- History of present symptoms
  - Onset, duration, and severity
  - Self-described issues or concerns
    - Feelings of being controlled or need for control
    - Family or social situation
    - Recent change or disruption
    - Rate and amount of weight loss/change
    - Nutritional status and BMI
    - Methods of weight control
      - Vomiting
      - Dieting
      - Excessive exercise
      - Inappropriate use of medications
        - Diet pills
        - Over-the-counter supplements
        - Laxatives
        - Emetics
        - Diuretics
        - Insulin
    - Dietary history and physical activity

- Neuropsychiatric history
  - Mood and anxiety disorders
  - Seizures
  - Memory loss or poor concentration
  - Insomnia or sleep disorder
  - Attempts or thoughts of self-harm
  - Suicidal ideation or suicide attempt
- Menstrual history and LMP
  - Frequency and duration of menses
  - Amenorrhea
- Medical history, including medications
- Family history
  - Symptoms or diagnosis of eating disorders or obesity
  - Mood and anxiety disorders
  - Alcohol or substance abuse
- Signs and symptoms of anorexia nervosa
  - Preoccupation with weight and food intake
  - Focus on control of food intake
  - Loss of more than 15% of body weight
  - Amenorrhea for at least three consecutive cycles
  - Denial
  - Self-repulsion
  - Distortion of body image
- Signs and symptoms of bulimia
  - Preoccupation with weight and food intake
  - Feelings of being out of control related to food intake
  - Binge eating
  - Purging
  - Fasting
  - Overexercising
  - Laxative or diuretic abuse
- Signs and symptoms of binge-eating disorder
  - Uncontrolled, compulsive, or continuous eating
  - Intermittent fasting or repetitive dieting
  - Anxiety, depression, and loneliness
- Review of systems
  - Cold intolerance
  - Weakness
  - Fatigue
  - Dizziness

- Syncope
- Chest pain or palpitations
- Epigastric discomfort
- Early satiety
- Gastroesophageal reflux
- Hematemesis
- Constipation
- Diminished libido

Physical Examination: Components of the Physical Exam to Consider

(Academy for Eating Disorders, 2011)

- Vital signs, including weight, height, and BMI
- Assess for physical findings associated with eating disorders
  - Head, eyes, ears, nose and throat
    - Oral trauma or lacerations
    - Dental erosion and dental caries
    - Parotid enlargement
  - Skin
    - Hair loss
    - Jaundice
    - Callus or scars on knuckles from self-induced vomiting
    - Poor healing
    - Development of lanugo hair
  - Cardiopulmonary
    - Signs of hypovolemia
    - Cardiac rhythm abnormalities
    - Shortness of breath
    - Edema
  - Gastrointestinal
    - Hemorrhoids or rectal prolapse
  - Musculoskeletal
    - Cachexia

Clinical Impression: Differential Diagnoses to Consider

(ICD-9Data.com, 2012)

- Anorexia nervosa
- Bulimia nervosa
- Eating disorders, unspecified

Diagnostic Testing: Diagnostic Tests and Procedures to Consider

(Academy for Eating Disorders, 2011)

- www Mental health assessment
  - Eating Disorder Inventory III
  - Beck Depression Inventory
- Laboratory testing
  - Complete blood count (CBC) with differential
  - Complete serum metabolic profile: Sodium, chloride, potassium, glucose, blood urea nitrogen (BUN), bicarbonate, creatinine, total protein, albumin, calcium, phosphate, magnesium, AST, amylase, lipase
  - Thyroid screen (T_3, T_4, TSH)
- Other testing
  - Electrocardiogram (ECG/EKG)
  - Holter monitor testing
  - Bone mineral density

Providing Treatment: Therapeutic Measures to Consider

(University of Maryland Medical Center, 2011a)

- Inpatient or outpatient therapy
- Medical stabilization of acute illness
  - Fluid and electrolytes
  - Nutritional support and rehabilitation
  - Monitoring for refeeding syndrome
- Treatment of mental health issues
  - Selective serotonin reuptake inhibitors (see "Care of the Woman with Affective (Mood) Disorder")
  - Cognitive-behavioral therapy
  - Family therapy
  - Eye movement desensitization and reprocessing
- Restoration of functional eating behaviors and ideation
  - Lifestyle changes
    - ◆ Moderate physical activity
    - ◆ Decrease intake of sugars and alcohol
    - ◆ Healthy food choices
  - Behavior repatterning
  - Social engagement and connection skills

Providing Treatment: Complementary and Alternative Measures to Consider

Integrated mind–body therapies may be helpful:

- Acupuncture
- Adventure therapy
- Biofeedback
- Bodywork
- Expressive arts therapy
- Hypnosis
- Yoga

Providing Support: Education and Support Measures to Consider

- Provide information and support for dietary and behavioral changes
- 🌐 Integrate nutritional education with cultural practices
- Engage the individual and her family in care and management plan
- Support and reinforce a positive self-image

Follow-up Care: Follow-up Measures to Consider

- Monitor weight and BMI
- Observe for signs or symptoms
  - Malnutrition syndromes
  - Relapse

Multidisciplinary Practice: Consider Consultation, Collaboration, or Referral

- Psychiatrist or mental health professional
- Registered dietician
- Eating disorder facility
- For diagnosis or treatment outside the midwife's scope of practice

ASSESSMENT OF THE WOMAN WITH MUSCULOSKELETAL SYMPTOMS

Key Clinical Information

The midwife assesses for musculoskeletal conditions during college, sports, or school physicals; before recommending that a client begin a vigorous exercise program; as a result of new-onset symptoms; or as part of a routine well-woman exam. The two most frequently diagnosed musculoskeletal problems in women are osteoarthritis and back strain (U.S. Bone and Joint Decade, 2008). Rheumatoid arthritis occurs two to three times more often in women than in men. Lupus and fibromyalgia also occur more frequently in women than in men. Lupus is three times more common in African American women than in white women. Obesity can result in increased complaints of musculoskeletal problems such as chronic pelvic, knee, or back pain. In addition, psychosocial stressors can result in somatic complaints related to the musculoskeletal system. For this reason, it is vital that the midwife pay attention not only to presenting physical symptoms but also to the circumstances surrounding the presentation of symptoms so as to make the correct diagnosis or referral.

Client History and Chart Review: Components of the History to Consider

- Primary indication for visit
- Evaluation of musculoskeletal symptoms
  - Location
    - Unilateral versus bilateral
    - Symmetric
    - Joint versus muscle
  - Onset
    - Precipitating factors
    - Mechanism of injury
    - Gradual versus sudden
    - Effect of time of day or weather
  - Duration
    - Chronic versus acute
    - Constant versus intermittent
  - Severity of symptoms
  - Relief measures used and their effects
    - Over-the-counter or prescription medications
    - Heat or ice
    - Rest
    - Compression
    - Brace or splint

- Associated symptoms
  - Atypical pain
  - Fever
  - Chills
  - Weight loss
- Medical/surgical history
  - Age (consider the client's life stage)
  - Allergies
  - Current medications
  - Last tetanus and diphtheria immunizations
  - History of GI upset or bleeding with prior NSAID use
  - Osteoporosis risk (see "Care of the Woman at Risk for Osteoporosis")
- Pregnancy history
  - Current reproductive status
  - LMP, GP TPAL
- Family history
  - Osteoarthritis
  - Osteoporosis
- Social history
  - Ethnic heritage
  - Physical activity patterns
    - Typical activity
    - Recent unusual activity
  - Nutritional status
  - Physical abuse/neglect/intimate-partner violence: Can present as somatic symptoms, aches and pains
  - Physical exertion or strain related to the following sources:
    - Job or child care
    - Hobby
    - School
    - Sports
    - Housework
  - Drug or alcohol use
- Review of systems

Physical Examination: Components of the Physical Exam to Consider

- Vital signs, including temperature
- BMI

- Overall muscle to fat ratio
- Posture and gait
- Evaluate for neurovascular status of tissues distal to the site of concern
- Evaluate affected area(s)
  - Heat, redness, or swelling
  - Range of motion, crepitus, or clicks
  - Muscle tension or limitation
- Palpation
  - Tenderness
  - Point tenderness
  - Soft-tissue spasm
  - Mass
- Neurologic assessment
  - Strength/weakness
  - Muscle wasting
  - Sensation
- Vascular assessment
  - Color
  - Pulses
  - Capillary refill
- Presence or absence of the following:
  - Ecchymosis
  - Hematoma
  - Limb or joint deformity

Clinical Impression: Differential Diagnoses to Consider

(ICD9Data.com, 2012)

- Osteoarthritis
- Back strain
- Physical abuse
- Joint strain or sprain
- Malignancy or tumor
- Systemic disorders
  - Multiple sclerosis
  - Chronic fatigue syndrome
  - Lupus erythematosus
  - Fibromyalgia
- Peripheral neuropathy and/or radiculopathy
- Fracture
- Carpal tunnel syndrome
- Rotator cuff tendonitis

Diagnostic Testing: Diagnostic Tests and Procedures to Consider

- Anticipated NSAID administration for more than 3 months: Baseline testing
  - Liver function
  - Platelets
- Inflammatory process versus infection
  - Complete blood count with differential
  - Erythrocyte sedimentation rate
  - C-reactive protein
  - Rheumatoid factor antibody
  - Creatinine
- Evaluation of mass or injury
  - Ultrasound
  - X-ray
  - Computed tomography
  - Magnetic resonance imaging

Providing Treatment: Therapeutic Measures to Consider

- Treatment is based on the client's diagnosis
- NSAIDs are frequently the first-line therapy
- RICE: Rest, ice, compression, elevation following acute injury

Providing Treatment: Complementary and Alternative Measures to Consider

- Treatment is based on the client's diagnosis
- Weight loss, as indicated
- Activities to maintain flexibility, balance, and strength
  - Yoga
  - Dance
  - Pilates
  - Resistance training
  - Swimming

Providing Support: Education and Support Measures to Consider

- Provide information related to the client's diagnosis
- Teach or reinforce proper body mechanics
  - Maintain a wide base of support
  - Lift with the object close to the body

- Encourage or reinforce maintaining a healthy weight for height
  - Well-balanced diet
  - Portion control
  - Adequate rest
  - Regular physical activity or exercise

Follow-up Care: Follow-up Measures to Consider

- Document
- Return for continued care
  - As needed within 7–14 days
  - If problem worsens or persists
  - Depression related to chronic pain syndrome(s)
  - As needed for medication management

Multidisciplinary Practice: Consider Consultation, Collaboration, or Referral

- Based on the diagnosis
  - Acupuncture
  - Chiropractic
  - Immunologist
  - Mental health services
  - Neurology
  - Physical therapy
  - Podiatry
  - Occupational therapy
  - Orthopedic services
  - Osteopath
  - Rheumatology
- For diagnosis or treatment outside the midwife's scope of practice

CARE OF THE WOMAN WITH ACUTE MUSCULOSKELETAL INJURY

Key Clinical Information

Injuries to muscles and joints occur frequently in women, particularly in women with a prior history of injury and those with nutritional deficiencies (Chorba, Chorba, Bouillon, Overmyer, & Landis, 2010; Thein-Nissenbaum, Rauh, Carr, Loud, & McGuine, 2011). Injury can occur as a result of impact trauma or muscle strain during sports, accident, or activities of daily living. Musculoskeletal injury results in inflammation, pain, and compensatory protective changes in patterns of movement; these compensatory changes, in turn, appear to increase the risk of future injury (Chorba et al., 2010). The inflammation seen early after muscle injury is thought to represent part of the healing process; thus use of anti-inflammatory agents is maintained at the minimum effective dose (Quintero, Wright, Fu, & Huard, 2009). Fibrotic scarring frequently occurs following injury, necessitating directed treatment to mobilize joints and rehabilitate atrophied muscle (Heiderscheit, Sherry, Silder, Chumanov, & Thelen, 2010; Quintero et al., 2009).

Client History and Chart Review: Components of the History to Consider

(Heiderscheit et al., 2010)

- Primary indication for the visit
- Mechanism of injury
  - Impact
  - Repetitive action
- Past injuries
- Evaluation of musculoskeletal symptoms
  - Location
    - Unilateral versus bilateral
    - Symmetric
    - Joint versus muscle
  - Onset
    - Precipitating factors
    - Mechanism of injury
    - Gradual versus sudden
    - Effect of time of day or weather
  - Duration
  - Severity of symptoms
  - Relief measures used and their effects
- Medical/surgical history
  - Age (consider the client's life stage)
  - Allergies
  - Current medications
  - History of GI upset or bleeding with prior NSAID use
- Pregnancy history
  - Current reproductive status
  - LMP, GP TPAL

- Social history
  - Physical activity patterns
    - Typical activity
    - Recent unusual activity
  - Physical exertion or strain related to the following sources:
    - Job or child care
    - Hobby
    - School
    - Sports
    - Housework
  - Drug or alcohol use
  - Intimate-partner violence
- Review of systems

Physical Examination: Components of the Physical Exam to Consider

(Heiderscheit et al., 2010)

- Vital signs, including height, weight, and BMI
- General affect and evidence of pain
- Posture and gait
- Palpation of the affected area
  - Pain and heat
  - Fluid collection
  - Crepitus
- Assessment of the affected area
  - Strength
  - Sensation
  - Reflexes
  - Neurologic function
  - Visible deformity
  - Erythema or rash
  - Ecchymosis
  - Range of motion
  - Pain with motion

Clinical Impression: Differential Diagnoses to Consider

(ICD9Data.com, 2012)

- Injury to muscles of the neck
- Injury to muscles of the lower back
- Injury to muscles of the shoulder and upper arm
- Injury to muscles of the elbow and forearm
- Injury to muscles of the wrist, hand, and fingers
- Injury to muscles of the hip and thigh
- Injury to muscles of the knee and lower leg
- Injury to muscles of the ankle and foot

Diagnostic Testing: Diagnostic Tests and Procedures to Consider

- Diagnostic imaging

Providing Treatment: Therapeutic Measures to Consider

- Protection from further injury
- Reduction of acute pain and inflammation (Quintero et al., 2009)
  - Rest
  - Cold therapy
    - 20-minute treatments
    - First 3 days
    - Protect skin from direct contact with the ice or cold pack
  - Compression to reduce swelling
  - Elevation of the affected area above the heart
  - Brace or splint for stability
  - Over-the-counter or prescription medications
    - Acetaminophen
    - NSAIDs
      - Naproxen sodium: Pregnancy Category B; Pregnancy Category D in third trimester
      - Ibuprofen: Pregnancy Category B; Pregnancy Category D in third trimester
- Rehabilitation of muscle strength and range
  - Physical therapy
  - Concentric/eccentric strength training
- Muscle relaxants
  - ⚠ Be alert for drug seekers complaining of chronic pain
  - Equagesic (meprobamate and aspirin): Musculoskeletal pain with anxiety (Pregnancy Category D)
    - Dose: 1–2 tablets TID or QID
    - Short-term use only

- Flexeril (cyclobenzaprine): Muscle spasm (Pregnancy Category B)
  - Dose: 10 mg TID; maximum 60 mg daily
  - Limit use to 21 days or less
- Robaxin (methocarbamol): Painful musculoskeletal conditions (Pregnancy Category C)
  - Dose: 1.5 mg QID for 2–3 days
  - Maintenance: 4 g daily in divided doses

Providing Treatment: Complementary and Alternative Measures to Consider

- Treatment is based on resting the affected area
- Gentle range-of-motion activities to maintain flexibility and strength
- Topical therapy
  - Comfrey compresses
  - Arnica montana
  - Capsaicin cream
- For soft-tissue injury
  - Comfrey leaf compresses
  - Castor oil warm packs
  - Homeopathic arnica montana
  - Massage therapy
  - Hydrotherapy
- Anti-inflammatory herbs: Tea, tincture, or capsule
  - Ginger
  - Tumeric
  - Feverfew
  - Rosehips
  - Flaxseed meal 2 Tbs daily with water

Providing Support: Education and Support Measures to Consider

- Provide information related to the diagnosis and injury prevention
  - Review the mechanism of injury, as applicable
  - Evaluation and treatment recommendations
  - Provide exercise recommendations
    - Limitations and restrictions
    - Range of motion

- Strengthening
- Aerobic and endurance
- Warning signs
- Medication information
- Encourage (Quintero et al., 2009)
  - Continued physical activity and early mobilization
  - Good body mechanics: Avoid favoring injured area
  - Warm-ups before physical activities
  - Activities that foster neuromuscular control

Follow-up Care: Follow-up Measures to Consider

- Document
  - Midwifery plan of care
  - Referrals for care
- Return for continued care
  - For no improvement within 7–14 days
  - If the problem worsens or persists

Multidisciplinary Practice: Consider Consultation, Collaboration, or Referral

- Orthopedic services: After limited results from treatment
  - Bursitis
  - Tendonitis
  - Carpal tunnel syndrome
  - Sprain or strain
  - Knee effusion
- Physical or occupational therapy
  - Evaluation of body mechanics
  - Strength training
  - Ergonomic training
- Based on the diagnosis and client preference
  - Acupuncture
  - Chiropractic
  - Neurology
  - Physical therapy
  - Orthopedic services
- For diagnosis or treatment outside the midwife's scope of practice

CARE OF THE WOMAN WITH ARTHRITIS

Key Clinical Information

The term *arthritis* refers to a wide range of rheumatic disorders and conditions that result in joint pain and, in some instances, inflammation (CDC, 2011a). The diagnosis of arthritis is based on symptoms of pain and stiffness in one or more joints, and encompasses osteoarthritis, rheumatoid arthritis, gout, lupus, and fibromyalgia. The diagnosis is based on the symptom profile, physical exam findings, and radiologic evidence of changes to joints and associated connective tissues (CDC, 2011a). As the condition progresses, pain becomes a primary symptom. Osteoarthritis, the most common form of arthritis, is a degenerative disorder in which use of the joint over time causes deterioration of its smooth articular surface. Rheumatoid arthritis and lupus are autoimmune disorders, while fibromyalgia has an unknown etiology. All four of these conditions occur more frequently in women than in men (CDC, 2011a).

Client History and Chart Review: Components of the History to Consider

(CDC, 2011a)

- Age
- Symptom profile
  - Onset, duration, and severity of arthritic symptoms
  - Symmetric versus asymmetric
  - Location(s)
  - Associated arthritis symptoms
    - Pain
    - Swelling
    - Fatigue
    - Morning stiffness
    - Difficulty with activities of daily living
- Medical/surgical history
  - Previous injury to the affected joint(s)
  - Psoriasis
- Pregnancy history
  - Current reproductive status
  - LMP, GP TPAL

- Family history
  - Arthritis
  - Thyroid disorders
- Common symptoms of rheumatoid arthritis
  - Swelling in one or more joints
  - Joint stiffness that lasts more than 1 hour on arising from sleep
  - Constant or recurring pain or tenderness in a joint
  - Difficulty using or moving a joint normally
  - Warmth and redness in a joint
- Common symptoms of osteoarthritis
  - Joint stiffness that lasts more than 1 hour on arising from sleep
  - Constant or recurring pain or tenderness in a joint
  - Difficulty using or moving a joint normally
- Common symptoms of lupus
  - Malar or butterfly rash
  - Joint stiffness that lasts more than 1 hour on arising from sleep
  - Constant or recurring pain or tenderness in a joint
  - Difficulty using or moving a joint normally
  - Warmth and redness in a joint
- Common symptoms of fibromyalgia
  - Non-restful sleep
  - Persistent fatigue
  - Constant or recurring pain or point tenderness

Physical Examination: Components of the Physical Exam to Consider

- Vital signs, including temperature, weight, and BMI
- Observation of posture and gait
- HEENT
  - Facial rash
  - Thyroid palpation
- Examination of affected joints
  - Swelling or deformity
  - Limited range of motion
  - Crepitus

- Skin changes
- Warmth and redness
- Palpation of muscles and soft tissues
  - Pain
  - Sensation
  - Strength
- Assessment of pain using a standardized tool

Clinical Impression: Differential Diagnoses to Consider

(ICD9Data.com, 2012)

- Osteoarthritis
- Rheumatoid arthritis
- Fibromyalgia
- Lupus
- Lyme disease

Diagnostic Testing: Diagnostic Tests and Procedures to Consider

- Complete blood count
- Erythrocyte sedimentation rate (ESR)
- C-reactive protein (CRP)
- Rheumatoid factor assay (RF)
- Antinuclear antibody assay (ANA)
- Urinalysis
- X-ray
- Physical or occupational therapy evaluation of functional status
- Bone mineral density testing
- Anticipated NSAID administration for more than 3 months: Baseline testing
  - Liver function
  - Platelets

Providing Treatment: Therapeutic Measures to Consider

- Active listening and validation of concerns
- Physical or occupational therapy
- NSAIDs are frequently the first-line therapy for inflammatory conditions
  - Naproxen sodium: Pregnancy Category B; Pregnancy Category D in third trimester

- Ibuprofen: Pregnancy Category B; Pregnancy Category D in third trimester
- Acetaminophen
- Trial of SSRI antidepressants for symptoms of fibromyalgia
- Steroids
- Cognitive-behavioral therapy

Providing Treatment: Complementary and Alternative Measures to Consider

- Very-low-fat vegan diet for rheumatoid arthritis (Elkan, Sjöberg, Kolsrud, Ringertz, Hafström, & Frostegård, 2008)
  - Reduction in symptoms
  - Decreased inflammatory markers
  - Improved CVD risk profile
- Chondroitin and glucosamine

Providing Support: Education and Support Measures to Consider

- Provide information regarding the type of arthritis
  - Chronic condition
  - Requires adaptation and lifestyle changes
  - Continue non-weight-bearing physical activity to maintain joint mobility
  - Continue weight-bearing physical activity to maintain muscle strength
  - Use splints and assistive aids as needed
- Maintain optimal weight through a healthy, low-fat diet
- Promote self-efficacy and self-management of lifestyle
  - Relaxation training
  - Self-pacing
  - Sleep hygiene
  - Stress reduction
  - Visualization
- Promote effective management of pain
  - Use nonpharmacologic therapies
    - Meditation
    - Yoga
    - Hydrotherapy
    - Massage

■ Take medications as instructed
   ◆ Avoid intermittent use
   ◆ Use the lowest effective dose

Follow-up Care: Follow-up Measures to Consider

- Document
  - ■ Midwifery plan of care
  - ■ 🕿 Referral of the client for a new diagnosis
- Return for continued care
  - ■ For no improvement within 7–14 days of beginning treatment
  - ■ If the problem worsens or persists
- Surgical joint replacement may be indicated

Multidisciplinary Practice: Consider Consultation, Collaboration, or Referral

- ⚠ Medical services for fever, rash, or neurologic involvement
- Based on the severity of the client's condition and response to treatment
  - ■ Acupuncture
  - ■ Chiropractic
  - ■ Mental health services
  - ■ Neurology
  - ■ Physical therapy
  - ■ Orthopedic services
  - ■ Rheumatology
- For diagnosis or treatment outside the midwife's scope of practice

CARE OF THE WOMAN WITH BACK PAIN

Key Clinical Information

Back and neck pain are generally classified as being either acute or chronic conditions that result in inflammatory or neuropathic pain. Injury resulting from muscle strain, overuse, or torque causes tissue damage and release of inflammatory mediators, which then stimulate an enhanced pain response (Scholz et al., 2009). Back pain is considered a multifactorial biopsychosocial condition affecting activities of daily living, including employment. A pessimistic attitude toward chronic back pain is associated with a greater perception of pain and of disability in women with this problem (Urquhart, Bell, Ciuttini, Cui, Forbes, & Davis, 2008). Nevertheless, many women have jobs or lives that require moderate to heavy lifting, tugging, or repetitious motion that can contribute to chronic back pain. Physical activity to provide muscular support to the spine is the most effective long-term treatment of back pain (Bigos, Holland, Holland, Webster, Battie, & Malmgren, 2009). Consultation or referral is indicated for women who present with apparent neuropathic pain such as might occur with a herniated or ruptured disc.

Client History and Chart Review: Components of the History to Consider

- Age
- Back pain symptom profile
  - ■ Onset, duration, and severity of symptoms
  - ■ Symmetric versus asymmetric
  - ■ Location(s): Sciatica
  - ■ Associated symptoms
    - ◆ Pain
      - ➤ Nature
      - ➤ Severity
      - ➤ Timing
    - ◆ Weakness in extremities
    - ◆ Tingling or numbness in extremities
    - ◆ Difficulty with activities of daily living
  - ■ Relief measures used and their effectiveness
- Medical/surgical history
  - ■ Medications
  - ■ Previous injury to back or neck
  - ■ Depression or anxiety
- Pregnancy history
  - ■ Current reproductive status
  - ■ LMP, GP TPAL
- Social history
  - ■ Effect of back pain on family and work
  - ■ Beliefs about back pain
  - ■ Contributing lifestyle factors
    - ◆ Attitude
    - ◆ Coping mechanism
    - ◆ Social support

◆ Heavy work or lifting

◆ Poor body mechanics

◆ Tension or muscle stress

◆ Fear of pain or re-injury

■ Alcohol or drug use

■ Employment status

Physical Examination: Components of the Physical Exam to Consider

(Koes, van Tulder, Lin, Macedo, McAuley, & Maher, 2010; Scholz et al., 2009)

- Vital signs, including weight and BMI
- Observation of posture and gait
- Assessment of affected area
  - Mobility
  - Sensation
  - Strength
  - Reflexes
  - Spinal mobility
  - Response to stimuli
    ◆ Touch
    ◆ Cold
    ◆ Pin prick
    ◆ Light and deep pressure
    ◆ Vibration
  - Proprioception (sense of position and passive movement)
  - Passive straight-leg–raising test
    ◆ Lift leg at the knee to a 90-degree angle
    ◆ Stop at less than 90 degrees if pain occurs
- Assessment of foot strength and flexibility: Note ankle flexion and extension
- Assessment of pain using a standardized tool
- [www] Assessment for anxiety or depression using a validated tool

Clinical Impression: Differential Diagnoses to Consider

(ICD9Data.com, 2012)

- Backache, unspecified
- Musculoskeletal disorders and symptoms referable to the neck
- Sciatica

- Thoracic or lumbosacral neuritis or radiculitis, unspecified

Diagnostic Testing: Diagnostic Tests and Procedures to Consider

(Scholz et al., 2009)

- MRI for women with back pain that meets the following criteria:
  - Persists beyond 4 weeks
  - Is associated with neurologic deficit
  - Raises suspicion of vertebral pathology
- Anticipated NSAID administration for more than 3 months: Baseline testing
  - Liver function
  - Platelets

Providing Treatment: Therapeutic Measures to Consider

(Furlan et al., 2010; Koes et al., 2010)

- For the pregnant woman, see "Care of the Pregnant Woman with Backache"
- Spinal manipulation or mobilization
- Pain relief
  - First-line drug therapy
    ◆ Acetaminophen (preferred)
    ◆ NSAIDs
  - For severe pain unresponsive to first-line therapy
    ◆ Aspirin
    ◆ Opioids
    ◆ Muscle relaxants
  - For persistent pain: SSRI
- Chronic pain
  - Multidisciplinary care
    ◆ Physical therapy
    ◆ Occupational therapy
    ◆ Back school
    ◆ Cognitive-behavioral therapy
  - Goal is to improve functional capacity
- Muscle relaxants
  - ⚠ Be alert for drug seekers complaining of chronic pain

- Equagesic: Musculoskeletal pain with anxiety (Pregnancy Category D)
  - Dose: 1–2 tablets TID or QID
  - Short-term use only
- Flexeril: Muscle spasm (Pregnancy Category B)
  - Dose: 10 mg TID; maximum 60 mg daily
  - Limit use to 21 days or less
- Robaxin: Painful musculoskeletal conditions (Pregnancy Category C)
  - Dose: 1.5 mg QID for 2–3 days
  - Maintenance: 4 g daily in divided doses

Providing Treatment: Complementary and Alternative Measures to Consider

(Furlan et al., 2010)
Consider the following measures for pain relief:

- Acupuncture
- Heat or cold
- Capsaicin cream
- Empathetic care practices
- Herbal therapy (Gagnier, van Tulder, Berman, & Bombardier, 2006)
  - Devil's claw: 50–100 mg harpagoside daily
  - Willow bark: 120–240 mg salicin daily
  - Cayenne: Poultice or plaster
- Massage
- Guided imagery
- Meditation
- Relaxation techniques
- Tai Chi

Providing Support: Education and Support Measures to Consider

- Provide information regarding back pain
  - Continue physical activity to maintain mobility
  - Use careful body mechanics
  - Avoid activities that cause stress and strain
    - Twisting
    - Favoring one side
    - Lifting with a bent back

- Following the acute phase, begin exercise to maintain muscle strength
- Maintain optimal weight through a healthy, low-fat diet
- Promote self-efficacy and self-management of lifestyle
  - Relaxation training
  - Self-pacing
  - Sleep hygiene
  - Stress reduction
  - Visualization
- Promote effective management of pain
  - Use nonpharmacologic therapies
    - Meditation
    - Yoga
    - Hydrotherapy
    - Massage
  - Take medications as instructed
    - Avoid intermittent use
    - Use the lowest effective dose
- Back pain can be a chronic condition: Address long-term sequelae
  - Depression resulting from chronic pain
  - Changes in activities of daily living
  - Warning signs

Follow-up Care: Follow-up Measures to Consider

- Document
- Return for continued care
  - For no improvement within 7–14 days of beginning treatment
  - If the problem worsens or neurologic symptoms occur
- Surgical treatment may be indicated

Multidisciplinary Practice: Consider Consultation, Collaboration, or Referral

(Koes et al., 2010)

- Neurologic services
  - Neurologic symptoms
  - Herniated disc
  - Suspicion of multiple sclerosis

- Physical or occupational therapy
  - Evaluation of body mechanics
  - Strength training
  - Ergonomic training
- Persistent back pain, without evidence of pathology: Consider referral
  - Acupuncturist
  - Chiropractor
  - Neurologist
  - Massage therapist
  - Osteopath
- Based on the severity of the client's condition and response to treatment
  - Back clinic
  - Mental health services
  - Neurology
  - Pain clinic
  - Orthopedic services
- For diagnosis or treatment outside the midwife's scope of practice

ASSESSMENT OF THE WOMAN WITH NEUROLOGIC SYMPTOMS

Key Clinical Information

Neurologic symptoms can present as indications of neurologic disease or injury, or as indicators of disorders or injury of other body systems. Neurologic symptoms occur with disorders and diseases such as chronic pain, dizziness, epilepsy, Lyme disease, migraine, multiple sclerosis, Parkinson's disease, spinal disorders, stroke, and trauma. As primary care providers, midwives are often women's first resource when such symptoms develop.

Neurologic assessment begins with the initial greeting, and many components are assessed as a matter of course during a routine exam. Focused evaluation of neurologic symptoms by the primary care practitioner is intended to assess the severity of symptoms, identify differential diagnoses, and arrange for specialist evaluation and treatment for all but the most common self-limiting conditions.

In caring for women across the life span, midwives will encounter women with preexisting neurologic disorders actively managed by neurologic specialists. Cyclical hormone changes, pregnancy, menopause, and other gender-related factors can make treating neurologic conditions in women a particular challenge. Coordinated multidisciplinary care offers women the best opportunity to manage their neurologic conditions in a way that meets their needs in the context of their lives, culture. and community.

Client History and Chart Review: Components of the History to Consider

(Critical Care Concepts, 2006)

- Report of symptoms documented using the client's own words
- History of the current problem:
  - Symptoms: Emotional, cognitive, and physical
    - Onset, duration, and cycles
    - Precipitating factors or events
    - Treatments used and their efficacy
  - Changes in the following aspects of functioning:
    - Weight
    - Appetite
    - Sleep patterns
    - Social activities
    - Relationships
- Mental status
  - General cognitive status
    - Orientation
    - Memory
    - Attention
    - Abstract thinking and reasoning
    - Speech patterns and use of language
    - Alterations in thought processes or responses
  - Previous mental health symptoms, diagnosis, or treatment
- Identify presence of new-onset neurologic symptoms
  - Headache
  - New-onset difficulty with speech

- Change in ability to read or write
- Alteration in memory
- Altered level of consciousness
- Confusion or change in thinking
- Difficulty hearing
- Change in vision or diplopia
- Altered gait or balance, falls
- Dizziness
- Disorientation
- Decreased sense of smell or taste
- Difficulty with swallowing or choking
- Decrease in sensation, tingling, or pain
- Motor weakness or decreased strength
- Tremors, twitches, or increased muscle tone
- Reproductive history
  - LMP, current menstrual status
  - GP TPAL, children at home
  - Current method of contraception
- Medical/surgical history
  - Allergies
  - Current medications
    - Hormones
    - Antidepressants
    - Analgesics
    - Other medications
    - Dietary supplements or herbal remedies
  - Medical conditions
    - Hypertension
    - Heart disease
  - Previous surgery
- Social history: Drug or alcohol use
- Related family history
- Review of systems

Physical Examination: Components of the Physical Exam to Consider

(Moses, 2012)

- Observe for gait and balance
- Vital signs
- Weight, height, and BMI
- Behavioral, cognitive and mental status assessment

- Age appropriate
- Developmentally appropriate
- Culturally appropriate
- Affect
- Alertness and level of consciousness
- Articulation of words
- Characteristics of voice
- Cooperation, participation, and eye contact
- Memory, logic, and reasoning
- Slow speech or movements
- Physical exam
  - Asymmetry
  - Involuntary motions
  - HEENT
    - Pupils and ocular movements
    - Hearing
    - Cranial nerve assessment
  - Cardiopulmonary status
    - Cardiac rate and rhythm
    - Respiratory rate, rhythm, and depth
  - Motor exam
    - Shoulders and arms
    - Hips and legs
    - Muscular atrophy
    - Range of motion
    - Strength, tone, and coordination
    - Symmetry of response
  - Reflexes
    - Deep tendon reflexes (DTRs)
    - Gag reflex
    - Plantar reflex
  - Sensory exam
    - Touch
    - Pain
    - Temperature
    - Proprioception

Clinical Impression: Differential Diagnoses to Consider

(ICD9Data.com, 2012)

- Chronic pain
- Headache

- Neurologic symptoms: Specify
- Neuropathy
- Meningitis
- Mental illness
- Substance abuse
- Seizure disorders

Diagnostic Testing: Diagnostic Tests and Procedures to Consider

- Evaluate for a physical disorder based on previous findings
  - History
  - Physical examination
- Laboratory values
  - Electrolytes
  - Toxicology
- 🕐 Imaging studies to evaluate for signs of neurologic disorders

Providing Treatment: Therapeutic Measures to Consider

Treatment is based on the client's symptom profile and diagnosis. When in doubt, consult with, or refer the client to, a mental health prescribing professional.

Providing Treatment: Complementary and Alternative Measures to Consider

⚠️ Alternative treatments are not intended as a substitute for medical care in the presence of a serious neurologic disorder.

- Dietary support
  - Gluten- and casein-free diet
  - Wheat germ
- Supplements
  - Minerals that enhance nerve function
    - Calcium
    - Magnesium
  - Omega-3 fatty acids
  - Evening primrose oil
  - Ginkgo biloba
- Support groups: Chosen based on the client's diagnosis

Providing Support: Education and Support Measures to Consider

- Engage the client in self-care (U.S. Department of Health and Human Services, 2006)
  - Eat a well-balanced, varied diet
  - Get regular rest and adequate sleep
  - Set attainable goals according to limitations
    - Set priorities
    - Break large tasks into smaller ones
    - Assume a tolerable amount of responsibility
- Provide information related to community resources
  - Health education services
  - Support groups
  - For women receiving medical treatment and/ or referrals, provide detailed information
    - Referral information and goal of referral
    - Medication
      - Name
      - Dosing instructions
      - Indication
      - Desired effects
      - Potential side effects
      - Interactions
      - Pregnancy category (as needed)
    - Midwifery plan for continued care and follow-up
- Signs and symptoms indicating a need for additional care
  - Return for care
  - Immediate care
  - Emergency care

Follow-up Care: Follow-up Measures to Consider

- Document
  - Client collaboration with the plan of care
  - Verify the client's attendance at the referral(s)
- Provide, as appropriate:
  - Support and education related to the diagnosis
  - Monitoring of the client's condition per the plan of care

- Routine women's health care
  - ◆ Annual women's health exam and screening as indicated
  - ◆ Contraception or prenatal care as needed

Multidisciplinary Practice: Consider Consultation, Collaboration, or Referral

- Neurology services
  - ■ Symptoms that suggest a complex or serious neurologic disorder
  - ■ Failure to respond to medication or prescribed treatment
- Emergency services: Potential life-threatening neurologic signs or symptoms
- Social services
  - ■ Concomitant substance abuse
  - ■ Concomitant psychosocial problems
  - ■ Counseling
  - ■ Nontraditional therapy options
- For diagnosis or treatment outside the midwife's scope of practice

CARE OF THE WOMAN WITH HEADACHE

Key Clinical Information

(American Headache Society, 2004)

Headache disorders are among the most common disabling conditions for women, and one of the most common symptoms that healthcare providers evaluate and treat. Headache is defined as "pain above the orbitomeatal line," which runs from the nasal bridge through the outer canthus of the eye to the center of the external auditory meatus (International Headache Society, 2005).

The differential diagnosis of headache includes more than 300 different types and etiologies. Headache disorders are classified into two general categories: primary and secondary headaches. Primary headache includes headaches that are not a symptom of, or caused by, another condition. They demonstrate several common patterns, including migraine, tension-type headache (TTH), and chronic daily headache. Most headache patients have primary headaches,

and many have more than one type of headache. It is important to integrate the information gained about the headaches with information known about the patient's other health problems.

Secondary headaches are rare and arise secondary to an underlying condition, such as a brain tumor or infection. These headaches are often characterized by abrupt onset of new headache, often described as the worst headache the patient ever had, and worsen over a period of days. Secondary-type headaches can be accompanied by fever, stiff neck, or vomiting.

Tension-type headache, previously called muscle tension or stress headache, is the most common type of headache in the general population. It is characterized by the absence of other associated features (Bendtsen et al., 2010).

Migraine is a recurrent headache disorder manifesting in attacks lasting 4 to 72 hours. Although a combination of features is required for making this diagnosis, not all features are present in every attack or in every patient (International Headache Society, 2005). Migraine is characterized by episodic attacks of severe headache and associated neurologic symptoms such as nausea, vomiting, photophobia, dizziness, cognitive impairment, and lethargy. The strongest predictors of migraine diagnosis are presence of nausea, disability, and photophobia.

Patients reporting headache who answer positively on two out of the three symptom questions have a 93% chance of being diagnosed with migraine. Because migraine is an illness of long duration, work productivity, family relationships, and quality of life are often affected by this condition. An estimated 18% of women experience migraine. Migraine increases in prevalence for women in their 20s and 30s, peaking around age 40, and then declining over the next few decades. Because these changes correspond with the childbearing years, it is theorized that estrogen and progesterone are involved in migraine etiology, but a causal relationship has not been established. The hormonal fluctuations that characterize the perimenopause period can result in worsening of migraine frequency for some women (Macgregor, 2008).

Client History and Chart Review: Components of the History to Consider

- Onset, severity, and frequency of symptoms
- Duration of pain (short-lived = cluster)
- Characteristics of pain
  - Tension-type headache
    - Pressing and tightening, described as a band around the head
    - Mild to moderate intensity
    - Not aggravated by routine activity such as climbing stairs or bending over
  - Migraine
    - Pulsating quality
    - Moderate or severe intensity
    - Aggravated by routine physical activity
    - Associated symptoms
- Location of pain
  - Bilateral: TTH
  - Unilateral: Cluster or migraine
- Preceding events
  - Menstruation: Menstrual migraines typically occur 2–3 days before or after the first day of menses
  - Sexual activity
  - Exercise
- Recent changes in the headache pattern
- Relief measures used and their results
- Associated symptoms
  - Presence of nausea and vomiting
  - Presence of light sensitivity
  - Aura
    - Blinking or flashing light
    - Blind spots
    - Speech difficulties
    - Tingling of the hands or face
- Degree of disability with headache
- Medication history
- Family history of headache
- Presence of additional neurologic symptoms
  - Cognitive changes
  - Changes in speech
  - Loss of strength or sensation
- Coexisting medical conditions

- Depression
- Anxiety

Physical Examination: Components of the Physical Exam to Consider

To evaluate for secondary headache, consider these elements of the physical exam:

- Vital signs: Pulse, blood pressure, and weight
- Ophthalmic exam
- Facial muscle strength
- Head and neck range of motion
- Pericranial tenderness
- Reflexes
- Balance

Clinical Impression: Differential Diagnoses to Consider

(ICD9Data.com, 2012)

- Tension-type headache
- Tension-type headache, unspecified
- Episodic tension-type headache
- Chronic tension-type headache
- Headache associated with sexual activity
- Other headache syndromes
- Migraine
- Variants of migraine, not elsewhere classified
- Menstrual migraine
- Persistent migraine aura without cerebral infarction
- Chronic migraine without aura
- Migraine, unspecified

Diagnostic Testing: Diagnostic Tests and Procedures to Consider

Diagnostic testing evaluates for secondary headache; it does not diagnose primary headache.

- Laboratory testing: Not useful
- Primary headache diagnosis: Based upon clinical symptoms
- Imaging studies to rule out secondary headache

Providing Treatment: Therapeutic Measures to Consider

(American Headache Society, 2004; King & Brucker, 2011)

There are many medication options from which to choose; a sampling is given here.

- Preemptive treatment is appropriate in the following circumstances:
  - When a time-limited trigger is expected, such as sexual activity or menstruation
  - For those experiencing migraine headaches two or more times per month
  - Those who perceive their headaches to be disabling and want preventive measures
- Migraine
  - Aspirin 900 mg or ibuprofen 200–800 mg q 4 hr, up to 1500 mg maximum daily
  - Oral or rectal antiemetic
    - Phenergan: 12.5–25 mg PO or rectally
    - Compazine: 25 mg rectally or 5–10 mg PO q 4–6 hr
    - Benadryl (OTC): 50–100 mg PO q 4–6 hr
  - Antimigraine medication
    - Almotriptan: 12.5 mg
    - Eletriptan: 40–80 mg
    - Rizatriptan: 10 mg
    - Sumatriptan: 50–100 mg with naproxen 500 mg for recurrent, prolonged attacks
    - Propranolol: 80–240 mg daily for migraine prevention
    - Paracetamol: 1000 mg for pregnant women
- Menstrual migraine
  - NSAID 1–2 days before the onset of expected headache: Ibuprofen 200–800 mg q 4 hr, up to 1500 mg maximum daily
  - Ergotamine tartrate HS or BID at the time of menses
- Tension-type headache
  - Aspirin: 250–1000 mg, up to 4000 mg maximum daily

- Ibuprofen: 200–800 mg q 4 hr, up to 3200 mg daily
- Acetaminophen: 1000 mg
- Amitriptyline: 30–75 mg daily for TTH prevention

Providing Treatment: Complementary and Alternative Measures to Consider

(Sun-Edelstein & Mauskop, 2011)

- Migraine
  - Dietary supplements
    - Magnesium: 600 mg daily
    - Coenzyme Q: 150 mg daily for 3 months
    - Riboflavin: 400 mg daily for 3 months
    - Butterbur root extract (Petadolex): 75 mg BID
    - Feverfew: Contraindicated in pregnancy
  - CAM therapies
    - Acupuncture
    - Transcutaneous electrical nerve stimulation (TENS)
    - Hydrotherapy
    - Massage
    - Relaxation training
    - Biofeedback
  - Cognitive-behavioral therapy (CBT)
- Tension-type headache
  - Biofeedback
  - Acupuncture
  - Physical therapy
  - Cervical spinal manipulation therapy
  - CBT

Providing Support: Education and Support Measures to Consider

- Provide information about the diagnosis, treatment options, and medication use
- Medications may take 2–3 months to demonstrate effectiveness in reducing headache frequency
- Discuss medication overuse and rebound headache

- Recommend keeping a headache diary
  - Date, time of onset, and resolution
  - Intensity using scale of 0 to 10
  - Preceding symptoms
  - Suspected triggers
  - Medication and dosage taken
  - Relief: Complete, partial, or none
- Avoid known triggers for headache
  - Smoke
  - Hot weather
  - Strong scents
  - Fatigue
  - Skipping meals
  - Stress
  - Caffeine withdrawal
- Research on migraine food triggers is inconclusive: Recommended to avoid strong, aged cheese and red wine
- Sleep hygiene: Avoid interrupted sleep or sleep deprivation
- Hormone replacement therapy (HRT): Can exacerbate migraine
- Use of oral contraceptives in women who have migraine with aura is controversial

Follow-up Care: Follow-up Measures to Consider

- Document
  - Symptoms
  - Evaluation and testing
  - Treatment recommendations and efficacy
  - Plan for continued care
  - Criteria for referral or consultation
- Review the client's headache diary
- Assess efficacy and use patterns of medication
- Engage the client in the plan of care

Multidisciplinary Practice: Criteria to Consider for Consultation, Collaboration, or Referral

- Neurology services or headache clinic
- Consider immediate referral for women with the following:
  - Papilledema
  - Presence of neurologic symptoms

- New persistent daily headache
- Headache with onset that is sudden and severe (thunderclap)
- Headache that changes with posture or Valsalva-type maneuvers such as sneezing or lifting
- Emergency or general medical services
  - Headache with additional features such as rash
  - Headache associated with hypertension
- CAM practitioners
- Physical therapy
- Chiropractic care
- Acupuncturist
- For diagnosis or treatment outside the midwife's scope of practice

ASSESSMENT OF THE WOMAN WITH RESPIRATORY SYMPTOMS

Key Clinical Information

Lung disease affects women of all ages and is a leading cause of illness and death. The provision of primary care to women who present with respiratory illness during pregnancy is not uncommon. Nasal mucosa and lung function can be affected by allergies, air quality, and environmental toxins, such as cigarette smoke, chemical fumes, or particulate matter. The respiratory disorders frequently seen in primary care include the common cold, sinusitis, bronchitis, asthma, and chronic cough. In addition, less common problems—such as tuberculosis, pneumonia, and respiratory malignancies—should be kept in mind when assessing the woman with respiratory symptoms (American Lung Association, 2010).

Client History and Chart Review: Components of the History to Consider

- Primary complaint
  - Symptom review
    - Onset, duration, and severity of symptoms
      - Cough
      - Sputum production
      - Color of sputum or nasal discharge

- ➤ Shortness of breath
- ➤ Difficulty with respiration or wheezing
- ➤ Frontal headache
- ➤ Fever and/or chills
- ▪ Other symptoms
  - ◆ Weight loss
  - ◆ Night sweats
  - ◆ Malaise
  - ◆ Loss of appetite
  - ◆ Weakness
  - ◆ Nasal congestion
  - ◆ Impaired or loss of sense of smell
  - ◆ Snoring or nasal obstruction
  - ◆ Bloody sputum
- ▪ Relief measures used and their effects
- • Medical and surgical history
  - ▪ Allergies
  - ▪ Medications
  - ▪ Medical conditions
    - ◆ Nasal polyposis
    - ◆ Heart disease
    - ◆ Respiratory disease
      - ➤ Asthma
      - ➤ Chronic obstructive pulmonary disease
      - ➤ Emphysema
      - ➤ Sinus infection(s)
      - ➤ Pneumonia
      - ➤ Cystic fibrosis
      - ➤ Cancer
      - ➤ HIV status, if known
- • Exposure to asthma triggers
  - ▪ Allergens
  - ▪ Irritants
  - ▪ Drugs
  - ▪ Exercise or cold air
- • Social history
  - ▪ Risk of type of lung disease varies with ethnicity (American Lung Association, 2010)
    - ◆ Higher rates of lung cancer in African Americans
    - ◆ Highest prevalence of asthma in Puerto Ricans
    - ◆ Highest death rate due to cystic fibrosis in Caucasians

- ◆ African Americans and Hispanics less likely to receive influenza immunizations
- ▪ IV drug, alcohol, or tobacco use
- ▪ Occupational exposure to respiratory irritants
- ▪ Air quality and living conditions (Hackley, 2007)
- ▪ Nutritional status
- • Review of systems

Physical Examination: Components of the Physical Exam to Consider

- • Vital signs
- • Color
  - ▪ Pallor
  - ▪ Rubor
  - ▪ Cyanosis
- • HEENT
  - ▪ Nasal septum and turbinates
  - ▪ Palpate sinuses
  - ▪ Palpation of lymph nodes
  - ▪ Throat
  - ▪ Tonsils
  - ▪ Tympanic membranes
- • Respiratory evaluation
  - ▪ Rate and pattern of breathing
  - ▪ Depth and symmetry of lung expansion
  - ▪ Auscultation
    - ◆ Quality and intensity of breath sounds
    - ◆ Adventitious breath sounds
      - ➤ Pneumonia: Crackles
      - ➤ Asthma
        - ◗ Diffuse wheezes or rhonchi
        - ◗ Prolonged expiratory phase
  - ▪ Percussion
    - ◆ Resonant: Normal, asthma, or interstitial lung disease
    - ◆ Dull: Consolidation or pleural effusion
    - ◆ Hyperresonant: Emphysema or pneumothorax
- • 🕐 Evidence of respiratory distress
  - ▪ Nasal flaring
  - ▪ Intercostal or supraclavicular retractions

- Peripheral cyanosis
- Elevated pulse and respiratory rate
- Grunting or wheezing

Clinical Impression: Differential Diagnoses to Consider

(ICD9Data.com, 2012)

- Asthma
- Bronchitis
- Chronic cough, due to the following causes:
  - Smoking
  - Postnasal drip
- Allergic rhinitis
- Sinusitis
- Influenza viruses: A, B, or C
- Nasal polyposis
- Deviated nasal septum
- *Pneumocystis carinii* pneumonia
- Tuberculosis
- Community-acquired pneumonia
- Acute upper respiratory infections
- Respiratory malignancies

Diagnostic Testing: Diagnostic Tests and Procedures to Consider

- Complete blood count (CBC)
- Nasal endoscopy
- Chest x-ray
  - Fever plus abnormal breath sounds
  - Suspicion of tuberculosis
- Gram stain and culture of purulent sputum: Suspected pneumonia
- HIV counseling and testing
- Pertussis serology
  - Afebrile client
  - Normal breath sounds
  - Cough greater than 2 weeks' duration
- Pulse oximetry and blood gases
- Peak flow or spirometry to assess
  - Lung function
    - Restrictive
    - Obstructive

- Progression of disorder
  - Severity
  - Medication effectiveness
- X-ray, MRI, or CT scan of sinuses: Chronic cough
- Tuberculosis testing: TB Mantoux (purified protein derivative [PPD])
  - 0.1 mL injected intradermally
  - [www] Two-step procedure indicated for select groups
  - For interpretation of PPD reaction, see "Care of the Woman with Tuberculosis"

Providing Treatment: Therapeutic Measures to Consider

- Treatment is based on the differential diagnosis
- For asthma, see "Care of the Woman with Asthma"
- For bronchitis, see "Care of the Woman with Bronchitis"
- For influenza, see "Care of the Woman with Influenza"
- For pneumonia, see "Care of the Woman with Pneumonia"
- For sinusitis, see "Care of the Woman with Sinusitis"
- For tuberculosis, see "Care of the Woman with Tuberculosis"
- For upper respiratory infection, see "Care of the Woman with Upper Respiratory Infection"
- Pertussis: Suspected or confirmed
  - Erythromycin: 1 g daily in divided doses for 14 days (Pregnancy Category B)
  - Sulfa-trimethoprim DS: 1 PO BID for 14 days (Pregnancy Category C/D in third trimester)

Providing Treatment: Complementary and Alternative Measures to Consider

- General measures to promote healing
  - Rest and adequate nutrition
  - Increased fluid intake, especially hot liquids

- High-protein, high-calorie diet
- Use positioning to aid drainage of secretions
- Saline nasal irrigation: Neti pot
- Eucalyptus steams
- Herbal remedies
  - Marshmallow root
  - Horehound
  - Mullein
- Astragalus: Safe for those with immune disorders

Providing Support: Education and Support Measures to Consider

- Provide information and recommendations
  - Diagnosis
  - Medication regimen(s)
    - Dosage and frequency
    - Potential side effects
  - Indications for cough suppressants
- Signs of improvement
  - Symptoms diminish within 1–3 days
  - Afebrile within 2–5 days (pneumonia)
- Warning signs and symptoms
  - Persistent cough
  - Fever with chills
  - Bloody sputum
  - Shortness of breath
- Environmental controls
  - Pets/allergens
  - Air conditioning
  - Mask or respirator
- Limitations
  - Isolation precautions with the client's family
  - Decreased activity

Follow-up Care: Follow-up Measures to Consider

- Document
- Return for continued care
  - Contact within 7–10 days (phone or visit)
  - As indicated by test results
  - Symptoms persist or worsen in spite of therapy
  - Persistent symptoms at revisit: Reevaluate for asthma

Multidisciplinary Practice: Consider Consultation, Collaboration, or Referral

- Medical services
  - Respiratory illness requiring hospitalization
  - Symptoms of respiratory distress
    - Respiratory rate greater than or equal to 30
    - Superclavicular or intercostal retractions
    - O_2 saturation of less than 95%
    - Cyanosis
  - Diagnosis of any of the following diseases:
    - Tuberculosis
    - Pertussis
    - *Pneumocystis carinii* pneumonia
    - Pneumonia
    - HIV/AIDS
- For diagnosis or treatment outside the midwife's scope of practices

CARE OF THE WOMAN WITH ASTHMA

Key Clinical Information

Asthma is a chronic respiratory condition characterized by inflammation of the pulmonary airways, leading to narrowing or obstruction of air exchange. Acute episodes can be triggered by numerous circumstances, such as infections, exercise, or exposure to allergens or airway irritants. Asthma affects children, women, African Americans, and economically disadvantaged individuals more than other populations. This disease is categorized based on the frequency and severity of its symptoms and signs. Use of asthma medications in pregnancy is safer for both mother and fetus than uncontrolled asthma and exacerbations (Hackley, 2007; King & Brucker, 2011).

Client History and Chart Review: Components of the History to Consider

- Asthma symptom review: See Table 8-7
  - Onset, duration, time of day, severity, and recurrence of symptoms
    - Chest tightness
    - Shortness of breath

Table 8-7 Determining Stage of Asthma by Symptoms

STAGE	SYMPTOMS
1: Mild	Daytime: 2 days or fewer per week
	Nighttime: 2 nights or fewer per month
2: Mild persistent	Daytime: more than 2 days per week but not daily
	Nighttime: more than 2 nights per month
3: Moderate persistent	Daytime: daily
	Nighttime: more than one night per week
4: Severe persistent	Daytime: continual
	Nighttime: frequent

Source: Adapted from Hackley, 2007.

- - ◆ Difficulty with respiration or wheezing
  - ◆ Nonproductive cough
  - ▪ Relief measures used and their effects
- Medical and surgical history
  - ▪ Allergies
  - ▪ Medications, including current asthma medication
    - ◆ Quick-relief medication and frequency of use
    - ◆ Longer-term asthma control medications
  - ▪ History of asthma
    - ◆ Childhood origin
    - ◆ Exercise induced
  - ▪ Other chronic diseases or disorders
  - ▪ Exposure to asthma triggers
    - ◆ Allergens
    - ◆ Irritants
    - ◆ Pet dander
    - ◆ Drugs
    - ◆ Exercise or cold air
- Social history
  - ▪ Race/ethnicity
  - ▪ Smoking or smoke exposure

- - ▪ Exposure to respiratory irritants at work
  - ▪ Air quality and living conditions at home
- Review of systems

Physical Examination: Components of the Physical Exam to Consider

- Vital signs
- Color
  - ▪ Pallor
  - ▪ Cyanosis
- HEENT: Pale nasal mucosa
- Respiratory evaluation
  - ▪ Rate and pattern of breathing
  - ▪ Depth and symmetry of lung expansion
  - ▪ Auscultation
  - ▪ Quality and intensity of breath sounds
  - ▪ Adventitious breath sounds
  - ▪ Findings common in asthma
    - ◆ Diffuse wheezes or rhonchi
    - ◆ Prolonged expiratory phase
    - ◆ Hyperinflated chest
    - ◆ Use of accessory muscles and retractions
    - ◆ Breathing easier in upright positions
  - ▪ Percussion
    - ◆ Resonant: Normal, asthma or interstitial lung disease
- Evidence of respiratory distress
  - ▪ Nasal flaring
  - ▪ Intercostal or supraclavicular retractions
  - ▪ Peripheral cyanosis
  - ▪ Elevated pulse and respiratory rate
  - ▪ Grunting or wheezing

Clinical Impression: Differential Diagnoses to Consider

(ICD9Data.com, 2012)

- Asthma

Diagnostic Testing: Diagnostic Tests and Procedures to Consider

- Peak flow: Diurnal variation of 20% or more
- Spirometry: Reversible airway obstruction

Providing Treatment: Therapeutic Measures to Consider

(King & Brucker, 2011)

See Table 8-8. Pregnant women on asthma medications should be maintained on these medications during pregnancy. It is safer for these women and their babies than asthma symptoms and exacerbations (ACOG, 2008).

- Quick-relief medications for asthma (fast-acting for acute attacks)
  - Short-acting beta$_2$ agonists: Albuterol
  - Anticholinergics: Ipratropium
  - Systemic corticosteroids: Methylprednisonolone
- Anti-inflammatory medications for long-term control
  - Inhaled corticosteroids: Beclomethasone and flunisolide
  - Mast cell stabilizers: Cromolyn sodium
  - Immunomodulators: Xolair
  - Leukotriene receptor antagonists: Accolate and Singulair
  - 5-Lipoxygenase inhibitors: Zyflo CR
  - Long-acting beta$_2$ agonists: Foradil and Serevent
  - Combination long-acting beta$_2$ agonist and steroid: Advair and Symbicort
  - Methylxanthines: Theophylline

Table 8-8 Determining Treatment of Asthma by Stage

STAGE	PREFERRED TREATMENT
1: Mild	No daily medications needed
2: Mild persistent	Low-dose inhaled corticosteroids
3: Moderate persistent	Low- to medium-dose inhaled corticosteroids and long-acting inhaled beta$_2$ agonists
4: Severe persistent	High-dose inhaled corticosteroids and long-acting inhaled beta$_2$ agonists

Source: Adapted from Hackley, 2007.

Providing Treatment: Complementary and Alternative Measures to Consider

- Herbal remedies should not be used in place of asthma medications
  - Licorice
  - Ginkgo biloba
  - Coltsfoot
- Yoga
- Acupuncture
- Biofeedback

Providing Support: Education and Support Measures to Consider

 Provide information and recommendations

- Have a written asthma action plan to manage symptoms (CDC, 2009b)
  - Medication regimen(s)
  - Dosage and frequency
  - When to contact the provider or come to the emergency room
- Environmental controls
  - Pets/allergens
  - Air conditioning
  - Mask or respirator
  - Avoid exposure to cold air
- Limitations
  - Decreased activity
  - Pre-exercise warm-up
  - Administration of a short-acting inhaled beta$_2$ agonist 15 minutes prior to exercise

Follow-up Care: Follow-up Measures to Consider

- Document
- Return for continued care if symptoms persist or worsen in spite of therapy

Multidisciplinary Practice: Consider Consultation, Collaboration, or Referral

- Medical services
  - Worsening of frequency and severity of asthma symptoms
  - Symptoms of respiratory distress

- For diagnosis or treatment outside the midwife's scope of practice

CARE OF THE WOMAN WITH BRONCHITIS

Key Clinical Information

Bronchitis is an inflammation of the bronchial epithelium of the tracheobronchial tree (Stemler, 2007). It can be acute or chronic in nature. Acute bronchitis is most often triggered by a viral infection, with its diagnosis and management based on the specific clinical findings. Chronic bronchitis is defined as a persistent cough that produces sputum and mucus for at least 3 consecutive months over the last 2 years. It is considered a form of chronic obstructive pulmonary disease (COPD); acute exacerbations of bronchitis in patients with chronic bronchitis require specialist care.

Client History and Chart Review: Components of the History to Consider

- Bronchitis symptom review
  - Onset, duration, severity, and persistence of symptoms
    - Cough: Often the dominant symptom
    - Sputum production
    - Color of sputum or nasal discharge
    - Shortness of breath
    - Chest discomfort
    - Frontal headache
    - Fever and/or chills
    - Throat pain
    - Postnasal drip
    - Fatigue
    - Malaise
  - Relief measures used and their effects
- Medical/surgical history
  - Allergies
  - Medications
  - Medical conditions
    - Chronic obstructive pulmonary disease
    - Recent "cold" or upper respiratory infection

- Social history
  - Tobacco use
  - Exposure to respiratory irritants
  - Air quality and living conditions
- Review of systems

Physical Examination: Components of the Physical Exam to Consider

- Vital signs
- HEENT
  - Nasal septum and turbinates
  - Palpate sinuses
  - Palpation of lymph nodes
  - Throat
  - Tonsils
  - Tympanic membranes
- Respiratory evaluation
  - Rate and pattern of breathing
  - Depth and symmetry of lung expansion
  - Auscultation: Quality and intensity of breath sounds
- Percussion

Clinical Impression: Differential Diagnoses to Consider

(ICD9Data.com, 2012)

- Bronchitis
- Chronic cough, due to the following causes:
  - Smoking
  - Postnasal drip

Diagnostic Testing: Diagnostic Tests and Procedures to Consider

- Chest x-ray: Fever plus abnormal breath sounds
- Gram stain and culture of purulent sputum: Suspected pneumonia
- Peak flow or spirometry to assess lung function

Providing Treatment: Therapeutic Measures to Consider

- Uncomplicated acute bronchitis treatment is directed to relief of cough: Use cough suppressants, expectorants, and mucolytics

- Tessalon perles: Pregnancy Category C
  - 100–200 mg PO TID as needed
  - Swallow capsules whole
  - Reduces the cough reflex by anesthetizing the respiratory passages
- Promethazine with codeine cough syrup: Pregnancy Category C
  - One tsp PO every 4 to 6 hours as needed
  - Drowsiness precautions
  - Narcotic precautions
- Antibiotics are generally not indicated, unless bacterial pneumonia is suspected
- Use beta$_2$ agonists, such as albuterol, in clients with abnormal breath sounds

Providing Treatment: Complementary and Alternative Measures to Consider

- General measures to promote healing
  - Rest and adequate nutrition
  - Increase fluids intake, especially hot liquids
  - Use positioning to aid drainage of secretions
- Eucalyptus steams
- Herbal remedies
  - Ginseng
  - Garlic
  - Echinacea
- Cough lozenges containing zinc

Herbal Cough Syrup Recipe

Mix 1 Tbs of slippery elm bark powder and ½ cup of honey in 1 cup of boiling water. Take 1 tsp of this syrup q 3–4 hours PRN hot or cold.

Providing Support: Education and Support Measures to Consider

Provide information and recommendations:

- Acute bronchitis
  - Cough suppression therapy
  - Reassurance that antibiotics are not always needed
  - Return for worsening symptoms

- Persistent cough
- Fever with chills
- Shortness of breath
- Chronic bronchitis: Explain the need for referral to specialist care

Follow-up Care: Follow-up Measures to Consider

- Document
- Return for continued care if symptoms persist or worsen in spite of therapy

Multidisciplinary Practice: Consider Consultation, Collaboration, or Referral

- Medical services
  - Respiratory illness requiring hospitalization
  - Symptoms of respiratory distress
- For diagnosis or treatment outside the midwife's scope of practice

CARE OF THE WOMAN WITH INFLUENZA

Key Clinical Information

Influenza, commonly referred to as the flu, is a contagious respiratory illness caused by influenza viruses. It can cause mild to severe illness and at times can lead to death (CDC, 2009a, 2011d; National Institute of Allergy and Infectious Diseases [NIAID], 2011). Influenza A and B viruses are responsible for seasonal flu epidemics that require development of a new vaccine each year, due to genetic changes that occur as the viruses replicate—a process known as antigenic drift. Influenza A undergoes an antigenic shift resulting in new subtypes of influenza A that occur when two different strains infect and exchange genetic material within the same cell. These subtypes are responsible for most severe epidemics or pandemics, as people have limited or no immunity to the new subtype. A recent example is the influenza pandemic that began in the spring of 2009 when a new influenza A (H1N1) virus emerged to cause illness in people and spread worldwide (American College of Nurse–Midwives [ACNM], 2009).

Every year in the United States, on average, 5% to 20% of the population gets the flu. In an average year, more than 200,000 people are hospitalized from flu-related complications, and approximately 36,000 people die from flu-related causes. Certain groups of people, such as older people, young children, pregnant women, and people with certain health conditions such as asthma, are at high risk for serious flu complications. Pregnant women should receive inactivated vaccine (flu shot) but should *not* receive the live attenuated vaccine (nasal spray).

Client History and Chart Review: Components of the History to Consider

- Influenza symptom review (CDC, 2011d): Onset, duration, time of day, severity, and recurrence of symptoms
  - Fever
  - Fatigue
  - Sore throat
  - Cough
  - Headache
  - Muscle or body aches
  - Runny or stuffy nose
  - Nausea
  - Diarrhea
  - Shortness of breath
  - Wheezing
- Relief measures used and their effects
- Pregnancy status and gestational age
- Medical/surgical history
  - Allergies
  - Current medications
  - Vaccination status
  - History of influenza
  - Other chronic diseases
- Social history
  - Exposure to others with influenza or influenza symptoms
  - Smoking
  - Nutritional status
- At-risk populations for serious morbidity/mortality with influenza
  - Pregnant women

- People younger than 5 years and older than 65 years of age
- Immunocompromised patients, such as those with HIV/AIDS
- Individuals with chronic diseases and disorders, such as diabetes and disabilities
- Native Americans/Alaskan natives
- Travelers to areas affected by H1N1
- Review of symptoms

Physical Exam: Components of the Physical Exam to Consider

(CDC, 2009a, 2011d)

- Vital signs
  - Fever
  - Tachypnea
  - Hypotension
- Color
  - Pallor
  - Cyanosis
- HEENT
  - Palpation of sinuses: Runny or stuffy nose
  - Palpation of lymph nodes
  - Throat: Sore throat
  - Tonsils
  - Tympanic membranes
- Respiratory evaluation
  - Rate and pattern or breathing
    - Shortness of breath
    - Cough
  - Depth and symmetry of lung expansion
  - Auscultation
    - Quality and intensity of breath sounds
      - Crackles
      - Wheezing
    - Adventitious breath sounds
- Emergent or warning signs (CDC, 2011d)
  - Difficulty breathing or shortness of breath
  - Pain or pressure in the chest or abdomen
  - Sudden dizziness
  - Confusion
  - Severe or persistent vomiting
  - Flu-like symptoms improve but then return with fever or worse cough

- Abdominal exam
  - Bowel sounds
  - Areas of pain or tenderness

Clinical Impression: Differential Diagnoses to Consider

(ICD9Data.com, 2012)

- Influenza viruses A, B, or C
- Influenza due to identified pandemic H1N1
- Influenza due to identified avian influenza virus H5N1
- Influenza with pneumonia
- Influenza with other respiratory manifestations

Diagnostic Testing: Diagnostic Tests and Procedures to Consider

(CDC, 2011d)

- Laboratory testing is of limited value in the management of influenza (Stemler, 2007)
- Nasopharyngeal or throat swab, nasal or bronchial wash, nasal aspirate, or sputum
  - Rapid influenza A and B diagnostic tests (RIDT)
    - Samples should be collected within first four days of illness
    - Most tests can be done in the care provider's office
    - Results are available in 15 minutes or less
    - Tests have 50–70% sensitivity for influenza detection and more than 90% specificity
  - Viral culture: Results in 3–10 days
  - Immunofluorescence DFA antibody staining: Results are available in 2–4 hours
  - Reverse transcriptase PCR (RT-PCR)
    - Recommended test for H1N1 diagnosis
    - Results are available in 2–4 hours
  - Enzyme immunoassay (EIA): Results are available in 2 hours
- Serology: Paired acute serum sample (collected within first week of illness) and convalescent serum sample (collected 2–4 weeks after the acute sample)
  - A fourfold or greater rise in antibody titer between the acute and convalescent samples indicates recent infection
  - Results are available in 2 weeks or more

Providing Treatment: Therapeutic Measures to Consider

(CDC, 2011d; King & Brucker, 2011)

- Prevention through vaccination (CDC, 2011d)
  - All persons older than 6 months of age should be vaccinated annually
  - Pregnant women are especially vulnerable
    - Encourage the flu shot
  - Check CDC sources annually for predicted flu types and vaccines for the ensuing season
- Antiviral medications: Begin within 48 hours of illness onset
  - Treatment of influenza
    - Oseltamivir (Tamiflu): Pregnancy Category C
      - 75-mg capsule twice daily for 5 days
      - Absorbed systemically
    - Zanamivir (Relenza): Pregnancy Category C
      - Two 5-mg inhalations (10 mg total) twice daily for 5 days
      - Limited systemic absorption
  - Chemoprophylaxis for individuals who cannot receive the vaccine or are immunosuppressed
    - Oseltamivir (Tamiflu): 75-mg capsule once daily for 10 days
    - Zanamivir (Relenza): Two 5 mg inhalations (10 mg total) once daily for 10 days
- Hydration
  - Oral fluids
  - IV therapy
- Fever reduction
  - Acetaminophen
    - 650–1000 mg every 4–6 hours
    - Daily maximum dose is 4 g
  - Cool, damp cloth on forehead
  - Tepid bath
  - Light blanket for chills

- Congestion
  - Warm washcloth over the face to ease sinus pain
  - Humidifier to moisturize the air
  - Decongestants
- Diarrhea, nausea, and vomiting
  - Clear liquids, then advance diet as tolerated
  - Antidiarrheal medications; see "Care of the Woman with Diarrhea"
  - Antiemetics; see "Care of the Woman with Nausea and Vomiting"
- Sore throat: Salt water throat gargle

Providing Treatment: Complementary and Alternative Measures to Consider

(Balch, 2010)

- Herbal remedies: Begin at the first signs of illness
  - Elderberry syrup: 1 tablespoon q 3–4 hours
  - Echinacea tincture: 1–2 droppers full q 3–4 hours in hot tea or juice
- Herbal teas: Use raw wild honey with bee propolis and boiling water
  - Lemon, ginger, echinacea, cayenne pepper, and honey
  - Chamomile, lavender, and honey
  - Peppermint
- Sleep and rest as much as possible in warm bed
  - Maintain dry bedclothing during times of feverish sweats
- Steam vaporizer with added oils
  - Tea tree oil (antiviral)
  - Eucalyptus oil
- Increased fluids intake
  - Hot herbal teas
  - Fresh fruit juices (especially orange juice)
  - Electrolyte drinks
  - Water
  - Broth soups with garlic and cayenne pepper to taste
- Hot baths with Epsom salts and eucalyptus oil (5 drops)
- Warm salt water gargle

- Vitamin C: 4000 mg daily (strengthens immune system by increasing white blood cells)
- Garlic (Kyolic): 2 capsules TID or eat raw cloves (antiviral properties)

Providing Support: Education and Support Measures to Consider

Provide information and recommendations:

- Diagnosis (from empirical evidence or lab testing)
- Medication regimen(s) if ordered
  - Dosage and frequency
  - Potential side effects
  - Indications for complementary and alternative therapies
- Signs of improvement
  - Symptoms usually diminish within 1 week
  - Fatigue can linger
- Warning signs and symptoms (CDC, 2011d)
  - Difficulty breathing
  - Cyanosis
  - Dehydration
  - Lethargy
  - Chest pressure
  - Dizziness
  - Confusion
  - Severe or persistent vomiting
  - Flu-like symptoms that improve and then return with fever or worse cough
- Limitations (CDC, 2011d)
  - Isolation for 24 hours after fever has subsided: Especially from children, pregnant women, and the elderly
  - Decreased activity
- Use of a facemask if in public
- Cough or sneeze into tissue or elbow to avoid transmission to others
- Frequent hand washing

Follow-up Care: Follow-up Measures to Consider

- Document
- Reevaluate in 24–48 hours: Phone or face-to-face consultation

- Return to office: For persistent or worsening symptoms

Multidisciplinary Practice: Consider Consultation, Collaboration, or Referral

- Medical services (CDC, 2009a)
  - Difficulty breathing or shortness of breath
  - Pain or pressure in the chest or abdomen
  - Sudden dizziness or confusion
  - Severe or persistent vomiting
  - Flu-like symptoms improve but then return with fever and worse cough
- Criteria for considering hospitalization (Morciano et al., 2009)
  - Age 65 or older
  - Pregnant woman, especially in the last 3 months of pregnancy
  - Concomitant pathologies
  - Abnormal chest x-ray findings
  - Signs of sepsis or organ damage
  - Patients of poor socioeconomic status with a lack of support systems
- For diagnosis or treatment outside of the practitioner's scope of practice

CARE OF THE WOMAN WITH PNEUMONIA

Key Clinical Information

Pneumonia is an inflammation of the lung tissues most often caused by bacterial or viral infection. As the microorganisms grow in the body, the lungs begin to fill with fluid and pus, producing areas of consolidation in the lung tissue. This consolidation is visible on x-ray. When pneumonia is present, airway exchange and oxygenation of the blood are compromised.

Pneumonia is the sixth leading cause of death in the United States. Globally, more than 1.5 million children younger than the age of 5 years die of pneumonia each year (CDC, 2011c). Pneumonia is categorized into two groups: community-acquired pneumonia (CAP) and hospital-acquired pneumonia (HAP).

Client History and Chart Review: Components of the History to Consider

(Stemler, 2007)

- Pneumonia symptom review: Onset, duration, and severity of symptoms
  - Cough: Productive or nonproductive
  - Pleuritic chest pain
  - Shortness of breath
  - Fever and/or chills
  - Night sweats
  - Malaise
  - Loss of appetite
  - Weakness
  - Myalgia
  - Lower right abdominal pain
- Relief measures used and their effects
- Medical and surgical history
  - Allergies
  - Medications
  - Medical conditions
    - Heart disease
    - Respiratory disease
- Social history and contributing factors
  - Smoking
  - Alcoholism
  - Native American and Alaskan Natives
- Review of systems

Physical Examination: Components of the Physical Exam to Consider

- Vital signs
  - Tachycardia
  - Tachypnea
  - Fever
- Respiratory evaluation
  - Rate and pattern of breathing: Depth and symmetry of lung expansion
  - Auscultation
    - Quality and intensity of breath sounds
    - Adventitious breath sounds: Crackles
- Percussion: Dull indicates consolidation or pleural effusion

- Evidence of respiratory distress
  - Nasal flaring
  - Intercostal or supraclavicular retractions
  - Peripheral cyanosis
  - Elevated pulse and respiratory rate
  - Grunting or wheezing

Clinical Impression: Differential Diagnoses to Consider

(ICD9Data.com, 2012)

- Community-acquired pneumonia

Diagnostic Testing: Diagnostic Tests and Procedures to Consider

- Chest x-ray
  - Anterior–posterior and lateral views
  - Posterior–anterior views for pregnant women: Reduces radiation exposure to fetus
- Gram stain and culture of purulent sputum: Suspected pneumonia

Providing Treatment: Therapeutic Measures to Consider

- Prevention through pneumococcal polysaccharide vaccination (King & Brucker, 2011): Recommended populations for vaccine
  - People older than 65 years of age
  - Immunocompromised patients, such as those with HIV/AIDS
  - Individuals with chronic diseases and disorders, such as diabetes and disabilities
  - Native Americans/Alaskan Natives
- Community-acquired pneumonia: Outpatient treatment (King & Brucker, 2011)
  - Erythromycin: 250–500 mg QID for 10 days
  - Azithromycin: 500 mg on day 1, then 250 mg every day for 4 additional days
  - Clarithromycin: 250 mg BID for 10 days

Providing Treatment: Complementary and Alternative Measures to Consider

- Alternative therapies are used to enhance immune function and do not replace antibiotics

- Rest
- Adequate nutrition
- Vitamin C
- Garlic

Providing Support: Education and Support Measures to Consider

Provide information and recommendations:

- Diagnosis
- Medication regimen(s)
  - Dosage and frequency
  - Potential side effects
- Afebrile within 2–5 days (pneumonia)
- Warning signs and symptoms
  - Respiratory distress
  - No improvement with treatment

Follow-up Care: Follow-up Measures to Consider

- Document
- Return for continued care
  - Contact within 7–10 days (phone or visit)
  - If symptoms persist or worsen in spite of therapy

Multidisciplinary Practice: Consider Consultation, Collaboration, or Referral

- Medical services
  - Respiratory illness requiring hospitalization
  - Symptoms of respiratory distress
    - Respiratory rate greater than 30
    - Superclavicular or intercostal retractions
    - O_2 saturation of less than 95%
    - Cyanosis
- For diagnosis or treatment outside the midwife's scope of practice

CARE OF THE WOMAN WITH SINUSITIS

Key Clinical Information

Sinusitis is inflammation or infection of the parana-sal sinuses. Acute sinusitis typically follows upper respiratory infection. When the nasal cavity is involved, the term *rhinosinusitis* is preferred. Chronic sinusitis is defined by a duration of symptoms for longer than 12 weeks. Acute sinusitis, by comparison, is often a self-limited viral infection. Chronic sinusitis is commonly seen in primary care offices for treatment; it affects more than 30 million Americans annually (King & Brucker, 2011; Stemler, 2007).

Client History and Chart Review: Components of the History to Consider

- ⬦ Sinusitis symptom review: Onset, duration, and severity of symptoms
  - Unilateral or bilateral mucopurulent nasal discharge: Color of sputum or nasal discharge
  - Unilateral maxillary, facial, or tooth pain
  - Unilateral sinus tenderness
  - Headache
  - Fever and/or chills
  - Postnasal drip
  - Cough
  - Nasal congestion
  - Impaired or loss of sense of smell
  - Itchiness of eyes or ears
- Relief measures used and their effects
- Medical/surgical history
  - Allergies
  - Medications
  - Recent respiratory infection
  - History of sinus infection(s)
- Review of systems

Physical Examination: Components of the Physical Exam to Consider

Focus on HEENT:

- Examine
  - Nasal septum and turbinates
  - Throat
  - Tonsils
  - Tympanic membranes
  - Eyes and conjunctiva
  - Teeth and gums

- Palpate
  - Sinuses
  - Lymph nodes
  - Jaw
- Transilluminate sinuses

Clinical Impression: Differential Diagnoses to Consider

(ICD9Data.com, 2012)

- Allergic rhinitis
- Sinusitis

Diagnostic Testing: Diagnostic Tests and Procedures to Consider

- Diagnosis is usually made based on the symptom review and clinical observation
- CT scan of the sinuses
- Aspiration of purulent secretions via sinus puncture

Providing Treatment: Therapeutic Measures to Consider

- Antibiotics should not be prescribed sooner than 7–10 days after the onset of symptoms
- For mild disease with no antibiotic use in past 4–6 weeks:
  - Ampicillin: 500 mg PO QID × 10 days
  - Bactrim DS: 1 tab PO BID × 10 days
- For moderate disease or mild disease with recent antibiotic use:
  - Augmentin: 500/125 mg PO QID × 10 days
- Inhaled nasal corticosteroids
  - Do not use long term
  - Atrovent: 2 sprays each nostril

Providing Treatment: Complementary and Alternative Measures to Consider

- Adequate fluids
- Saline nasal spray
- Eucalyptus steams
- Warm compresses to the sinuses

Providing Support: Education and Support Measures to Consider

- Provide information and recommendations
  - Diagnosis
  - Medication regimen(s)
  - Dosage and frequency
  - Reassurance if no medications are indicated
- Check the client's environment for potential allergen triggers

Follow-up Care: Follow-up Measures to Consider

- Document
- Return for continued care if symptoms persist or worsen in spite of therapy

Multidisciplinary Practice: Consider Consultation, Collaboration, or Referral

- ENT services
  - Rhinosinusitis symptoms that last longer than 8 weeks
  - Recurrent sinusitis
  - No improvement with treatment
  - Worsening symptoms
- For diagnosis or treatment outside the midwife's scope of practice

CARE OF THE WOMAN WITH TUBERCULOSIS

Key Clinical Information

Tuberculosis (TB) is an infectious disease caused by the bacterium *Mycobacterium tuberculosis* (CDC, 2011e; Stemler, 2007). The infection primarily affects the lungs, although other organ systems can become infected. The bacteria are spread through respiratory droplets. Most TB infections begin as a latent infection with no symptoms. While TB is confined to particularly high-risk populations in the United States, it remains an important public health problem globally; in fact, an estimated one third of the world's population is infected with *M. tuberculosis*. Active disease, if left untreated, is lethal in approximately 50% of infected individuals. Antibiotic resistance is a growing problem that has resulted in the emergence of multidrug-resistant tuberculosis.

Client History and Chart Review: Components of the History to Consider

- Tuberculosis symptom review
  - Onset, duration, and severity of symptoms
    - Chronic cough
    - Blood-tinged sputum
    - Weight loss
    - Night sweats
    - Fever
    - Weakness
    - Chest pain
    - Shortness of breath
    - Can be asymptomatic with latent infection
  - Relief measures used and their effects
- Medical conditions, especially those that weaken the immune system
  - HIV status, if known
- Social history
  - IV drug use
  - Recent travel abroad
  - Immigrant or refugee status
  - Housing arrangements
- Risk factors for TB (CDC, 2011e)
  - Close contact with a TB-infected person
  - Immigration from TB-endemic areas
  - Travel to TB-endemic areas
  - Groups with high rates of TB transmission
    - Homeless persons
    - IV drug users
    - Persons with HIV infection
  - Persons who work with or reside with people at high risk, such as at these locations:
    - Hospitals
    - Homeless shelters
    - Correctional facilities
    - Nursing homes
    - Drug rehabilitation centers
- Review of systems

Physical Examination: Components of the Physical Exam to Consider

(Stemler, 2007)

- Physical findings can be minimal in latent TB
- HEENT
  - Nasal septum and turbinates
  - Palpation of lymph nodes
- Respiratory evaluation
  - Rate and pattern of breathing
  - Depth and symmetry of lung expansion
  - Auscultation
    - Quality and intensity of breath sounds
    - Adventitious breath sounds
  - Percussion: Dullness indicates consolidation or pleural effusion

Clinical Impression: Differential Diagnoses to Consider

(ICD9Data.com, 2012)

- Tuberculosis

Diagnostic Testing: Diagnostic Tests and Procedures to Consider

- www Tuberculosis testing: TB Mantoux (purified protein derivative [PPD])
  - 0.1 mL injected intradermally
  - Two-step procedure indicated for selected groups
  - For interpretation of purified protein derivative, see Table 8-9
- Chest x-ray for positive PPD
- Gram stain and culture of purulent sputum
- HIV counseling and testing
- Baseline lab tests for patients with chronic comorbidities
  - CBC with platelets
  - Liver function studies
  - Renal function studies
  - Hepatitis panel

Providing Treatment: Therapeutic Measures to Consider

(CDC, 2003; King & Brucker, 2011; Stemler, 2007)

Table 8-9 PPD Interpretation

GREATER THAN OR EQUAL TO MILLIMETERS OF INDURATION	CONSIDERED POSITIVE IN THE FOLLOWING CONDITIONS
5 mm	HIV-infected patients
	Close contact of a newly diagnosed patient with active tuberculosis
	Scars on x-ray suggest prior healed active tuberculosis
	Organ transplant recipients
	Immunosuppressed persons
10 mm	Immigrants from areas with endemic tuberculosis prevalence
	Low-income and/or medically underserved population
	IV drug users
	Residents and employees of high-risk facilities
	Laboratory personnel in mycobacteriology labs
	Chronic illness or exposure that may increase risk of contracting tuberculosis
	Infants and young children
15 mm	No known risk factors for tuberculosis

Source: CDC, 2011e.

- Bacille Calmette-Guerin (BCG) vaccine
  - Commonly given in TB-endemic countries
  - Not recommended for use in the United States for the following reasons:
    - Low risk of infection with *M. tuberculosis*
    - Interference with TB testing
    - Variable effectiveness against pulmonary TB
- Latent tuberculosis infection (LTBI): Long-term course of drugs
  - Isoniazid (INH)
  - Rifampin (Rifadin)
  - Rifampin plus pyrazinamide (RZ)
- Active tuberculosis infection
  - 10 drugs approved for use in the United States
  - Varying schedules of treatment based on the following factors:
    - Culture and sensitivity results
    - Client comorbidities
  - Respiratory isolation precautions

Providing Treatment: Complementary and Alternative Measures to Consider

- Alternative therapies are used to enhance immune function and do not replace antibiotics
- Rest
- Adequate nutrition
- Vitamin C
- Garlic

Providing Support: Education and Support Measures to Consider

- Provide information and recommendations
  - TB test results
  - Follow-up testing as needed
- Diagnosis of TB, if made
  - Method of testing and result
  - Warning signs and symptoms
    - Persistent cough
    - Fever with chills
    - Bloody sputum
    - Shortness of breath

- Need for specialist care
  - Referral to TB specialist
  - Public health department: Screening of contacts
- Respiratory isolation precautions
  - At home and in public
  - Use of special mask

Follow-up Care: Follow-up Measures to Consider

- Document
- Return for continued care: Follow-up testing
- Appointment with a specialist

Multidisciplinary Practice: Consider Consultation, Collaboration, or Referral

- Infectious disease or pulmonary services: Tuberculosis diagnosis
- Public health department: Screening and follow-up of contacts of infected person
- For diagnosis or treatment outside the midwife's scope of practice

CARE OF THE WOMAN WITH UPPER RESPIRATORY INFECTION

Key Clinical Information

Upper respiratory infection (URI), also known as the common cold, is a viral infection of the upper airways. More than 200 viruses may lead to a URI, with the rhinovirus serotypes causing 80% of all cases (Stemler, 2007). Onset of URI symptoms begins within 1 to 3 days after exposure to, and colonization with, the microorganism. Symptoms typically follow a pattern that begins with a sore throat and malaise, and then peaks with nasal congestion and cough in 2 to 3 days. Symptoms gradually subside over the next 5 to 7 days. Spread of URI viruses is primarily by the hands; thus hand washing serves as a valuable preventive measure. Healthy adults develop URIs on average two or three times each year, making this infection a leading cause of healthcare visits and missed days of school and work (King & Brucker, 2011).

Client History and Chart Review: Components of the History to Consider

- URI symptom review
    - Onset, duration, and severity of symptoms
        - Cough
        - Sneezing
        - Nasal congestion
        - Color of nasal discharge
        - Postnasal drip
        - Headache
        - Sore throat
        - Facial pressure
        - Hoarseness
        - Malaise
    - Relief measures used and their effects
- Medical/surgical history
    - Allergies
    - Medications
    - Medical conditions
- Social history
    - Exposure to an infected individual
    - Smoking or secondhand exposure to smoke
- Review of systems

Physical Examination: Components of the Physical Exam to Consider

- Vital signs, including temperature
- HEENT
    - Nasal septum and turbinates
    - Palpation of sinuses
    - Palpation of lymph nodes
    - Throat
    - Tonsils
    - Tympanic membranes
    - Conjunctiva
- Respiratory evaluation
    - Rate and pattern of breathing
    - Auscultation
        - Quality and intensity of breath sounds
        - Upper airway congestion

Clinical Impression: Differential Diagnoses to Consider

(ICD9Data.com, 2012)

- Acute upper respiratory infections

Diagnostic Testing: Diagnostic Tests and Procedures to Consider

There are currently no clinically useful laboratory tests for URI (Stemler, 2007).

Providing Treatment: Therapeutic Measures to Consider

- Treatment is directed toward relief and management of symptoms
- Antibiotics are not indicated in the treatment of URI
- A wide variety of OTC cold medicines are available
    - Are of limited value
    - Provide symptomatic relief
- Tincture of time and supportive measures are the first-line treatment measures

Providing Treatment: Complementary and Alternative Measures to Consider

- General measures to promote healing
    - Rest and adequate nutrition
    - Increase fluids intake, especially hot liquids
    - Use positioning to aid drainage of secretions
- Saline nasal irrigation: Neti pot
- Eucalyptus steams
- Herbal remedies
    - Marshmallow root
    - Horehound
    - Mullein
- Astragalus

Providing Support: Education and Support Measures to Consider

- Provide information and recommendations
    - Diagnosis of URI
    - Antibiotics not indicated
    - Reassurance and review timeline of the URI

- Review OTC medicines available
- Supportive measures
- Warning signs and symptoms
  - Persistent cough
  - Fever with chills
  - Symptoms lasting longer than 2 weeks
- Isolation precautions
  - Meticulous hand washing
  - Cough into elbow or tissue

Follow-up Care: Follow-up Measures to Consider

- Document
- Return for continued care if symptoms persist or worsen after 2 weeks

Multidisciplinary Practice: Consider Consultation, Collaboration, or Referral

- Medical services: Symptoms of respiratory illness that persist or worsen
- For diagnosis or treatment outside the midwife's scope of practice

ASSESSMENT OF THE WOMAN WITH URINARY TRACT SYMPTOMS

Key Clinical Information

Urinary symptoms are a frequent presenting problem in primary care settings. One in three women will experience a urinary tract infection (UTI) by age 24, with more than half of all women experiencing a UTI in their lifetime (Dason, Dason, & Kapoor, 2011). Symptomatic urinary tract problems include bladder infections, pyelonephritis, renal lithiasis, incontinence issues, overactive bladder, and structural problems such as cystocele. Lower urinary tract symptoms create significant discomfort for women, including alterations in physical, sexual, emotional, and social functioning (Humburg, Frei, Wight, & Troeger, 2011; Morgan, Cardoza, Guire, Fenner, & DeLancey, 2010). Thoughtfully worded questions during the history can encourage discussion of urinary symptoms and exploration of potential solutions.

Client History and Chart Review: Components of the History to Consider

(Hawn et al., 2009; Kodner & Gupton, 2010; Morgan et al., 2010)

- Age
- Urinary history
  - Frequency, volume, and timing of voids
  - Changes in lifestyle related to the urinary tract
  - Urogenital hygiene habits
  - Onset, duration, type, and severity of symptoms
    - Incontinence
    - Urgency or frequency
    - Flank pain and/or dysuria
    - Fever and chills
    - Malaise
    - Odor to urine
    - Color of urine: Any blood noted
    - Other associated symptoms
  - Relief measures used and results
  - Previous UTI or problem with urination
- Reproductive history
  - GP TPAL
  - LMP, current method of birth control, or age at menopause
  - Vaginal or cesarean births
  - Sexually transmitted infections
  - Sexual activity
    - Anal/vaginal intercourse
    - Lubrication
    - Use of sex toys
  - Vasomotor symptoms
- Medical/surgical history
  - Allergies
  - Current medications
  - Neurologic disorders
  - Medical conditions
    - Lung disease
    - Elevated BMI
    - Diabetes
  - Genital or pelvic surgery

- Social history
  - Dietary patterns
  - Smoking
  - Caffeine and alcohol intake
  - Fluid intake
  - Heavy lifting
- Family history
  - Urinary tract infections
  - Pelvic prolapse
  - Renal calculi
- Review of systems

Physical Examination: Components of the Physical Exam to Consider

(Kodner & Gupton, 2010; Wennberg, Molander, Fall, Edlund, Peeker, & Milsom, 2009)

- Vital signs, including temperature
- Weight, height, and BMI
- Thorax
  - Costovertebral angle tenderness (CVAT)
  - Flank pain
- Abdominal palpation: Suprapubic pain
- Pelvic examination with focus on the following:
  - Urethra
  - Presence of cystocele or rectocele
  - Signs or symptoms
    - Reproductive tract infection (RTI)
    - Genital atrophy
    - Genital trauma
  - Evaluation of pelvic floor strength and function

Clinical Impression: Differential Diagnoses to Consider

(ICD9Data.com, 2012)

- Lower urinary tract symptoms
- Urinary tract infection
- UTI in pregnancy
- Urinary incontinence
- Interstitial cystitis
- Sexually transmitted infection affecting the urinary tract
- Vaginitis

Diagnostic Testing: Diagnostic Tests and Procedures to Consider

- Testing is based on the symptom profile (Humburg et al., 2011; Kodner & Gupton, 2010)
- Urine analysis (dip and/or microscopic)

Providing Treatment: Therapeutic Measures to Consider

- Treatment is based on the differential diagnosis
- For UTI in pregnancy, see "Care of the Pregnant Woman with Urinary Tract Infection"

Providing Treatment: Complementary and Alternative Measures to Consider

- Measures to support urinary health:
  - Cranberry tablets, capsules, or juice
  - Flush urinary system
    - Drink water or herbal tea
    - Avoid caffeine, sugar, and alcohol
  - Vitamin C: 250–500 mg BID
  - Beta-carotene: 25,000–50,000 IU daily
  - Zinc: 30–50 mg daily

Providing Support: Education and Support Measures to Consider

- Provide information based on differential diagnosis
  - Diagnosis
  - Treatment options
  - Lifestyle modifications
  - Urinary tract hygiene
  - Medication instructions and side effects
- Signs and symptoms requiring return for continued care
  - Hematuria
  - Pain
  - Renal calculi
  - Fever
  - Worsening symptoms

Follow-up Care: Follow-up Measures to Consider

- Document
- Plan for continued care

- Test of cure or other follow-up testing as indicated
- Indications for cystoscopy (Dason et al., 2011)
  - Recurrent UTIs
  - Persistent hematuria
  - Obstructive symptoms
  - Unusual cells in the urine sample
  - Persistent dysuria or pelvic pain
  - Suspected interstitial cystitis
  - Urinary stricture
  - Bladder or kidney stones
  - History of abdominopelvic malignancy

Multidisciplinary Practice: Consider Consultation, Collaboration, or Referral

- OB/GYN or urogynecologic services
- Urology services
- For diagnosis or treatment outside the midwife's scope of practice

CARE OF THE WOMAN WITH URINARY INCONTINENCE

Key Clinical Information

Urinary incontinence is the complaint of involuntary leakage of urine, causing distress in the individual. It is a challenging condition to address and has a significant effect on women's lives. Incontinence takes several forms and can result from increased intra-abdominal pressure, abnormal functioning of the detrusor muscle, or structural changes such as occur with cystocele. Overactive bladder symptoms without dysuria can result from urinary tract infection by atypical bacteria, such as *Mycoplasma*. Stress urinary incontinence occurs in 15% to 35% of all women, while urge incontinence occurs in 5% to 10% of women (Hantoushzadeh, Javadian, Shariat, Salmanian, Ghazizadeh, & Aghssa, 2011; Richter et al., 2010). Stress incontinence can occur during pregnancy but resolves in most women in the 12 months following the birth (Hantoushzadeh et al., 2011).

Urinary incontinence creates significant embarrassment for the woman, affecting her physically, emotionally, and socially. Many women restrict their activities due to this condition and may be reluctant to address the issue of incontinence with their midwife out of either embarrassment or the erroneous belief that urine leakage is an expected consequence of aging or childbearing (Morgan et al., 2010; Richter et al., 2010). The midwife who can ask clear, matter-of-fact, thoughtfully worded questions during the health history can encourage disclosure and discussion of the problem, and explore potential solutions with the affected individual.

Client History and Chart Review: Components of the History to Consider

(Hantoushzadeh et al., 2011; Morgan et al., 2010; Nygaard, 2010)

- Age
- Urinary history
  - Frequency, volume, and timing of voids
  - Changes in lifestyle related to the urinary tract
  - Urogenital hygiene habits
  - Onset, duration, type, and severity of symptoms
    - Frequency and volume of incontinence
    - Urinary urgency, urinary frequency, or both
    - Progression of incontinence symptoms
    - Other associated symptoms
      - Triggers (coughing, lifting, laughter)
      - Dysuria, or bladder spasm
      - Nocturia
      - Dizziness
      - Gait disturbance
      - Memory dysfunction
      - Any restriction of activities of daily living due to this issue
    - Relief measures used and results
- Reproductive history
  - GP TPAL
  - LMP, potential for pregnancy
  - Age at menopause

- Vaginal or cesarean births
- Sexually transmitted infections
- Sexual activity
- Vasomotor symptoms
- Medical/surgical history
  - Allergies
  - Current medications
  - Medical conditions
    - Lung disease/COPD
    - Elevated BMI
    - Diabetes
    - Neurologic disorders
  - Genital or pelvic surgery
- Social history
  - Caffeine and alcohol intake
  - Fluid intake patterns
  - Heavy lifting or exercise
  - Travel to developing countries
- Urge incontinence
  - Characterized by involuntary bladder contractions
  - Can be neurologic or caused by a urinary tract irritant
  - Results in overactive bladder symptoms with or without urine leakage
- Stress incontinence
  - Occurs when the intra-abdominal pressure is greater than the urethra's closing pressure
  - Contributing factors
    - Decreased tissue elasticity due to age or heredity
    - Childbearing, regardless of the mechanism of birth
    - Repetitive high-impact activities
    - Structural changes in the bladder neck
    - Insufficient pelvic floor muscle tone
- Mixed incontinence: Combines stress and urge incontinence
- Overflow incontinence
  - Urinary tract obstruction
  - Detrusor muscle dysfunction
  - Urethral torsion
- Iatrogenic incontinence

- Surgical scarring or trauma
- Medications
- Review of systems

Physical Examination: Components of the Physical Exam to Consider

(Nygaard, 2010)

- Vital signs, including temperature
- Weight, height, and BMI
- Observation of gait and posture
- Abdominal palpation: Suprapubic pain
- Pelvic examination
  - Evaluation of pelvic floor strength and function
  - Presence of the following:
    - Cystocele or rectocele
    - Leakage with cough or Valsalva maneuver
    - Pelvic mass
  - Signs or symptoms
    - Genital atrophy
    - Neurologic dysfunction
    - Reproductive tract infection

Clinical Impression: Differential Diagnoses to Consider

(ICD9Data.com, 2012)

- Urinary incontinence
  - Urge
  - Stress
  - Mixed
  - Overflow
  - Iatrogenic
- Pelvic prolapse

Diagnostic Testing: Diagnostic Tests and Procedures to Consider

(Nygaard, 2010)

- Urinalysis (dip and/or microscopic)
- Culture for *Mycoplasma*
- Incontinence
  - Postvoid catheterization to determine residual
  - Cough stress test
  - Urodynamic testing

Providing Treatment: Therapeutic Measures to Consider

(Morgan et al., 2010; Nygaard, 2010; Richter et al., 2010)

- Lifestyle changes
  - Smoking cessation
  - Limiting caffeine intake
  - Moderating fluid intake
  - Scheduled toileting
  - Weight loss of 5–15% of total body weight if the client has a high BMI
- Urge incontinence
  - Treatment of any underlying infection
  - Bladder retraining (biofeedback)
  - Pelvic muscle rehabilitation
  - Kegel exercises
  - Medications, for nonpregnant women (Nygaard, 2010)
    - Darifenacin: 7.5 or 15 mg PO daily (Pregnancy Category C)
    - Fesoterodine fumarate: 4 or 8 mg PO daily (Pregnancy Category C)
    - Oxybutynin chloride: 5 mg 3–4 times daily (Pregnancy Category B)
    - Oxybutynin chloride XL: 5, 10, or 15 mg QD (Pregnancy Category B)
    - Solifenacin succinate: 5 or 10 mg PO daily (Pregnancy Category C)
    - Tolterodine tartrate: 2 mg PO BID (Pregnancy Category C)
    - Tolterodine tartrate LA: 4 mg PO daily (Pregnancy Category C)
    - Trospium chloride: 20 mg BID (Pregnancy Category C)
    - Trospium chloride ER: 60 mg PO daily (Pregnancy Category C)
- Stress incontinence
  - Bladder retraining (biofeedback)
  - Pelvic muscle rehabilitation
  - Kegel exercises
  - Hormonal treatment for urogenital atrophy
    - Estring
    - Vaginal estrogen cream
  - Medications: Pseudoephedrine HCl (Pregnancy Category C)
  - Pessary fitting
    - Ring
    - Ring with support
    - Gellhorn
    - Use a vaginal cream with the pessary
      - Trimo-san
      - Acigel
      - Estrogen cream

Providing Treatment: Alternative Measures to Consider

- www Voiding diary
- Acupuncture

Providing Support: Education and Support Measures to Consider

(Nygaard, 2010; Richter et al., 2010)

- Provide information
  - Diagnosis
  - Treatment options
  - Medication instructions
- Voiding diary
- Urge incontinence
  - Manage voiding pattern
    - Frequently
    - With initial urge
    - Do not limit fluids
  - Kegel exercises daily: 3 sets of 15 10-second contractions
  - Medication instructions
- Stress incontinence
  - Kegel exercises daily: 3 sets of 15 10-second contractions
  - Biofeedback plan
  - Pessary use and fitting instructions as indicated
  - Limit increased intra-abdominal pressure
    - Heavy lifting
    - Straining at stool
    - Coughing

- Signs and symptoms requiring return for continued care
  - Signs of infection or stones
  - Worsening symptoms
- Option for referral for surgical evaluation and treatment

Follow-up Care: Follow-up Measures to Consider

- Document
- Plan for continued care
  - UTI: Reculture after treatment
    - Acute pyelonephritis
    - Recurrent symptoms
    - Pregnancy
  - Urge/stress incontinence
    - Keep a 2- to 5-day urinary diary
    - Follow-up
      - Biofeedback
      - Reevaluation
        - Pelvic floor strength
        - Response to medications
        - Need for a pessary
        - Need for a surgical consult
  - Pessary use
    - Check every 3 months
    - Clean the pessary
    - Evaluate for tissue breakdown

Multidisciplinary Practice: Consider Consultation, Collaboration, or Referral

- OB/GYN or urogynecologic services
  - Evaluation of persistent urinary incontinence
  - Pelvic prolapse
  - Pessary fitting
  - Surgical treatment
- For diagnosis or treatment outside the midwife's scope of practice

CARE OF THE WOMAN WITH URINARY TRACT INFECTION

Key Clinical Information

Acute urinary tract infections affect 30% of women during their lifetime, with recurrent infections affecting many of these individuals (Dason et al., 2011; Kodner & Gupton, 2010). New research indicates that some women have a genetic predisposition for UTI (Hawn et al., 2009). The highest incidence of UTIs occurs in young, healthy, sexually active women and in women with comorbid conditions such as structural or functional abnormalities of the urinary tract that predispose them to ascending infection (Kodner & Gupton, 2010). Urinary tract infections include simple cystitis, pyelonephritis, infection complicated by renal lithiasis, and infections resulting from inability to effectively empty the bladder during micturition. Such infections are the most common cause of overactive bladder symptoms, and urinary frequency without dysuria can be the result of infection with atypical bacteria such as *Mycoplasma* (Lee, Kim, Park, Choo, & Lee, 2010). While uncomplicated UTIs can be a self-limiting condition, most practitioners provide treatment with antibiotic therapy to alleviate symptoms and prevent ascending infection (Bleidorn, Gágyor, Kochen, Wegscheider, & Hummers-Pradier, 2010).

Client History and Chart Review: Components of the History to Consider

(Dason et al., 2011)

- Age
- Urinary history
  - Frequency, volume, and timing of voids
  - Changes in lifestyle related to the urinary tract
  - Urogenital hygiene habits
  - Onset, duration, type, and severity of symptoms
    - Incontinence
    - Urgency or frequency
    - Flank pain and/or dysuria
    - Fever and chills
    - Malaise
    - Relief measures used and results
  - Previous UTI or problem with urination
- Risk factors for UTI
  - Diabetes

- Family history of UTI
- History of UTI in past 6 months
- Incomplete voiding
- More frequent or intense intercourse
- New sex partner or multiple partners
- Pregnancy
- Postmenopausal status
- Use of irritating products or devices
  - Skin cleansers
  - Diaphragms
  - Pessary
  - Spermicides
- Reproductive history
  - GP TPAL, LMP
  - Vaginal or cesarean births
  - Sexually transmitted infections
  - Sexual activity
    - Frequency of intercourse
    - Anal/vaginal intercourse
    - Lubrication
    - Sex toys
    - Spermicide use
    - Voiding pre- and post-sexual activity
- Medical/surgical history
  - Allergies
  - Current medications and supplements
  - Medical conditions
    - Diabetes
    - Neurologic disorders
  - Genital or pelvic surgery
- Social history
  - Smoking
  - Caffeine and alcohol intake
  - Fluid intake
- Review of systems

Physical Examination: Components of the Physical Exam to Consider

(Dason et al., 2011; Kodner & Gupton, 2010)

- Vital signs, including temperature
- Weight, height, and BMI

- Thorax
  - Costovertebral angle tenderness (CVAT)
  - Flank pain
- Abdominal palpation: Suprapubic pain
- Pelvic examination
  - Urethral redness, edema, or trauma
  - Presence of cystocele or rectocele
  - Urethral or vaginal discharge
  - Genital lesions
  - Genital atrophy

Clinical Impression: Differential Diagnoses to Consider

(ICD9Data.com, 2012)

- Urinary tract infection
  - Cystitis
  - Urethritis
  - Pyelonephritis
- Interstitial cystitis
- Sexually transmitted infection affecting the urinary tract

Diagnostic Testing: Diagnostic Tests and Procedures to Consider

- UTIs (Kodner & Gupton, 2010; Lee et al., 2010)
  - Urinalysis (dip and/or microscopic)
    - Leukocyte esterase: Associated with frequent false-positive results
    - Nitrites: First morning urine yields a more accurate result
    - Positive leukocytes plus positive nitrites: Predictive of UTI
  - Culture and sensitivities
    - Pregnancy
    - Presence of urinary calculi
    - Recurrent or persistent symptoms
    - Diagnosis is considered positive if the colony count is more than 100,000 in a clean-catch specimen
    - Most common pathogens (routine culture)
    - *Escherichia coli*

- ◆ *Staphylococcus*
- ◆ *Proteus*
- ◆ *Enterococcus*
- ▪ Less common organisms (require specific test kits)
  - ◆ *Chlamydia*
  - ◆ *Mycoplasma*
  - ◆ *Ureaplasma*
- • Human chorionic gonadotropin (HCG): Serum or urine
- • Ultrasound: Suspected urinary calculi

Providing Treatment: Therapeutic Measures to Consider

For UTI in pregnancy, see "Care of the Pregnant Woman with Urinary Tract Infection."

- • UTI
  - ▪ Phenazopyridine for pain relief: 200 mg TID for 2 days (Pregnancy Category B)

- ▪ Methenamine or flavoxate for bladder spasms
- ▪ Cranberry tablets, capsules, or juice (McMurdo, Argo, Phillips, Daly, & Davey, 2009)
- ▪ Appropriate antibiotic therapy (see Table 8-10)
- ▪ Atypical bacteria (Lee et al., 2010)
  - ◆ Azithromycin: 1 g for one dose
  - ◆ Treat sexual partner
  - ◆ Recommend condom use
- • Pyelonephritis
  - ▪ IV fluids
  - ▪ Pain relief
  - ▪ Appropriate IV antibiotic therapy
- • Postmenopausal women with recurrent UTI (Dason et al., 2011): Hormonal treatment for urogenital atrophy
  - ▪ Estring
  - ▪ Vaginal estrogen cream

Table 8-10 Medications for Uncomplicated Urinary Tract Infections

Medication	Dose	Side Effects
Amoxicillin/clavulanate	500/125 mg q 12 hr × 3–5 days	Rash, GI upset
Cefaclor	250–500 mg q 8 hr × 3 days	Caution if penicillin allergic
Cephalexin	250 mg q 6 hr or 500 mg q 8 hr × 3 days	Caution if penicillin allergic
Ciprofloxacin	250–500 mg BID × 3 days	Dizziness, headache, GI upset
Fosfomycin (first-line therapy)	3 g, single dose	Diarrhea, headache
Levofloxacin	250 mg QD × 3 days	GI upset, headache
Nitrofurantoin (first-line therapy)	50–100 mg q 6 hr × 5 days	Nausea, pulmonitis, neuropathy
Ofloxacin	400 mg BID × 3 days	Dizziness, headache, GI upset
Pivmecillinam (first-line therapy)	400 mg BID × 5 days	GI upset, skin reactions
Sulfa-trimethoprim (first-line therapy)	800/160 mg BID × 3 days	Rash, Stevens-Johnson syndrome

Source: Gupta et al., 2011.

Providing Treatment: Complementary and Alternative Measures to Consider

- Beta-carotene: 25,000–50,000 IU daily
- Flush urinary system
  - Drink water or herbal tea
  - Avoid caffeine, sugar, and alcohol
- Ibuprofen: 400 mg TID × 3 days (Bleidorn, 2010)
- Vitamin C: 250–500 mg BID
- Zinc: 30–50 mg daily
- Herbal therapies (Romm, 2010)
  - Echinacea
  - Urinary antiseptics
    - Pipsissewa
    - Bearberry (uva-ursi): Not for use in pregnancy
    - Thyme
    - Marshmallow root
  - Topical treatment for urethral inflammation
    - Calendula: 7 g
    - Lavender: 4 g
      - Steep in 1 L boiling water for 30 minutes
      - Strain, then add 1 tsp sea salt
      - Rinse the perineal area and pat dry

Providing Support: Education and Support Measures to Consider

- Provide information
  - Diagnosis
  - Treatment options
  - Medication instructions
  - ⚠ Indications to return for care
    - Signs of infection or stones
    - Worsening symptoms
- UTI self-care
  - Avoid caffeine, alcohol, and sugar
  - Blot from front to back after voiding
  - Drink plenty of water
  - Void frequently
  - Void after intercourse

Follow-up Care: Follow-up Measures to Consider

- Document clinical findings
- Plan for continued care
  - Culture for atypical bacteria with persistent symptoms (Lee et al., 2010)
  - Reculture two weeks after treatment
    - Atypical bacteria, if positive
      - Retreat with doxycycline 100 mg BID × 7 days
      - Retest in 2 weeks
    - Acute pyelonephritis
    - Recurrent symptoms
    - Pregnancy
  - Recurrent infection (Dason et al., 2011)
    - Consider self-start antibiotics: Return for care if no improvement in 48 hours
    - Consider prophylactic antibiotics
      - Daily
      - Postcoital

Multidisciplinary Practice: Consider Consultation, Collaboration, or Referral

- OB/GYN services
  - Acute pyelonephritis
  - Persistent UTI during pregnancy
- Urology services
  - Unresolved, recurrent, or persistent infection
  - Persistent renal calculi
  - Suspected conditions
    - Urinary tract obstruction
    - Interstitial cystitis
- For diagnosis or treatment outside the midwife's scope of practice

Web Resources for Clinicians

- Risk assessment tool for estimating 10-year risk of CVD: http://hin.nhlbi.nih.gov/atpiii/calculator.asp?usertype=prof
- DASH diet plan: http://www.nhlbi.nih.gov/health/public/heart/hbp/dash/new_dash.pdf
- Mediterranean diet guidelines: http://www.mayoclinic.com/health/mediterranean-diet/CL00011

[www] WEB RESOURCES FOR CLINICIANS

RESOURCE	URL
Skin Disorders	
Dermatology Image Atlas: Pictures and clinical descriptions of dermatologic conditions	http://www.dermatlas.com/derm/
Skin rashes and other changes: Diagnostic tool for common skin conditions	http://familydoctor.org/online/famdocen/home/tools/symptom/545.printerview.html
How to do a skin self-examination	http://www.skincancer.org/Self-Examination/
Endocrine Disorders	
American Diabeties Association: Clinical practice recommendations (2011)	http://professional.diabetes.org/CPR_Search.aspx
American Thyroid Association: Guidelines of the American Thyroid Association for the diagnosis and management of thyroid disease during pregnancy and postpartum (2011)	http://www.liebertpub.com/contentframe.aspx?code=nh31x7M2VXcDkUK2yLHKgCdvvaMD4fwLwbhPWLtSBQ7GuKZ1Y8ps%2fbmdWZnnT%2b5hKTt9qG7wZdquP12B0QftTcEwXzs8DPQ%2fHYCSN%2fCfACw%3d
American Thyroid Association and American Association of Clinical Endocrinologists: Management guidelines for hyperthyroidism and other causes of thyrotoxicosis (2001)	http://www.liebertonline.com/toc/thy/21/6
Gastroenterology Disorders	
Bristol Stool Scale	http://www.ibsgroup.org/bristolstool
American Gastroenterological Association	http://www.gastro.org/practice/medical-position-statements
Mental Health Disorders	
Depression	http://www.depression-primarycare.org/
Screening tools	http://psychcorp.pearsonassessments.com/hai/SimpleProductListing.aspx?Mode=title&sCommunity=
WHO guide to mental and neurologic health in primary care	http://www.mentalneurologicalprimarycare.org/index.asp
Musculoskeletal Disorders	
CDC arthritis resource pages	http://www.cdc.gov/arthritis/index.htm
Merck Manual: Professional Musculoskeletal Injuries	http://www.merckmanuals.com/professional/injuries_poisoning/fractures_dislocations_and_sprains/overview_of_musculoskeletal_injuries.html
Spinal conditions from A–Z	http://www.spineuniverse.com/conditions

Respiratory Disorders

American Lung Association: Lung disease finder	http://www.lungusa.org/lung-disease/list.html
Centers for Disease Control and Prevention: Tuberculosis	http://www.cdc.gov/tb/
National Heart, Lung, and Blood Institute: Asthma, Expert Panel Report 3.	http://www.nhlbi.nih.gov/guidelines/asthma/index.htm

Headache

American Headache Society: Brainstorm: Diagnosing and treating migraine (2004)	http://www.americanheadachesociety.org/assets/Book_-_Brainstorm_Syllabus.pdf
American Headache Society and American Council for Headache Education: Headache diary	http://www.achenet.org/prevention/understanding/diary.php
Journal of the American Medical Association: Migraine Information Center	http://www.ama-assn.org/special/migraine/support/educate/diary.htm
National Headache Foundation	http://www.headaches.org/professional/educationresources/PDF/headache diary.pdf

Neurologic Disorders

National Institute of Neurologic Disorders and Stroke	http://www.ninds.nih.gov/index.htm
Neurologic exam	http://medinfo.ufl.edu/year1/bcs/clist/neuro.html
Women's neurology specialists	http://www.brighamandwomens.org/Departments_and_Services/neurology/services/WomensNeurology/default.aspx

Urologic Disorders

Voiding diary	http://content.revolutionhealth.com/contentfiles/form_aa137606.pdf

REFERENCES

Academy for Eating Disorders. (2011). Eating disorders: Critical points for early recognition and medical risk management in the care of individuals with eating disorder (2nd ed.). Retrieved from http://www.aedweb.org/AM/Template.cfm?Section=Medical_Care_Standards&Template=/CM/ContentDisplay.cfm&ContentID=2413

Agency for Healthcare Research and Quality. (2007). Comparative effectiveness of second-generation antidepressants in the pharmacologic treatment of adult depression. AHRQ Pub. No. 07-EHC007-1. Retrieved from http://effectivehealthcare.ahrq.gov/ehc/products/7/61/Antidepressants_Executive_Summary

Agency for Healthcare Research and Quality. (2009). Aspirin for the prevention of cardiovascular disease. AHRQ Pub. No. 09-05129-EF-2. Retrieved from http://www.uspreventiveservicestaskforce.org/uspstf09/aspirincvd/aspcvdrs.htm

American Academy of Dermatology. (2011). Skin cancer detection. Retrieved from http://www.aad.org/skin-conditions/skin-cancer-detection

American College of Nurse–Midwives (ACNM). (1997). *Certified nurse–midwives and certified midwives as primary care providers/case managers.* Silver Spring, MD: Author.

American College of Nurse–Midwives (ACNM). (2009). H1N1 flu (swine flu). *Journal of Midwifery & Women's Health, 54*(6), 517–518.

American College of Obstetrics and Gynecology (ACOG). (2006). Committee on Obstetric Practice: Treatment with selective serotonin reuptake inhibitors during pregnancy. *Obstetrics & Gynecology, 108,* 1601–1603.

American College of Obstetrics and Gynecology (ACOG). (2007). Practice Bulletin No. 87: Use of psychiatric medications during pregnancy and lactation. *Obstetrics & Gynecology, 110,* 1179–1198.

American College of Obstetrics and Gynecology (ACOG). (2008). Practice Bulletin No. 90: Asthma in pregnancy. *Obstetrics & Gynecology, 111*, 457–464.

American Diabetes Association (ADA). (2011a). Diagnosis and classification of diabetes mellitus. Retrieved from http://care.diabetesjournals.org/content/34/Supplement_1/S62.full.pdf+html

American Diabetes Association (ADA). (2011b). Standards of medical care in diabetes—2011. Retrieved from http://care.diabetesjournals.org/content/34/Supplement_1/S11.full

American Headache Society. (2004). Brainstorm: Diagnosing and treating migraine. Retrieved from http://www.americanheadachesociety.org/assets/Book_-_Brainstorm_Syllabus.pdf

American Heart Association (AHA). (2004). Women and coronary heart disease. Retrieved from http://www.americanheart.org/presenter.jhtml?identifier=2859

American Heart Association (AHA). (2011). Statements and guidelines. Retrieved from http://my.americanheart.org/professional/StatementsGuidelines/Statements-Guidelines_UCM_316885_SubHomePage.jsp

American Lung Association. (2010). State of lung disease in diverse communities. Retrieved from http://www.lungusa.org/assets/documents/publications/lung-disease-data/solddc_2010.pdf

American Psychiatric Association. (2006). Practice guideline for the psychiatric evaluation of adults (2nd ed.). doi:10.1176/appi.books.9780890423363.137162.Retrieved from http://www.psychiatryonline.com/pracGuide/PracticePDFs/PsychEval2ePG_04-28-06.pdf

Angelini, D., Hodgman, D., & McConaughey, E. (2007). Gastrointestinal. In B. Hackley, J. M. Kriebs, & M. E. Rousseau (Eds.), *Primary care of women: A guide for midwives and women's health providers* (pp. 597–678). Sudbury, MA: Jones and Bartlett.

Avery, M. D., & Baum, K. D. (2007). Endocrine. In B. Hackley, J. M. Kriebs, & M. E. Rousseau (Eds.). *Primary care of women: A guide for midwives and women's health providers* (pp. 559–596). Sudbury, MA: Jones and Bartlett.

Balch, P. (2010). *Prescription for nutritional healing* (5th ed.). New York, NY: Penguin Group.

Barry, D., Pietrzak, R. H., & Petry, N. M. (2008). Gender differences in associations between body mass index and DSM-IV mood and anxiety disorders: Results from the National Epidemiologic Survey on Alcohol and Related Conditions. *Annals of Epidemiology, 18*, 458–466.

Bendtsen, L., Evers, S., Linde, M., Mitsikostas, G., Sandrini, J., & Schoenen, J. (2010). EFNS guideline on the treatment of tension-type headache: Report of an EFNS task force. *European Journal of Neurology, 17*, 1318–1325.

Bhate, C., & Schwartz, R. (2011). Lyme disease: Part II: Management and prevention. *Journal of the American Academy of Dermatology, 64*(4), 639–653.

Bigos, S. J., Holland, J., Holland, C., Webster, J. S., Battie, M., & Malmgren, J. A. (2009). High-quality controlled trials on preventing episodes of back problems: Systematic literature review in working-age adults. *Spine Journal, 9*, 147–168.

Bleidorn, J., Gágyor, I., Kochen, M. M., Wegscheider, K., & Hummers-Pradier, E. (2010). Symptomatic treatment (ibuprofen) or antibiotics (ciprofloxacin) for uncomplicated urinary tract infection? Results of a randomized controlled pilot trial. *BMC Medicine, 8*, 30. doi:10.1186/1741-7015-8-30. Retrieved from http://www.biomedcentral.com/content/pdf/1741-7015-8-30.pdf

Boyce, P., & Barriball, E. (2010). Circadian rhythms and depression. *Australian Family Physician, 29*, 307–310.

Brown, A. C., Hairfield, M., Richards, D. G., McMillin, D. L., Meine, E. A., & Nelson, C. D. (2004). Medical nutritions therapy as a potential complementary treatment for psoriasis: Five case reports. *Alternative Medicine Review, 9*(3), 297–307. Retrieved from http://www.anaturalhealingcenter.com/documents/Thorne/articles/psoriasis.pdf

Butarro, T., Trybulski, J., Bailey, P., & Sandberg-Cook, J. (2007). *Primary care: A collaborative practice*. St. Louis, MO: Mosby.

Centers for Disease Control and Prevention (CDC). (2003). Treatment of tuberculosis. Retrieved from http://www.cdc.gov/mmwr/pdf/rr/rr5211.pdf

Centers for Disease Control and Prevention (CDC). (2009a). H1N1 flu (swine flu): General information. Retrieved from http://www.cdc.gov/h1n1flu/general_info.htm

Centers for Disease Control and Prevention (CDC). (2009b). Written action asthma plan. Retrieved from http://www.cdc.gov/asthma/actionplan.html

Centers for Disease Control and Prevention (CDC). (2010a). Health, United States, 2010. Retrieved from http://www.cdc.gov/nchs/data/hus/hus10.pdf#067

Centers for Disease Control and Prevention (CDC). (2010b). Lice. Retrieved from http://www.cdc.gov/parasites/lice/body/index.html

Centers for Disease Control and Prevention (CDC). (2011a). Arthritis. Retrieved from http://www.cdc.gov/arthritis/index.htm

Centers for Disease Control and Prevention (CDC). (2011b). Lyme disease. Retrieved from http://www.cdc.gov/lyme/healthcare/clinicians.html

Centers for Disease Control and Prevention (CDC). (2011c). Pneumonia can be prevented: Vaccines can help. Retrieved from http://www.cdc.gov/Features/Pneumonia/

Centers for Disease Control and Prevention (CDC). (2011d). Seasonal influenza (flu). Retrieved from http://www.cdc.gov/flu/

Centers for Disease Control and Prevention (CDC). (2011e). Tuberculin skin testing. Retrieved from http://www.cdc.gov/tb/publications/factsheets/testing/skintesting.htm

Chorba, R. S., Chorba, D. J., Bouillon L. E., Overmyer, C. A., & Landis, J. A. (2010). Use of a functional movement screening tool to determine injury risk in female collegiate athletes. *North American Journal of Sports Physical Therapy, 5*, 47–54.

Cordain, L. (2002). Acne vulgaris: A disease of western civilization. *Archives of Dermatology, 138*, 1584–1590.

Critical Care Concepts. (2006). Neurological assessment. Retrieved from http://lane.stanford.edu/portals/cvicu/HCP_Neuro_Tab_4/Neuro_Assessment.pdf

Dason, S., Dason, J. T., & Kapoor, A. (2011). Guidelines for the diagnosis and management of recurrent urinary tract infection in women. *Canadian Urology Association Journal, 5*, 316–322. doi: 10.5489/cuaj.11214. Retrieved from http://www.ncbi.nlm.nih.gov/pmc/articles/PMC3202002/pdf/cuaj-5-316.pdf

Deligiannidis, K. M., & Freeman, M. P. (2010). Complementary and alternative medicine for the treatment of depressive disorders in women. *Psychiatric Clinics of North America, 33*, 441–463.

Donaldson, M., Yordy, K., & Vanselow, N. (Eds.). (1994). *Defining primary care: An interim report*. Washington, DC: National Academy Press.

Elkan, A. C., Sjöberg, B., Kolsrud, B., Ringertz, B., Hafström, I., & Frostegård, J. (2008). Gluten-free vegan diet induces decreased LDL and oxidized LDL levels and raised atheroprotective natural antibodies against phosphorylcholine in patients with rheumatoid arthritis: a randomized study. *Arthritis Research & Therapy, 10*, R34. doi: 10.1186/ar2388. Retrieved from http://www.ncbi.nlm.nih.gov/pmc/articles/PMC2453753/pdf/ar2388.pdf

Farley, C. L., Tharpe, N., Miller, L., & Ruxer, D. (2006). Women's health care minimum data set: Pilot testing and validation for use in clinical practice. *Journal of Midwifery & Women's Health, 51*, 493–501.

Fava, M. (2010). Using complementary and alternative medicines for depression. *Journal of Clinical Psychiatry, 71*, e24.

Ferdowsian, H., & Levin, S. (2010). Does diet really affect acne? *Skin Therapy Letter, 15*(3), 1–2.

Frank, E., Maggi, L., Miniati, M., & Benvenuti, A. (2009). The rationale for combining interpersonal and social rhythm therapy and pharmacotherapy for the treatment of bipolar disorders. *Clinical Neuropsychiatry, 6*, 63–74.

Frosch, P., & John, S. (2011). Clinical aspects of irritant contact dermatitis. In P. Frosch, T. Menne, & J. P. Lepoittevin (Eds.), *Contact dermatitis* (4th ed., p. 255). New York, NY: Springer.

Furlan, A., Yazdi, F., Tsertsvadze, A., Gross, A., Van Tulder, M., & Santaguida, L. (2010). *Complementary and alternative therapies for back pain. II. Evidence report/technology assessment No. 194*. Prepared by the University of Ottawa Evidence-based Practice Center under Contract No. 290-2007-10059-I (EPCIII). AHRQ Publication No. 10(11) E007. Rockville, MD: Agency for Healthcare Research and Quality. Retrieved from http://www.ahrq.gov/downloads/pub/evidence/pdf/backpaincam/backcam2.pdf

Gagnier, J. J., van Tulder, M. W., Berman, B. M., & Bombardier, C. (2006). Herbal medicine for low back pain. *Cochrane Database of Systematic Reviews, 2*, CD004504. doi: 10.1002/14651858.CD004504.pub3

Goldbacher, E. M., Bromberger, J., & Matthews, K. A. (2009). Lifetime history of major depression predicts the development of the metabolic syndrome in middle-aged women. *Psychosomatic Medicine, 71*, 266–272. doi: 10.1097/PSY.0b013e318197a4d5

Goldgar, C., Keahey, D., & Houchins, J. (2009). Treatment options for acne rosacea. *American Family Physician, 80*(5), 461–468.

Grant, T. M., Jack, D. C., Fitzpatrick, A. I., & Ernst, C. C. (2008). Carrying the burdens of poverty, parenting, and addiction: Depression symptoms and self-silencing among ethnically diverse women. *Community Mental Health Journal*, 1–5. doi: 10.1007/s10597-009-9255-y. Retrieved from http://faculty.wwu.edu/djack/publications/Carrying_the_Burdens_of_Poverty.pdf

Gupta, K., Hooton, T. M., Naber, K. G., Wullt, B., Colgan, R., & Miller, L. G. (2011). International clinical practice guidelines for the treatment of acute uncomplicated cystitis and pyelonephritis in women: A 2010 update by the Infectious Diseases Society of America and the European Society for Microbiology and Infectious Diseases. *Clinical Infectious Diseases,* 52(5), e103–e120. Retrieved from http://www.uphs .upenn.edu/bugdrug/antibiotic_manual/idsa-cystitispyelo-2010.pdf

Hackley, B. (2007). Asthma and allergy. In B. Hackley, J. M. Kriebs, & M. Rousseau (Eds.), *Primary care of women: A guide for midwives and women's health providers* (pp. 383–428). Sudbury, MA: Jones and Bartlett.

Haisley-Royster, C. (2011). Cutaneous infestations and infections. *Adolescent Medicine: State of the Art Reviews,* 22(1), 129–145.

Hantoushzadeh, S., Javadian, P., Shariat, M., Salmanian, B., Ghazizadeh, S., & Aghssa, M. (2011). Stress urinary incontinence: Pre-pregnancy history and effects of mode of delivery on its postpartum persistency. *International Urogynecology Journal, 22,* 651–655. doi: 10.1007/s00192-010-1335-6. Retrieved from http:// www.springerlink.com/content/g033206g33w62px3 /fulltext.pdf

Hawn, T. R., Scholes, D., Li, S. S., Wang, H., Yang, Y., & Roberts, P. L. (2009). Toll-like receptor polymorphisms and susceptibility to urinary tract infections in adult women. *PLoS ONE, 4*(6), e5990. doi: 10.1371/ journal.pone.0005990. Retrieved from http://www .plosone.org/article/info%3Adoi%2F10.1371%2Fjournal .pone.0005990

Heiderscheit, B. C., Sherry, M. A., Silder, A., Chumanov, E. S., & Thelen, D. G. (2010). Hamstring strain injuries: Recommendations for diagnosis, rehabilitation and injury prevention. *Journal of Orthopaedic & Sports Physical Therapy, 40,* 67–81. doi: 10.2519 /jospt.2010.3047

Hlebowicz, J., Darwiche, G., Björgell, O., & Almér, L. O. (2007). Effect of cinnamon on postprandial blood glucose, gastric emptying, and satiety in healthy subjects. *American Journal of Clinical Nutrition, 85,* 1552–1556.

Hofmann, S. G., & Smits, J. A. (2008). Cognitive-behavioral therapy for adult anxiety disorders: A meta-analysis of randomized placebo-controlled trials. *Journal of Clinical Psychiatry, 69,* 621–632.

Humburg, J., Frei, R., Wight, E., & Troeger, C. (2011). Accuracy of urethral swab and urine analysis for the detection of *Mycoplasma hominis* and *Ureaplasma urealyticum* in women with lower urinary tract symptoms. *Archives of Gynecology and Obstetrics, 10,* 1–5. doi: 10.1007/s00404-011-2109-1

Hyde, J. S., Mezulis, A. H., & Abramso, L. Y. (2008). The ABCs of depression: Integrating affective, biological, and cognitive models to explain the emergence of the gender difference in depression. *Psychological Review, 115,* 291–231.

ICD9Data.com. (2012). Free 2012 ICD-9 medical coding data. Retrieved from http://www.ICD9Data.com/

Institute of Medicine (IOM). (2010). IOM Report Brief 2010: The future of nursing: Focus on scope of practice. Retrieved from http://www.iom.edu/Reports/2010 /The-Future-of-Nursing-Leading-Change-Advancing-Health.aspx

International Headache Society (IHS). (2005). Retrieved from http://ihs-classification.org/en/

King, T., & Brucker, M. (Eds.). (2011). *Pharmacology in women's health.* Sudbury, MA: Jones & Bartlett Learning.

Kodner, C. M., & Gupton, E. K. T. (2010). Recurrent urinary tract infections in women: Diagnosis and management. *American Family Physician, 82,* 638–643. Retrieved from http://journals.dev.aafp.org/XML-journal-files /afp/2010/0915/.svn/text-base/afp20100915p638.pdf .svn-base

Koes, B. W., van Tulder, M., Lin, C. W. C., Macedo, L. G., McAuley, J., & Maher, C. (2010). An updated overview of clinical guidelines for the management of non-specific low back pain in primary care. *European Spine Journal, 19,* 2075–2094. doi: 10.1007/s00586-010-1502-y. Retrieved from http://www.ncbi.nlm.nih .gov/pmc/articles/PMC2997201/?tool=pmcentrez

Lee, Y. S., Kim, J. Y., Park, W. H., Choo, M. S., & Lee, K. S. (2010). Prevalence and treatment efficacy of genitourinary mycoplasmas in women with overactive bladder symptoms. *Korean Journal of Urology, 51,* 625–630. Retrieved from http://www.ncbi.nlm.nih.gov /pmc/articles/PMC2941811/pdf/kju-51-625.pdf

Lobo, R. (2009). The risk of stroke in post menopausal women receiving hormone therapy. *Climacteric, 12-S*(1), 81–85.

Louik, C., Lin., A., Werler, M., Hernandez-Diaz, S., & Mitchell, A. (2007). First trimester use of selective serotonin-reuptake inhibitors and the risks of birth defects. *New England Journal of Medicine, 356,* 2675–2683.

Lucas, M., Mirazaei, F., O'Reilly, E. J., Pan, A., Willett, W., Kawachi, I., . . . Aschiero, A. (2011). Dietary intake of n−3 and n−6 fatty acids and the risk of clinical depression in women: A 10-y prospective follow-up study. *American Journal of Clinical Nutrition, 93*(6): 1337-134. doi: 10.3945/ ajcn.111.011817

Maas, A., & Franke, H. (2009). Women's health in menopause with a focus on hypertension. *Netherlands Heart, 17*(2), 68–72.

Macgregor, A. (2008). Estrogen and migraine: Correlations and prevention. *Headache, 48,* S99–S107.

McMurdo, M. E. T., Argo, I., Phillips, G., Daly, F., & Davey, P. (2009). Cranberry or trimethoprim for the prevention of recurrent urinary tract infections? A randomized controlled trial in older women. *Journal of Antimicrobial Chemotherapy, 63,* 389–395. doi: 10.1093/jac/dkn489. Retrieved from http://jac.oxfordjournals.org/content/63/2/389.full.pdf

Medline Plus. (2009). Dermatitis. Retrieved from http://www.nlm.nih.gov/medlineplus/ency/article/000869.htm

Medline Plus. (2011). Fungal infections. Retrieved from http://www.nlm.nih.gov/medlineplus/fungalinfections.html

Menter, A., Korman, N., Elmets, C., Feldman, S., Gelfand, J., Gordon, K., . . . Bhushan, R. (2009). Guidelines for the management of psoriasis and psoriatic arthritis. *Journal of the American Academy of Dermatology, 60*(4), 643–659.

Mitchell, A. M., & Bulik, C. M. (2006). Eating disorders and women's health: An update. *Journal of Midwifery & Women's Health, 51,* 193–201.

Morciano, C., Vitale, A., De Masi, S., Sagliocca, L., Sampaolo, L., Lacorte, E., & Mele, A. (2009). Italian evidence-based guidelines for the management of influenza-like syndrome in adults and children. *Annali dell'Istituto Superiore di Sanita, 45*(2), 185–92.

Morgan, D. M., Cardoza, P., Guire, K., Fenner, D. E., & DeLancey, J. O. L. (2010). Levator ani defect status and lower urinary tract symptoms in women with pelvic organ prolapse. *International Urogynecology Journal, 21,* 47–52. doi: 10.1007/s00192-009-0970-2. Retrieved from http://www.ncbi.nlm.nih.gov/pmc/articles/PMC2866151/pdf/nihms190382.pdf

Mosca, L., Banka, C. L., Benjamin, E. J., Berra, K., Bushnell, C., Dolor, R. J., . . . Wenger, N. K. (2007). Evidence based guidelines for cardiovascular disease prevention in women: 2007 update. *Circulation, 115,* 1481–1501.

Moses, S. (2012). Neurologic exam. Retrieved from http://www.fpnotebook.com/neuro/exam/NrlgcExm.htm

National Cancer Institute at the National Institute of Health. (2011). Skin cancer screening. Retrieved from http://www.cancer.gov/cancertopics/types/skin

National Heart, Lung, and Blood Institute (NHLBI). (2003). The seventh report of the Joint National Committee on Prevention, Detection, Evaluation, and Treatment of High Blood Pressure. Retrieved from http://www.nhlbi.nih.gov/guidelines/hypertension/express.pdf

National Heart, Lung, and Blood Institute (NHLBI). (2004). National Cholesterol Education Program: Detection, evaluation and treatment of high blood cholesterol in adults (Adult Treatment Panel III). Retrieved from http://www.nhlbi.nih.gov/guidelines/cholesterol/atp3xsum.pdf

National Heart, Lung, and Blood Institute (NHLBI). (2006). Your guide to lowering your blood pressure with DASH. Retrieved from http://www.nhlbi.nih.gov/health/public/heart/hbp/dash/new_dash.pdf

National Institute of Allergy and Infectious Diseases (NIAID). (2011). Understanding flu. Retrieved from http://www.niaid.nih.gov/topics/flu/pages/default.aspx?wt.ac=bcFlu

National Institute of Mental Health (NIMH). (2007). The numbers count: Mental disorders in America. Retrieved from http://www.nimh.nih.gov/health/publications/the-numbers-count-mental-disorders-in-america.shtml

National Institutes of Health (NIH). (2010). Women's health initiative. Retrieved from http://www.nhlbi.nih.gov/whi/

National Psoriasis Foundation. (2012). About psoriasis. Retrieved from http://www.psoriasis.org/about-psoriasis

Nygaard, I. (2010). Idiopathic urgency urinary incontinence. *New England Journal of Medicine, 363,* 1156–1162. Retrieved from http://medres.med.ucla.edu/Education/syllabus/Geri/pdf/Urgency.pdf

Ogg, B., & Cochran, S. (2006). Managing head lice safely. University of Nebraska. Retrieved from http://lancaster.unl.edu/pest/lice/headlice018.shtml

Oni-Orisa, A., Hiersteine, D., & Swett, A. (2010). Fact sheet: Women's health disparities and midwifery care. University of Massachusetts Center for Women in Politics and Public Policy. Retrieved from http://www.mccormack.umb.edu/centers/cwppp/documents/NE_Sept2010.pdf

Patten, S. B. (2009). Canadian Network for Mood and Anxiety Treatments (CANMAT) clinical guidelines for the management of major depressive disorder in adults. V. Complementary and alternative medicine treatments. *Journal of Affective Disorders, 117*(Suppl. 1), S54–S64.

Pimenta, E., Amodeo, C., & Oparil, S. (2008). Hypertension in women. *International Journal of Atherosclerosis, 3*(3), 138–145.

Powell, D. L. (2005). Anxiety. In *Louisiana State University family medicine outpatient manual.* Retrieved from http://www.sh.lsuhsc.edu/fammed/OutpatientManual/Anxiety.htm

Powell, F. (2005). Rosacea. *New England Journal of Medicine, 352*(8), 793–803.

Pye, L. (2010). Bacterial skin infections. *InnovAit, 3*(7), 388–395.

Quintero, A. J., Wright, V. J., Fu, F. H., & Huard, J. (2009). Stem cells for the treatment of skeletal muscle injury. *Clinical Sports Medicine, 28*(1), 1–11. doi: 10.1016/j.csm.2008.08.009

Raiput, M. S., Sinha, S., Mathur, V., & Agrawal, P. (2011). Herbal antidepressants. *International Journal of Pharmaceutical Frontier Research, 1*, 159–169.

Rao, S. S., Camilleri, M., Hasler, W. L., Mauer, A. H., Parkman, H. P., Saad, R., . . . Szarka, L. (2011). Evaluation of gastrointestinal transit in clinical practice: Position paper of the American and European Neurogastroenterology and Motility Societies. *Neurogastroenterology and Motility, 23*(1), 8–23.

Ravindran, A. V., Lam, R. W., Filteau, M. J., Lespérance, F., Kennedy, S. H., Parikh, S. V., &

Richter, H. E., Burgio, K. L., Brubaker, L., Nygaard, I. E., Weidner, A., & Bradley, C. S. (2010). A trial of continence pessary vs behavioral therapy vs combined therapy for stress incontinence. *Obstetrics & Gynecology, 115*(3), 609–617. doi: 10.1097/AOG.0b013e3181d055d4

Romm, A. (2010). *Botanical medicine for women's health.* St. Louis, MO: Churchill Livingstone.

Rousseau, M. E. (2007). Dermatology. In B. Hackley, J. M. Kriebs, & M. E. Rousseau (Eds.), *Primary care of women: A guide for midwives and women's health providers* (pp. 809–864). Sudbury, MA: Jones and Bartlett.

Sackeim, H., Dillingham, E. M., Prudic, J., Cooper, T., McCall, W. V., Rosenquist, P., . . . Haskett, R. F. (2009). Effect of concomitant pharmacotherapy on electroconvulsive therapy outcomes. *Archives of General Psychiatry, 66*, 729–737.

Sagud, M., Mihaljevic-Peles, A., Pivac, N., Jakovljevic, M., &, Muck-Seler, D. (2009). Lipid levels in female patients with affective disorders. *Psychiatry Research, 168*, 218–221.

Sanders, L. B. (2006). Assessing and managing women with depression: A midwifery perspective. *Journal of Midwifery & Women's Health, 51*, 185–192.

Scholz, J., Mannion, R. J., Hord, D. E., Griffin, R. S., Rawal, B., & Zheng, H. (2009). A novel tool for the assessment of pain: Validation in low back pain. *PLoS Medicine, 6*(4), e1000047. doi: 10.1371/journal.pmed.1000047

Sharkansky, E. (2010). Sexual trauma: Information for women's medical providers. Retrieved from http://www.ptsd.va.gov/professional/pages/ptsd-womens-providers.asp

Skin Cancer Foundation. (2011). Actinic keratosis and other precancers. Retrieved from http://www.skincancer.org/

Stemler, K. A. (2007). Respiratory conditions. In B. Hackley, J. M. Kriebs, & M. Rousseau (Eds.), *Primary care of women: A guide for midwives and women's health providers* (pp. 429–526). Sudbury, MA: Jones and Bartlett.

Strauss, J., Krowchuk, D., Leyden, J., Lucky, A., Shalita, A., Seigfried, E., . . . Bhushan, R. (2007). Guidelines of care for acne vulgaris management. *Journal of the American. Academy of Dermatology, 56*(4), 651–663.

Ströhle A. (2009). Physical activity, depression, and anxiety disorders. *Journal of Neural Transmission, 116*(6): 777–784.

Sun-Edelstein, C., & Mauskop, A. (2011). Alternative headache treatments: Nutraceuticals, behavioral and physical therapy. *Headache: The Journal of Head and Face Pain, 51*(3), 469–483.

Tambs, K., Czajkowsky, N., Roysamb, E., Neale, M. C., Reichborn-Kjennerud, T., Aggen, S. H., . . . Kendler, K. S. (2009). Structure of genetic and environmental risk factors for dimensional representations of DSM-IV anxiety disorders. *British Journal of Psychiatry, 195*, 301–307.

Thein-Nissenbaum, J. M., Rauh, M. J., Carr, K. E., Loud, K. J., & McGuine, T. A. (2011). Associations between disordered eating, menstrual dysfunction, and musculoskeletal injury among high school athletes. *Journal of Orthopaedic & Sports Physical Therapy, 41*, 60–69.

U.S. Bone and Joint Decade: *The burden of musculoskeletal diseases in the United States.* (2008). Rosemont, IL: American Academy of Orthopaedic Surgeons. Retrieved from http://www.boneandjointburden.org/

U.S. Department of Health and Human Services. (2006). Caregiver stress. Retrieved from http://www.4women.gov/faq/caregiver.htm

U.S. Department of Health and Human Services. (2012). The health care law and you. Retrieved from http://www.healthcare.gov/law/index.html

U.S. Preventive Services Task Force (USPSTF). (2008). Screening for lipid disorders in adults. Retrieved from http://www.uspreventiveservicestaskforce.org/uspstf08/lipid/lipidrs.htm

University of Maryland Medical Center. (2011a). Anorexia nervosa. Retrieved from http://www.umm.edu/altmed/articles/anorexia-nervosa-000012.htm

University of Maryland Medical Center. (2011b). Lyme disease. Retrieved from http://www.umm.edu/altmed /articles/lyme-disease-000102.htm

Urquhart, D. M., Bell, R. J., Ciuttini, F. M., Cui, J., Forbes, A., & Davis, S. R. (2008). Negative beliefs about low back pain are associated with high pain intensity and high level disability in community-based women. *BMC Musculoskeletal Disorders, 9*, 148. doi: 10.1186 /1471-2474-9-148. Retrieved from http://www.ncbi .nlm.nih.gov/pmc/articles/PMC2587466/pdf /1471-2474-9-148.pdf

van der Watt, G., Laugharne, J., & Janca, A. (2008). Complementary and alternative medicine in the treatment of anxiety and depression. *Current Opinion in Psychiatry, 21*, 37–42.

Wennberg, A. L., Molander, U., Fall, M., Edlund, C., Peeker, R., & Milsom, I. (2009). A longitudinal population-based survey of urinary incontinence, overactive bladder, and other lower urinary tract symptoms in women. *European Urology, 55*(4), 783–791. doi: 10.1016/j.eururo.2009.01.007

Whang, W., Kubzansky, L. D., Kawachi, I., Rexrode, R. M., Kroenke, C. H., Glynn, R. J., . . . Albert, C. M. (2009). Depression and risk of sudden cardiac death and coronary heart disease in women. *Journal of the American College of Cardiology, 53*, 950–958. doi:10.1016/j. jacc.2008.10.060

Wier, F., & Farley, C. L. (2006). Clinical controversies in screening for thyroid disorders in women during childbearing years. *Journal of Midwifery & Women's Health, 51*(3), 152–158.

World Health Organization (WHO). (2004). *WHO guide to mental and neurologic health in primary care: Diagnostic checklists.* From http://www.mentalneuro-logicalprimarycare.org/index.asp

Wyner, E., Marfell, J., Karsnitz, D., & Rousseau, M. E. (2007). Cardiovascular disease in women. In B. Hackley, J. Kriebs, & M. E. Rousseau (Eds.), *Primary care of women* (pp. 481–526). Sudbury, MA: Jones and Bartlett.

An Herbal Primer

Plants and herbs provide not only medicines but also vitamins, minerals, and micronutrients for optimal benefits.

Plants and botanical medicines have been used for women's health and healing for centuries, as preventive and therapeutic treatments during pregnancy, birth, and breastfeeding. Natural medicines have been shown, through traditional wisdom and modern science, to relieve symptoms, promote health, and provide support for the childbearing year.

Natural medicines are often less toxic and safer than many pharmaceuticals, but that does not mean that all natural medicines are safe. As in nature, there are both helpful and harmful commercially prepared and wildcrafted herbal products. Many botanicals have side effects or may be toxic if not used wisely. The most common side effects that occur with herbal use are headaches, rash, indigestion and nausea, vomiting, or allergic reaction to the plant. Education on safe herbal use is imperative for practitioners and patients alike.

HERBAL PREPARATIONS

There are many sources of herbal medicines: plants, including the aerial parts and roots; trees; shrubs; seeds; berries; fruits; and vegetables. Most herbs can be used in several forms; the most common are teas, tinctures, syrups, decoctions, capsules, compresses, infused oils, and herbal baths.

Teas (Infusions)

Teas are the traditional way of taking herbal medicines. One to two teaspoons of fresh or dried plant material is steeped in 6–8 oz hot water for 5–10 minutes. For children, a lower "dose" can be accomplished by steeping the herbs for only 2–3 minutes. The plant material is then strained from the liquid, and the tea can be sweetened with honey or other sweetener. Organic plants are preferred, and many medicinal teas include a blend of several herbs. For a medicinal dose, usually two to three cups a day should be consumed. Teas or infusions may also be applied topically.

Decoction

A decoction is a tea (or infusion) made from the bark or woody parts of plants. The plant part is broken or crushed and simmered in water for 20–30 minutes to extract the medicinal qualities and then strained and used as a tea or topical application.

Tincture

Another way of preparing and storing botanical medicines is to take fresh or dried plant material and soak it in an alcohol base for 2 weeks. A clean clear glass jar should be used and sealed tightly during the soaking process. The formula for tincture preparation is to create a ratio of 1:4 plant-to-liquid (with fresh plant materials, use half the amount):

- One part plant material
- One part distilled water
- Three parts 80-proof vodka

A "part" can be 1 tablespoon, ½ cup, or any desired amount.

Label the jar with the herb name and date. Seal it tightly, and set the jar out of sunlight. Gently shake it twice daily for 2 weeks. Strain the plant material from the liquid, and store the tincture in an amber glass jar, out of direct sunlight.

Tinctures maintain their potency for 2–3 years. The medicinal dose of a tincture is 20–30 drops in water or juice taken two to three times daily. Nonalcoholic forms of tinctures for children or others preferring not to have the alcohol base are prepared with glycerin or vinegar in place of alcohol.

Syrup

A syrup is produced when a prepared infusion or decoction is heated and honey is added to the desired thickness and taste to make it more palatable.

Capsules

Plant material may be dried or flash frozen, ground into a fine powder, and placed in gelatin or vegetable-based capsules. In commercial products, doses vary; label directions should be followed.

Compress (Poultice)

Dry or moistened herb is placed in a gauze pad, cheesecloth, or soft porous fabric; folded into a "packet"; and placed directly onto the affected area for 10–20 minutes three to four times daily. Gauze or fabric compresses may also be soaked in an infusion and placed directly on the affected area.

Infused Oil

An infused oil is an extract of the plant's medicinal quality in an oil-based form. To prepare an oil infusion, tightly pack plant material in a clean, clear jar. Completely cover the herbs with a base or carrier oil such as olive, sweet almond, apricot kernel, jojoba, or wheat germ oil. Seal the jar and place it in a sun-exposed window for 2 weeks. Strain the plant material from the oil, and store the infused oil in an amber jar out of direct sunlight. Apply the infused oil to affected area two to three times daily.

Salve (Ointment)

Warm (do not boil) two to three cups of infused oil. Add 1 oz of beeswax and slowly warm the mixture until the beeswax is melted. Pour the salve into clean jars and allow it to cool before sealing. Apply a small amount to the affected area two to four times daily. For a softer ointment, use three cups oil to 1 oz beeswax. For a firmer ointment, use two cups oil to 1 oz beeswax.

HERBS IN PREGNANCY: SAFETY GUIDELINES

1. Use smaller doses.
2. Use milder herbs.
3. Use only herbs and essential oils deemed safe for pregnancy.
4. Use 12 drops of 2% or 6 drops of 4% dilution of essential oils.
5. Avoid herbal preparations in the first trimester.
6. Avoid uterine stimulant herbs (emmenagogues) before 37 weeks' gestation.

7. Tea or infusion forms may be better tolerated and cause less indigestion.
8. Discontinue essential oils if headache or nausea occurs.
9. Discontinue herbs if nausea, vomiting, rash, or headache occurs.

Herbs Not Recommended in Pregnancy

Barberry	Licorice
Bladderwack	Lobelia
Cascara	Mandrake
Chaparral	Pennyroyal
Damiana	Pleurisy root
Ephedra	Rue
Fenugreek	Saw palmetto
Gentian	Sage
Ginseng (caution)	Tansy
Goldenseal	Uva ursi
Juniper	Yarrow

Herbs Generally Regarded as Safe in Pregnancy

Alfalfa	Hawthorn
Arnica (external only or homeopathic)	Horehound
	Horse chestnut
Astragalus	Lemon balm
Bilberry	Marshmallow
Black haw	Meadowsweet
Burdock	Milk thistle
Calendula	Mullein
Catnip	Nettle
Chamomile	Oatstraw
Corn silk	Parsley
Dandelion	Passionflower
Echinacea	Peppermint
Elderberry	Red raspberry
Evening primrose oil	Slippery elm
Fennel	St. John's wort
Feverfew (after first trimester)	Skullcap
	Wild yam
Flax	Valerian
Garlic	Yellow dock
Ginger	Vitex

Emmenagogues (Uterine Stimulants)

Use only after 37 weeks' gestation:

Birthwort	Dong quai
Black cohosh	Motherwort
Blue cohosh	Shepherd's purse
Cottonroot	Squaw vine (partridgeberry)

AROMATHERAPY

How to Use Essential Oils

Inhalation: The essential oil can be infused with electric, battery, reed, or candle diffusers or by placing a small amount on fabric or a cotton ball. This option is good for relaxation and calming essential oils.

Topical: Pure essential oils should not be used undiluted on the skin. Dilute the essential oil with a base oil (olive, sweet almond, jojoba, apricot kernel, or any cold-pressed oil) or distilled water for direct application or misting of the skin.

Hydrotherapy: Essential oils are added as drops to baths, including foot or sitz baths.

Most healthy adults should use the 4% dilution for most topical applications. Children, the elderly, or health-compromised people should use the 1% dilution. Pregnant women should use 12 drops of 2% or 6 drops of 4% dilutions.

Essential Oils Considered Toxic and Harmful

Bitter melon	Rue
Buchu	Sassafras
Camphor	Tansy
Cassia	Thuja
Mugwort	Wintergreen
Pennyroyal	Wormwood

Essential Oils to Avoid in Pregnancy

Ginger (do not use in first trimester)	Pennyroyal
	Tansy
Juniper	Thuja
Mugwort	Thyme
Nutmeg	Wormwood

Essential Oils Generally Regarded as Safe in Pregnancy

Bergamot	Marjoram
Cedarwood	Neroli
Chamomile	Patchouli
Citrus (in small amounts)	Rose
Clary sage	Rose geranium
Cypress	Rosemary
Eucalyptus	Sandalwood
Jasmine	Tea tree
Lavender	Ylang ylang

BIBLIOGRAPHY

Balch, P. (2010). *Prescription for nutritional healing* (5th ed.). New York: Penguin Group.

Cooksley, V. (2002). *Aromatherapy natural healing essential oils.* Upper Saddle River, NJ: Prentice Hall.

Keville, K. (2008). *Aromatherapy: A complete guide to the healing art.* Langhorne, PA: Crossing Press.

Low Dog, T., & Micozzi, M. (2005). *Women's health in complementary and integrative medicine: A clinical guide.* St. Louis, MO: Elsevier.

McCaleb, R. S., Leigh, E., & Morien, K. (2000). *The encyclopedia of popular herbs.* Boulder, CO: Herb Research Foundation.

Murray, M. T. (2004). *The healing power of herbs: The enlightened person's guide to the wonders of medicinal plants.* New York, NY: Gramercy Books.

Romm, A. (2010). *Botanical medicine for women's health.* St. Louis, MO: Churchill Livingstone.

Walls, D. (2007). *Natural families—healthy homes.* LaVergne, TN: Ingram.

Walls, D. (2009). Herbs and natural therapies for pregnancy, birth and breastfeeding. *International Journal of Childbirth Education, 24*(2), 28–37.

A Nutritional Primer

Caring for clients provides midwives with a perfect opportunity to address the very basic, yet often overlooked need for good nutrition information.

There are so many other issues to address with clients that attention to nutritional habits may be given short shrift or delayed. A brief nutritional assessment and counseling session takes just a few minutes, and can positively influence women's lives in profound ways. A well-balanced and healthy diet affects not only physical well-being but also mental health. Straightforward nutritional assessment and counseling strategies are presented here that are easy for providers to incorporate into practice and hold the potential to influence both short- and long-term health of women and their families.

In addition to nourishing the body, eating and drinking have strong emotional and sociocultural links that must be considered when assessing and counseling women about diet. From the first suckles at the breast, emotions are associated with food. While in times past, women traditionally did the meal planning, grocery shopping, and food preparation, social changes, including the industrialization of food and the entry of women into the workplace, have altered these patterns in recent decades. Even so, for many families, the responsibility of feeding the family disproportionately remains a woman's job. In many instances, women will subordinate their own dietary preferences to those of the family, making family structure and dietary patterns important to understand.

Many food preferences, prohibitions, and habits are rooted in individuals' cultural, religious, and ethnic backgrounds ("Food in Every Country," 2011). Money available for food purchase influences food choices; however, the price of a food is not indicative of its nutritional value. Cooking skills and food preparation and storage facilities are other factors that come into play. Holidays and special religious observations often have traditional meals or periods of fasting as features of their observances. Clearly, dietary decisions are influenced by many and varied factors.

Preconception, pregnancy, and lactation are times of altered nutritional needs for women; fortunately, these are also times when women are often more receptive to making changes in their dietary patterns. Appropriate and timely vitamin and mineral supplementation is useful, but the quality of the daily diet is the key to health promotion and maintenance (American Dietetic Association [ADA], 2008). Recommended pregnancy weight gain should be determined according to prepregnancy body mass index (BMI) and Institute of Medicine guidelines (see Table B-1). Certain prohibitions are emphasized during this time, such as the consumption of alcohol, and the use of tobacco and recreational drugs.

Midwives are fully capable of providing sound nutritional advice and recommendations within their scope of practice based on current best evidence as well as and their knowledge of nutrition. Study of nutrition, including cultural variations in food choices, is helpful to the practicing midwife when providing nutritional counseling to clients. Frequent brief counseling has been demonstrated to be effective when repeated consistently over the course of several appointments and visits. Short and focused discussion is best for this type of assessment and client education.

The conversation can begin with an exploration of the client's present overall nutritional choices and habits. Be specific in determining typical food choices. Explore how the woman feels about her food choices and recommendations for modification of her diet. Is she willing to make changes? If the answer is no, then the counseling session will be extremely brief. Provide general information about the importance of a healthy diet to women who need to improve their diets, along with concrete examples of healthy food choices based on their preferences, but without pushing the issue. It is important to acknowledge that changing one's eating habits may be difficult, and it can take time and practice to make necessary adjustments. Keep in mind that not all clients have the financial resources or desire to purchase expensive, high-end organic foods. There are ways to incorporate healthy eating habits within any budget, such as increasing protein intake through increased use of peanut butter, canned chicken or tuna, cheese, yogurt, or beans.

Once an assessment has been made, review with the client food sources high in nutrients deemed deficient in her diet (see the Food Source charts that follow), and help her to explore how to incorporate these foods in her diet in ways that are palatable to her.

A very brief nutrition practice guideline is presented here for incorporation into routine prenatal or well-woman care. It is recommended that dietary patterns be reviewed at each routine prenatal visit and at annual exams. Additionally, some problem-oriented visits can have diet or nutritional deficiencies as key features in the etiology or treatment of the condition. Certain diet-related conditions are addressed in other practice guidelines throughout this book. Through use of short, structured tools, midwives can confidently address the basic nutritional recommendations supported by current evidence in the short time frames dictated by the clinical setting (see Tables B-2 and B-3 and Figure B-1).

Table B-1   The Institute of Medicine's (IOM) Gestational Weight Gain Recommendations (2009)

PRE-PREGNANCY BMI CATEGORY	TOTAL WEIGHT GAIN
Underweight (< 18.5 kg/m²)	28–40 lb or 12.5–18 kg
Normal Weight (18.5–24.9 kg/m²)	25–35 lb or 11.5–16 kg
Overweight (25.0–29.9 kg/m²)	15–25 lb or 7–11.5 kg
Obese (≥ 30 kg/m²)	11–20 lb or 5–9 kg

Table B-2	Starting the Conversation: A Brief Dietary Assessment Tool (Paxton et al., 2011).

Over the past few months:

1) How many times a week did you eat fast food meals or snacks?

      a) Less than 1 time   b) 1-3 times   c) 4 or more times

2) How many servings of fruit did you eat each day?

      a) 5 or more   b) 3-4   c) 2 or less

3) How many servings of vegetables did you eat each day?

      a) 5 or more   b) 3-4   c) 2 or less

4) How many regular sodas or glasses of sweet tea did you drink each day?

      a) Less than 1   b) 1-2   c) 3 or more

5) How many times a week did you eat beans (like pinto or black beans), chicken, or fish?

      a) 3 or more times   b) 1-2 times   c) Less than 1 time

6) How many times a week did you eat regular snack chips or crackers (not low-fat)?

      a) 1 time or less   b) 2-3 times   c) 4 or more times

7) How many times a week did you eat desserts and other sweets (not the low-fat kind)?

      a) 1 time or less   b) 2-3 times   c) 4 or more times

8) How much margarine, butter, or meat fat do you use to season vegetables or put on potatoes, bread, or corn?

      a) Very little   b) Some   c) A lot

Table B-3	The Fruit and Vegetable Questionnaire (FV-Q) (Godin et al., 2008)

Fruit and vegetable portion size definition

One portion of fruit or vegetable equals:

      1 medium-size fruit or vegetable

      ½ cup of cut fruit or vegetables (125 ml)

      ½ cup of fruit juice (125 ml)

      1 cup of green salad (250 ml)

All of these foods can be fresh, frozen, or canned

In the **last seven days**, how many servings of these foods did you eat?

Example: *If you drank 8 ounces of fruit juice during the two weekend days only, enter 0 in all weekday boxes and 2 in the Saturday and Sunday boxes.*

	MONDAY	TUESDAY	WEDNESDAY	THURSDAY	FRIDAY	SATURDAY	SUNDAY
Fruit juice	<u>0</u> servings	<u>0</u> servings	<u>0</u> servings	<u>0</u> servings	<u>0</u> servings	<u>2</u> servings	<u>2</u> servings

Please indicate the appropriate number of servings in each box…

(continues)

Table B-3	The Fruit and Vegetable Questionnaire (FV-Q) (Godin et al., 2008) (Continued)						
	MONDAY	TUESDAY	WEDNESDAY	THURSDAY	FRIDAY	SATURDAY	SUNDAY
Fruit juice	__ servings	__ servings	__ servings	__ servings	__ servings	__ servings	__ servings
Vegetable juice	__ servings	__ servings	__ servings	__ servings	__ servings	__ servings	__ servings
Fruit	__ servings	__ servings	__ servings	__ servings	__ servings	__ servings	__ servings
Potatoes (excluding French-fried potatoes)	__ servings	__ servings	__ servings	__ servings	__ servings	__ servings	__ servings
Green salads	__ servings	__ servings	__ servings	__ servings	__ servings	__ servings	__ servings
Other vegetables	__ servings	__ servings	__ servings	__ servings	__ servings	__ servings	__ servings

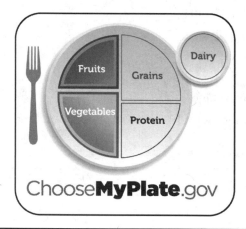

Figure B-1   Food Plate: USDA's new image for nutrition counseling

CARE OF WOMEN ACROSS THE LIFE SPAN: NUTRITIONAL ASSESSMENT AND COUNSELING

Client History and Chart Review: Components of the History to Consider

- Age
- Reproductive cycle status
  - Well woman
  - Preconception
  - Pregnancy
  - Lactation
- Physical activity

- Dietary preferences or prohibitions
  - Cultural
  - Individual taste
  - Portion size
  - Vegetarian
    - Vegan
    - Lacto-ovo
- Dietary supplement use
- Past medical/surgical history
  - Diabetes
  - Anemia
  - Eating disorders
  - Bariatric surgery
  - Other diet-related conditions

Physical Examination: Components of the Physical Exam to Consider

- Height, weight, and BMI
- Interval weight gain or loss
- Selected body measures
  - Abdominal girth
  - Hip-to-waist ratio

Clinical Impression: Differential Diagnoses to Consider

- Inappropriate diet and eating habits
- Body mass index

- Symptoms concerning nutrition metabolism and development
- Unspecified nutritional deficiency

Diagnostic Testing: Diagnostic Tests and Procedures to Consider

(Godin, Belanger-Gravel, Paradis, Vohl, & Perusse, 2008; Paxton, Strycker, Toobert, Ammerman, & Glasgow, 2011)

- Nutritional assessment
  - Twenty-four-hour diet recall
  - Diet diary
  - Other assessment tools (see Tables B-2 and B-3)
- Laboratory testing
  - Vitamin B_{12}
  - Vitamin D
  - Iron
  - Serum albumin

Providing Treatment: Therapeutic Measures to Consider

(Skerrett & Willett, 2010)

- Nutritional counseling:
  - Eat a variety of foods from each food group each day
  - Drink 8–10 glasses of water each day
  - Limit or avoid high-calorie drinks
  - Limit foods with high dietary saturated fat, sugar, and salt content
  - Limit processed and refined foods
- Preconception nutritional counseling (see "Care of the Woman Interested in Preconception Care"):
  - Attain healthy weight prior to pregnancy
  - Avoid cigarettes, secondhand smoke, alcohol, and recreational drugs
  - Avoid excesses in vitamin A, vitamin D, and caffeine intake
  - Folic acid supplementation
    - ◆ 0.4 mg PO daily

- ◆ 4.0 mg PO daily for women with prior pregnancy affected by neural tube defect
- Prenatal nutritional counseling (see "Care of the Woman During Pregnancy"):
  - Achieve healthy weight gain during pregnancy (Institute of Medicine [IOM], 2009)
  - Avoid cigarettes, secondhand smoke, alcohol, and recreational drugs
  - Moderation in caffeine intake (200 mg or less per day) (March of Dimes, 2010)
  - Prenatal vitamin and mineral supplementation with adequate folic acid and omega-3 fatty acids
  - Eat regularly throughout the day

Providing Treatment: Complementary and Alternative Measures to Consider

- Daily multivitamin and mineral supplement as needed
- Omega-3 fatty acid supplement as needed
- Increased daily physical activity as needed
- Regular exercise

Providing Support: Education and Support Measures to Consider

(Institute of Medicine [IOM], 2006)

- Recommend reputable sources for nutrition advice:
  - http://www.choosemyplate.gov/
  - http://www.choosemyplate.gov /mypyramidmoms/index.html
  - http://health.gov/dietaryguidelines/
- Praise intention and progress

Follow-up Care: Follow-up Measures to Consider

- Document
- Reinforce prior teaching
- Repeat the brief assessment and counseling at the client's next visit for care

Multidisciplinary Practice: Consider Consultation, Collaboration, or Referral

- Dietician referral
  - Eating disorders
  - Postbariatric surgery
  - Diabetes
  - Obesity
  - Other chronic diet-related disorders
- WIC or food stamps referral
- Classes for exercise
- Weight-control programs, such as Weight Watchers
- For diagnosis or treatment outside the midwife's scope of practice

REFERENCES

American Dietetic Association (ADA). (2008). Position of the American Dietetic Association: Nutrition and lifestyle for a healthy pregnancy outcome. *Journal of the American Dietetic Association, 108*(3), 553–561.

Food in every country. (2011). Retrieved from http://www.foodbycountry.com

Godin, G., Belanger-Gravel, A., Paradis, A., Vohl, M., & Perusse, L. (2008). A simple method to assess fruit and vegetable intake among obese and non-obese individuals. *Canadian Journal of Public Health, 99*(6), 494–498.

ICD9Data.com. (2012). The Web's free 2012 ICD-9 medical coding data. Retrieved from http://www.icd9data.com/

Institute of Medicine (IOM). (2006). *Dietary reference intakes: The essential guide to nutrient requirements.* Washington, DC: National Academies Press.

Institute of Medicine (IOM). (2009). *Weight gain during pregnancy: Reexamining the guidelines.* Washington, DC: National Academies Press.

Jordan, R. (2010). Prenatal omega-3 fatty acids: Review and recommendations. *Journal of Midwifery & Women's Health, 55*(6), 520–528.

March of Dimes. (2010). Caffeine in pregnancy. Retrieved from http://www.marchofdimes.com/pregnancy/nutrition_caffeine.html

Paxton, A., Strycker, L., Toobert, D., Ammerman, A., & Glasgow, R. (2011). Starting the conversation: Performance of a brief dietary assessment and intervention tool for health professionals. *American Journal of Preventive Medicine, 40*(1), 67–71.

Skerrett, P., & Willett, W. (2010). Essentials of healthy eating: A guide. *Journal of Midwifery & Women's Health, 55*(6), 492–501.

U.S. Department of Health and Human Services & U.S. Department of Agriculture. (2005). *Dietary guidelines for Americans* (6th ed.). Washington, DC: U.S. Government Printing Office.

APPENDIX B-1   DAIRY FOOD SOURCES OF CALCIUM

Dairy food sources of calcium are ranked by milligrams of calcium per standard amount of the food; calories are also based on the standard amount. The Adequate Intakes (AI) for adults aged 19–50 is 1000 mg/day.

FOOD, STANDARD AMOUNT	CALCIUM (MG)	CALORIES
Plain yogurt, nonfat (13 g protein/8 oz), 8-oz container	452	127
Romano cheese, 1.5 oz	452	165
Pasteurized process Swiss cheese, 2 oz	438	190
Plain yogurt, low fat (12 g protein/8 oz), 8-oz container	415	143
Fruit yogurt, low fat (10 g protein/8 oz), 8-oz container	345	232
Swiss cheese, 1.5 oz	336	162
Ricotta cheese, part skim, ½ cup	335	170
Pasteurized process American cheese food, 2 oz	323	188
Provolone cheese, 1.5 oz	321	150
Mozzarella cheese, part skim, 1.5 oz	311	129
Greek yogurt, nonfat (20 g protein/8 oz), 8-oz container	151	121

Source: U.S. Department of Health and Human Services & U.S. Department of Agriculture, 2005.

APPENDIX B-2   NONDAIRY FOOD SOURCES OF CALCIUM

Nondairy food sources of calcium are ranked by milligrams of calcium per standard amount of the food; calories are also based on the standard amount. The bioavailability may vary. The Adequate Intakes (AI) for adults is 1000 mg/day.*

FOOD, STANDARD AMOUNT	CALCIUM (MG)	CALORIES
Fortified ready-to-eat cereals (various), 1 oz	236–1043	88–106
Soy beverage, calcium fortified, 1 cup	368	98
Sardines, Atlantic, in oil, drained, 3 oz	325	177
Tofu, firm, prepared with nigari,† ½ cup	253	88
Pink salmon, canned, with bone, 3 oz	181	118
Collards, cooked from frozen, ½ cup	178	31
Molasses, blackstrap, 1 Tbsp	172	47
Spinach, cooked from frozen, ½ cup	146	30
Soybeans, green, cooked, ½ cup	130	127
Turnip greens, cooked from frozen, ½ cup	124	24

*Both calcium content and bioavailability should be considered when selecting dietary sources of calcium. Some plant foods have calcium that is well absorbed, but the large quantity of plant foods that would be needed to provide as much calcium as in a glass of milk may be unachievable for many. Many other calcium-fortified foods are available, but the percentage of calcium that can be absorbed from them is variable.

†Calcium sulfate and magnesium chloride.

Source: U.S. Department of Health and Human Services & U.S. Department of Agriculture, 2005.

APPENDIX B-3   FOOD SOURCES OF VITAMIN C

Food sources of Vitamin C are ranked by milligrams of Vitamin C per standard amount of the food; calories are also based on the standard amount. The Recommended Daily Allowance (RDA) for adult women who are not pregnant is 75 mg/day.

FOOD, STANDARD AMOUNT	VITAMIN C (MG)	CALORIES
Guava, raw, ½ cup	188	56
Red sweet pepper, raw, ½ cup	142	20
Red sweet pepper, cooked, ½ cup	116	0.19
Kiwi fruit, 1 medium	70	46
Orange, raw, 1 medium	70	62
Orange juice, ¾ cup	61–93	79–84
Green pepper, sweet, raw, ½ cup	60	15
Green pepper, sweet, cooked, ½ cup	51	19
Grapefruit juice, ¾ cup	50–70	71–86
Vegetable juice cocktail, ¾ cup	50	34
Strawberries, raw, ½ cup	49	27

Source: U.S. Department of Health and Human Services & U.S. Department of Agriculture, 2005.

APPENDIX B-4   FOOD SOURCES OF DIETARY FIBER

Food sources of dietary fiber are ranked by grams of dietary fiber per standard amount of the food; calories are also based on the standard amount. The Adequate Intakes (AI) for adult women is 25 g/day.

FOOD, STANDARD AMOUNT	DIETARY FIBER (G)	CALORIES
Flax seed, 3.5 ounces	27.3	534
Navy beans, cooked, ½ cup	9.5	128
Bran ready-to-eat cereal (100%), ½ cup	8.8	78
Kidney beans, canned, ½ cup	8.2	109
Split peas, cooked, ½ cup	8.1	116
Lentils, cooked, ½ cup	7.8	115
Black beans, cooked, ½ cup	7.5	114
Pinto beans, cooked, ½ cup	7.7	122
Lima beans, cooked, ½ cup	6.6	108
Artichoke, globe, cooked, 1 each	6.5	60
White beans, canned, ½ cup	6.3	154
Chickpeas, cooked, ½ cup	6.2	135

Source: U.S. Department of Health and Human Services & U.S. Department of Agriculture, 2005.

APPENDIX B-5   FOOD SOURCES OF IRON

Food sources of iron are ranked by milligrams of iron per standard amount of the food; calories are also based on the standard amount. The Recommended Daily Allowance (RDA) for teen and adult females is 18 mg/day.

FOOD, STANDARD AMOUNT	IRON (MG)	CALORIES
Clams, canned, drained, 3 oz	23.8	126
Fortified ready-to-eat cereals (various), ~1 oz	1.8–21.1	54–127
Oysters, eastern, wild, cooked, moist heat, 3 oz	10.2	116
Organ meats (liver, giblets), various, cooked, 3 oz*	5.2–9.9	134–235
Fortified instant cooked cereals (various), 1 packet	4.9–8.1	Varies
Soybeans, mature, cooked, ½ cup	4.4	149
Pumpkin and squash seed kernels, roasted, 1 oz	4.2	148
White beans, canned, ½ cup	3.9	153
Blackstrap molasses, 1 Tbsp	3.5	47
Lentils, cooked, ½ cup	3.3	115
Spinach, cooked from fresh, ½ cup	3.2	21

*High in cholesterol.

Source: U.S. Department of Health and Human Services & U.S. Department of Agriculture, 2005.

APPENDIX B-6 FOOD SOURCES OF OMEGA-3 FATTY ACIDS

Approximate DHA plus EPA is given in milligrams per 6 oz uncooked serving, unless otherwise noted. The Adequate Intakes (AI) for adult women who are not pregnant is 1.1 g/day.

FOOD	DHA (MG)	EPA (MG)
Atlantic salmon, farmed	2477	1173
Atlantic salmon, wild	2429	699
Sockeye salmon, canned	1190	901
Sardines (3.75-oz can)	468	435
Atlantic herring (3 oz)	939	773
Farmed catfish	653	250
Atlantic/Pacific halibut	636	154
Canned light tuna	1137	240
Rainbow trout, farmed	1394	568
Atlantic cod	262	7
Alaskan king crab	602	1504
Blue crab (1 cup)	230	261
Shrimp	245	291

Source: Jordan, 2010.

Index